Amsler's Grid

The chart on the opposite page is patterned after the grid devised by Professor Marc Amsler. It can provide for the rapid detection of small irregularities in the central 20° of the field of vision. The chart is composed of a grid of lines containing a central white fixation spot. The squares on the grid are 5 mm in size and subtend a visual angle of 1° at 30 cm viewing distance.

The chart is to be viewed in modest light monocularly at a distance of 28-30 cm utilizing the correct refraction for this distance. Viewing should be accomplished without previous ophthalmoscopy and without instillation of any drugs affecting pupillary size or accommodation.

A series of questions should be asked while the patient is viewing the central white spot.

1) Is the center spot visible? The absence of the spot may indicate the presence of a central scotoma.

2) While viewing the center white spot can you see all four sides? The inability to perceive these areas may indicate the presence of an arcuate scotoma of glaucoma encroaching upon the central area or a centrocecal scotoma.

3) Do you see the entire grid intact? Are there any defects? If an area of the grid is not visible, then a paracentral scotoma is present.

4) Are the horizontal and vertical lines straight and parallel? If not, then metamorphopsia is present. The parallel lines may "bend" inwards giving rise to micropsia or "bend" outwards giving rise to macropsia.

5) Do you see any blur or distortion in the grid? Any movement? A color aberration? These changes may be present prior to the appearance of a definite scotoma.

FOREWORD TO THE TWENTY-THIRD EDITION

Welcome to the 1995 edition of *Physicians' Desk Reference For Ophthalmology®*. Long the profession's leading source of FDA-approved prescribing information, PDR For Ophthalmology® also brings you the latest contact lens specifications directly from the files of *Frames*, the nation's leading source of contact lens and eyeglass information. You'll also find a wealth of reference material on lens care products, plus key facts about a variety of specialized ophthalmic equipment and a wide array of fundamental clinical reference data to aid in your daily practice.

Near the beginning of the book, you'll find a convenient set of tables summarizing the major therapeutic alternatives available in ophthalmology today, as well as a handy bank of information on low vision. For your convenience, the complete chapter on the visual system from the just-released fourth edition of *Guides to the Evaluation of Permanent Impairment* is also included; and you'll find a full-color product identification section augmented with reproductions of the Rosenbaum Vision Screener and a Color Vision Screening Chart. Five detailed indices help you locate products by manufacturer, trade name, active ingredient, therapeutic category, and — for instrumentation — by type of device.

The special reference sections near the beginning of the book have been prepared with the assistance of Clement A. Weisbecker, RPh, Michael Naidoff, MD, and Richard Tippermann, MD of Wills Eye Hospital in Philadelphia, Pennsylvania. Our thanks also go to F.T. Fraunfelder, MD, author of the section on ocular toxicology, and to Arthur Gold, MD, who prepared the commentary on ophthalmic lenses. The opinions expressed in these sections are those of the authors and are not necessarily endorsed by the publisher, Medical Economics Data.

Under the federal Food, Drug & Cosmetics (FD&C) Act, a drug approved for marketing may be labeled, promoted, and advertised by the manufacturer for only those uses for which the drug's safety and effectiveness have been established. The Code of Federal Regulations 201.100(d)(1) pertaining to labeling for prescription products requires that for content of *Physicians' Desk Reference For Ophthalmology* "indications, effects, dosages, routes, methods, and frequency and duration of administration and any relevant warnings, hazards, contraindications, side effects, and precautions" must be in the *"same language and emphasis"* as the approved labeling for the products. FDA regards the words *same language and emphasis* as requiring VERBATIM use of the approved labeling providing such information. Furthermore, information in the approved labeling that is emphasized by the use of type set in a box or in capitals, boldface, or italics must also be given the same emphasis in *Physicians' Desk Reference For Ophthalmology.*

The FDA has also recognized that the FD&C Act does not, however, limit the manner in which a physician may use an approved drug. Once a product has been approved for marketing, a physician may prescribe it for uses or in treatment regimens or patient populations that are not included in approved labeling. The FDA also observes that accepted medical practice often includes drug use that is not reflected in approved drug labeling. For products that do not have official package circulars, the publisher has emphasized the necessity of describing such products comprehensively, so that physicians have access to all information essential for intelligent and informed decision making.

The function of the publisher is the compilation, organization, and distribution of this information. Each product description has been prepared by the manufacturer, and edited and approved by the manufacturer's medical department, medical director, and/or medical consultant. In organizing and presenting the material in *Physicians' Desk Reference For Ophthalmology,* the publisher does not warrant or guarantee any of the products described, or perform any independent analysis in connection with any of the product information contained herein. *Physicians' Desk Reference For Ophthalmology* does not assume, and expressly disclaims, any obligation to obtain and include any information other than that provided to it by the manufacturer. It should be understood that by making this material available the publisher is not advocating the use of any product described herein, nor is the publisher responsible for misuse of a product due to typographical error. Additional information on any product may be obtained from the manufacturer.

We at Medical Economics Data stand ready to provide you with as much assistance as possible. For customer service, please call 1-800-232-7379, or fax 201-573-4956.

PART II/PRODUCT NAME INDEX

A

B

C

D

E

◆ Shown in Product Identification Guide

Italic Page Number Indicates Brief Listing

◆ Shown in Product Identification Guide

Italic Page Number Indicates Brief Listing

PART III/PRODUCT CATEGORY INDEX

Italic Page Number **Indicates Brief Listing**

PART V/ INSTRUMENTATION AND EQUIPMENT INDEX

MEDICAL ECONOMICS

SECTION 2

PHARMACEUTICALS IN OPHTHALMOLOGY

Clement A. Weisbecker, RPh, Michael Naidoff, MD, and Richard Tippermann, MD (Wills Eye Hospital, Philadelphia, Pa), with a section on ocular toxicology by F. T. Fraunfelder, MD

Once again we are pleased to present an updated and expanded overview of pharmaceuticals in ophthalmology. New in this edition are sections on viscoelastic materials and off-label drug uses. The discussion of unapproved uses is intended to alert clinicians to both the potential benefits and, in some cases, the substantial risks associated with the drugs in question.

This section now offers 23 reference tables presenting therapeutic alternatives in all major categories of ophthalmic treatment, as well as a survey of recently identified adverse drug reactions encountered in ophthalmology. The material is divided into 13 parts as follows:

1. Mydriatics and Cycloplegics
2. Antimicrobial Therapy
3. Ocular Anti-inflammatory Agents
4. Anesthetic Agents
5. Agents for Treatment of Glaucoma
6. Medications for Dry Eye
7. Ocular Decongestants
8. Ophthalmic Irrigating Solutions
9. Hyperosmolar Agents
10. Diagnostic Agents
11. Viscoelastic Materials Used in Ophthalmology
12. Off-Label Drug Applications in Ophthalmology
13. Ocular Toxicology

There are a large number of excellent references related to pharmacology and treatment regimens in ophthalmology. Listed below are some of the ones we regard as particularly useful.

GENERAL REFERENCES

1. American Medical Association. *Drug Evaluations Annual 1991*. Milwaukee, Wis: AMA Department of Drugs, Division of Toxicology.
2. Fraunfelder FT, Roy FH. *Current Ocular Therapy*, ed 3. Philadelphia, Pa: WB Saunders; 1989.
3. Fraunfelder FT. *Drug-Induced Ocular Side Effects and Drug Interactions*. Philadelphia, Pa: Lea & Febiger; 1989.
4. Reynolds L, Closson R. *Extemporoneous Ophthalmic Preparations: Applied Therapeutics,* 1993.
5. Lerman S, Tripathi R. *Ocular Toxicology*. New York, NY: Marcel Dekker, Inc; 1990.
6. Olin B (editor-in-chief). *Ophthalmic Drug Facts*. St. Louis, Mo: JB Lippincott; 1992.
7. Vaughan D, Asbury T, Riordan-Eva P. *General Ophthalmology*, ed 13. Norwalk, Conn: Appleton & Lange; 1992.

1. MYDRIATICS AND CYCLOPLEGICS

The autonomic drugs that produce mydriasis (pupillary dilation) and cycloplegia (paralysis of accommodation) are among the most frequently used topical medications in ophthalmic practice. The most commonly used mydriatic is the direct-acting adrenergic agent, phenylephrine hydrochloride. The other mydriatic, the indirectly acting adrenergic hydroxyamphetamine, is available only in combination with tropicamide.

Phenylephrine is used alone or, more commonly, in combination with a cycloplegic agent for refraction or for pupillary dilation. The 2.5% concentration is favored for cases in which there is a possibility of severe adverse systemic effects from the use of the 10% solution.

Hydroxyamphetamine hydrobromide, which will become commercially available in late 1994, or early 1995, is most commonly used as a diagnostic in Horner's syndrome.

Anticholinergic agents have both cycloplegic and mydriatic activity. They are usually used for refraction, pupillary dilation, and relief of inflammation.

It is important to remember that the effect of these medications depends on many factors, including age, race, and eye color. For example, the mydriatics and cycloplegics tend to be less effective in dark-eyed individuals than in blue-eyed ones.

The recently introduced drug dapiprazole hydrochloride (Rēv-Eyes) can be used to reverse the effects of phenylephrine and, to a lesser extent, tropicamide. Activity against phenylephrine is excellent: 88% reversal at the end of 1 hour. Against tropicamide, results are significantly lower: 38% at the end of 2 hours. It therefore remains important, when using both drugs, to instruct the patient to use sunglasses and avoid driving or operating dangerous machinery.

TABLE 1

MYDRIATICS AND CYCLOPLEGICS

GENERIC NAME	TRADE NAMES	CONCENTRATION (%)	ONSET/DURATION OF ACTION
Phenylephrine hydrochloride	AK-Dilate	Soln, 2.5%, 10%	30–60 min/3–5 h
	Mydfrin	Soln, 2.5%	
	Neo-Synephrine	Soln, 2.5%, 10%	
	Available generically	Soln, 2.5%, 10%	
Hydroxyamphetamine hydrobromide*	Paremyd	Soln, 1%	15–60 min/3–4 h
Atropine sulfate	Atropisol	Soln, 0.5%, 1%, 2%	45–120 min/7–14 days
	Atropine-Care	Soln, 1%	
	Isopto Atropine	Soln, 0.5%, 1%, 2%, 3%	
	Available generically	Soln, 1%	
		Ointment, 0.5%, 1%	
Cyclopentolate hydrochloride	AK-Pentolate	Soln, 1%	30–60 min/2 days
	Cyclogyl	Soln, 0.5%, 1%, 2%	
	Available generically	Soln, 1%	
Homatropine hydrobromide	Isopto Homatropine	Soln, 2%, 5%	30–60 min/3 days
	Available generically	Soln, 2%, 5%	
Scopolamine hydrobromide	Isopto Hyoscine	Soln, 0.25%	30–60 min/4–7 days
Tropicamide	Mydriacyl	Soln, 0.5%, 1%	20–40 min/4–6 h
	Tropicacyl	Soln, 0.5%, 1%	
	Available generically	Soln, 0.5%, 1%	

* In combination with Tropicamide

2. ANTIMICROBIAL THERAPY

Antibiotics are routinely used in ophthalmology for both treatment and prophylaxis. They are used prophylactically in the management of foreign bodies and corneal abrasions and in pre- and postoperative care, administered as an ointment or by subconjunctival injection. (see **Table 2**).

Recently, many ophthalmic institutions have been using a solution of 5% povidone-iodine (Betadine) preoperatively to "sterilize" the eye, lids, and brow. Another recent development is the use of collagen shields (usually 12-hour) soaked in antibiotic, with or without steroid, in place of a patch and/or subconjunctival injection. While more expensive, the shields do have the advantage of being more comfortable for the patient and are less likely to cause tissue degeneration.

When treating an active or suspected external or intraocular infection, slides for gram and Giemsa stain and aerobic and anaerobic cultures should be secured prior to initiating therapy. When fungal involvement is a possibility, additional stains to consider are: methenamine silver, acridine orange, and calcofluor white.

Corneal ulcers and intraocular infections require vigorous management. Most physicians and hospitals have protocols for their treatment. One such protocol for treating endophthalmitis, from Mandelbaum and Forster, is given in **Table 3**. Serious ocular infections are usually treated by the topical, subconjunctival, and intravenous routes of administration (see **Table 4**). Corneal ulcers are usually treated with one or more of the topical solutions listed in **Table 4**, usually given every $^1/_2$ to 1 hour, in alternating doses if more than one solution is used. In severe cases, such as impending or actual perforation and scleral extension, medication is given by the topical, subconjunctival, and/or intravenous route.

Fungal keratitis (keratomycosis) is relatively uncommon, but should be suspected in patients who have previously received topical steroids and/or antibiotics, and in patients whose corneal ulcer does not respond to antibiotics. Corneal scraping often permits correct clinical diagnosis. Natamycin 5% ophthalmic suspension (Natacyn) is recognized as the most potent broad-spectrum antifungal agent available for use in the eye.

Incidence of endogenous fungal endophthalmitis can be seen in intravenous drug users and patients with compromised immune systems. For these infections, amphotericin B has been used subconjunctivally, intravenously, and, where indicated, intravitreally. Sterile operating room technique and a coaxially illuminated operating microscope should be used when administering the medication intravitreally. Prior to intravitreal use, a small portion of the vitreous abscess should be aspirated for microbiologic study. Flucytosine and miconazole have also been used to treat fungal endophthalmitis. For more on treatment of fungal infections, see **Table 5**.

There has been an increase, within the last decade, in the incidence of *Acanthamoeba* keratitis. This has been linked, in many cases, to use of contaminated solutions for soft contact lenses — especially homemade saline solutions. Current therapy includes the use of polymyxin/neomycin/bacitracin ophthalmic solution.

In bacterial endophthalmitis, the use of intraocular and periocular antimicrobial therapy has significantly improved the final visual outcome. A diagnosis of bacterial endophthalmitis should be strongly suspected in a patient who is postoperative or posttraumatic, or when the intraocular inflammation is out of proportion to the situation. Ocular pain is often present before obvious inflammation. Preoperative antibiotics may decrease the incidence of postoperative endophthalmitis.

Once endophthalmitis is suspected, prompt intervention is required. Samples of the aqueous and vitreous humors must be promptly secured and treatment quickly initiated with antimicrobials appropriate to the suspected organism(s). When inflammation occurs several weeks or more after surgery or in cases of trauma or in immunosuppressed patients, fungal or anaerobic organisms should be considered.

Once the aqueous and vitreous humors have been cultured, antimicrobial agents should be directly injected into these cavities. To prevent retinal toxicity, medications should be injected slowly into the anterior vitreous cavity, with particular caution after vitrectomy. Vitrectomy and intravitreal antibiotics should always be considered when treating endophthalmitis.

REFERENCES

Axelrod AJ, Peyman GA. Intravitreal amphotericin B treatment of experimental fungal endophthalmitis. *Am J Ophthalmol.* 1973;76:584.

Barza M. Antibacterial agents in the treatment of ocular infections. *Infect Dis Clin North Am.* 3:533-551.

Baum JL. Initial therapy of suspected microbial corneal ulcers. I. Broad antibiotic therapy based on prevalence of organisms. *Surv Opthalmol.* 1979; 24:97.

Baum JL. Antibiotic use in ophthalmology. In: Tasman W, Jaeger EA, eds. *Duane's Clinical Ophthalmology.* Philadelphia, Pa: JB Lippincott; 1989; vol 4, chap 26.

Ellis P. *Ocular Therapeutics and Pharmacology.* 7th ed. St. Louis, Mo: CV Mosby; 1985.

Forster RK. Endophthalmitis. In: Tasman W, Jaeger EA, eds. *Duane's Clinical Ophthalmology.* Philadelphia, Pa: JB Lippincott; 1989, vol 4, chap 24.

Gardner S. Treatment of bacterial endophthalmitis. In: *Ocular Therapeutics and Management.* Atlanta, Ga: 1991; vol 2, no. 1.

Havener WH. *Ocular Pharmacology.* 5th ed. St. Louis, Mo: CV Mosby; 1983.

Lamberts DW, Potter DE, eds. *Clinical Ocular Pharmacology.* Boston, Mass: Little, Brown; 1987.

Lemp MA, Blackman HJ, Koffler BH. Therapy for bacterial and fungal infections. *Int Ophthalmol Clin.* 1980; 20(no. 3):135-145.

Pavan PR, Brinser JH. Exogenous bacterial endophthalmitis treated without systemic antibiotics. *Am J Ophthalmol.* 1987; 104:121.

Peyman GA. Antibiotic administration in the treatment of bacterial endophthalmitis. II. Intravitreal injections. *Surv Ophthalmol.* 1977; 21: 332,339.

Tabbara KF, Hyndiuk RA, eds. *Infections of the Eye.* Boston, Mass: Little, Brown; 1986.

TABLE 2

COMMERCIALLY AVAILABLE OPHTHALMIC ANTIBACTERIAL AGENTS

GENERIC NAME	TRADE NAME	CONCENTRATION OPH. SOLN (%)	OPH OINT
INDIVIDUAL AGENTS			
Bacitracin zinc	AK-Tracin	Not available	500 units/g
Chloramphenicol	AK-Chlor	0.5%	1%
	Chloromycetin	0.5%	1%
	Chloroptic	0.5%	1%
	Ocu-Chlor	0.5%	1%
	Available generically	0.5%	1%
Chlortetracycline hydrochloride	Aureomycin	Not available	1%
Ciprofloxacin hydrochloride	Ciloxan	0.3%	Not available
Erythromycin	AK-Mycin	Not available	0.5%
	Ilotycin	Not available	0.5%
	Available generically	Not available	0.5%
Gentamicin sulfate	Garamycin	0.3%	0.3%
	Genoptic	0.3%	0.3%
	Gentacidin	0.3%	0.3%
	Gentak	0.3%	0.3%
	Available generically	0.3%	0.3%
Norfloxacin	Chibroxin	0.3%	Not available
Ofloxacin	Ocuflox	0.3%	Not available
Sulfacetamide sodium	AK-Sulf	10%	10%
	Bleph-10	10%	10%
	Cetamide	Not available	10%
	Isopto Cetamide	15%	Not available
	Ophthacet	10%	Not available
	Sulamyd sodium	10%, 30%	10%
	Sulf-10	10%	Not available
	Available generically	10%, 15%, 30%	10%
Sulfisoxazole diolamine	Gantrisin	4%	4%
Tetracycline hydrochloride	Achromycin	1%	Not available
Tobramycin sulfate	Defy	0.3%	0.3%
	Tobrex	0.3%	Not available
	Available generically	0.3%	0.3%
MIXTURES			
Polymyxin B/Bacitracin	AK-Poly-Bac Polysporin	Not available	10,000 units 500 units/g
Polymyxin B/Neomycin	Statrol	16,250 units 3.5 mg/mL	10,000 units 3.5 mg/g
Polymyxin B/Neomycin/Bacitracin	Neotal	Not available	5,000 units 5 mg 400 units/g
Polymyxin B/Neomycin/Bacitracin	AK-Spore Neosporin Available generically	Not available	10,000 units 3.5 mg 400 units/g
Polymyxin B/Neomycin/Gramicidin	AK-Spore Neosporin Available generically	10,000 units 1.75 mg 0.025 mg/mL	Not available
Polymyxin B/Oxytetracycline	Terramycin	Not available	10,000 units 5 mg/g
Polymyxin B/Trimethoprim	Polytrim	10,000 units 1 mg/mL	Not available

TABLE 3

AN INTRAOCULAR THERAPEUTIC REGIMEN FOR ENDOPHTHALMITIS

1. Diagnostic anterior chamber and vitreous aspiration; diagnostic vitrectomy when liquid vitreous fails to aspirate or in cases of suspected fungal endophthalmitis.

2. Initial therapy (in operating room after diagnostic technique).

   A. Intraocular
   gentamicin 100 μg or amikacin 400 μg and vancomycin 1000 μg or cefazolin 2250 μg

   B. Subconjunctival
   gentamicin 40 mg and triamcinolone diacetate (Aristocort) 40 mg*

   C. Topical
   gentamicin 9.1 or 13.4 mg/mL and cefazolin 50 mg/mL and prednisolone acetate 1%

   D. Systemic
   cefazolin (Ancef or Kefzol) 1000 mg every 6 to 8 hours. (Ceftriaxone has good penetration of the blood ocular barrier and may be used as an alternative.)

3. If cultures are *positive* for virulent bacteria, consider repeating the above intraocular injections at the bedside on the second and fourth postoperative days. Continue topical treatment every half hour, subconjunctival treatment daily, and systemic therapy. Consider therapeutic vitrectomy with repeat intraocular antibiotics.

4. If cultures are negative after 48 hours, do not repeat intraocular antibiotics. Consider tapering topical, subconjunctival, and systemic antibiotic therapy while continuing topical and subconjunctival corticosteroids.

5. If the endophthalmitis presents as a *delayed inflammation* in which a fungal etiology is considered, the vitreous sample should be obtained by a vitreous instrument using membrane filters; intraocular amphotericin B (Fungizone) at a dosage of 5 μg or miconazole at a dosage of 10 to 25 μg should be considered.

6. If the endophthalmitis presents as a delayed inflammation or chronic indolent infection, a *Propionibacterium acnes* infection should be considered.

Source: Mandelbaum S, Forster RK.

*Subconjunctival corticosteroids should be deferred 48 to 72 hours to await culture growth and confirmation if a fungal etiology is suspected or the inflammation is delayed.

TABLE 4

CONCENTRATIONS AND DOSAGE OF PRINCIPAL ANTIBIOTIC AGENTS

DRUG NAME*	TOPICAL	SUBCONJUNCTIVAL	INTRAVITREAL	INTRAVENOUS†
Amikacin sulfate	10 mg/mL	25 mg	400 μg	15 mg/kg daily in 2–3 doses
Ampicillin sodium	50 mg/mL	50–150 mg	500 μg	4–12 g daily in 4 doses
Bacitracin zinc	10,000 units/mL	5,000 units	. . .	. . .
Carbenicillin disodium	4–6 mg/mL	100 mg	250–2000 μg	8–24 g daily in 4–6 doses
Cefazolin sodium	50 mg/mL	100 mg	2250 μg	2–4 g daily in 3–4 doses
Ceftazidime	. . .	200 mg	2200 μg	1 g daily in 2–3 doses
Clindamycin	50 mg/mL	15–50 mg	1000 μg	900–1800 mg daily in 2–3 doses
Colistimethate sodium	10 mg/mL	15–25 mg	100 μg	2.5–5 mg/kg daily in 2–4 doses
Erythromycin	50 mg/mL	100 mg	500 μg	. . .
Gentamicin sulfate	8–15 mg/mL	10–20 mg	100–200 μg	3–5 mg/kg daily in 2–3 doses
Imipenem/Cilastatin sodium	5 mg/mL	. . .	. . .	2 g daily in 3–4 doses
Kanamycin sulfate	30–50 mg/mL	30 mg	. . .	. . .
Methicillin sodium	50 mg/mL	50–100 mg	1000–2000 μg	6–10 g daily in 4 doses
Neomycin sulfate	5–8 mg/mL	125–250 mg	. . .	. . .
Penicillin G	100,000 units/mL	0.5–1.0 million units	. . .	12–24 million units daily in 4–6 doses
Polymyxin B sulfate	10,000 units/mL	100,000 units	. . .	. . .
Ticarcillin disodium	6 mg/mL	100 mg	. . .	200–300 mg/kg daily 3 x in 4–6 doses
Tobramycin sulfate	8–15 mg/mL	10–20 mg	100–200 μg	3–5 mg/kg daily in 2–3 doses
Vancomycin hydrochloride	20–50 mg/mL	25 mg	1000 μg	15–30 mg/kg daily in 1–2 doses

*Most penicillins and cephalosporins are physically incompatible when combined in the same bottle with aminoglycosides such as amikacin, gentamicin, or tobramycin.
†Adult doses.

TABLE 5

ANTIFUNGAL AGENTS

GENERIC (TRADE) NAME	ROUTE	DOSAGE	SPECTRUM
Amphotericin B	Topical Subconjunctival Intravitreal Intravenous	0.1–0.5% solution; dilute with water for injection or dextrose 5% in water 0.8–1.0 mg 5 μg Because of side effects and toxicity, see main *PDR* for dosing instructions	*Blastomyces* *Candida* *Coccidioides* *Histoplasma*
Fluconazole (Diflucan)	Oral	800 mg on day 1, then 400 mg daily in divided doses	*Candida*
Flucytosine (Ancobon)	Oral Topical	50–150 mg/kg daily in 4 divided doses* 1% solution	*Candida* *Cryptococcus*
Natamycin (Natacyn)	Topical	5% suspension	*Candida* *Aspergillus* *Cephalosporium* *Fusarium* *Penicillium*
Miconazole nitrate (Monistat)	Topical Subconjunctival Intravitreal	1% solution 5–10 mg 10 μg	*Candida* *Cryptococcus* *Aspergillus*
Ketoconazole (Nizoral)	Oral	200–400 mg daily*	*Candida* *Cryptococcus* *Histoplasma*

*Because of potential side and toxic effects, the practitioner should consult the main PDR for possible dosage adjustments and warnings.

TABLE 6

ANTIVIRAL AGENTS

GENERIC (TRADE) NAME	TOPICAL CONC (%)	INTRAVIT DOSE	SYSTEMIC DOSAGE*
Idoxuridine (Herplex)	0.1% (oph solution)	. . .	. . .
Trifluridine (Viroptic)	1.0% (oph solution)	. . .	. . .
Vidarabine monohydrate (Vira-A)	3.0% (oph ointment)	. . .	. . .
Acyclovir sodium (Zovirax)	. . .	. . .	* Oral–*Herpes simplex* keratitis–200 mg 5 times daily for 7–10 days. Oral–*Herpes zoster ophthalmicus*–600–800 mg 5 times daily for 10 days * IV†
Foscarnet sodium (Foscavir)	. . .	. . .	* IV–by controlled infusion only, either by central vein or by peripheral vein–Induction: 60 mg/kg (adjusted for renal function) given over 1 h every 8 h for 14–21 days Maintenance: 90–120 mg/kg given over 2 hours once daily
Ganciclovir sodium (Cytovene)	. . .	200 μg	* IV–Induction: 5 mg/kg every 12 h for 14–21days Maintenance: 5 mg/kg daily for 7 days.

*Because of potential side and toxic effects, the practitioner should consult the main PDR for possible dosage adjustments and warnings.
†IV therapy should be considered if the patient is immunocompromised.

3. OCULAR ANTI-INFLAMMATORY AGENTS

A wide variety of medications are available to treat ocular inflammation. They are listed in **Table 7**. Corticosteroids are the most commonly used. Many are available in combination with antibiotics and/or other medications.

At one time, it was felt that corticosteroids were contraindicated in infectious disease states. However, it is now appreciated that steroids, when used in conjunction with appropriate antimicrobial, antifungal, or antiviral agents, may help prevent more serious ocular damage.

TABLE 7

TOPICAL ANTI-INFLAMMATORY AGENTS

NAME AND DOSAGE FORM	TRADE NAME	CONCENTRATION
Dexamethasone Ophthalmic Suspension	Maxidex	0.1%
Dexamethasone Sodium Phosphate Ophthalmic Ointment	AK-Dex Decadron Maxidex Available generically	0.05% 0.05% 0.05% 0.05%
Dexamethasone Sodium Phosphate Ophthalmic Solution	AK-Dex Decadron Available generically	0.1% 0.1% 0.1%
Fluorometholone Ophthalmic Ointment	FML S.O.P.	0.1%
Fluorometholone Ophthalmic Suspension	Fluor-Op FML FML Forte	0.1% 0.1% 0.25%
Fluorometholone Acetate Ophthalmic Suspension	Flarex	0.1%
Medrysone Ophthalmic Suspension	HMS	1%
Prednisolone Acetate Ophthalmic Suspension	Pred Mild Econopred Econopred Plus Pred Forte	0.12% 0.125% 1% 1%
Prednisolone Sodium Phosphate Ophthalmic Solution	AK-Pred Inflamase Available generically AK-Pred Inflamase Forte Available generically	0.125% 0.125% 0.125% 1% 1% 1%
NONSTEROIDAL ANTI-INFLAMMATORY DRUGS		
Diclofenac Ophthalmic Solution	Voltaren	0.1%
Flurbiprofen Ophthalmic Solution*	Ocufen	0.03%
Ketorolac Ophthalmic Solution	Acular	0.5%
Suprofen Ophthalmic Solution*	Profenal	1%

*Indicated for intraoperative miosis only.

Steroids may be administered by four different routes in the treatment of ocular inflammation. **Table 8** lists the preferred route in various conditions.

Topical corticosteroids can elevate intraocular pressure and, in susceptible individuals, can induce glaucoma. Some corticosteroids, such as fluorometholone, fluorometholone acetate, and medrysone, cause less elevation of intraocular pressure than others. Corticosteroids may also cause cataract formation, a complication more likely with high-dose, long-term systemic use.

There are also four nonsteroidal anti-inflammatory drugs (NSAIDs) available. They are: diclofenac (Voltaren); flurbiprofen (Ocufen); ketorolac (Acular); and suprofen (Profenal). Flurbiprofen and suprofen are indicated solely for inhibition of intraoperative miosis. They are very similar in activity and some hospitals use them interchangeably. Diclofenac has an official indication for the postoperative prophylaxis and treatment of ocular inflammation. Ketorolac has FDA approval for relief of ocular itching due to seasonal allergic conjunctivitis. Both diclofenac and ketorolac have also been used successfully to prevent and treat cystoid macular edema. NSAIDs cause little, if any, rise in intraocular pressure.

Other useful agents include 4% sodium cromolyn (Opticrom) to treat vernal conjunctivitis or allergic keratoconjunctivitis. Tetracycline, taken orally, in doses of 250 mg four times daily for 4 weeks, then 250 mg once daily, is useful in treating ocular rosacea.

Other agents useful in treatment of seasonal allergic conjunctivitis are listed in **Table 9.**

TABLE 8

USUAL ROUTE OF STEROID ADMINISTRATION IN OCULAR INFLAMMATION

CONDITION	ROUTE
Blepharitis	Topical
Conjunctivitis	Topical
Episcleritis	Topical
Scleritis	Topical and/or systemic
Keratitis	Topical
Anterior uveitis	Topical and/or periocular
Posterior uveitis	Systemic and/or periocular
Endophthalmitis	Systemic/periocular, intravitreal
Optic neuritis	Systemic or periocular
Cranial arteritis	Systemic
Sympathetic ophthalmia	Systemic and topical

TABLE 9

AGENTS FOR RELIEF OF SEASONAL ALLERGIC CONJUNCTIVITIS

GENERIC NAME	TRADE NAME	CLASS
Ketorolac	Acular	N.S.A.I.D.
Levocabastin	Livostin	H_1-Antagonist
Lodoxamide	Alomide	Mast-cell Inhibitor
Naphazoline/antazoline	Vasocon-A	Antihistamine/ decongestant
Naphazoline/pheniramine	Naphcon-A	Antihistamine/ decongestant

4. ANESTHETIC AGENTS

A. Topical anesthetics

The agents listed in **Table 10** permit the clinician to perform ocular procedures such as tonometry, removal of foreign bodies from the surface of the eye, and lacrimal canalicular manipulation and irrigation. Cocaine, the prototype topical anesthetic, is a natural compound; the others are synthetic.

Cocaine is rarely used as an anesthetic agent because it causes damage to the corneal epithelium, produces pupillary dilation, and may affect intraocular pressure. However, it is considered useful when removal of the corneal epithelium is desired, as in epithelial debridement for dendritic keratitis.

The Table lists available agents and concentrations. Most begin working within a minute and continue acting for 10 to 20 minutes. A transient, superficial punctate keratitis may develop rapidly after instillation of the agent.

B. Regional anesthetics

The actions, benefits, and drawbacks of the most common regional anesthetic agents used in ophthalmic surgery are summarized in **Table 11**.

TABLE 10

TOPICAL ANESTHETIC AGENTS

USP OR NF NAME	TRADE NAME	CONCENTRATION (%)
Cocaine hydrochloride	. . .	1% to 4%
Proparacaine hydrochloride	AK-Taine	0.5%
	Alcaine	0.5%
	Ophthaine	0.5%
	Ophthetic	0.5%
Tetracaine hydrochloride	AK-T-Caine	0.5%
	Pontocaine hydrochloride	0.5%

TABLE 11

REGIONAL ANESTHETICS*

USP OR NF NAME	CONCENTRATION (%)/ MAXIMUM DOSE	ONSET OF ACTION	DURATION OF ACTION	MAJOR ADVANTAGES/ DISADVANTAGES
Procaine†	1%–4%/500 mg	7–8 min	30–45 min 60 min (with epinephrine)	Short duration. Poor absorption from mucous membranes
Tetracaine†	0.25%	5–9 min	120–140 min (with epinephrine)	
Hexylcaine†	1%–2%	5–10 min	60 min	
Bupivacaine††, **	0.25%–0.75%	5–11 min	480–720 min (with epinephrine)	
Lidocaine††	1%–2%/500 mg	4–6 min	40–60 min 120 min (with epinephrine)	Spreads readily without hyaluronidase
Mepivacaine††	1%–2%/500 mg	3–5 min	120 min	Duration of action greater without epinephrine[1]
Prilocaine††	1%–2%/600 mg	3–4 min	90–120 min (with epinephrine)	As effective as lidocaine
Etidocaine††	1%	3 min	300–600 min	

*Retrobulbar injection has been reported to cause apnea.
† Ester type compound
††Amide type compound
** A mixture of bupivacaine, lidocaine, and epinephrine has been shown to be effective in retinal detachment surgery under local anesthesia.

REFERENCES:

1. Everett WG, Vey EK, Finlay JW. Duration of oculomotor akinesia of injectable anesthetics. *Trans Am Acad Ophthalmol.* 1961; 65:308.
2. Holekamp TLR, Arribas NP, Boniuk I. Bupivacaine anesthesia in retinal detachment surgery. *Arch Ophthalmol.* 1979; 97:109.

5. AGENTS FOR TREATMENT OF GLAUCOMA

A. Miotics — see **Table 12**
Parasympathomimetic agents (miotics) are used primarily as topical therapy for glaucoma. A secondary use is the control of accommodative esotropia. This class of agents mimics the effect of acetylcholine on parasympathomimetic postganglionic nerve endings within the eye. The class is subdivided into direct-acting (cholinergic) agents and indirect-acting (anticholinesterase) agents, based on their respective abilities to bind acetylcholine receptors and inhibit the enzymatic hydrolysis of acetylcholine. **Table 12** lists the parasympathomimetics approved for topical use in this country. In addition, two agents are available for intraocular use: Miochol, a 1% solution of acetylcholine, and Miostat, a 0.01% solution of carbachol.

B. Sympathomimetics — see **Table 13**
These medications work by improving aqueous outflow and, to a lesser extent, improving uveoscleral output. The prodrug dipivefrin causes fewer systemic side effects than epinephrine and can sometimes be used in patients who have developed a sensitivity to epinephrine.

C. β-Adrenergic blocking agents — see **Table 14**
These medications work by blocking β-adrenergic receptor sites, decreasing aqueous production, and, thereby, reducing intraocular pressure. Because β-adrenergic receptors occur in a number of organ systems, systemic side effects of these drugs may include slowed heart rate, decreased blood pressure, and exacerbation of intrinsic bronchial asthma and emphysema. These agents can also enhance the effects of a number of systemic medications including β-blockers, digitalis alkaloids, and reserpine. Since betaxolol is a cardioselective β-blocker, it has significantly less effect on the respiratory system and can be used in some patients with respiratory illnesses.

D. Hyperosmotic agents — see **Table 15**
These medications decrease intraocular pressure by creating an osmotic gradient between the blood and intraocular fluid, causing fluid to move out of the aqueous and vitreous humors into the bloodstream. Though not usually used in open-angle glaucoma, these medications are employed to decrease pressure in an attack of angle-closure glaucoma, and to give a "soft" eye during surgery.

E. Carbonic anhydrase inhibitors —see **Table 16**.
These systemic drugs decrease the formation and secretion of aqueous humor. They are usually used as a supplement to topical agents in the treatment of open-angle glaucoma. Their use is limited by their side effects, which include paresthesias, anorexia, gastrointestinal disturbances, headaches, altered taste and smell, sodium and potassium depletion, ureteral colic, a predisposition to form renal calculi, and, rarely, bone marrow suppression.

F. β_2 Adrenoreceptor agonist —Aproclonidine is the only FDA approved drug in this class. It is available as a single dose applicator of a 1% solution for suppression of the acute intraocular pressure spikes that occur after laser treatments. Recently, a multiple dose container (5 ml) of the 0.5% concentration has been approved to be used with other glaucoma medications to control pressure in patients who are not responding adequately to traditional therapy.

TABLE 12

MIOTICS

GENERIC NAME	TRADE NAME	STRENGTHS (%)	SIZES
CHOLINERGIC AGENTS			
Carbachol	Isopto Carbachol	0.75%, 1.5%, 2.25%, 3%	15, 30 mL
Pilocarpine hydrochloride	Akarpine	1%, 2%, 4%	15 mL
	Isopto Carpine	0.25, 0.5, 1, 2, 3, 4, 5, 6, 8, 10%	15 & 30 mL
	Ocusert-Pilo	20, 40	Box of 8 inserts
	Pilocar	0.5%, 1%, 2%, 3%, 4%, 6%	15 & 2 x 15 mL
	Pilopine-HS gel	4%	3.5 g
	Piloptic	0.5%, 1%, 2%, 3%, 4%, 6%	15 mL
	Pilostat	1%, 2%, 4%	15 mL
	Storzine	1%, 2%, 4%	15 mL
	Available generically	0.5%, 1%, 2%, 3%, 4%, 6%	15 mL
Pilocarpine nitrate	Pilagan	1%, 2%, 4%	15 mL
CHOLINESTERASE INHIBITORS			
Physostigmine	Isopto Eserine	0.25%, 0.5%	15 mL
	Available generically as		
	Eserine Oph Oint	0.25%	3.5 g
Demecarium	Humorsol	0.25%, 0.5%	5 mL
Echothiophate iodide	Phospholine Iodide	0.03%, 0.06%, 0.125%, 0.25%	5 mL
Isofluorphate	Floropryl	0.025%	3.5 g

TABLE 13

SYMPATHOMIMETICS

GENERIC NAME	TRADE NAME	CONCENTRATION (%)	SIZE(S) (mL)
Dipivefrin hydrochloride	Propine AK PRO	0.1%	5,10, 15
Epinephrine bitartrate	Epitrate	2.0%	7.5
Epinephrine borate	Epinal Eppy/N	0.5%, 1% 1%, 2%	7.5 7.5
Epinephrine hydrocloride	Epifrin Glaucon	0.5%, 1%, 2% 1%, 2%	5, 10, & 15 10

TABLE 14

β-ADRENERGIC BLOCKING AGENTS

GENERIC NAME	TRADE NAME	CONCENTRATION (%)	SIZE(S) (mL)
Betaxolol hydrochloride	Betoptic-S Betoptic	0.25% 0.5%	2.5, 5, 15 2.5, 5, 10, 15
Carteolol hydrochloride	Ocupress	1.0%	5 & 10
Levobunolol hydrochloride	Betagan Available generically	0.25%, 0.5% 0.25%, 0.5%	2, 5, 10, 15 5, 10 & 15
Metipranolol	OptiPranolol	0.3%	5 & 10
Timolol maleate	Timoptic	0.25%, 0.5%	2.5, 5, 10, 15
Timolol maleate (preservative-free)	Timoptic in OCUDOSE	0.25%, 0.5%	0.45 , box of 60 units

TABLE 15

HYPEROSMOTIC AGENTS

USP OR NF NAME	TRADE NAME	PREPARATION	DOSE	ROUTE	ONSET/DURATION OF ACTION
Glycerin	Osmoglyn	50%	1–1.5 g/kg	Oral	. . .
Isosorbide*	Ismotic	45%	1.5 g/kg	Oral	30 min/5–6 h
Mannitol†	Osmitrol	5%–20%	0.5–2 g/kg	IV	30–60 min/6 h
Urea	Ureaphil	Powder or 30% soln	0.5–2 g/kg	IV	30–45 min/5–6 h

*Do not confuse with isosorbide dinitrate, an antianginal agent.
†Do not confuse with mannitol hexanitrate, an antianginal agent.

TABLE 16

CARBONIC ANHYDRASE INHIBITORS

USP OR NF NAME	TRADE NAME	PREPARATION	ONSET/DURATION OF ACTION
Acetazolamide	Diamox Available generically	125, 250 mg tablets 500 mg (timed-release) capsules 250 mg tablets	2 h/4–6 h
Acetazolamide Sodium	Diamox Parenteral	500 mg	5–10 min/2 h
Dichlorphenamide	Daranide	50 mg tablets	30 min/6 h
Methazolamide	Glauctabs MZM Neptazane Available generically	25, 50 mg tablets 25, 50 mg tablets 25, 50 mg tablets 25, 50 mg tablets	2 h/4–6 h

6. MEDICATIONS FOR DRY EYE

Dry eye refers to a deficiency in either the aqueous or mucin components of the precorneal tear film. The most commonly encountered aqueous-deficient dry eye in the United States is keratoconjunctivitis sicca, while mucin-deficient dry eyes may be seen in cases of hypovitaminosis A, Stevens-Johnson syndrome, ocular pemphigoid, extensive trachoma, and chemical burns.

Dry eye is treated with artificial tear preparations (see **Table 17**) and ophthalmic lubricants (see **Table 18**). The lubricants form an occlusive film over the ocular surface and protect the eye from drying. Administered as a nighttime medication, they are useful both for dry eye and in cases of recurrent corneal erosion.

TABLE 17

ARTIFICIAL TEAR PREPARATIONS

MAJOR COMPONENT(S)	CONCENTRATION (%)	TRADE NAME	PRESERVATIVE/EDTA*
Carboxymethyl cellulose	0.5%	Refresh Plus	None
	1%	Celluvisc	None
Hydroxyethyl cellulose		Comfort Tears	Benzalkonium chloride, EDTA
		TearGard	Sorbic acid, EDTA
Hydroxyethyl cellulose, polyvinyl alcohol		Neo-Tears	Thimerosal, EDTA
Hydroxyethyl cellulose, povidone		Adsorbotear	Thimerosal, EDTA
Hydroxypropyl cellulose		Lacrisert (biodegradable insert)	None
Hydroxypropyl methylcellulose	0.5%	Isopto Plain	Benzalkonium chloride
		Isopto Tears	Benzalkonium chloride
		Tearisol	Benzalkonium chloride, EDTA
	1%	Isopto Alkaline	Benzalkonium chloride
		Ultra Tears	Benzalkonium chloride
Hydroxypropyl methylcellulose, dextran 70		Bion Tears	None
		Tears Naturale II	Polyquad
		Tears Naturale Free	None
		Tears Renewed	Benzalkonium chloride, EDTA
Hydroxypropyl methylcellulose, gelatin A		Lacril	Chlorobutanol, polysorbate 80
Methylcellulose	1%	Murocel	Methyl-, propylparabens
Polycarbophil, PEG-400, dextran 70		AquaSite	EDTA
		AquaSite multi-dose	EDTA, Sorbic acid
Polyvinyl alcohol	1.4%	AKWA Tears	Benzalkonium chloride, EDTA
		Just Tears	Benzalkonium chloride, EDTA
		Liquifilm Tears	Chlorobutanol
	3%	Liquifilm Forte	Thimerosal, EDTA
Polyvinyl alcohol, PEG-400, dextrose	1%	HypoTears	Benzalkonium chloride, EDTA
		HypoTears PF	EDTA
		Puralube Tears	Benzalkonium chloride, EDTA
Polyvinyl alcohol, povidone	1.4%	Murine	Benzalkonium chloride, EDTA
	0.6%	Refresh	None
		Tears Plus	Chlorobutanol

*EDTA = ethylenediaminetetraacetic acid.

TABLE 18

OPHTHALMIC LUBRICANTS

TRADE NAME	COMPOSITION OF STERILE OINTMENT
AKWA Tears Ointment	White petrolatum, liquid lanolin, and mineral oil
Duolube	White petrolatum and mineral oil
Duratears Naturale	White petrolatum, liquid lanolin, and mineral oil
HypoTears	White petrolatum and light mineral oil
Lacri-Lube S.O.P.	42.5% mineral oil, 55% white petrolatum, lanolin alcohol, and chlorobutanol
Refresh P.M.	41.5% mineral oil, 55% white petrolatum, petrolatum, and lanolin alcohol

7. OCULAR DECONGESTANTS

These topically applied adrenergic medications are commonly used to whiten the eye. Three types are available. Those containing naphazoline and tetrahydrozoline are more stable than those with phenylephrine. Usual dosage is 1 or 2 drops no more than 4 times a day (see **Table 19**).

TABLE 19

OCULAR DECONGESTANTS

DRUG	TRADE NAME	ADDITIONAL COMPONENTS
Naphazoline hydrochloride	AK-Con*	Benzalkonium chloride, edetate disodium
	Albalon*	Benzalkonium chloride, edetate disodium
	Clear Eyes	Benzalkonium chloride, edetate disodium
	Degest 2	Benzalkonium chloride, edetate disodium
	Naphcon*	Benzalkonium chloride, edetate disodium
	Opcon*	Benzalkonium chloride, edetate disodium
	Vasoclear	Benzalkonium chloride, edetate disodium
	Vasocon Regular*	Phenylmercuric acetate
Phenylephrine hydrochloride	AK-Nefrin	Benzalkonium chloride, edetate disodium
	Efricel	Benzalkonium chloride, edetate disodium
	Eye Cool	Thimerosal, edetate disodium
	Isopto Frin	Benzalkonium chloride, edetate disodium
	Prefrin Liquifilm	Benzalkonium chloride, edetate disodium
	Relief	—
	Tear-Efrin	Benzalkonium chloride, edetate disodium
	Velva-Kleen	Thimerosal, edetate disodium
Tetrahydrozoline hydrochloride	Collyrium	Benzalkonium chloride, edetate disodium
	Murine Plus	Benzalkonium chloride, edetate disodium
	Soothe*	Benzalkonium chloride, edetate disodium
	Tetracon	Benzalkonium chloride, edetate disodium
	Visine	Benzalkonium chloride, edetate disodium
DECONGESTANT/ASTRINGENT COMBINATIONS		
Naphazoline hydrochloride plus zinc sulfate	Clear Eyes ACR (allergy/cold relief)	Benzalkonium chloride, edetate disodium
Phenylephrine hydrochloride plus zinc sulfate	Prefrin-Z	Thimerosal
	Zincfrin	Benzalkonium chloride
Tetrahydrozoline plus zinc sulfate	Visine A.C.	Benzalkonium chloride, edetate disodium

*Prescription medication.

8. OPHTHALMIC IRRIGATING SOLUTIONS

Listed in **Table 20** are sterile isotonic solutions for general ophthalmic use. They are all over-the-counter products. There are also intraocular irrigating solutions available for use during surgical procedures. They include prescription medications such as Bausch & Lomb's Balanced Salt Solution, Alcon's BSS and BSS Plus, and Iolab's Iocare Balanced Salt Solution.

TABLE 20

OPHTHALMIC IRRIGATING SOLUTIONS

TRADE NAME	COMPONENTS	ADDITIONAL COMPONENTS
AK-Rinse	Sodium, potassium, calcium, and magnesium chlorides, sodium acetate, and sodium citrate	Benzalkonium chloride
Blinx	Boric acid and sodium borate	Phenylmercuric acetate
Collyrium	Antipyrine, boric acid, and borax	Thimerosal
Dacriose	Sodium and potassium chlorides, and sodium phosphate	Benzalkonium chloride, edetate disodium
Eye-Stream	Sodium, potassium, magnesium and calcium chlorides, sodium acetate, and sodium citrate	Benzalkonium chloride
Irigate	Boric acid, potassium chloride, and sodium carbonate	Benzalkonium chloride, edetate disodium
Lavoptik Eye Wash	Sodium chloride, sodium biphosphate, and sodium phosphate	Benzalkonium chloride
M/Rinse	Sodium and potassium chlorides, sodium borate, and boric acid	Thimerosal, edetate disodium

9. HYPEROSMOLAR AGENTS

Hyperosmolar (hypertonic) agents are used to reduce corneal edema therapeutically or for diagnostic purposes. They act through osmotic attraction of water through the semipermeable corneal epithelium.

TABLE 21

HYPEROSMOLAR AGENTS

GENERIC NAME	TRADE NAME	CONCENTRATION (%)
A. Therapeutic preparations		
Sodium chloride	Adsorbonac Ophthalmic	2% or 5% (solution)
	AK-NaCl	5% (solution and ointment)
	Muro-128	5% (solution and ointment)
Glucose	Glucose 40 Ophthalmic	40% (ointment)
B. Diagnostic preparation		
Glycerin	Ophthalgan	

10. DIAGNOSTIC AGENTS

Some of the more common diagnostic agents and tests used in ophthalmologic practice are listed below.

A. Examination of the Conjunctiva, Cornea, and Lacrimal Apparatus

Fluorescein, applied primarily as a 2% alkaline solution, and with impregnated paper strips, is used to examine the integrity of the conjunctival and corneal epithelia. Defects in the corneal epithelium will appear bright green in ordinary light and bright yellow when a cobalt blue filter is used in the light path. Similar lesions of the conjunctiva appear bright orange-yellow in ordinary illumination.

Fluorescein has also come into wide use in the fitting of rigid contact lenses, though it cannot be used for soft lenses, which absorb the dye. Proper fit is determined by examining the pattern of fluorescein beneath the contact lens.

In addition, fluorescein is used in performing applanation tonometry and one test of lacrimal apparatus patency (Jones test) uses 1 drop of 1% fluorescein instilled into the conjunctival sac. If the dye appears in the nose, drainage is normal.[1]

Rose bengal, as a 1% solution, is particularly useful for demonstrating abnormal conjunctival or corneal epithelium. Devitalized cells stain bright red, while normal cells show no change. The abnormal epithelial cells present in dry eye disorders are effectively revealed by this stain.

The Schirmer test is a valuable method of assessing tear production. It employs prepared strips of filter paper 5 by 30 mm in size. The strips are inserted into the topically anesthetized conjunctival sac at the junction of the middle and outer third of the lower lid, with approximately 25 mm of paper exposed. After 5 minutes, the strip is removed and the amount of moistening measured. The normal range is 10 to 25 mm. If inadequate production of tears is found on the initial test, a Schirmer II test can be performed by repeating the procedure while stimulating the nasal mucosa.[2] A number of variations of the Schirmer test can be found in textbooks and journals.

B. Examination of Acquired Ptosis or Extraocular Muscle Palsy

To confirm myasthenia gravis as the cause of ptosis or muscle palsy, an intravenous injection of 2 mg of *edrophonium chloride* is administered, followed 45 seconds later by an additional 8 mg if there is no response to the first dose. (In case of a severe reaction to the edrophonium, immediately give atropine sulfate, 0.6 mg intravenously.)

C. Examination of the Retina and Choroid

Sodium fluorescein solution, in concentrations of 5%, 10%, and 25%, is injected intravenously to study the retinal and choroidal circulation. It has been used primarily in examination of lesions at the posterior pole of the eye, but anterior segment fluorescein angiography (wherein the vessels of the iris, sclera, and conjunctiva are studied) is also a useful clinical tool.

Intravascular fluorescein is normally prevented from entering the retina by the intact retinal vascular endothelium (blood-retinal barrier) and the intact retinal pigment epithelium. Defects in either the retinal vessels or the pigment epithelium will allow leakage of fluorescein, which can then be studied by either direct observation or photography. For good results, appropriate filters are needed to excite the fluorescein and exclude unwanted wavelengths. The peak frequencies for excitation lie between 485 and 500 nm and, for emission, between 520 and 530 nm.

Fluorescein has proved to be a safe diagnostic agent, the most common side effects being nausea and vomiting. However, occasional allergic and vagal reactions do occur, so oxygen and emergency equipment should be readily available when angiography is performed. Patients should also be warned that the dye will temporarily stain their skin and urine; in the average patient this lasts no more than a day.

D. Examination of Abnormal Pupillary Responses

Methacholine, as a 2.5% solution instilled into the conjunctival sac, will cause the tonic pupil (Adie's pupil) to contract, but will leave a normal pupil unchanged. A similar pupillary response is seen following instillation of 2.5% methacholine in patients with familial dysautonomia (Riley-Day syndrome).

Table 22 shows the effects of several drugs on miosis due to interruption of the sympathetic system (Horner's syndrome). The effect depends on the location of the lesion in the sympathetic chain.

TABLE 22

HORNER'S SYNDROME

TOPICAL DROP	NEURON III (POST-GANGLIONIC)	NEURON II (PRE-GANGLIONIC)	NEURON I (CENTRAL)
Cocaine 2%–10%	–	–	+/–
Epinephrine (Adrenalin) 1:1000	+++	+	–
Phenylephrine 1%	+++	+	+/–
Hydroxy-amphetamine 1%	–	+	+

Pilocarpine may be used to determine whether a fixed dilated pupil is due to an atropinelike drug or interruption of the pupil's parasympathetic innervation.[3] If an atropine-like drug is involved, the pupil will not react to pilocarpine. If dilation is due to interruption of the parasympathetic innervation (compression by aneurysm, Adie's tonic pupil) instillation of pilocarpine will cause the pupil to constrict.

REFERENCES

1. Thompson HS, Mensher JH. Adrenergic mydrisis in Homer's syndrome: hydroxyampheta mine test for diagnosis of post-ganglionic defects.*Am J Ophthalmol.* 1971;72:472.
2. Hecht SD. Evaluation of the lacrimal drainage system. *Ophthalmology.* 1978;85:1250.
3. Thompson HS, Newsome DA, Lowenfeld I E. The fixed dilated pupil. Sudden iridoplegia or mydriatic drops; a simple diagnostic test. *Arch Ophthalmol.* 1971;86:12.

11. VISCOELASTIC MATERIALS USED IN OPHTHALMALOGY

Viscoelastic substances are used in ophthalmic surgery to maintain the anterior chamber, hydraulically dissect tissues, act as a vitreous substitute/tamponade, and prevent mechanical damage to tissue, especially the corneal endothelium. The individual characteristics of the various viscoelastic materials are the result of the chain length and intra- and interchain molecular interactions of the compounds comprising the viscoelastic substance. All viscoelastic materials have the potential to produce a large postoperative increase in pressure if they are not adequately removed from the anterior chamber following surgery.

HEALON (Kabi Pharmacia Ophthalmics)–Composed of sodium hyaluronate with a molecular weight of approximately 3.8 million. Viscosity is 26,250 cp.*

AMVISC PLUS (IOLAB)–A 1.6% sodium hyaluronate product with a viscosity of 40,125 cp. The greater viscosity is obtained by increasing total concentration and using sodium hyaluronate of lower molecular weight.

OCCUCOAT (Storz)–A 2% hydroxypropyl methylcellulose material with a molecular weight greater than 80,000 daltons. Occucoat is termed a viscoadherent rather than a viscoelastic because of its coating ability, which is related to its contact angle and low surface tension. Its viscosity is 4,000 cp.

VISCOAT (Alcon)–A 1:3 mixture of 4% chondroitin sulfate (molecular weight 22,500) and 3% sodium hyaluronate (molecular weight greater than 500,000). The viscosity is 51,000 cp.

*Dynamic viscosity at 25°C with a Brookfield digital viscometer, shear rate 2/second.

12. OFF-LABEL DRUG APPLICATIONS IN OPHTHALMOLOGY

A. Acetylcysteine

This agent is used to treat corneal conditions such as alkali burns, corneal melts, and keratoconjunctivitis sicca. It is thought to improve healing by inhibiting the action of collagenase, which may contribute to delay in healing. The drug is available generically or under the trade name Mucomyst in 10% and 20% solutions. Though none of the commercially available solutions are approved for use in ophthalmology, they have been administered as frequently as hourly in acute cases, and up to 4 times a day in maintenance therapy.

B. Alteplase (tissue plasminogen activator)

This thrombolytic agent, trade-named Activase, is used to treat fibrin formation in postvitrectomy patients. Though initial studies were based on intraocular injections of 25 µg, more recent work has shown the drug to be effective in doses of as little as 3 to 6 µg. Because by-products of alteplase activity may mediate endothelial cell toxicity, the lower doses are preferred.

C. Antimetabolites

5-Fluorouracil (5-FU). This drug inhibits fibroblasts and therefore diminishes scarring after glaucoma filtering surgery. Initial recommendations called for subconjunctival injection of 5 mg twice daily for 7 days postoperatively and once daily for the succeeding 7 days. However, many physicians today are achieving positive results with as little as 4 mg administered 4 to 6 times during a 10-day period. Use of this drug is associated with a number of complications, including conjunctival wound leak, corneal epithelial defects, hypotony associated with permanently reduced vision acuity, serious corneal infections in eyes with preexistent corneal epithelial edema, and increased susceptibility to late-onset bleb infections. The drug should be considered only when there is a high risk of surgical failure.

Mitomycin. This potent chemotherapeutic agent, trade-named Mutamycin, is being used in filtering surgery for the same purpose and on the same type of patients as 5-FU. It is applied once during surgery on a small piece of Gelfilm or Weck Cell in a concentration of 0.2 to 0.4 mg/mL. Reported side effects are similar to those of 5-FU. However, some serious side effects may go unreported, since there is a possibility of delayed reactions 6 to 24 months after surgery. Mitomycin has also been administered in a 0.02% to 0.04% solution 2 to 4 times a day to prevent recurrence after pterygium surgery. Serious side effects associated with this therapy include corneal melts and scleral ulceration and calcification.

Physicians should bear in mind the possibility of major side effects from all antineoplastic agents and carefully weigh the risks and benefits of the use. Remember, too, that these agents should always be handled and discarded in accordance with OSHA, AMA, ASHP, and/or hospital policies regarding the safe use of antineoplastics.

D. Cyclosporine

This potent immunosuppressant has a high degree of selectivity for T lymphocytes. Available under the trade name Sandimmune, it has been used in a 2% topical solution as prophylaxis against rejection in high-risk, penetrating keratoplasty and for treatment of severe vernal conjunctivitis resistant to more conventional therapy, ligneous conjunctivitis unresponsive to other topical therapy, and noninfectious peripheral ulcerative keratitis associated with systemic autoimmune disorders. All contraindications for systemic use also apply to topical administration, since blood levels of up to 64 ng/mL have been observed after topical application. All patients receiving this medication should have blood work that includes cyclosporine levels, blood urea nitrogen, creatinine, lactate dehyrogenase, alkaline phosphatase, and total bilirubin.

E. Edetate disodium

This chelating agent plays a role in the treatment of band keratopathy. After removal of the corneal epithelium, it is used to remove calcium from Bowman's membrane.

REFERENCES

Nesburn A. Trauma topics: small corneal perforations. *Audio Digest: Ophthalmol.* 1983;12:21.

Ralph R. Chemical burns of the eye. In: Tasman W, Jaeger E, eds. *Duane's Clinical Ophthalmology.* Philadelphia, Pa: JB Lippincott; 1989 vol. 4, chap 28:14.

Jaffe G, Abrams G, et al. Tissue plasminogen activator for post vitrectomy fibrin formation. *Opthalmology.* 1990;97:189.

McDermott M, Edelhauser H, et al. Tissue plasminogen activator and corneal endothelium. *Am J Ophthalmol.* 1989;108.

Williams D, Benett S, et al. Low-dose intraocular tissue plasminogen activator for treatment of postvitrectomy firbrin formations. *Am J Opthalmol.* 1990;109:606.

Williams G, Lambrou F, et al. Treatment of postvitrectomy fibrin formation with intraocular tissue plasminogen activator. *Arch Ophthalmol.* 1988;106:1055.

Ando H, Tadayoshi I, et al. Inhibition of corneal epithelial wound healing. A comparative study of mitomycin C and 5-fluorouracil. *Ophthalmology.* 1992;99:1809.

Falck F, Skuta G, Klein T. Mitomycin versus 5-fluorouracil antimetabolite therapy for glaucoma filtration surgery. *Semin in Ophthalmol.* 1992;7:97.

Who should receive antimetabolites after filtering surgery? *Arch Ophthalmol.* 1992;110:1069. Editorial.

Welsh R, Palmer S. Mitomycin in trabeculectomy: alter your technique. *Ocular Surgery News*; May 1, 1992:67.

Dunn J, Seamone S, Ostler H. Development of scleral ulceration and calcification after pterygium excision and mitomycin therapy. *Am J Ophthalmol.* 1991;112:343.

Rubinfeld R, Pfister R, et al. Serious complications of topical mitomycin-C after pterygium surgery. *Ophthalmology.* 1992;99:1647.

Bonomi L. Medical treatment of glaucoma. *Current Science.* 1992;1040:70.

Lish A, Camras C, Podos S. Effect of apraclonidine on intraocular pressure in glaucoma patients receiving maximally tolerated medications. *Glaucoma* 1992;1:19.

Holland E, Chan C, et al. Immunohistologic findings and results of treatment with cyclosporine in ligneous conjunctivitis. *Am J Ophthalmol* 1989;107:160.

Bouchard C, Belin M, Letter to Editor concerning above article, with reply by author. *Am J Ophthalmol* 1989;108:210.

Secchi A, Tognan M, Leonardi A. Topical use of cyclosporine in the treatment of vernal conjunctivitis. *Am J Ophthalmol* 1990;110:641.

BenEzra D, Matamoros N, Cohen E. Treatment of severe vernal keratoconjunctivitis with cyclosporine A eyedrops. *Transplant Proc.* 1988;20,No.2(suppl 2):644.

Zierhut H, Thiel E, et al. Topical treatment of severe corneal ulcers with cyclosporine A. *Graefe's* Arch *Clin Exp Opthalmol.* 1989;227:30.

Hill J. The use of cyclosporin in high-risk keratoplasty. *Am J Ophthalmol* 1989;107:506.

Belin M, Bouchard C, Frantz S, et al. Topical cyclosporine in high-risk corneal transplants. *Ophthalmology.* 1989;96:1144.

13. OCULAR TOXICOLOGY — F. T. Fraunfelder, MD

The table on the following pages recounts some of the more recently published findings on ocular side effects of drugs in general, as well as systemic side effects of drugs commonly used by ophthalmologists. It is not a catalog of all such reactions, since the data would be too lengthy for this format.

The volume of ocular toxicology in the medical literature is overwhelming. However, much is based on soft data, since, in most practices, the number of patients on a particular drug falls short of providing an adequate sample. Even in a controlled experimental environment, it is often difficult to prove a cause-and-effect relationship. In clinical practice, with its multitude of variables, a definitive finding is nearly impossible. It was to alleviate this problem that the National Registry of Drug-Induced Ocular Side Effects was founded.

Established by the federal Food and Drug Administration, with endorsement of the American Academy of Ophthalmology, the National Registry works on the supposition that, if the suspicions of practicing clinicians can be pooled in a large-enough database, they can be used as a flagging system to decrease the lag time in recognizing a possible adverse ocular response.

The registry welcomes communications from all concerned clinicians. To report a suspected adverse drug response, or to obtain references for the information listed below, please contact:

F.T. Fraunfelder, MD, Director, National Registry of Drug-Induced Ocular Side Effects
Casey Eye Institute
Oregon Health Sciences/University
3375 SW Terwilliger Blvd
Portland, OR 97201-4197

REFERENCE

Fraunfelder, FT. *Drug-Induced Ocular Side Effects and Drug Interactions.* 3rd ed. Philadelphia, Pa: W.B. Saunders; 1989.

TABLE 23

ADVERSE DRUG EFFECTS

GENERIC NAME	PRINCIPAL GENERAL USE	POSSIBLE ADVERSE EFFECTS
I. MEDICATION BY INJECTION		
a. Adrenal Corticosteroids		
Depo-steroids	Allergic disorders Anti-inflammatory disorders	If injected into a blood vessel, eg, the tonsillar fossa, may cause unilateral or bilateral retinal arterial occlusions due to emboli of depo-steroid. Permanent bilateral blindness may ensue.
Triamcinolone	Allergic disorders Anti-inflammatory disorders	Fatty atrophy in area of injection, ie, enophthalmus if given retrobulbar or, if given in periocular skin, some deformity can occur in area due to loss of fat.
b. Anesthetics		
Ketamine hydrochloride	Adjunct to anesthesia Short-term diagnostic or surgical procedures	Reversible nystagmus
c. Antifungals		
Amphotericin B	Aspergillosis, blastomycosis, candidiasis, coccidioidomycosis, histoplasmosis	Ischemic necrosis after subconjunctival injection Subconjunctival nodule
d. Antineoplastics		
Carmustine	Brain tumors Multiple myeloma	Optic neuritis Retinal vascular disorders
Cisplatin	Metastatic testicular or ovarian tumors. Advanced bladder carcinoma	Cortical blindness Papilledema, retrobulbar or optic neuritis
Fluorouracil	Carcinoma of the colon, rectum, breast, stomach, and pancreas	Ocular irritation with tearing, conjunctival hyperemia, canalicular fibrosis
e. Miscellaneous		
Skin Tests	Tests for allergies	Recurrence or aggravation of episcleritis or scleritis
f. Ophthalmic Dyes		
Fluorescein	Ocular diagnostic tests	Nausea, vomiting, urticaria, rhinorrhea, dizziness, hypotension, pharyngoedema, anaphylactic reaction
g. Parasympathomimetics		
Acetylcholine	Produces prompt, short-term miosis	Hypotension and bradycardia with intraocular injection
II. ORAL		
a. Amebicides		
Iodochlorhydroxyquin	Acrodermatitis enteropathica *Entamoeba histolytica*	Optic atrophy—may be due to a zinc deficiency of the optic nerve
b. Anthelminthics		
Levamisol hydrochloride	Connective tissue disorders Ascaris infestation	Patients with Sjögren's syndrome and possibly keratitis sicca have marked increase in systemic side effects, including pruritus and muscle weakness
c. Antianxiety Agents		
Diazepam	Acute alcohol withdrawal Preoperative medication Psychoneurotic anxiety, depression, tension, or agitation Skeletal muscle spasms	Allergic conjunctivitis Extraocular muscle paresis Nystagmus
d. Antiarrhythmics		
Amiodarone hydrochloride	Cardiac abnormalities Ventricular arrhythmias	Keratopathy Lens opacities, optic neuropathy, optic neuritis
Oxprenolol	Cardiovascular abnormalities Certain hypertensive states	Conjunctival hyperemia Decreased lacrimation, nonspecific ocular irritation, photophobia
Propranolol	Cardiovascular abnormalities Certain hypertensive states	May precipitate latent myotonia May mask hyperthyroidism; when taken off drug, thyroid stare and exophthalmos may occur

GENERIC NAME	PRINCIPAL GENERAL USE	POSSIBLE ADVERSE EFFECTS
e. Antibiotics and Antituberculars		
Chloramphenicol		Aplastic anemia
Ethambutol hydrochloride	Pulmonary tuberculosis	Optic neuropathy
Rifampin	Asymptomatic carriers of meningococcus Many gram-negative and gram-positive cocci, including *Neisseria* and *Hemophilus influenzae* Pulmonary tuberculosis	Conjunctival hyperemia Exudative conjunctivitis Increased lacrimation
Tetracycline hydrochloride	Useful against gram-negative and gram-positive bacteria Members of lymphogranuloma-psittacosis group *Mycoplasma*	Pseudotumor cerebri and papilledema as early as 3 days after onset of medication in infants and in young adults Transient myopia
f. Antihypertensives		
Sodium nitroprusside	Provides controlled hypertension during anesthesia Management of severe hypertension	Contraindicated in Leber's hereditary optic atrophy and tobacco amblyopia
g. Antileprotics		
Clofazimine	Dermatologic diseases—psoriasis, pyoderma gangrenosum Leprosy	Conjunctival, corneal, and macular pigmentation
h. Antimalarials and Anti-inflammatories		
Hydroxychloroquine	Malaria Lupus erythematosus Rheumatoid arthritis	Disturbance of accommodation Corneal changes Bull's-eye maculopathy—central, pericentral, or paracentral scotomas
i. Antineoplastics		
Busulfan	Chronic myelogenous leukemia	Cataracts Decreased lacrimation
Tamoxifen	Metastatic breast carcinoma	Corneal opacities Refractile retinal deposits
j. Antipsychotics		
Haloperidol	Acute and chronic schizophrenia Manic/depressive psychosis	Capsular cataracts with chronic use Cycloplegia and mydriasis
Lithium carbonate	Manic phase of manic/depressive exophthalmos psychosis	Oculogyric crisis Myoclonus
k. Antispasmodics		
Baclofen	Muscle spasms in multiple sclerosis and disorders associated with increased muscular tone	Blurred vision Hallucinations
l. Carbonic Anhydrase Inhibitors		
Acetazolamide Dichlorphenamide Ethoxzolamide	Centrencephalic epilepsies Congestive heart failure edema Drug-induced edema	Aggravation of metabolic acidosis, primarily in known CO_2-retaining diseases such as emphysema and bronchiectasis, and in patients with poor vital capacity
Methazolamide	Glaucoma	Aplastic anemia Decreased libido Impotency
m. Chelating Agents		
Penicillamine	Cystinuria Heavy metal antagonist—iron, lead, copper, mercury poisoning Wilson's disease	Facial or ocular myasthenia, including extraocular muscle paralysis, ptosis, and diplopia Ocular pemphigoid Optic neuritis and color-vision problems
n. Hormonal Agents		
Oral contraceptives	Amenorrhea Dysfunctional uterine bleeding Dysmenorrhea Hypogonadism Oral contraception Premenstrual tension	Contraindicated in patients with preexisting retinal vascular diseases Decrease in color vision with chronic use Macular edema

GENERIC NAME	PRINCIPAL GENERAL USE	POSSIBLE ADVERSE EFFECTS
o. Hydantoins		
Phenytoin	Chronic epilepsy	Optic nerve hypoplasia in infants with epileptic mothers on the drug Ocular teratogenic effects, including strabismus, ptosis, hypertelorism, epicanthus
p. Nonsteroidal Anti-inflammatory Drugs		
Ibuprofen	Rheumatoid arthritis Osteoarthritis	Decreased color vision Optic neuritis Visual field defects
Naproxen	Rheumatoid arthritis Osteoarthritis Ankylosing spondylitis	Corneal opacity Periorbital edema
Sulindac	Rheumatoid arthritis Osteoarthritis Ankylosing spondylitis	Keratitis Stevens-Johnson syndrome
q. Psychedelics		
Marijuana	Cerebral sedative or narcotic	Conjunctival hyperemia Decreased lacrimation Decreased intraocular pressure Dyschromatopsia with chronic long-term use
r. Red Blood Cell Sickling Inhibitors		
Sodium cyanate	Sickle cell hemoglobinopathy	Partially reversible posterior subcapsular cataracts
s. Sedatives and Hypnotics		
Ethanol	Antiseptic Used as a beverage	Fetal alcohol syndrome: offspring of alcoholic mothers may have epicanthus, small palpebral fissures, and microphthalmia
t. Synthetic Retinoids		
Etretinate Isotretinoin	Cystic acne and other keratinizing skin disorders	Dark eye, abnormal dark adaptation, electro-oculography (EOG) and electroretinography (ERG), cataracts, optic neuritis, pseudotumor cerebri and papilledema
III. TOPICAL		
a. Anticholinergics		
Cyclopentolate hydrochloride	Used as a cycloplegic and mydriatic	Central nervous system toxicity, including slurred speech, ataxia,hallucinations, hyperactivity, seizures, syncope, and paralytic ileus
Tropicamide	Used as a cycloplegic and mydriatic	Cyanosis, muscle rigidity, nausea, pallor, vomiting, vasomotor collapse
b. Parasympathomimetics or Anticholinesterases		
Demecarium bromide Echothiophate iodide Isofluorphate Pilocarpine	Glaucoma	Retinal detachments primarily in eyes with peripheral retinal or retinal-vitreal disease. (Patients need to be warned of this possible effect when first placed on this medication.) Miotic upper respiratory infection—rhinorrhea, sensation of chest constriction, cough, conjunctival hyperemia; seen primarily in young children on anticholinesterase agents
c. Sympathomimetics		
Dipivefrin	Open-angle glaucoma	Follicular blepharoconjunctivitis, keratitis
Epinephrine	Used as a bronchodilator Open-angle glaucoma Used as a vasoconstrictor to prolong anesthetic action	Cicatricial pemphigoid Stains soft contact lenses black Hypertension, headache
10% Phenylephrine	Used as a mydriatic and vasoconstrictor	Cardiac arrhythmias and cardiac arrests with pledget form or subconjunctival injection, possible myocardial infarcts, systemic hypertension
Betaxolol Levobunolol hydrochloride Timolol	Glaucoma	Cardiac syncope, bradycardia, light-headedness, fatigue, congestive heart failure; In diabetics—hyperglycemia; In myasthenia gravis—severe dysarthria

SECTION 3

SUTURE MATERIALS

There is perhaps no other discipline that requires as many specialized needles and suture materials as ophthalmic surgery. To meet this need, manufacturers offer the ophthalmologist a comprehensive array of precisely manufactured reverse-cutting and spatula needles swaged to suture materials of collagen (plain and chromic), silk (black and white braided), virgin silk (black and white twisted), Nylon, Dacron, and synthetics.

Suture material intended for use in ophthalmic surgery can be either nonabsorbable or absorbable. Following is a list of various suture materials available for ophthalmology, with a brief description of each.

Absorbable

Plain Catgut—Prepared from the submucosal or mucosal layers of sheep or beef intestine, respectively, this material consists primarily of collagen—a fibrous protein—which is absorbed by the body. The material is chemically purified to minimize tissue reaction. Available in sizes 4–0 through 6–0.

Chromic Catgut—same as plain catgut except that it is treated with chromium salts to delay the absorption time. Available in sizes 4–0 through 7–0.

Plain Collagen—prepared from bovine deep flexor tendon. The tendon is purified and converted to a uniform suspension of collagen fibril. This fibrillar suspension is then extruded into suture strands and chemically treated to accurately control absorption rate. Available in sizes 4–0 through 7–0.

Chromic Collagen—prepared in the same way as plain collagen except that chromium salts are added during the chemical treatment to further delay absorption. Available in sizes 4–0 through 8–0.

TABLE 1

COMPARISON OF OPHTHALMIC SUTURE MATERIALS

SUTURE MATERIAL	RELATIVE TENSILE STRENGTH*	RELATIVE HOLDING DURATION†	RELATIVE TISSUE REACTION‡	EASE OF HANDLING	SPECIAL KNOT REQUIRED	BEHAVIOR OF EXPOSED ENDS	AVAILABLE SIZES§
Surgical gut or collagen							
Plain	6	1 week	4+	Fair	No	Stiff	4–0 to 6–0
Chromic	6	<2 weeks	3+	Fair	No	Stiff	4–0 to 8–0
Polyglactin 910							
Braided	9	2 weeks	2+	Good	Yes	Stiff	4–0 to 9–0
Monofilament	9	2 weeks	2+	Good	Yes	Stiff	9–0 to 10–0
Polyglycolic acid	9	2 weeks	2+	Good	Yes	Stiff	
Silk							
Virgin	7	2 months	3+	Excellent	No	Softest	8–0 to 9–0
Braided	8	2 months	3+	Good	No	Soft	4–0 to 9–0
Polyamide (Nylon)	9	6 months	1+	Fair	Yes	Stiff, sharp	8–0 to 11–0
Polypropylene	10	>12 months	1+	Fair	Yes	Stiff, sharp	4–0 to 6–0 9–0 to 10–0

Adapted from Spaeth GL. *Ophthalmic Surgery, Principles and Practice*. Philadelphia, Pa: WB Saunders; 1982:64.

*The higher the number, the greater the relative tensile strength. Strength varies with size of material; estimates apply mainly to size 8–0 sutures.

† Holding duration will vary with location and size of suture, health of patient, medications employed, etc. The time given in this table is an average of the time at which about 30% of tensile strength is lost.

‡ 1+ indicates least inflammatory response, 4+ greatest.

§ With needles appropriate for ophthalmic use. Sizes available will vary from time to time.

Synthetic Absorbable Sutures–Products include Vicryl (Polyglactin 910, a copolymer of lactide and glycolide) and Dexon (polyglycolic acid). These materials offer high tensile strength and minimal tissue reaction during the critical postoperative healing period, followed by predictable absorption. Coated Vicryl sutures are also available. Manufactured in size 4–0 through 10–0 (coated 4–0 through 8–0).

It is interesting to note that the absorption of sutures occurs in two distinct phases. After implantation, the suture's tensile strength diminishes during the early postoperative period. When most of the strength is lost, the remaining suture mass begins to decrease in what may be termed the second phase of absorption. The mass-loss phase then proceeds until the entire suture has been absorbed.

Nonabsorbable

Monofilament Nylon Sutures (Ethilon, Dermalon, and Supramid). These sutures offer high tensile strength and minimal tissue reaction. Nylon has been reported to lose tensile strength postoperatively at a rate of approximately 15% per year. Available in sizes 8–0 through 14–0.

Polypropylene Suture (Prolene)—a monofilament suture with high tensile strength and minimal tissue reaction. The material is not degraded or weakened by tissue enzymes. Available in sizes 5–0, 9–0, and 11–0.

Black Braided Silk Suture—braided under controlled conditions to maximize strength and assure resistance to breaking while knots are tied. Gums and other impurities are removed, resulting in a suture that remains tightly braided, with virtually no loose filaments and minimal tendency to broom. Available in sizes 4–0 and 6–0 through 9–0.

Virgin Silk—twisted with the individual silk filaments still embedded in their natural sericin coating, providing a smooth, uniform suture in very fine sizes. The suture is offered in black or white, permitting optimum contrast with tissues. Available in sizes 8–0 and 9–0.

Polyester Fiber Sutures–Products include Mersilene and Ti Cron. They exhibit minimal tissue reaction and are braided by a special method for tightness, uniformity, and a smooth surface that minimizes trauma. Available in sizes 4–0 through 6–0.

A variety of physical characteristics of different sutures have been published. In addition, the United States Pharmacopeia has established specifications for various suture materials. Some of the useful parameters measured have been: (1) tensile strength; (2) elasticity; (3) suture diameters; (4) weight per unit length. Data are summarized in **Tables 1** through **3.**

REFERENCE

1. Middleton DG, McCulloch C. An enquiry into characteristics of sutures, particularly fine sutures. *Adv Ophthalmol.* 1970;22:35.

TABLE 2

ELASTICITY OF SUTURES

SUTURE MATERIAL	ELONGATION OF STANDARD 30.5-cm SEGMENT	INCREASE IN LENGTH	WEIGHT AT BREAKING POINT
6–0 plain gut	4.7 cm	15.4%	264 g
6–0 chromic gut	4.3 cm	14.1%	257 g
6–0 Mersilene	1.9 cm	6.3%	254 g
6–0 braided silk	1.2 cm	3.9%	237 g
7–0 chromic gut	3.6 cm	1.8%	118 g
7–0 braided silk	0.9 cm	3.0%	126 g
8–0 virgin silk	0.8 cm	2.6%	53 g
10–0 Nylon	8.7 cm	28.5%	23 g

From Middleton DG, McCulloch C. *Adv Ophthalmol.* 1970;22:35.

TABLE 3

WEIGHT OF SUTURE MATERIAL

SUTURE MATERIAL	WEIGHT/LENGTH (mg/cm)
6–0 plain gut (wet)	0.170
6–0 chromic gut (wet)	0.176
6–0 Mersilene	0.116
6–0 braided silk	0.165
7–0 chromic gut (wet)	0.062
7–0 braided silk	0.065
8–0 virgin silk	0.025
10–0 Nylon	0.007

SECTION 4

OPHTHALMIC LENSES

Arthur A. Gold, MD

The array of options in ophthalmic lenses continues to increase. Though glass remains in use, there is an ever-increasing trend toward plastics, particularly CR-39, the polycarbonates, and high-index plastic. The number of specialized tints and coatings continues to grow as well, further extending our range of choices. Among the more significant developments:

- Scratch-resistant coatings for CR-39 and polycarbonate lenses (Antireflection coatings have been developed, too.)
- New lenses with UV-blocking protection ranging from 395 to 400 nm; plus UV-protective tints for existing spectacle lenses (Existing plastic lenses can be tinted through a dipping process.)
- 1.80-index glass and similar high-index plastic that permit a new generation of lighter, thinner lenses, tintable and impact-resistant
- CR-39 aphakic lens corrections that provide wider fields and reduced magnification, yet are still much thinner
- Polarized glass and plastic for use in single-vision, multifocal, and progressive lenses
- New progressive lens designs that reduce distortion and provide wider progressive corridors

The following tables and charts offer a sampling of the many advanced and specialized options these new technological developments have made possible.

1. ABSORPTIVE AND TINTED LENSES

These lenses provide protection against radiation—either excessive light or harmful wavelengths in the long and short bands of the spectrum. **Tables 1** and **2** summarize some types and functions.

TABLE 1

ABSORPTIVE AND TINTED LENSES

TYPE (TRANSMISSION)	PURPOSE
1. Ordinary-tint lighter shades	Cosmetic; slight reduction in light intensity.
2. Sunglasses	
a. Neutral gray (20% to 30%)	Reduce intensity of light (designed to transmit the spectrum nonselectively, ie, without altering the relative proportions of the various wavelengths).
b. Colored green (30% to 70%)	Transmission curve follows sensitivity curve of the eye; absorb most of ultraviolet and nearly all of the infrared in heat-producing range.
c. Yellow (77%)	Minimize haze; no effect on glare. Filter out blue light. Absorb ultraviolet. No effect on infrareds.
d. Brown Polaroid (21%)	Absorb blue light. Transmission of plane polarized light.
e. Photochromic	Change density by decomposition of a silver halide crystal in presence of ultraviolet or deep ultraviolet light.
3. Antireflecting (about 6%)	Increase transmission.
4. Special-use lenses	
a. Ultraviolet absorption	Almost all glass absorptive lenses absorb strongly in the ultraviolet. (Neutral gray and green absorb strongly throughout the spectrum and in the ultraviolet.)
b. Infrared absorption	Relatively few glass absorptive lenses are good absorbers of infrared radiation alone. (Green absorbs large amounts of visible and infrared.)
c. Laser protection	Didymium.
d. X-ray protection	Radiglasses offer significant protection to the eye lens of the physician, technologist, and other personnel against direct and scattered radiation during use of x-ray equipment. Shielding is equivalent to 0.25 mm of lead and provides radiation dose reduction up to 90%. Optically clear, optional sideshields provide protection from scatter radiation without restricting peripheral vision. *Range of available foci: plano to ±8.00 +0.25 to +8.00 ≈ −0.25 to −5.00 cylinder −0.25 to −8.00 ≈ −0.25 to −5.00 cylinder Bifocals (flat-top, laminated), 22-mm segment. Additions to 4.00.

*Foci beyond standard range may be obtained by inquiry from Nuclear Associates, Carle Place, NY 11514.
From Borish IM. *Clinical Refraction.* 3rd ed. The Professional Press; and manufacturers' data. 1970:1123.

TABLE 2

LENSES FOR INDUSTRIAL USE

SHADE NUMBER	USE	LUMINOUS TRANSMITTANCE	MAXIMUM INFRARED	MAXIMUM ULTRAVIOLET (% AT 365 nm)
14	Carbon arc welding, furnace operation	0.00027	0.3	0.05
12	Metallic electric arc welding over 250 amp	0.0019	0.5	0.5
10	Metal arc welding 75–250 amp	0.0139	0.6	0.1
8	Heavy acetylene cutting and welding	0.1	1.0	0.1
6	Acetylene welding, electrical welding, firebox observation	0.72	1.5	0.1
5	Acetylene buming, brazing, cutting	1.93	2.5	0.2
3	Light brazing	13.9	9.0	0.5

Adapted from Borish IM. *Clinical Refraction.* 3rd ed. The Professional Press; 1970:1123.

2. MULTIFOCAL LENSES

TABLE 3

MULTIFOCAL LENSES, PRINCIPAL TYPES

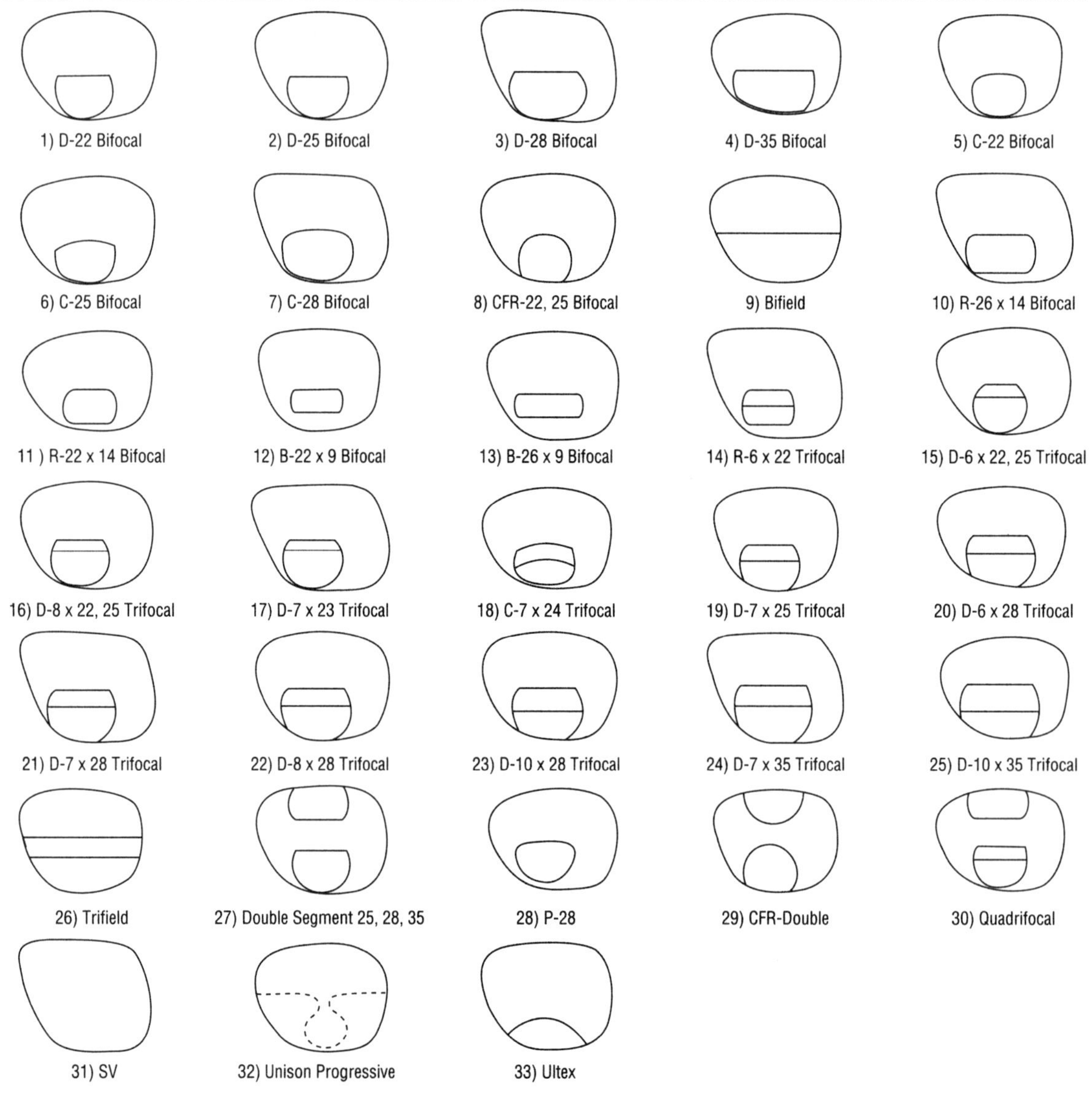

3. INVISIBLE-SEGMENT LENSES

These lenses are available in bifocal and progressive-power formats. The bifocals provide distance and near powers; progressive-power lenses add an intermediate correction. Both formats offer a cosmetic advantage to the many patients who dislike lenses with visible segments and sharp dividing lines. However, their improved appearance is not necessarily accompanied by improved optics.

In the case of bifocal lenses, the blend area surrounding the reading segment can reduce the area of clear vision to an extent noticeable to the patient. With progressive-power lenses, astigmatic distortion can occur on either side of both the reading segment and the intermediate zone or corridor, though a new design has minimized this problem, according to the manufacturer of the Varilux 2.

Invisible bifocals can be fitted in the same manner as ordinary bifocals. However, invisible progressive-power lenses demand much more care. Pupillary distance measurements must be precise in both the horizontal and vertical meridians; and the prescription must be fitted as close as possible, with proper pantoscopic tilt. The range of available foci for both types of lenses is generally less than that of standard multifocals.

4. FRESNEL LENSES AND PRISMS

TABLE 4

FRESNEL LENSES AND PRISMS

PRISMS (MINUS)	SEGMENT ADDITIONS	SPHERES (PLUS)	SPHERES
0.5 Δ	+0.50	+0.50	
1.00 Δ	+1.00	+1.00	
1.50 Δ	+1.25 to +2.50[a]	+1.25 to +2.50[a]	
2 Δ to 10 Δ[c]	+3.00 to +4.00[b]	+3.00 to +4.00[b]	−1.00 to −14.00[c]
12 Δ	+5.00 to +8.00[c]	+5.00 to +14.00[c]	
15 Δ	segments greater than	+16.00	
20 Δ	+3 have incorporated prism	+20.00	
25 Δ, 30 Δ			

Prism bars: 1–40 Δ horizontal; 1–25 Δ vertical. Prism trial set: 12, 15, 20, 25, 30, 35, 40 ΔD.
Increments: a = 0.25, b = 0.50, c = 1.00 step in either prism diopters or lens.

5. SOFT CONTACT LENSES

The table in this year's edition has been expanded and enhanced through the courtesy of *Contact Lens Quarterly*, a publication of the Frames Data subsidiary of Medical Economics Data. Reproduced from the Summer 1994 issue, the table provides additional specifications for each product, including center thickness and the size of the optic zone. Also included are separate sections for the increasingly popular programmed replacement systems and for disposable extended-wear lenses.

Because rigid gas-permeable lenses can be ordered in standard or custom designs from more than 200 independent laboratories, it is impractical to provide a comprehensive table here, and of little value to present a selective list. However, one development worth noting in this area is the recent introduction of rosilfocon A — a "hybrid" rigid lens material with a hydrophilic surface. As this and other new materials gain widespread use, they will be added to this section as necessary.

TABLE 5

EXTENDED WEAR SPHERICAL

MFR.	LENS	MATERIAL, % H_2O, PROCESS	DIAMETER (mm)	BASE CURVE (mm)	POWER (D)	CENTER THICKNESS (mm)	OPTIC ZONE (mm)	dK+ VALUE
BAUSCH & LOMB	**B&L 70**	lidofilcon A, 70%, lathe-cut	14.3	8.4, 8.7, 9.0 (–); 8.7, 9.0 (+)	–5.00 to ±5.00 in 0.25 steps; ±5.50, ±6.00 plano	0.14 (–); 0.16 to 0.25 (+)	8.0 to 12.0 (–); 8.0 (+)	33.8
	Optima FW Visibility Tint	polymacon, 38.6%, spin-cast front, lathe-cut back	14	8.4, 8.7, 9.0	+4.00 to –9.00 includes plano	0.035	8.0	9.2
	Soflens 03®/04® Series	polymacon, 38.6%, spin-cast	03®: 13.5 ——— 04®: 14.5	varies	–1.00 to –5.00; –5.50, –6.00	0.035	12.4 (03) ——— 13.6 (04)	9.2
BIOCURVE SOFT LENSES	**BioCurve EW Spheres EW**	methafilcon A, 55%	14.0 ——— 14.5	8.4 ——— 8.4, 8.6, 8.8, 9.0	–20.00 to +10.00 in 0.25 steps	0.06	7.8 to 8.3	18.8
BREGER-MUELLER WELT	**Q&E 70**	lidofilcon A, 70%, lathe-cut	14.3	8.4, 8.7, 9.0	+8.00 to –12.00 (in 0.50 steps above ±5.00)	.14 to .17	8 to 12	31.0
CIBA VISION CORP.	**CIBATHIN®**	tefilcon, 37.5%	13.8	8.6, 8.9	Plano to –6.00	.035 @ –3.00D	Varies with power (7.0 to 9.8)	8.9
	SOFTCON® EW	vifilcon A, 55%	14.0 ——— 14.5	8.1, 8.4, 8.7 ——— 8.7 in minus powers only	–8.00 to +5.00 in 0.25 steps ——— +5.50 to +9.50 in 0.50 steps Plano to –8.00 in 0.25 steps	.10 @ –3.00D .15 @ +3.00D	7.5	16.0
COASTVISION	**Hydrasoft® XW**	methafilcon A, 55%, lathe-cut, Pitch polished	15.0 ——— 14.2	8.6, 8.9 ——— 8.3, 8.6	+10.00 to –20.00 (in 0.50 steps after –10.00) ——— +10.00 to –12.00 (in 0.50 steps after ±8.00)	.06	8.0	18.8
	Hydrasoft® Aphakic	methafilcon A, 55%, lathe-cut, Pitch polished	15.0 14.2	8.6, 8.9 8.3, 8.6	+10.50 to +20.00 (in 0.50 steps)	varies	8.0	18.8
COOPERVISION INC.	**Permaflex® Naturals Flexible Wear**	surfilcon A, 74%, cast-molded construction	14.4 ——— 14.4	8.7 ——— 8.9	–0.25 to –6.00 in 0.25 steps; –6.50 to –10.00 in 0.50 steps ——— +0.50 to +5.00 in 0.25 steps; +5.50, +6.00 ——— –1.00 to –6.00 in 0.25 steps	0.10 to 0.18 ——— 0.22 to 0.41 ——— 0.14 to 0.24	7.0 to 8.5 AOZ ——— 7.9 to 8.1 AOZ ——— 7.0 to 8.5	38.9

EXTENDED WEAR SPHERICAL (CONTINUED)

MFR.	LENS	MATERIAL, % H_2O, PROCESS	DIAMETER (mm)	BASE CURVE (mm)	POWER (D)	CENTER THICKNESS (mm)	OPTIC ZONE (mm)	dK+ VALUE
COOPERVISION INC.	**Permaflex® UV Naturals Flexible Wear**	vasurfilcon A, 74%, cast-molded	14.4	8.7	−0.25 to −6.00 in 0.25 steps; −6.50,−10.00 to 0.50 steps;	0.10 to 0.18		38.9
					+0.50 to +6.00 in 0.25 steps; +5.50, +6.00	0.22 to 0.32		
	Permalens®	perfilcon A, 71%, lathe-cut	13.5	7.7, 8.0, 8.3	−0.25 to −20.00 (0.50 steps above −6.00)	0.10 to 0.26	7.0	34
			14.2	8.6	−0.25 to −10.00 (0.50 steps above −6.00)			
	Permalens® Low Plus	perfilcon A, 71%, lathe-cut	14.0	8.0, 8.3, 8.6	+0.25 to +5.00 (0.25 steps); +5.50 to +8.00 (0.50 steps)	0.27 to 0.40	7.0	34
	Permalens® XL	perfilcon A, 71%, cast-molded	14.5	8.3	−0.25 to −6.00 in 0.25 steps; −6.50 to −10.00 in 0.50 steps	0.11 to 0.26	8.0 AOZ	34
KONTUR KONTACT LENS CO.	**Kontur 55 EW**	methafilcon A, 55%, lathe-cut	15.0	8.3, 8.6, 8.9	+10.00 to −20.00	.08 to .40	8.0	18.8
OCULAR SCIENCES/ AMERICAN HYDRON	**Zero–4 Softints Flexible Wear**	polymacon, 38%, cast-molded	13.8	8.6	Plano to −10.00	.04	8-11	8.4
	Zero–4F Colors: Clear or Visibility Blue.	polymacon, 38%, cast-molded	14.0	8.8	Plano to −5.25D	.04	8-11	8.4
	Zero–4	polymacon, 38%, cast-molded	14.0	8.6	Plano to −10.00	.04	8-11	8.4
PBH	**CSI® Clarity Flexible Wear**	crofilcon A, 38.6%, lathe-cut	13.8	8.0, 8.3, 8.6, 8.9	Plano to −10.00	.035	10.9 to 6.5	13
			14.8	8.6, 8.9, 9.35	Plano to −7.00			
	Gentle Touch	netrafilcon A, 65%, lathe-cut w/spc	14.5	8.2, 8.5	−0.500 to −6.00D	.10	9.6	38
	Hydrocurve II 55% Custom tints available	bufilcon A, 55%, lathe-cut	14.5	8.8, 9.1	−12.00 to +7.00 (0.50 steps above +5.00 & 8.00)	0.04 to 0.48 varies with power	8.0 to 8.5	16
			14.0	8.5				
	Soft Mate I	bufilcon, 45%, lathe-cut	14.3	8.7	Plano to −6.00 in 0.25 steps	.05 (−3.00)	8.0 to 8.5	12
			14.8	9.0				
	Soft Mate II	bufilcon A, 55%, lathe-cut	14.3	8.7	−12.00 to +7.00 in 0.25 steps (0.50D steps above +5.00 & −8.00)	.05 (−3.00)	8.0 to 8.5	16
			14.8	9.0				
SALVATORI OPHTHALMICS	**Sof-form® 55 Flexible Wear**	methafilcon A, 55%, lathe-cut	14.0	8.3, 8.6, 8.9	−20.00 to +9.75	.10 (minus)	8.2	18.8
			15.0	8.6, 8.9, 9.2				
SUNSOFT	**Revolution Light Blue Visibility Tint**	methafilcon A, 55%, patented molding process	14.0	8.5	Plano to −10.00 in 0.25 steps	varies by power	8.0	18.8
				8.7	+4.00 to −6.00			
	Sportsoft Light Blue Visibility Tint	methafilcon A, 55%, patented molding process	15.0	8.9, 9.2	Plano to −6.00 in 0.25 steps	varies by power	8.0	18.8

EXTENDED WEAR SPHERICAL (CONTINUED)

MFR.	LENS	MATERIAL, % H_2O, PROCESS	DIAMETER (mm)	BASE CURVE (mm)	POWER (D)	CENTER THICKNESS (mm)	OPTIC ZONE (mm)	dK+ VALUE
SUNSOFT	**Sunflex**	methafilcon A, 55%, lathe-cut	14.0 15.0	8.3, 8.6, 8.9	+5.00 to −10.00 +10.00 to −20.00 in 0.50 steps above −10.00	.10	8.0	18.8
	Sunsoft Aphakic EW	methafilcon A, 55%, lathe-cut	15.0	8.3, 8.6, 8.9	+10.50 to +20.00 in 0.50 steps	.26	8.0	18.8
WESLEY-JESSEN	**Durasoft® 3 Colors**	phemfilcon A, 55%, lathe-cut	14.5	8.6 median 8.3 steep 9.00 flat	−8.00 to +6.00 −8.00 to +6.00 Plano to −4.00	.05 @ −3.00D	5.0 (clear pupil zone)	16.1
	Colors: Baby Blue-Opaque, Emerald Green-Opaque, Aqua-Opaque, Hazel-Opaque, Sapphire Blue-Opaque, Jade Green-Opaque, Violet-Opaque, Misty Gray-Opaque, Chestnut Brown-Opaque (8.6 to pl −4.0), Baby Blue-Enhance (8.6 b.c. only).							
	Durasoft® 3 Complements Colors	phemfilcon A, 55%, lathe-cut	14.5	8.6 median	−8.00 to +6.00	.05 @ −3.00D	5.0 (clear pupil zone)	16.1
	Colors: Complements Blue, Complements Green, Complements Brown, Complements Shadow Gray (available only in plano to −4.00), Complements Blue-Violet (available only in plano to −4.00)							
	Durasoft® 3 Flexiwear	phemfilcon A, 55%, lathe-cut	D3-X3: 13.5 D3-X4: 14.5	8.5 median, 8.2 steep 8.6 median, 8.3 steep, 9.0 flat	±6.00 in 0.25 steps ±20.00 in 0.25 steps to ±10.00, in 0.50 steps over ±10.00	.05 @ −3.00D	8.0	16.1
	Durasoft® 3 Lite Tint	phemfilcon A, 55%, lathe-cut	14.5	8.3, 8.6, 9.0	±20.00 in 0.25 steps to ±10.00, in 0.50 steps over ±10.00	.05 @ −3.00D	8.0	16.1
WESTCON	**Horizon EW**	methafilcon A, 55%, lathe-cut	14.0, 14.5, 15.0 15.0	8.0, 8.3, 8.6, 8.9 8.6, 8.9, 9.2	+10.00 to −20.00	varies	varies	18.8
	Horizon Specialty	methafilcon A, 55%, lathe-cut	14.0, 14.5, 15.0 14.5 15.0	8.0, 8.3, 8.6, 8.9, 9.2 8.3, 8.6, 8.9 8.6, 8.9, 9.2	+20.00 to −20.00	varies	varies	18.8
	Horizon Sports Lens	methafilcon A, 55%, lathe-cut	15.0 to 18.0 in 5 mm steps	8.6 to 10.1 in 3mm steps	+6.00 to −12.00	varies	varies	
	Avoid: potassium sorbate, sorbic acid and papain.							
	Horizon Custom	Any parameters not listed above including Non-Aphakic Extended Wear up to 7 days.						

EXTENDED WEAR TORIC

MFR.	LENS	MATERIAL, % H_2O, PROCESS	DIAMETER (mm)	BASE CURVE (mm)	SPHERE POWER (mm)	CYLINDER POWER (mm)	AXIS	CENTER THICKNESS (mm)	OPTIC ZONE (mm)	dK+ VALUE
COAST-VISION	**Hydrasoft® Toric XW Div. I Std. Toric**	methafilcon B, 55%, lathe-cut, pitch polished	15.0	8.9	+3.00 to −6.00 in 0.25 steps	−0.75 to −2.00 in 0.25 steps	180° ±20° 90° ±20° in 1° steps	.035 to .20	8.0	18.8
	Hydrasoft® Toric XW Div. II Spec. Toric	methafilcon B, 55%, lathe-cut, pitch polished	15.0	8.6, 8.9	+10.00 to −20.00 in 0.25 steps	−0.75 to −5.00 in 0.25 steps	any 1° steps	0.35 to .20	8.0	18.8
	Hydrasoft® Toric XW Div. III Custom Toric	methafilcon B, 55%, lathe-cut,	15.0	8.3, 8.6, 8.9, 9.2	+10.00 to −20.00 in 0.25 steps	−0.50 to −5.00 in 0.25 steps	any 1° steps	0.35 to .20	8.0	18.8

EXTENDED WEAR TORIC (CONTINUED)

MFR.	LENS	MATERIAL, % H_2O, PROCESS	DIAMETER (mm)	BASE CURVE (mm)	SPHERE POWER (mm)	CYLINDER POWER (mm)	AXIS	CENTER THICKNESS (mm)	OPTIC ZONE (mm)	dK+ VALUE
COAST-VISION	Hydrasoft® Toric XW Div. III Aphakic Toric	methafilcon B, 55%, lathe-cut,	15.0	8.6, 8.9	+10.25 to +20.00	–0.75 to –5.00 in 0.25 steps	any 1° steps	0.35 to .20	8.0	18.8
PBH	Hydrocurve II 55%	bufilcon A, 55%, lathe-cut	14.5 (non-core) 14.5	8.5 8.8	Plano to –6.00 +4.00 to –8.00	90°+/- 20° 180° +/- 20° 10° around the clock (180° ± 20°, 90° ± 20° in 5° steps)	–1.25, –0.75 –1.25 –2.00	.07	8.0	16
	Custom tints: Blue, Green, Aqua, Lavender									
	Hydrocurve III	bufilcon A, 55%, lathe-cut	14.5	8.8	+4.00 to –8.00D	–0.75D –1.25D –2.00D	1° steps	0.06 (–3.00)	8.2	16
SUNSOFT	Eclipse	methafilcon A, 55%, lathe-cut	14.5	standard	+2.00 to –6.00 in 0.25 steps	–0.75 to –2.50 in 0.25 steps	90° ±30° 180° ±30° (5° steps)	varies by power	8.0	18.8
	Sunsoft Toric 15.0 Div. I	methafilcon A, 55%, lathe-cut	15.0	8.9	+3.00 to –6.00 in 0.25 steps	–0.75 to –2.00 in 0.25 steps	180°±20 90°±20 (5° inc. in stock)	varies by power	8.0	18.8
	Sunsoft Toric 15.0 Div. II	methafilcon A, 55%, lathe-cut	15.0	8.3, 8.9	+10.00 to –20.00 in 0.25 steps	–0.75 to –7.00 in 0.25 steps	Any	varies by power	8.0	18.8
WESLEY-JESSEN	Durasoft® 3 Optifit Toric Colors Flexiwear	phemfilcon A, 55%, lathe-cut (back-toric)	14.5	8.6 median (fits equivalent to an 8.6)	pl to –4.00	–1.25, –1.75	180° ±20°, 90° ±20° 5° increments	.07	8.0	16.1
	Colors: Baby Blue – Opaque, Emerald Green – Opaque, Hazel – Opaque									
	Durasoft® 3 Optifit Toric Flexiwear	phemfilcon A, 55%, lathe-cut (back-toric)	14.5	8.6 median (fits equivalent to an 8.6)	–8.00 to +4.00 in 0.25 steps	–0.75 to –2.25 in 0.50 steps	180° ±30°, 90° ±30° 5° increments	.07	8.0	16.1

EXTENDED WEAR THERAPEUTIC

MFR.	LENS	MATERIAL, % H_2O, PROCESS	DIAMETER (mm)	BASE CURVE (mm)	POWER (D)	CENTER THICKNESS (mm)	OPTIC ZONE (mm)	dK+ VALUE
ADVENTURES IN COLORS, INC.	Custom Made Prosthetic Lenses	bufilcon A, 48.5%	15	8.3 8.6 8.9	varies	varies	varies	
COOPERVISION INC.	Permalens Therapeutic	perfilcon A, 71%, lathe-cut	13.5 14.2 15.0	7.7, 8.0, 8.3 8.6 9.0	Plano Plano Plano	.24		34

EXTENDED WEAR DISPOSABLE

MFR.	LENS	MATERIAL, % H_2O, PROCESS	DIAMETER (mm)	BASE CURVE (mm)	POWER (D)	CENTER THICKNESS (mm)	OPTIC ZONE (mm)	dK+ VALUE
BAUSCH & LOMB	**SeeQuence**	polymacon, 38.6%	14.0		+4.00 to −9.00 in 0.25D steps	.035 varies w/power .032 to .038	13.6	
	SeeQuence 2	polymacon, 38%	14.0	8.4, 8.7, 9.0	+4.00 to −9.00 in 0.25D steps	.035	8.0 to 10.0	
CIBA VISION CORP.	**NewVues®**	vifilcon A, 55%	14.0	8.4, 8.8	+4.00 to−6.00 in 0.25 steps; −6.50 to −10.00 in 0.50 steps	.06 @ −3.00 0.12 @ +3.00D	7.2	16.0
	NewVues® SOFTCOLORS® **Colors:** Aqua, Royal Blue, Evergreen	vifilcon A, 55%	14.0	8.4, 8.8	Plano to −6.00 in 0.25 steps	.06 @ −3.00	7.2	16.0
OCULAR SCIENCES/ AMERICAN HYDRON	**Hydron Biomedics** **Colors:** Visi blue	polymacon, 38%, cast-molded	14.0	8.6	−0.25 to −8,00D	.04	8.0 min.	8.4
VISTAKON	**ACUVUE®** Conversion to Visibility Tint begins in May.	etafilcon A, 58%, stabilized soft molding	14.0 (-)	8.4, 8.8	−0.50 to −6.00 in 0.25 steps −6.50 to −9.00 in 0.50 steps	.07 at −3.00D	8.0	28.0
			14.4 (+)	9.3	+0.50 to +6.00 in 0.25 steps −6.50 to −9.00 in 0.50 steps			

EXTENDED WEAR TINTED

MFR.	LENS	MATERIAL, % H_2O, PROCESS	DIAMETER (mm)	BASE CURVE (mm)	POWER (D)	CENTER THICKNESS (mm)	OPTIC ZONE (mm)	dK+ VALUE
CIBA VISION CORP.	**CIBATHIN® SOFTCOLORS®** **Colors:** Aqua, Blue, Royal Blue, Green, Amber	tefilcon, 37.5%	13.8	8.6, 8.9	Plano to −6.00	.035 all minus powers	varies w/power (7.0 to 12.8)	8.9
Colors: Royal Blue, Aqua, Evergreen	**Focus® SOFTCOLORS®**	vifilcon A, 55%, CIBACAST® molding	14.0	8.6, 8.9	−8.00 to +6.00 in 0.25 steps	.10 @ −3.00 .15 @ +3.00	7.8	16.0
	Focus® VISITINT® Light Blue Visibility Tint	vifilcon A, 55%	14.0	8.6, 8.9	−8.00 to +6.00 in 0.25 steps	.10 @ −3.00 .15 @ +3.00	7.8	16.0
	SPECTRUM® VISITINT® Light Blue Visibility Tint	vifilcon A, 55%	14.0	8.3, 8.6, 8.9	−8.00 to +5.00 in 0.25 steps +5.50 to +9.50 in 0.50 steps	0.10 @ −3.00 0.15 @ +3.00D	7.8	16.0
			14.5	8.9, 9.2	Plano to −8.00 in 0.25 steps	.15 @ +3.00D	8.0	
OCULAR SCIENCES/ AMERICAN HYDRON	**Zero–4F**	polymacon, 38%, cast-molded	14.0	8.8	Plano to −5.25	.04	8–11	8.4
	Zero–4 Softints	polymacon, 38%, cast-molded	14.0	8.6	Plano to −10.00	.04	8–11	8.4

EXTENDED WEAR BIFOCAL

MFR.	LENS	MATERIAL, % H_2O, PROCESS	DIAMETER (mm)	BASE CURVE (mm)	POWER (D)	CENTER THICKNESS (mm)	OPTIC ZONE (mm)	dK+ VALUE
CIBA VISION CORP.	**SPECTRUM® Bifocal**	vifilcon A, 55%	14.0	8.6, 8.9	Sphere: +6.00 to −6.00 in 0.25 steps Add: +1.50 to +3.00 in 0.50 steps	.10 all minus powers, .16 @ +3.00D	Sm: 2.3/7.8 Lg. 3.0/7.8	16.0

DAILY WEAR SPHERICAL

MFR.	LENS	MATERIAL, % H_2O, PROCESS	DIAMETER (mm)	BASE CURVE (mm)	POWER (D)	CENTER THICKNESS (mm)	OPTIC ZONE (mm)	dK+ VALUE
ACCUGEL LABS	**Accugel Spherical Div. A**	droxifilcon, 46.6%, lathe-cut	13.5, 14.0	8.3, 8.6, 8.9	Pl to ±10.00	all lenticular	8.0	18.7
	Accugel Spherical Div. P	droxifilcon, 46.6%, lathe-cut	13.0	7.6 to 8.6 in 0.2 steps	+20.25 to +36.00 in 1.00 steps	all lenticular	7.0	18.7
	Accugel Spherical Div. I	droxifilcon, 46.6%, lathe-cut	13.5, 14.0	7.8 to 9.2 in 0.1 steps	Pl to ±10.00	all lenticular	8.0	18.7
	Accugel Spherical Div. 2	droxifilcon, 46.6%, lathe-cut	13.5, 14.0	7.8 to 9.2	±10.25 to ±20.00	all lenticular	8.0	18.7
	Accugel Spherical Div. 4	droxifilcon, 46.6%, lathe-cut	any	any	over ±20.00	all lenticular	8.0	18.7
ALDEN OPTICAL LABS	**AL-47** Custom lenses available upon request.	isofilcon, 35.5%, lathe-cut	12.5, 13.0, 13.5, 14.0	7.7, 7.9, 8.1, 8.3, 8.5, 8.7, 8.9	Pl to ±30.00	0.12 (–3.00)	7.5	3.7
AQUA SITE	**Aqua-Sphere 53**	ocufilcon-B, 53%, lathe-cut	14.5 or custom	8.6, 8.8, 9.0, or custom	–25.00 to + 10.00 or custom	varies with power	minus lenses 8.6, plus lenses 7.4, or custom	15.4
BAUSCH & LOMB	**Occasions™ Multifocal**	polymacon, 38%, shape-cast	14.0	8.6	+6.00 to –9.00 in 0.25 diapter steps	.08 to .61	8.0 to 9.0	9.2
	Optima 38 Visibility Tint available	polymacon, 38%, spin-cast front, lathe-cut back	14.0	3.6, 3.82 (sag. depths), 8.7, 8.4	+5.00 to –9.00 in 0.25 steps –9.00 to –12.00 in 0.50 steps	.06 (–), .095 to .19 (+)	8.0	9.2
	Soflens® Series B3	polymacon, 38.6%, spin-cast	13.5	varies w/power	+6.00 to –12.00 in 0.50 steps above ±5.00	.12 to .21	12.1	9.2
	Soflens® Series B4	polymacon, 38.6%, spin-cast	14.5	varies w/power	+6.00 to –9.00 in 0.50 steps above ±5.00	.12 to .21	13.4 (–), 10.0 (+)	9.2
	Soflens® Series H4	polymacon, 38.6%, spin-cast	14.5	varies w/power	+6.50 to +20.00 in 0.50 steps	.49 to .60	9.0	9.2
	Soflens® Series HO3	polymacon, 38.6%, spin-cast	13.5	varies w/power	–8.00 to –20.00 in 0.50 steps	.035	9.0	9.2
	Soflens® Series HO4	polymacon, 38.6%, spin-cast	14.5	varies w/power	–8.00 to –20.00 in 0.50 steps	.035	9.0	9.2
	Soflens® Series N	polymacon, 38.6%, spin-cast	13.5	varies w/power	+6.50 to +18.50 in 0.50 steps	.34 to .66	7.8	9.2
	Soflens® Series Sofspin	polymacon, 38.6%, spin-cast	14.0	varies w/power	–0.25 to –5.00, –5.50, –6.00	.05 to .09	13.2	9.2
	Soflens® Series U3	polymacon, 38.6%, spin-cast	13.5	varies w/power	+6.00 to –9.00 in 0.50 steps above ±5.00	.07 (–), .12 (+)	12.4 (–), 7.8 (+)	9.2

DAILY WEAR SPHERICAL (CONTINUED)

MFR.	LENS	MATERIAL, % H_2O, PROCESS	DIAMETER (mm)	BASE CURVE (mm)	POWER (D)	CENTER THICKNESS (mm)	OPTIC ZONE (mm)	dK+ VALUE
BAUSCH & LOMB	**Soflens® Series U4**	polymacon, 38.6%, spin-cast	14.5	varies w/power	+6.00 to −9.00 in 0.50 steps above ±5.00	.07 (−), .12 (+)	13.6 (−), 7.8 (+)	9.2
BIOCURVE SOFT LENSES	**Biocurve Aphakic Spheres**	methafilcon A, 55%	14.0 14.5 15.0	8.4 8.4, 8.6, 8.8, 9.0 8.9	+10.50 to +20.00 in .050 steps	.06–.30	7.8–8.3	18.8
	Biocurve Aphakic Spheres	methafilcon A, 55%	14.0 14.5 15.0	8.4 8.4, 8.6, 8.8, 9.0 8.9	+10.50 to +20.00 in .050 steps	.10–.60	7.8–8.3	18.8
	Biocurve Spheres	methafilcon A, 55%	14.0 14.5 15.0	8.4 8.4, 8.6, 8.8, 9.0 8.9	−20.00 to +10.00 in 0.25 steps	.06–.30	7.8–8.3	18.8
BREGER-MUELLER WELT	**Q & E**	deltafilcon B, 43% lathe-cut	13.8 13.5	8.3, 8.6, 8.9 8.1, 8.4, 8.7	−25 to −12.00 Plano to + 5.00 (on special order)	0.06	13.0	8.4
CIBA VISION CORP.	**AOSOFT®**	tetrafilcon A, 42.5%	13.2	Vault 1: 8.8 Vault 2: 8.5 Vault 3: 8.2 Vault 4: 7.9	Plano to −9.75	.13 @ −3.00D	varies w/power (9.0 to 12.0)	8.5
	CIBASOFT®	tefilcon, 37.5%	13.8 14.5	8.3, 8.6, 8.9 8.6, 8.9, 9.2	+6.00 to −6.00 in 0.25 steps; −6.50 to −10.00 in 0.50 steps Plano to −6.00 in 0.25 steps; −6.50 to −10.00 in 0.50 steps	.07 @ −3.00 .14 @ +3.00	varies w/ power (7.0 to 12.0)	8.9
	SOFTCON® *Not available +5.50 to +9.50 **Plus powers only	vifilcon A, 55%	14.0 14.5	7.8*, 8.1, 8.4, 8.7** 8.1, 8.4, 8.7	−8.00 to +5.00 in 0.25 steps +5.50 to +9.50 in .50 steps	.17 to .46	7.55	16.0
	SOFTCON® Aphakic	vifilcon A, 55%	14.5	8.1, 8.4	+10.00 to +18.0 in 0.50 steps	.47 to .61	7.55	16.0
	STD™ Clear	tefilcon, 37.5%	13.8	8.3, 8.6, 8.9	+6.00 to −6.00	.10 @ −3.00D .17 @ +3.00D	varies w/ power (7.0 to 12.0)	8.9
COAST-VISION	**Hydrasoft® Standard**	methafilcon B, 55%, lathe-cut, pitch polished	14.2 15.0	8.3, 8.6 8.6, 8.9, 9.2	+10.00 to −12.00 (in 0.50 steps after ±8.00) +10.00 to -20.00 (in 0.50 steps after −10.00)	.10 .12	8.5	18.8
CONTACT LENS CORP. OF AMERICA	**Softact II**	polymacon, 38%, lathe-cut	14.0	8.4, 8.7, 9.0	−20.00 to +20.00 in 0.25 steps to ±12.00, 0.50 steps over ±12.00	0.06 to .32	varies	8.4
CONTACT LENS LABS, INC. OF GREATER CINCINNATI	**CLL-38**	polymacon, 38%, lathe-cut pitch polished	14.0	8.3, 8.5, 8.7, 8.9	Plano to −15.00 in 0.25D steps Plano to +10.00			8.4
CONTINENTAL SOFT LENS INC.	**Continental Spherical**	ocufilcon B, 53%, lathing	13.0 to 17.5		±30.00	varies with power	8.0	16.5

DAILY WEAR SPHERICAL (CONTINUED)

MFR.	LENS	MATERIAL, % H_2O, PROCESS	DIAMETER (mm)	BASE CURVE (mm)	POWER (D)	CENTER THICKNESS (mm)	OPTIC ZONE (mm)	dK+ VALUE
COOPERVISION INC.	**Cooper™ Clear**	tetrafilcon A, 43%, lathe-cut	14.0 14.4	8.3, 8.6 8.7	Plano to −6.50 in 0.25 steps; −6.50 to −10.00 in 0.50 steps	0.06 to 0.15	9.0 to 11.5	8.5
			14.4 14.0	8.7 8.3, 8.6	Plano to +6.00 in 0.25 steps	0.10 to 0.25		
	CooperThin®	polymacon, 38%, cast-molded	14.0	8.4	−0.25 to −5.00 in 0.25 steps, −5.50 to −10.00 in 0.50 steps	0.06	12.75 to 7.5	8.4
			14.5	8.6	−0.25 to −5.00 in 0.25 steps, −5.50 to 6.50 in 0.50 steps			
	Vantage® Light Blue Handling Tint	tetrafilcon A, 43% water lathe-cut	14.0	8.3, 8.6, 8.9	Plano to −6.50 in 0.25 steps −6.50 to −10.00 in 0.50 steps	0.06 to 0.9	9.0 to 11.5	8.5
			14.4	8.7	Plano to +6.00 in 0.25 steps			
	Vantage® Accents	tetrafilcon A, 43%, lathe-cut	14.0 14.4	8.3, 8.6 8.7	Plano to −6.50 in 0.25 steps	0.06 to 0.09	5.0 pupil zone clear	8.5
	Colors: Sky Blue, Violet Blue, Spring Green, Turquoise, Auburn, Misty Brown							
EPCON LABS	**Epcon Soft**	polymacon 38% lathe-cut	14.0	8.4, 8.7, 9.0	−20.00 to +9.00	.05 @−3.00	varies with power	8.4
FLEXLENS	**Flexlens Custom**	hefilcon A, 45%, lathe-cut	12.5 to 22.0 in 0.50 steps	8.3, 8.6, 8.9, 9.2	6.0 to 11.0 in 0.25 steps	+50.00 to −50.00	varies	11.3
	Flexlens Custom Keratoconus	hefilcon A, 45%, lathe-cut	13.5, 14.5	9.0/7.7, 8.7/7.1, 8.4/6.7 or 8.1/6.3	Plano to −20 in 0.50 steps	+20.00 to −20.00	varies	11.3
	Flexlens Custom Piggyback	hefilcon A, 45%, lathe-cut	12.5 to 14.5 in 0.50 steps	6.2 to 9.8 in 0.3 steps	Groove 8.6mm	varies	varies	11.3
GREAT LAKES	**ProSoft**	methafilcon 55, 55%, lathe cut	14.0	8.3, 8.6	+2.50 to +6.00; −2.50 to −9.00	.08		
IDEAL OPTICS	**Ideal Soft**	polymacon, 38.6%, lathe-cut	14.0	8.6, 8.9	−20.00 to +20.00	.06	12.4 to 11.4	
				8.3	−20.00 to Plano			
KONTUR KONTACT LENS CO.	**Kontur 55 Sphere**	methafilcon A, 55%, lathe-cut	15.0	8.3, 8.6, 8.9	+10.00 to −20.00	.10 to .40	8.0	18.8
METRO OPTICS	**Metro 55**	methafilcon A, 55%, lathe-cut	14.2	8.4, 8.7, 9.0	Pl. to −10.00 in 0.50 steps above −7.00	.14 (−3.00)	9.0	18.8
				8.7	Pl. to +10.00 in 0.50 steps above +7.00			
	Metro Soft II	polymacon, 38%, lathe-cut	13.5	8.3, 8.6, 8.9	−20.00 to +20.00 in 0.50 steps above ±7.00	.10 (−3.00)	9.0	8.4
	Metro Soft II Series M	polymacon, 38%, lathe-cut	14.0	Series M	Pl to −7.00 in 0.25 steps	.06 (−3.00)	9.0	8.4

DAILY WEAR SPHERICAL (CONTINUED)

MFR.	LENS	MATERIAL, % H_2O, PROCESS	DIAMETER (mm)	BASE CURVE (mm)	POWER (D)	CENTER THICKNESS (mm)	OPTIC ZONE (mm)	dK+ VALUE
OCU-EASE OPTICAL PRODUCTS	Ocuflex 53	ocufilcon B, 53%, lathe-cut	14.0, 14.5, 15.0	8.2, 8.4, 8.6, 8.8 (interchangeable)	−20.00 to +12.00	.13 (−); .18 (+)	8.0	18.1
	Ocuflex 53	ocufilcon B, 53%, lathe-cut •other parameters available upon request	14.0, 14.5, 15.0	8.2, 8.4, 8.6, 8.8	+12.25 to + 20.00	varies	8.0	18.1
	Ocuflex 65 Spherical	ocufilcon B, 65%, lathe-cut	14.5, 15.0	8.45, 8.65, 8.85	−20.00 to +12.00		8.0	22.0±2.0
OCULAR SCIENCES/ AMERICAN HYDRON	EDGE® III	polymacon, 38%, cast-mold	14.0	8.7 8.3, 8.6, 8.9	+0.25 to +5.00 in 0.25 steps −0.25 to −8.00	.10	8.0 to 12.5	8.4
	EDGE® III Thin	polymacon, 38%, cast-mold	14.5	8.4, 8.7, 9.0	Plano to −8.00 in 0.25 steps	.07	8.0 to 13.0	8.4
	Edge® III XT	polymacon, 38%, cast-mold	14.0	8.7 8.3, 8.9	+0.25 to +5.00 in 0.25 steps −0.25 to −8.00	.07	8.0 to 12.5	8.4
	Hydron Custom Lens	Available in Mini, Zero-6, Semi Scleral. Please call for parameters.						
	Hydron Spin-Cast	polymacon, 38%, spin-cast	14.5	8.5 (P.A.R.)	Plano to 8.00	.07	6.5	8.4
	Mini-Lens	polymacon, 38%, lathe-cut	13.0	8.1 - 8.9 (in .2mm steps)	Plano to ±20.00 (in .50 steps above ±10.00)	.10 (minus) .12 (plus)	8-11	8.4
	ULTRAFLEX™	polymacon, 38%, cast-mold	14.0	8.7 8.3, 8.6, 8.9	+0.25 to +5.00 in 0.25 steps −0.25 to −8.00	.10	8.0 to 12.5	8.4
	ULTRAFLEX™ Thin	polymacon, 38%, cast-mold	14.5	8.4, 8.7, 9.0	Plano to −8.00 in 0.25 steps	.07	8.0 to 13.0	8.4
	Ultra Flex® XT	polymacon, 38%, cast-mold	14.0	8.7 8.3, 8.6, 8.9	+0.25 to +5.00 in 0.25 steps −0.25 to −8.00	.07	8.0 to 12.5	8.4
	Zero-6	polymacon, 38%, lathe-cut	14.0	8.4, 8.7, 9.0	Plano to −10.00	.06	8.11	8.4
	Z-Plus	polymacon, 38%, lathe-cut	14.0	8.4, 8.7, 9.0	Plano to +10.00	.10	8.0	8.4
OPTECH, INC.	Fre–Flex Custom	focofilcon A, 55%, lathe-cut	10.0 to 17.0	6.0 to 11.0	−40.00 to +40.00	varies	varies	15.5
	Fre–Flex Stock	focofilcon A, 55%, lathe-cut	14.0 15.0	8.6 9.2	−20.00 to +20.00	.10 at −3.00D .13 at −3.00D	8.0 at -3.00D	15.5

DAILY WEAR SPHERICAL (CONTINUED)

MFR.	LENS	MATERIAL, % H_2O, PROCESS	DIAMETER (mm)	BASE CURVE (mm)	POWER (D)	CENTER THICKNESS (mm)	OPTIC ZONE (mm)	dK+ VALUE
PBH	**CSI Clarity Daily Wear Clear**	crofilcon A, 38.6%, lathe-cut	13.8 14.8	8.0, 8.3, 8.6 8.6, 8.9, 9.35	+8.00 to −20.00 in 0.50D steps above −10.00 Plano to −20.00	.06 (−3.00) .06 (−3.00)	10.9 to 6.5 10.9 to 6.5	13
	CTL Clear	polymacon, 38%, molded	14.0	8.4, 8.7	+5.00 to −8.00 in 0.50 steps above +0.50 & −6.00D	0.5		8.4
	CTL Lite	polymacon, 38%, molded	14.0	8.4, 8.7	+5.00 to −8.00 in 0.50 steps above +0.50 &−6.00D	0.03 to 1.0 varies with power		8.4
	Gentle Touch	netrafilcon A, 65%, lathe-cut w/spc	14.5	8.2, 8.5	−5.00 to −6.00D	.10	9.6	38
	Hydrocurve II	bufilcon A, 45%, lathe-cut	13.5 14.5	8.3, 8.6 8.9	+7.00 to −12.00 in 0.50 steps above +5.00 & −8.00	.05 @ −3.00	7.5 - 8.0	12.0
	SOFT MATE B	bufilcon A, 45%, lathe-cut	14.3 14.8	8.7 9.0	+7.00 to −12.00 in 0.50 steps above +5.00 & −8.00	.07 @ −3.00	8.0	12.0
	Sportmate Light Blue Handling Tint	bufilcon A, 45%, lathe-cut	15.5	9.2 9.5 9.8 10.1	Pl to −12.00 +6.00 to −12.00 in 0.50 steps above −6.0 +6.00 to −12.00 in 0.50 steps above −6.00 Plano to −12.00	.05	7.5–8.0	12.0
PLATT CONTACT LENS SERVICE	**LL – 38**	polymacon, 38.6%, embryo molded	14.0 14.5	8.3, 8.6, 8.9 8.4, 8.7, 9.0	Plano to −8.00			
	SOFT FORM II	polymacon, 38%	14.0	8.3 8.5, 8.7, 8.9	−0.25 to −8.00 in 0.25 steps +20.00 to −20.00 in 0.25 steps			
PREFERRED OPTICS, INC.	**Vision 38**	polymacon, 38 %, lathe-cut sphere corrected	14.0	8.7	−6.00 to +6.00 (in 0.25D steps)	.11 (minus) .14 (plus)	7.5	8.4
SALVATORI OPHTHALMICS	**Sof-Form II** custom lenses available for pediatric or special needs	polymacon, 38%, lathe-cut	14.0	8.3, 8.5, 8.7, 8.9 (8.3 not available in +powers)	Div. I +4.25 to −6.00 in 0.25 steps Div. II +4.50 to +10.00, −6.50 to −20.00 in 0.50 steps Div. III +11.00 to +20.00 in 0.50 steps Div. IV any custom design	.07 at −3.00	8.0	

DAILY WEAR SPHERICAL (CONTINUED)

MFR.	LENS	MATERIAL, % H_2O, PROCESS	DIAMETER (mm)	BASE CURVE (mm)	POWER (D)	CENTER THICKNESS (mm)	OPTIC ZONE (mm)	dK+ VALUE
SALVATORI OPHTHALMICS	**Sof-Form 55 Spherical** *Custom lenses available for pediatric or special needs*	methafilcon A, 55%, lathe-cut	14.0 15.0	8.3, 8.6,8.9, 8.6, 8.9, 9.2	Div. I +6.25 to −10.00 in 0.25 steps Div. II +6.50 to +10.50 in 0.25 steps, −10.50 to −20.00 in 0.50 steps Div. III +11.00 to +20.00 in 0.50 steps Div. IV any custom design	.10 (minus)	8.2	18.8
SUNSOFT	**Revolution** Light Blue Visibility Tint	methafilcon A, 55%, patented molding process	14.0	8.5, 8.7	Plano to −10.00 in 0.25 steps +4.00 to −6.00	varies by power	8.0	18.8
	Sportsoft Light Blue Visibility Tint	methafilcon A, 55%, patented molding process	15.0	8.9, 9.2	Plano to −6.00 in 0.25 steps	varies by power	8.0	18.8
	Sunflex	methafilcon A, 55%, lathe-cut	14.0 15.0	8.3, 8.6, 8.9	+5.00 to −10.00 +10.00 to −20.00 in 0.50 steps above −10.00	.10	8.0	18.8
	Sunsoft Aphakic	methafilcon A, 55%, lathe-cut	15.0	8.3, 8.6, 8.9	+10.50 to +20.00 in 0.50 steps	.26	8.0	18.8
UNITED CONTACT LENS	**UCL 55%**	ocufilcon C, 55%	14.0, 14.5, 15.0	8.3, 8.6 to 8.9	sph: +20.00 to −20.00 0.50 after ±9.00D			
WESLEY-JESSEN	**Aquaflex® Spheres**	tetrafilcon A, 43%	13.2 (Standard Minus)	Vault 0: 9.1 I: 8.8 II: 8.5 III: 8.2 IV: 7.9	Plano to −9.75 in 0.25 steps	.14 @ −3.00D	11.4	9.3
	Aquaflex® Spheres	tetrafilcon A, 43%	13.8 (Super Thin™ Minus)	Vault I: 9.1 II: 8.8 III: 8.5 IV: 8.2	−0.25 to −20.00 in 0.25 steps	.06 @ −3.00D	12.0	9.3
	Aquaflex® Spheres	tetrafilcon A, 43%	13.8 (Super Thin™ Low Plus)	Vault I: 9.1 II: 8.8 III: 8.5 IV: 8.2	+0.25 to +9.75 in 0.25 steps	.21 @ +3.00D	9.0	9.3
	DuraSoft 2® Colors **Colors:** Opaque Blue, Opaque Green, Opaque Hazel, Opaque Gray	phemfilcon A, 38%, lathe-cut	14.5	8.3, 8.6	+4.00 to −6.00	.07 @ −3.00D	8.0 (pupil opening 5)	9.03
	DuraSoft 2® LiteTint	phemfilcon A, 38%, lathe-cut	14.5 13.8	8.3, 8.6, 9.0 8.0, 8.3, 8.6 (median)	+20.00 to −20.00 in 0.25 steps to ±10.00, 0.50 steps over ±10.00	.07 @ −3.00D	8.0	9.03

DAILY WEAR SPHERICAL (CONTINUED)

MFR.	LENS	MATERIAL, % H_2O, PROCESS	DIAMETER (mm)	BASE CURVE (mm)	POWER (D)	CENTER THICKNESS (mm)	OPTIC ZONE (mm)	dK+ VALUE
WESLEY-JESSEN	DuraSoft 2® Thinair™ D_2-T3 D_2-T4	phemfilcon A, 38%, lathe-cut	13.5 (D_2-T3) / 14.5 (D_2-T4)	8.2 steep, 8.5 median / 8.3 steep, 8.6 median, 9.0 flat	+20.00 to −20.00 in 0.25 steps to ±10.00, 0.50 steps over ±10.00	.07 at −3.00D	8.0	9.3
WESTCON	Horizon 38 Sphere™	polymacon, 38%, lathe-cut	14.0, 14.5	8.0, 8.3, 8.6, 8.9, 9.2	+10.00 to −10.00	varies	varies	8.4
	Horizon DW	methafilcon A, 55%, lathe-cut	14.0, 15.0	8.0 8.3, 8.6, 8.9, 9.2	+10.00 to −20.00	varies	varies	18.8
	Horizon Specialty	methafilcon A, 55%, lathe-cut	14.0, 14.5, 15.0	8.0, 8.3, 8.6, 8.9, 9.2	+20.00 to −20.00	varies	varies	18.8
	Horizon Custom	methafilcon A, 55%, lathe-cut	10.00 to 16.0 .5 steps	6.8 to 10.1 .3 steps	+40.00 to −40.00	varies	varies	18.8
	Avoid potassium sorbate, sorbic acid and papain.							
	Prism Sphere	methafilcon A, 55%, lathe-cut	14.5	8.6	+2.00 to −6.00 in 0.25 steps	varies	varies	18.8

DAILY WEAR TORIC

MFR.	LENS	MATERIAL, % H_2O, PROCESS	DIAMETER (mm)	BASE CURVE (mm)	SPHERE POWER (mm)	CYLINDER POWER (mm)	AXIS	CENTER THICKNESS (mm)	OPTIC ZONE (mm)	dK+ VALUE
ACCUGEL LABS	Accugel Toric Division I	droxifilcon, 46.6%, lathe-cut	14.0	9.0	+3.00 to −6.00	−.75 to −2.00	90° & 180° ±25°	all lenticular	8.0	18
	Accugel Toric Division 2	droxifilcon, 46.6%, lathe-cut	14.0	7.8 to 9.2 in 0.1 steps	+10.00 to −20.00	−.75 to −5.00	any	all lenticular	8.0	18
	Accugel Toric Division 3	droxifilcon, 46.6%, lathe-cut	<14.0 >14.0	<7.8 >9.2	>+ 10.00 or >−20.00	> −5.00	any	all lenticular	any	18
ACRO CONTACT LENS	Torisoft	tefilcon, 37.5%	14.5	8.6, 8.9, 9.2* *minus only	+4.00 to −6.00 in 0.25 steps, −6.50 & −7.00	−1.00, −1.75, −2.50*	8.6 & 8.9: 0° to 180°; 9.2: 180° ± 20; 90° ± 20 (10° steps)	.095 @ -3.00 .17 @ +3.00		
AQUA-SITE	Aqua-Cyl	ocufilcon-B, 53%, lathe-cut	14.5 or custom	8.6, 8.8, 9.0, or custom	-25.00 to +10.00 or custom	-0.25 to -4.50 or custom	0° & 180°	varies with power	8.2	15.4
BAUSCH & LOMB	Optima™ Toric Stock	hefilcon B, 45%	14.0	8.3, 8.6, 8.9	+4.00 to −9.00D (in 0.25D steps)	−0.75, −1.25, −1.75D	10° full circle	.10 – .28	8.0	
	Optima™ Toric Custom				+4.00 to +6.00	−2.25, −2.75D	5° full circle	.10 – .33	8.0	

DAILY WEAR TORIC (CONTINUED)

MFR.	LENS	MATERIAL, % H_2O, PROCESS	DIAMETER (mm)	BASE CURVE (mm)	SPHERE POWER (mm)	CYLINDER POWER (mm)	AXIS	CENTER THICKNESS (mm)	OPTIC ZONE (mm)	dK+ VALUE
BIOCURVE SOFT LENSES	**Biocurve Custom Toric**	methafilcon A, 55%	14.0, 14.5	any	–20.00 to +10.00 in 0.25 steps	–3.25 to –5.00 in 0.25 steps	any in 1° steps	.08 –.30	8.0	18.8
	Biocurve Standard Toric	methafilcon A, 55%	14.0, 14.5	8.4, 8.6, 8.8, 9.0	–20.00 to +10.00 in 0.25 steps	–0.75 to –3.00 in 0.25 steps	any in 1° steps	.08 –.30	8.0	18.8
	Biocurve Stock Toric	methafilcon A, 55%	14.5	8.8	–6.00 to +3.00 in 0.25 steps	–0.75 to –2.00 in 0.25 steps	180 ± 20° in 5° steps, 90 ± 20° in 5° steps	.08 –.30	8.0	18.8
CIBA VISION CORP.	**Focus® Toric**	vifilcon A, 55%, CIBACAST® molding	14.5	8.9, 9.2	–6.00 to +4.00 in 0.25 steps	–1.00, –1.75	180° ± 20°& 90° ± 20° (10° steps)	0.147 @ –3.00 0.264 @ +3.00	8.0	16.0
	TORISOFT®	tefilcon, 37.5%	14.5	8.6, 8.9, 9.2* *Minus powers only	Plano to –6.00 (0.25 steps) –6.50, –7.00 Plus: 0.25 to +4.00 in 0.25 steps	–1.00, –1.75,	8.6 & 8.9: 0° to 180° 9.2: B.C. 180°±20°, 90° ±20° (10° steps)	.095 @ –3.00 .175 @ +3.00	8.0	
				8.6, 8.9	Plano to –8.00D (0.50D steps), –6.50D, –7.00D	–2.50	180°±90°, 90° ±20°			
	TORISOFT® Softcolors® **Colors:** Aqua Blue, Green, Amber, Royal Blue, Evergreen	tefilcon 37.5 %	14.5	8.6, 8.9, 9.2*	Plano to –6.00 (0.25 steps) –6.50, –7.00	–1.00, –1.75	8.6 & 8.9 BC: 0° to 180° 9.2 BC: 180° ±20°	.095 @ –3.00 .175 @ +3.00	8.0	
				*Minus powers only	Plus: 0.25 to +4.00 in 0.25 steps		90° ±20° (10° steps)			
COAST–VISION	**Hydrasoft® Toric Div. I Standard Toric**	methafilcon B, 55%, lathe-cut, pitch polished	15.0	8.9	+3.00 to –6.00	–0.75 to –2.00 (in 0.25 steps)	180° ±20°, 90° ±20° (1° steps)	.07 to .40	8.0	18.8
	Hydrasoft® Toric Div. II Specialty Toric	methafilcon B, 55%, lathe-cut, pitch polished	15.0	8.6, 8.9	+10.00 to –20.00	–0.75 to –5.00 (in 0.25 steps)	any (1° steps)	.07 to .40	8.0	18.8
	Hydrasoft® Toric Div. III Custom Toric	methafilcon B, 55%, lathe-cut, pitch polished	14.2	8.3, 8.6	+10.00 to –20.00	–0.50 to –10.00 (in 0.25 steps)	any (1° steps)	.07 to .40	8.0	18.8
			15.0	8.3, 8.6, 8.9, 9.2						
	Hydrasoft® Toric Aphakic	methafilcon B, 55%, lathe-cut pitch polished	15.0	8.6, 8.9	+10.25 to +20.00 (in 0.25 steps)	–0.75 to –10.00	any (1° steps)	varies	8.0	18.8
CONTINENTAL SOFT LENS INC.	**Continental Torric**	ocufilcon B, 53%, lathing	13.5 to 15.0	7.8 to 10.0 min.	±20.00	–11.00	any	varies with power	8.0	16.5

DAILY WEAR TORIC (CONTINUED)

MFR.	LENS	MATERIAL, % H_2O, PROCESS	DIAMETER (mm)	BASE CURVE (mm)	SPHERE POWER (mm)	CYLINDER POWER (mm)	AXIS	CENTER THICKNESS (mm)	OPTIC ZONE (mm)	dK+ VALUE
GREAT LAKES CONTACT LENSES	**Technicon Custom Soft Toric**	methafilcon A, 55%, lathe-cut	14.5 & 15.0	8.3, 8.6, 8.9	+1.00 to +10.00, –1.00 to –10.00	–0.75 to –5.00	any			
KONTUR KONTACT LENS CO.	**Kontur 55 Toric Div. I**	methafilcon A, lathe-cut back surface toric zone	15.0	8.6, 8.9	+4.00 to –6.00	–0.75 to –2.00	any in 1° steps	.10 to .25	8.0	18.8
			Do not use potassium sorbate or sorbic acid.							
	Kontur 55 Toric Div. II	methafilcon A, lathe-cut back surface toric zone	15.0	8.6, 8.9	+4.25 to +10.00 –6.25 to –10.00	–2.25 to –3.50	any in 1° steps	.10 to .45	8.0	18.8
	Kontur 55 Toric Div. III	methafilcon A, lathe-cut back surface toric zone	15.0	8.6, 8.9	–10.00 to –20.00	–3.75 to –5.00	any in 1° steps	.10 to .45	8.0	18.8
	Kontur 55 Toric Div. IV Custom	methafilcon A, lathe-cut back surface toric zone	15.0	8.6, 8.9	over +10.00 or –20.00	over –5.00	any in 1° steps	.10 to .45	8.0	18.8
METRO OPTICS	**Metro Soft II Toric**	polymacon, 38%, lathe-cut	14.0	8.7	–10.00 to +10.00 in 0.25 steps	–0.75 to –4.00 in 0.25 steps	any in 5° steps	.14	9.0	8.4
OCU-EASE OPTICAL PRODUCTS	**Ocuflex 53 Custom**	ocufilcon B, 53%, lathe-cut	14.5 / 15.0 (No interchangaes)	8.6 / 8.8	+4.00 to –7.00	–0.50 to –2.50	any	.13 (–), .18 (+)	8.0 Other parameters available on request	18.1
	Ocuflex 53 Special Custom	ocufilcon B, 53%, lathe-cut	14.0 to 15.0 (interchangeable)	8.4, 8.6, 8.8, 9.0	–20.00 to +20.00	–0.50 to –6.00	any	.13 (–), .18 (+)	8.0	18.1
OCULAR SCIENCE/ AMERICAN HYDRON	**Hydron Ultra T**	polymacon, 43%, spin-cast front surface	14.5	varies with power	Plano to –6.00	–1.00, –1.50, –2.00	full circle in 10° steps, scribe marks at 5.30, 6.00, 6.30	.15 (–3.00)	8.0 (–3.00)	11.2
	Custo Toric	polymacon, 38%, lathe-cut (optional truncation with .50 to 2.0 pd BD front surface toric)	13.0, 13.5, 14.0, 14.5, 15.0, 15.5	7.2 – 9.3 in .1 steps	Plano to ±25.00 in –.25 steps	Plano to –10.00 in .25D steps	any	.14 to .52	8 to 11	8.4
OPTECH, INC.	**Fre-Flex Custom Toric**	focofilcon A, 55%, lathe-cut	15.0	9.0	–20.00 to +20.00	–0.50 to –8.00	any	.14 @ –3.00	8.0	15.5
	Fre-Flex Special Design Toric	focofilcon A, 55%, lathe-cut	10.00 to 17.0	6.0 to 11.0	–30.00 to +30.00	–0.50 to –16.00	any	.14 @ –3.00	8.0	15.5
PBH	**CSI Clarity Toric** **Notes:** Edge to Edge Visibility Tint	crofilcon A, 38.6%, lathe-cut	14.0	8.3, 8.6	+4.00 to –8.00	–1.00, –1.75	10° around the clock; (180° ± 20°, 90° ± 20° in 5° steps)	0.02 to 0.40 varies with power	7.6	13

DAILY WEAR TORIC (CONTINUED)

MFR.	LENS	MATERIAL, % H_2O, PROCESS	DIAMETER (mm)	BASE CURVE (mm)	SPHERE POWER (mm)	CYLINDER POWER (mm)	AXIS	CENTER THICKNESS (mm)	OPTIC ZONE (mm)	dK+ VALUE
PBH	**Hydrocurve II 45%**	bufilcon A, 45%, lathe-cut	14.5	8.9	+3.00 to −8.00	−1.25, −2.00	10° around the clock 180° ± 20°, 90° ± 20° in 5° steps	0.08 (−3.00)	8.0	12.0
	Custom tints: Blue, Green, Aqua, Lavender		14.5	8.9	Plano to −6.00	−0.75	90° ±20°, 180° ±20°			
			13.5 (non-core)	8.6	−6.25 to +3.00	−1.25, −2.00	90° ±20°, 180° ±20°			
	Signature Toric	bufilcon A, 45%, lathe-cut	14.5	8.9	+4.00 to −8.00	−1.00, −1.75	10° around the clock (180° ± 20°, 90° ± 20° in 5° steps)	0.05 (−3.00)		12.0
SALVATORI OPH-THALMICS	**Sof-Form® 55 Toric**	methafilcon A, 55%, lathe-cut	15.0	Div I 8.9	+4.00 to −6.00	−0.50 to −2.00	any	1.5D prism	8.0	
				Div II 8.6 8.9	+10.00 to −20.00	−0.50 to −5.00				
			13.0 to 15.5	Div III Any parameter not listed above						
SUNSOFT	**Eclipse**	methafilcon A, 55%, lathe-cut	14.5	standard	+2.00 to −6.00 in 0.25 steps	−0.75 to −2.50 in 0.25 steps	180 ± 30°, 90 ± 30° 5° incre-ments	varies by power	8.0	18.8
	Sunsoft Toric 15.0 Div. I	methafilcon A, 55%, lathe-cut	15.0	8.9	+3.00 to −6.00 in 0.25 steps	−0.75 to −2.00 in 0.25 steps	180° ±20° 90 ±20° (5° incre-ments in stock)	varies by power	8.0	18.8
	Sunsoft Toric 15.0 Div. II	methafilcon A, 55%, lathe-cut	15.0	8.3, 8.9	+10.00 to −20.00 in 0.25 steps	−0.75 to −5.00 in 0.25 steps	any	varies by power	8.0	18.8
	Sunsoft Toric 15.0 Div. III Custom	methafilcon A, 55%, lathe-cut	15.0	8.3, 8.9	+10.00 to −20.00 in 0.25 steps	−5.25 to −7.00 in 0.25 steps	any	varies by power	8.0	18.8
UNITED CONTACT LENS	**UCL Toric**	ocufilcon C, 55%	14.5 – 15.0	8.6, 8.9	any	any	any			55
	UCL Custom	ocufilcon C, 55%	any	any	any	any	any			
WESLEY-JESSEN	**DuraSoft® 2 OptiFit® Toric**	phemfilcon A, 38%, lathe-cut (back toric)	14.5	median (fits equivalent to an 8.6 sph.)	−12.00 to +4.00 in 0.50 steps over −8.00	−0.75 to −3.75 in 0.50 steps	5° incre-ments (full circle)	.07	8.0	9.03
WESTCON	**Horizon 55 Toric ™ (STD)**	methafilcon A, 55%, lathe-cut prism ballast	14.5	8.6	+2.00 to −6.00 in 0.25 steps	−0.75 to −2.50 in 0.25 steps	180° ± 30° in 1° steps 90° ± 30° in 1° steps	varies	varies	18.8
	Horizon F.S. (Front Surface Toric)	polymacon 38% or methafilcon A, lathe-cut	14.5	8.3, 8.6, 8.9	Div I +4.00 to −6.00 in 0.25 steps Div.II +10.00 to −20.00 in 0.25 steps	.50 to −1.50 in 0.25 steps	any 1° steps		8	18.8
	Avoid potassium sorbate, sorbic acid, and papain.									
	Horizon Toric Division I	methafilcon A, 55%, lathe-cut prism ballast	14.5, 15.0	8.3, 8.6, 8.9	+4.00 to −8.00 in 0.25 steps	−0.75 to −2.50 in 0.25 steps	any steps	varies	varies	18.8
			Avoid potassium sorbate, sorbic acid, and papain.							

DAILY WEAR TORIC (CONTINUED)

MFR.	LENS	MATERIAL, % H_2O, PROCESS	DIAMETER (mm)	BASE CURVE (mm)	SPHERE POWER (mm)	CYLINDER POWER (mm)	AXIS	CENTER THICKNESS (mm)	OPTIC ZONE (mm)	dK+ VALUE
WESTCON	**Horizon Toric Division II**	methafilcon A, 55%, lathe-cut prism ballast	14.5, 15.0	8.3, 8.6, 8.9, 9.2	+10.00 to –10.00 in 0.25 steps	–0.75 to –5.00 in 0.25 steps	any in 1° steps	varies	varies	18.8
	Horizon Toric Division III	methafilcon A, 55%, lathe-cut prism ballast	14.5, 15.0	8.3, 8.6, 8.9, 9.2	+20.00 to –20.00 in 0.25 steps	–0.50 to –10.00 in 0.25 steps	any in 1° steps	varies	varies	18.8
	Horizon Toric Custom	methafilcon A, 55%, lathe-cut prism ballast	Please call for any parameters not listed above.							
	Westhin Toric Div I	polymacon*, 38%, lathe-cut, back, toric double slab-off	14.2	8.6	+4.00 to –7.00	–.75 to –2.00		varies	varies	8.0
	Div II		14.2	8.2, 8.6, 8.9	9.75 to 12.00	–2.25 to –4.00		varies	varies	8.0
	Div III		14.3	8.3, 8.6, 8.9	+20.00 to –22.00	–4.25 to –6.00		varies	varies	8.0

*Also available in methafilcon A, 55%, with dk+ value of 18.8.
Use only peroxide and chemical disinfection.
Avoid potassium sorbate, sorbic acid and papain.

DAILY WEAR MULTIFOCAL

MFR.	LENS	MATERIAL, % H_2O, PROCESS	DIAMETER (mm)	BASE CURVE (mm)	POWER (mm) CYLINDER	AD POWER (mm)	CENTER THICKNESS (mm)	OPTIC ZONE (mm)	dK+ VALUE
BAUSCH & LOMB	**Bi-Tech Bifocal Visibility Tint**	polymacon, 38%, spin-cast front, lathe-cut back	13.5 vert., 14.5 horiz.	Sag I 9.0 Sag II 8.7	+6.00 to –6.00D (in 0.50D steps above –5.00D includes Plano)	+2.00, +2.50	0.16 (–6.00D) to 0.22 (plano); 0.22 (+0.25D) to 0.36 (+6.00D).		
	Bifocal P.A. I Series	polymacon, 38%, spin-cast	13.5	8.6	+6.00 to –6.00D (in 0.50D steps above –5.00D)	nominal + 1.50D	.08 – .21		
	Occasions™ Multifocal	polymacon, 38%, shape-cast	14	8.6	+6.00 to –9.00D (in 0.25D steps)		.08 to –16	8.0 to 9.0	
CONTACT LENS CORP. OF AMERICA	**FULFOCUS**	polymacon, 38%, lathe	14.2	8.4	+4.00 to–6.50 in 0.25 steps	1.00 to +3.00	.06 to .32	varies with power Add. type aspheric	8.6
				8.7	+6.00 to –12.50 in 0.25 steps				8.4
				9.0	+4.00 to –6.50				
ESSTECH	**ESSTECH PS**	polymacon, 38%, lathe-cut	14.0	8.7 and 9.1		up to +2.00	.14(–) .15(+)	9.0 to 11.5	
OCULAR SCIENCES/ AMERICAN HYDRON	**Hydron Echelon** light blue visibility tint with clear pupil	polymacon, 38%, cast-molded	13.8	8.7	+4.00 to –6.00	+1.50, +2.00, +2.50	.08 (–3.00)	8.7 to 6.4 aspheric with phase plate (4.55 + 4.21)	8.4
PBH	**Hydrocurve II** Custom tint available	bufilcon A, 45%, lathe-cut aspheric	14.8	9.0	+4.00 to–6.00	(progressive add up to +1.50)*	.05@–3.00	dist.4	12

*effective add up to +2.50D may be achieved depending upon pupil size and asphericity of cornea.

DAILY WEAR MULTIFOCAL (CONTINUED)

MFR.	LENS	MATERIAL, % H_2O, PROCESS	DIAMETER (mm)	BASE CURVE (mm)	POWER (mm) CYLINDER	AD POWER (mm)	CENTER THICKNESS (mm)	OPTIC ZONE (mm)	dK+ VALUE
PBH	**Hydrocurve II** Bifocal Custom Tint Available	bufilcon A, 45%, lathe-cut aspheric	14.8	9.0	+4.00 to −6.00	progressive to +1.50	.05 @−3.00	dist. 4	12
PREFERRED OPTICS INC.	**PS 45**	polymacon, 38%, lathe-cut aspheric	14.0	8.7	+7.00 to −5.00 .25D steps	ADD up to +2.00	.20		8.4
	Multi-Vue 53 High ADD series	ocufilcon B, 53%, lathe-cut	14.5	8.6	+7.00 to −7.00 .25D steps	progressive ADD +2.00 to +3.00	.15	8.0	18.2
	Multi-Vue 53 Low ADD series	ocufilcon B, 53%, lathe-cut	14.5	8.6, 8.3	+7.00 to −7.00 .25D steps	progessive ADD +1.00 to +2.00	.15	8.0	18.2
SALVATORI OPH-THALMICS	**ALLVUE™ Multifocal**	polymacon, 38%, lathe-cut	14.0	8.5, 8.7, 8.9	+4.00 to −6.00 in 0.25 steps	+1 to +3 inclusive	varies	varies	varies
UNILENS CORP. USA	**Unilens™**	hefilcon A, 45%, lathe-cut aspheric	14.0, 14.5 14.5	8.4, 8.7, 9.0 9.3	−8.00 to +6.00 in 0.25 steps	varies up to +2.00 through aspheric optics	0.16	9.0	11.6
	SimulVue™	hefilcon A, 45%, lathe-cut	14.5	8.7, 9.0	−8.00 to +6.00 in 0.25 steps	+2.00, +2.50, +3.00 seg sizes: 2.35, 2.55	0.14	9.0	11.6
	ALGES® Bifocal	hefilcon A, 45%, lathe-cut	14.0	8.6, 8.9	+4.00 to −4.00 in 0.25 steps; ±4.00 to ±6.00 in 0.50 steps	1.50*, 2.00, 2.50, 3.00, 3.50* Seg Sizes: 2.12*, 2.35, 2.55, 3.00*, 3.50*	.14	8.5	11.3

•Indicates nonstandard parameters.

DAILY WEAR TINTED

MFR.	LENS	MATERIAL, % H_2O, PROCESS	DIAMETER (mm)	BASE CURVE (mm)	POWER (D)	CENTER THICKNESS (mm)	OPTIC ZONE (mm)	dK+ VALUE
BAUSCH & LOMB	**Optima 38 Natural Tint** **Colors:** Aqua, Blue, Green	polymacon, 38%, spin-cast front, lathe-cut back	14.0	3.6, 3.82 (sag. depths), 8.4, 8.7 also available in plano	+5.0 to −5.00 in 0.25 steps +5.50 to −9.00 in 0.50 steps	.06 (−)	8.0	9.2
	Soflens® Series Natural Tint-B3 **Colors:** Aqua, Blue, Green, Brown (tint. dia. 11mm solid)	polymacon, 38.6%, spin-cast front	13.5		−0.25 to −5.00, −5.50, −6.00	.12	12.1	9.2
	Soflens® Series Natural Tint-U3 **Colors:** Aqua, Blue, Green, Brown (tint. dia. 11mm solid)	polymacon, 38.6%, spin-cast front	13.5		Plano to −5.00, −5.50, −6.00	.07	12.4	9.2
	Soflens® Series Natural Tint-U4 **Colors:** Aqua, Blue, Green, Brown (tint. dia. 11mm solid)	polymacon, 38.6%, spin-cast front	14.5		−0.25 to −5.00, −5.50, −6.00	.07	13.6	9.2

DAILY WEAR TINTED (CONTINUED)

MFR.	LENS	MATERIAL, % H_2O, PROCESS	DIAMETER (mm)	BASE CURVE (mm)	POWER (D)	CENTER THICKNESS (mm)	OPTIC ZONE (mm)	dK+ VALUE
CIBA VISION CORP.	**CIBASOFT® Softcolors®**	tefilcon, 37.5%	13.8	8.3, 8.6, 8.9	+6.00 to –6.00 in 0.25 steps;–6.50 to –10.00 in 0.50 steps	.07 @ –3.00 .14 @ +3.00	varies w/ power (7.0 to 12.0)	8.9
			14.5	8.6, 8.9, 9.2	Plano to –6.00 in 0.25 steps; –6.50 to –10.00 in 0.50 steps			
	Colors: Aqua Blue, Royal Blue, Green, Amber, Evergreen							
	CIBASOFT® Visitint® Light Blue Visibility Tint	tefilcon, 37.5%	13.8	8.3, 8.6, 8.9	+6.00 to –6.00 in 0.25 steps;–6.50 to –10.00 in 0.25 steps	.07 @ –3.00 .14 @ +3.00	varies w/ power (7.0 to 12.0)	8.9
			14.5	8.6, 8.9, 9.2	Plano to –6.00 in 0.25 steps; –6.50 to –10.00 in 0.50 steps			
	ILLUSIONS® Opaque	tefilcon, 37.5%	13.8	8.3, 8.6, 8.9	+4.00 to –6.00 in 0.25D steps	.10 @ –3.00 .17 @ +3.00	varies with power (7.0 to 12.8)	8.9
	Colors: Deep Blue, Soft Blue, Deep Green, Soft Green, Soft Amber, Grey							
	STD™ Softcolors®	tefilcon, 37.5%	13.8	8.3, 8.6, 8.9	+6.00 to –6.00 in 0.25D steps	.10 @ –3.00 .17 @ +3.00		8.9
	Colors: Aqua, Evergreen, Royal Blue							
	STD™ Visitint® Light Blue Visibility Tint	tefilcon, 37.5%	13.8	8.3, 8.6, 8.9	+6.00 to –6.00 in 0.25D steps	.10 @ –3.00 .17 @ +3.00	(7.0 to 12.8)	8.9
METRO OPTICS	**Metro Lite**	polymacon, 38%, lathe-cut	13.5	8.3, 8.6, 8.9	–20.00 to +20.00 in 0.50 steps above ±7.00	.10	9.0	8.4
	Colors: Light Blue		14.0	Series M	Pl to –7.00	.06		
	Metro Tint	polymacon, 38%, lathe-cut	13.5	8.3, 8.6, 8.9	–20.00 to +20.00 in 0.50 steps above ±7.00	.10	9.0	8.4
	Colors: Blue, Green, Aqua		14.0	Series M	Pl to –7.00	.06		
OCULAR SCIENCES/ AMERICAN HYDRON	**Zero–6 Softints**	polymacon, 38%, lathe-cut	14.0	8.4, 8.7, 9.0	to ±10.00	.06(–) .10(+)	8–11	8.4
	Colors::Sapphire Aqua, Emerald, Smokey Quartz, Clear Pupil, 4.5 mm tint, diam. 11mm (in matrix tint)							
PBH	**Cosmetic Tint**	Polymacon, 38%	14.0	8.4, 8.7	–8.00 to +5.00 (0.50 steps above +0.50 & –6.00D)	.06	8 to 11	8.4
	Colors: Aquamarine, Cocoa, Emerald, Sapphire							
	CSI® Clarity Daily Wear Colours	crofilcon A, 38.6%, lathe-cut	13.8	8.3, 8.6	Plano to –6.00	.07 (-3.00)	10.9 to 6.5	13
	Colors: Blue, Green, Violet Blue, Aqua							
	CSI® Clarity Daily Wear Locator Tint	crofilcon A, 38.6%, lathe-cut	13.8	8.0, 8.3, 8.6	+8.00 to –6.00	0.02 to 0.40 varies with power	10.9 to 6.5	13
	*Note: Edge to edge visibility tint							
	Natural™ Touch	polymacon, 38%, molded	13.8	8.4, 8.7	+6.00 to –10.00	.06 –3.00D	5.3	8
	Colors: Willow Green, Baby Blue, Sophisticated Blue, Aqua Seas, Sultry Gray, Hazel							
	Soft Mate B Locator	bufilcon A, 45%	14.3 14.8	8.7 9.0	–4.00 to +4.00 –6.00 to +6.00	.06 (–3.00)	8.0 to 8.5	12

DAILY WEAR TINTED (CONTINUED)

MFR.	LENS	MATERIAL, % H_2O, PROCESS	DIAMETER (mm)	BASE CURVE (mm)	POWER (D)	CENTER THICKNESS (mm)	OPTIC ZONE (mm)	dK+ VALUE
WESLEY-JESSEN	Durasoft® 2 Colors	phemfilcon A, 38%, lathe-cut	14.5	8.3, 8.6	+4.00 to –6.00	.07	8.0	9.03
	Colors: Opaque Blue, Opaque Green, Opaque Hazel, Opaque Gray							
	Durasoft® 2 Colors for Light Eyes	phemfilcon A, 38%, lathe-cut	14.5	8.3 steep 8.6 median 9.0 flat	Plano to –4.00 +4.00 to –8.00 Plano to –4.00 all in 0.25 steps	.07 @ –3.00D	5.00 (clear pupil zone)	9.03
	Colors: Enhance-Sky Blue, Enhance-Jade Green, Enhance-Aquamarine, Enhance-Violet Blue							

DAILY WEAR THERAPEUTIC

MFR.	LENS	MATERIAL, % H_2O, PROCESS	DIAMETER (mm)	BASE CURVE (mm)	POWER (D)	CENTER THICKNESS (mm)	OPTIC ZONE (mm)	dK+ VALUE
KONTUR	Kontur 55 Sphere*	methafilcon A, 55%, lathe-cut	16.0 to 24.0	8.30 to 9.80	+.50	.16	8.0	18.8
	*Intended for post-schlerostomy use.							
NARCISSUS	Custom Made Prosthetic lenses	ocufilcon B	varies	varies	varies	varies	varies	varies

DAILY WEAR BIFOCAL

MFR.	LENS	MATERIAL, % H_2O, PROCESS	DIAMETER (mm)	BASE CURVE (mm)	POWER (D)	CENTER THICKNESS (mm)	OPTIC ZONE (mm)	dK+ VALUE
BAUSCH & LOMB	Bi-Tech Visibility Tint	polymacon, 38%	14.5 (horiz.) 13.5 (vert.)	Sag I 9.0 Sag II 8.7	+6.00 to –6.00 in 0.50 steps above ±5.00 (includes plano)	0.16 (6.00) to 0.22 (plano); 0.22 (+0.25) to 0.36 (+6.00)		+2.00 +2.50
	P.A. 1	polymacon, 38%	13.5	8.6	+6.00 to –6.00 in 0.50 steps above ±5.00	.08 to .21		nominal +1.50
CIBA VISION CORP.	BI-SOFT®	tefilcon, 37.5%	13.8	8.3, 8.6, 8.9* *plus powers only	+6.00 to –6.00 in 0.25 steps	.07 @ –3.00 .12 @ +3.00	2.3/7.0 to 12.8	+1.50 to+3.00 in 0.50 steps

PROGRAMMED REPLACEMENT LENSES

MFR.	LENS	MATERIAL, % H_2O, PROCESS	DIAMETER (mm)	BASE CURVE (mm)	POWER (D)	CENTER THICKNESS (mm)	OPTIC ZONE (mm)	dK+ VALUE
BAUSCH & LOMB	Medalist Toric	lidofilcon A, 70%		8.7, 9.0	Sphere: Plano to –6.00 in 0.25 steps; Cyl: –0.75, –1.25, –1.75; Axis: 90+/–20° to 180+/–20° in 10° increments	0.12	8.0	
	03/04 Blister	polymacon, 38%	13.5, 14.5	spin-cast	–1.00 to –6.00 in 0.50 steps above –5.00 DW above –6.00	0.035	12.4, 13.6	
	Medalist Visibility Tint	polymacon, 38%	14.0	8.4, 8.7, 9.0	+4.00 to –9.00 in 0.25 steps	.026 to .035	8.0 to 10.0	8.0
CIBA VISION CORP.	Focus® SOFT-COLORS®	vifilcon A, 55%, CIBACAST® molding	14.0	8.6, 8.9	–8.00 to +6.00 (0.25 steps)	.10 @ –3.00 .15 @ +3.00	7.8	16.0
	Colors: Royal Blue, Aqua, Evergreen							

PROGRAMMED REPLACEMENT LENSES

MFR.	LENS	MATERIAL, % $H^2$0, PROCESS	DIAMETER (mm)	BASE CURVE (mm)	POWER (D)	CENTER THICKNESS (mm)	OPTIC ZONE (mm)	dK+ VALUE
CIBA VISION CORP.	**Focus® Toric**	vifilcon A, 55%, CIBACAST® molding	14.5	8.9, 9.2	sphere: –6.00 to +4.00 in 0.25 steps; cyl: –1.00, –1.75 180° + 20° & 90° ± 20° (10° steps)	0.147 @ –3.00 0.264 @ +3.00	8.0	16.0
	Focus® Visitint®	vifilcon A, 55%, CIBACAST® molding	14.0	8.6, 8.9	–8.00 to +6.00 (0.25 steps)	.10 @ –3.00 .15 @ +3.00	7.8	16.0
COOPERVISION INC.	**Preference™ Standard** Planned Replacement Light Blue Handling Tint Edge to Edge Daily Wear	tetrafilcon A, 43%, lathe-cut	14.0 14.4	8.3, 8.6 8.7	–0.25 to –6.50 in 0.25 steps; –6.50 to –10.00 in 0.50 steps; Plano to +4.00 in 0.25 steps	0.03 to 0.12 (–) 0.08 to 0.23 (+)	12.8 13.2	9.3
OCULAR SCIENCES/ AMERICAN HYDRON	**EDGE® III ProActive**	polymacon, 38%, mold-cast	14.0	8.7 8.3, 8.6, 8.9	+0.25 to +5.00 –0.25 to –8.00	.07	8.00 to –12.50	
PBH	**Gentle Touch**	netrafilcon A, 65%, lathe-cut w/spc	14.5	8.2, 8.5	–0.500 to –6.00D	.10	9.6	38
VISTAKON	**Acuvue®** conversion to Visibility Tint begins in May	etafilcon A, 58%, stabilized soft molding	14.0 (–) 14.4 (+)	8.4, 8.8 9.3	–0.50 to –6.00 in 0.25 steps –6.50 to –9.00 in 0.50 steps +0.50 to +6.00 in 0.25 steps –6.50 to –9.00 in 0.50 steps	.07 at –3.00D	8.0	28.0
	Surevue® Visibility Tint as of 3/1/94	etafilcon A, 58%, stabilized soft molding	14.0	8.8, 8.4 B.C./ 14.0 Diam minus lenses only, 9.1B.C 14.4 Diam, plus lenses only	–0.50 to –6.00 in 0.25 steps; –6.50 to –9.00 in 0.50 steps +0.50 to +6.00 in 0.25 steps	0.105 at –3.00		28.0

FLEXIBLE WEAR

MFR.	LENS	MATERIAL, % $H_2$0, PROCESS	DIAMETER (mm)	BASE CURVE (mm)	SPHERE POWER (mm)	CYLINDER POWER (mm)	CENTER THICKNESS (mm)	OPTIC ZONE (mm)	dK+ VALUE
COOPER VISION	**Vantage® Thin** (Clear)	tetrafilcon A, 43%, lathe-cut	14.0 14.4	8.4 8.7		Plano to –6.50 in 0.25 steps; –6.50 to –10.00 in 0.50 steps	0.03-0.082	12.8 13.2	9.3
	CooperClear ™FW	tetrafilcon A, 43%, lathe-cut	14.4 14.4	8.4 8.7		–0.25 to –10.00 (in .50 steps above –6.50)	0.03-0.082	13.2	9.3
GREAT LAKES	**Pro Soft**	methafilcon, 55%, lathe-cut	14.0	8.3, 8.6	+.25 to +6.00; –.25 to –9.00		.06		

FLEXIBLE WEAR (CONTINUED)

MFR.	LENS	MATERIAL, % H_2O, PROCESS	DIAMETER (mm)	BASE CURVE (mm)	SPHERE POWER (mm)	CYLINDER POWER (mm)	CENTER THICKNESS (mm)	OPTIC ZONE (mm)	dK+ VALUE
SUNSOFT	**Revolution** Light Blue Visibility Tint	methafilcon A, 55%, patented molding process	14.0	8.5 8.7	Plano to –10 in 0.25 steps +4.00 to –6.00		varies by power	8.0	18.8
	Sportsoft Light Blue Visibility Tint	methafilcon A, 55%, patented molding process	15.0	8.9, 9.2	Plano to –6.00 in 0.25 steps		varies by power	8.0	18.8
	Sunflex	methaflicon A, 55%, lathe-cut	14.0 15.0	8.3, 8.6, 8.9	+5.00 to –10.00 +10.00 to –20.00 in 0.50 steps above –10.00		.10	8.0	18.8
	Sunsoft Aphakic	methafilcon A, 55%, lathe-cut	15.0	8.3, 8.6, 8.9	+10.50 to +20.00 in 0.50 steps		.26	8.0	18.8
WESTCON	**Horizon FW Custom Sphere**	methafilcon A, 55%	10.00 to 16.00 in 5mm steps	6.80 to 10.10 in 3mm steps	+20.00 to –20.00		varies	varies	18.8
	Horizon FW Specialty	methafilcon A, 55%, lathe-cut, pitch polished	14.0, 14.5, 15.0	8.0, 8.3, 8.6, 8.9	+20.00 to –20.00		varies	varies	18.8
	Horizon 55 FW Sphere	methafilcon A, 55%, lathe-cut pitch polished	14.0, 14.5, 15.0 Avoid potassium sorbate, sorbic acid, and papain	8.0, 8.3, 8.8, 8.9, 9.2	+10.00 to –20.00		varies	varies	18.8
	Prism Spheres	methafilcon A, 55%, lathe-cut	14.5 Avoid potassium sorbate, sorbic acid, and papain	8.6	+2.00 –6.00		varies	varies	18.8

FLEXIBLE WEAR HANDLING TINTS

MFR.	LENS	MATERIAL, % H_2O, PROCESS	DIAMETER (mm)	BASE CURVE (mm)	POWER (D)	CENTER THICKNESS (mm)	OPTIC ZONE (mm)	dK+ VALUE
COOPER VISION	**Preference™ Planned Replacement** Light Blue Handling Tint Edge to Edge	tetrafilcon A, 43%, lathe-cut	14.4	8.4, 8.7	–0.25 to –6.50 in 0.25 steps; –6.50 to –10.00 in 0.50 steps	0.03 to 0.082	13.2	9.3
	Vantage® Thin Light Blue Handling Tint	tetrafilcon A, 43%, lathe-cut	14.0 14.4	8.4 8.7	Plano to –6.50 in 0.25 steps; –6.50 to –10.00 in 0.50 steps	0.03 to 0.082	12.8 13.2	9.3

FLEXIBLE WEAR ENHANCEMENT TINTS

MFR.	LENS	MATERIAL, % H²O, PROCESS	DIAMETER (mm)	BASE CURVE (mm)	POWER (D)	CENTER THICKNESS (mm)	OPTIC ZONE (mm)	dK+ VALUE
BAUSCH & LOMB	Natural Tint–03	polymacon, 38%	13.5		Plano (Daily Wear) –1.00 to –5.00, –5.50, –6.00	.035	12.4	
	Natural Tint–04	polymacon, 38%,	14.5				13.6	
	Colors: Crystal Blue, Aqua, Jade Green, Sable Brown							
	Optima FW Natural Tint	polymacon, 38%	14.0	8.7	–0.25 to –9.00 (in 0.50 steps above –5.00)	.026 to .035	8.0	
	Colors: Crystal Blue, Aqua, Jade Green							
	Optima FW Visibility Tint	polymacon, 38%	14.0	8.4, 8.7, 9.0	+4.00 to –9.00 includes Plano	.026 to .035	8.0	
	Colors: Light Blue							
CIBA VISION CORP	Cibathin® Soft Colors®	tcfilcon, 37.5%	13.8	8.6, 8.9	Plano to –6.00	.035 at –3.00D	varies with power (7.0 to 12.8)	8.9
	Colors: Aqua Blue, Royal Blue, Green, Amber							
	Focus® Soft Colors®	vifilcon A, 55% CIBACAST® molding	14.0	8.6, 8.9	–8.00 to +6.00 (0.25 steps)	.10@ –3.00 .15@ +3.00	7.8	16.3
	Colors: Royal Blue, Aqua, Evergreen							
COOPERVISION	Vantage® Thin Accemts (Enhancement Tint)	tetrafilcon A, 43%, lathe-cut	14.0	8.4	Plano to –6.50 in 0.25 steps	0.03 to 0.12	12.8	9.3
			14.4	8.7			13.2	
	Colors: Sky Blue, Violet Blue, Spring Green, Turquoise, Auburn, Misty Brown							

FLEXIBLE WEAR TORIC

MFR.	LENS	MATERIAL, % H_2O, PROCESS	DIAMETER (mm)	BASE CURVE (mm)	SPHERE POWER (D) (if toric)	CYLINDER POWER (mm)	AXIS	CENTER THICKNESS (mm)	OPTIC ZONE (mm)	dK+ VALUE
PBH	Hydrocurve 3	bufilcon A, 55%, lathe-cut	14.5	8.8	+4.00D to –8.00D	–0.75D –1.25D –2.00D	1° steps	.06@ –3.00	8.2mm	16
SUNSOFT	Eclipse	methafilcon A, 55%, lathe-cut	14.5	standard	+2.00 to –6.00 in 0.25 steps	–0.75 to –2.50 in 0.25 steps	180 ± 30°, 90 ± 30° 5° increments	varies by power	8.0	18.8
	Sunsoft Toric 15.0 DIV.I	methafilcon A, 55%, lathe-cut	15.0	8.9	+3.00 to –6.00 in 0.25 steps	–0.75 to –2.00 in 0.25 steps	180 ± 20°, 90 ± 20° (5° increments in stock)	varies by power	8.0	18.8
	Sunsoft Toric 15.0 DIV.II	methafilcon A, 55%, lathe-cut	15.0	8.3, 8.9	+10.00 to –20.00 in 0.25 steps	–0.75 to –7.00 in 0.25 steps	any	varies by power	8.0	18.8

6. APHAKIC LENSES

A. Recent Methods of Correcting Aphakia

To enjoy useful visual acuity, aphakic patients generally require optical correction. Spectacles have been the most common, safest, and generally most acceptable way to correct aphakia. However, other useful methods have been developed in the past few decades. These include daily-wear contact lenses both hard and soft, long-term-wear soft lenses, and intraocular lenses. Long-term-wear lenses with FDA approval are listed in **Table 6**.

Intraocular lenses were pioneered by Dr. Harold Ridly of England more than 50 years ago. In the United States, at present, more than 50% of patients undergoing cataract extraction will receive some type of intraocular lens. There are now more than 300 intraocular lenses available in various sizes, shapes, and powers. However, some are considered investigational and, to implant them, a surgeon must have investigator status from the manufacturer in order to comply with FDA regulations.

Proponents claim specific merits for each type of lens. However, many lack sufficient data to support their claims. Differences in manufacture or fabrication can have significant impact in the incidence of complications following lens implantation.

B. 4-Drop Aphakic Corrective Lenses

In contrast to those in aspheric aphakic lenses, the curves in the 4-drop lenses are spherical. Instead of a transition from maximum lens power centrally to lesser power peripherally, the 4-drop lens has 4 zones of diminishing spherical power. These powers can be measured by a Geneva lens measure–type device. This optical design is claimed to minimize ring scotoma and the distortions experienced with aspheric lenses. The field of view is also increased.

TABLE 6

DAILY WEAR APHAKIC

MFR.	LENS	MATERIAL, % H_2O, PROCESS	DIAMETER (mm)	BASE CURVE (mm)	POWER (D)	CENTER THICKNESS (mm)	OPTIC ZONE (mm)	dK+ VALUE
BAUSCH & LOMB	Soflens® Series B3	polymacon, 38.6%, spin-cast	13.5		+11.00 to +20.00	.55	7.8	
	Soflens® Series F3	polymacon, 38.6%, spin-cast	13.5		+6.50 to +20.00 in 0.50 steps	.52	7.8	
	Soflens® Series H3, H4	polymacon, 38.6%, spin-cast	13.5		+6.50 to + 20.00 in 0.50 steps	.52	9.0	9.2
			14.5			.49 to .60	9.0	9.2
	Soflens® Series N	polymacon, 38.6%, spin-cast	13.5		+6.50 to +18.50	.48 (+12.00), .34 – .66		
COASTVISION	Hydrasoft® Aphakic	methafilcon B, 55%, lathe-cut pitch polished	15.0	8.6, 8.9, 9.2	+10.50 to +20.00 (in 0.50 steps)	varies	8.5	18.8
PBH	Hydrocurve II Aphakic Custom Tints Available	bufilcon A, 45%, lathe-cut	13.5	8.9	+12.00 to +16.00		7.1	12
			13.5	8.3, 8.6	+7.50 to +20.00			
			14.5	8.9	+7.50 to +20.00			

EXTENDED WEAR APHAKIC SOFT LENSES

MFR.	LENS	MATERIAL, % H_2O, PROCESS	DIAMETER (mm)	BASE CURVE (mm)	POWER (D)	CENTER THICKNESS (mm)	OPTIC ZONE (mm)	dK+ VALUE
BAUSCH & LOMB	CW 79	lidofilcon B, 79%, lathe-cut	14.4	8.1, 8.4, 8.7	+10.00 to +20.00 in 0.50 steps	.49 to .79	8.0	38.0
	Silsoft	elastofilcon A, 0.2%, cast molded	11.3 (available in super plus), 12.5	7.5, 7.7, 7.9 (all available in super plus); 8.1, 8.3	+12.00 to +20.00 in 1.00 steps; +23.00 to +32.00 in 3.00 steps (super plus)	.32 to .71	at least 7.0	340

EXTENDED WEAR APHAKIC SOFT LENSES (CONTINUED)

MFR.	LENS	MATERIAL, % H_2O, PROCESS	DIAMETER (mm)	BASE CURVE (mm)	POWER (D)	CENTER THICKNESS (mm)	OPTIC ZONE (mm)	dK+ VALUE
CIBA VISION CORP.	**SOFTCON® EW Aphakic**	vifilcon A, 55%	14.0	7.8, 8.1, 8.4, 8.7	+10.00 to +18.00 in 0.50 steps	0.36 @ +14.00D	7.5	16.0
			14.5	8.1, 8.4				
COOPER-VISION INC.	**Permalens®**	perfilcon A, 71%, lathe-cut	14.0	8.0, 8.3	+8.50 to +20.00 in 0.50 steps	.40 to .52	7.9 to 6.4	34
			14.5	8.3, 8.6, 8.9				
PBH	**Hydrocurve II Aphakic**	bufilcon A, 55%. lathe-cut	14.0	8.5	+7.50 to +20.00	min. plus .10	7.1	16
	Custom Tints Available		14.5	8.8	+7.50 to +20.00			
			15.5	9.5, 9.8	+7.50 to +20.00			
				9.2	+12.00 to +16.00			
SUNSOFT	**Sunsoft Aphakic**	methafilcon A, 55%, lathe-cut	15.0	8.3, 8.6, 8.9	+10.50 to +20.00 in 0.50 steps	.26	8.0	18.8

7. COMPARISON AND CONVERSION TABLES

TABLE 7

RELATIVE MAGNIFICATION PRODUCED BY CONTACT AND SPECTACLE LENSES

The percentage increase (or decrease) in the size of the retinal image afforded by contact lenses in comparison with orthodox spectacles fitted at 12 mm from the cornea.

SPECTACLE REFRACTION	EQUIVALENT POWER OF CONTACT LENS SYSTEM	PERCENTAGE INCREASE AFFORDED BY CONTACT LENS	SPECTACLE REFRACTION	EQUIVALENT POWER OF CONTACT LENS SYSTEM	PERCENTAGE INCREASE AFFORDED BY CONTACT LENS	SPECTACLE REFRACTION	EQUIVALENT POWER OF CONTACT LENS SYSTEM	PERCENTAGE INCREASE AFFORDED BY CONTACT LENS
−20	−15.73	27.2	−8	−7.07	12.9	+6	+6.10	−4.7
−18	−14.41	24.8	−6	−5.42	10.5	+8	+8.29	−7.4
−16	−13.06	22.5	−4	−3.69	7.8	+10	+10.62	−10.3
−14	−11.65	20.1	−2	−1.88	5.4	+12	+13.07	−13.8
−12	−10.19	17.8	+2	+1.96	1.2	+14	+15.64	−17.3
−10	−8.66	15.3	+4	+3.99	−1.7			

Bennet AG. *Optics of Contact Lenses.* 4th ed. London: Hatton Press; 1966.

TABLE 8

LENS EFFECTIVITY

The power of equivalent lens at reduced or increased vertex distance can be approximated by the formula:

$$> F = sD^2$$

Where: s = change in vertex distance in meters
D = power of lens

Example: 10.00 D lens fitted at vertex distance 15 mm.
(1) Lens is refitted at 10 mm. vertex distance
$> F = 0.005(10)^2 = 0.005(100) = 0.50$ D
(2) Lens is fitted as a contact lens.
$> F = 0.015(10)^2 = 0.015(100) = 1.50$ D

If lens is replaced by one closer to eye, plus power must be increased, minus power must be decreased by > F. If lens is replaced by one further from eye, plus power must be reduced, minus power must be increased by > F.

Bennet AG. *Optics of Contact Lenses.* 4th ed. London: Hatton Press; 1966.

TABLE 9

AVAILABLE STOCK BASE CURVES

POWER OF LENS (DIOPTERS)	NEAREST STANDARD BASE CURVE
0.0 to + 7.0	− 6.0 (back surface)
− 0.12 to − 5.0	+ 6.0 (front surface)
− 5.0 to − 9.0	+ 3.0 (front surface)
− 10.0 to − 15.0	+ 1.25 (front surface)
− 15.0 to − 20.0	plano (front surface)

TABLE 10

INDEX OF REFRACTION OF LENS MATERIAL

	CROWN GLASS	1.6-INDEX CROWNLITE GLASS	HILITE GLASS	8-INDEX GLASS	CR–39 PLASTIC	HIRI PLASTIC	1.6-INDEX PLASTIC	POLY–CARBONATE THIN–LITE PLASTIC
INDEX OF REFRACTION The higher the number, the thinner the material	1.523	1.601	1.701	1.805	1.498	1.56	1.6	1.586
SPECIFIC GRAVITY The higher the number, the heavier the material	2.5	2.67	2.99	3.37	1.32	1.216	1.34	1.20
DISPERSION The higher the number, the less chromatic aberration (Abbe value)	59	42.24	31	25	58	38	37	31
PERSONALITY	temperable, coatable, ease in handling, vast availability	chemically temperable, ease in handling, limited availability	chemically temperable, fairly easy to handle, SV and multifocals; vacuum coatings cause lens to become highly sensitive to scratching	SV, difficult to temper, highly reflective so A/R coatings recommended, but have same problems as hilite; mfrs suggest having patient sign liability waiver when ground thin. Multifocal available in laminate.	strong, tintable, coatable, ease in handling, vast availability	SV and bifocal, tints well before SRC, edges well, must be SRC, extremely brittle	SV only, tints well before SRC, edges well, must be SRC	SV and multifocal, strongest lens material available, limited tintability, must be SPC, no fast fabrication, special edging equipment needed, a must for children and athletes

SV = single-vision lenses. A/R = antireflective. SRC = scratch-resistant coating.

TABLE 11

CYLINDER POWER IN OFF-AXIS MERIDIAN

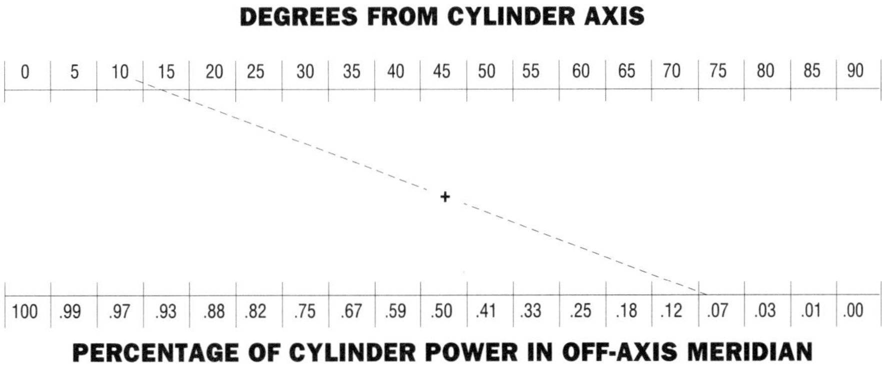

To determine cylinder power in an off–axis meridian, place straightedge on diagram above so that it intersects center dot and upper-scale position for number of degrees that the meridian sought is off axis. Percentage of cylinder power in the meridian sought is indicated on lower scale at point of intersection with straightedge.

Example: 2.00 D cyl × 75° What is the power at 90° that is 15° off axis?
Reading on lower scale is 0.07; therefore, power in 90th meridian is 0.14 D.

TABLE 12

CORNEAL RADIUS EQUIVALENCE DIOPTERS/MILLIMETERS

DIOPTERS	mm	DIOPTERS	mm	DIOPTERS	mm	DIOPTERS	mm	DIOPTERS	mm	DIOPTERS	mm	DIOPTERS	mm	DIOPTERS	mm
20.00	16.875	36.00	9.375	39.00	8.653	42.00	8.035	45.00	7.500	48.00	7.031	51.00	6.617	54.00	6.250
22.00	15.340	36.12	9.343	39.12	8.627	42.12	8.012	45.12	7.480	48.12	7.013	51.12	6.602	54.12	6.236
24.00	14.062	36.25	9.310	39.25	8.598	42.25	7.988	45.25	7.458	48.25	6.994	51.25	6.585	54.25	6.221
26.00	12.980	36.37	9.279	39.37	8.572	42.37	7.965	45.37	7.438	48.37	6.977	51.37	6.569	54.37	6.207
27.00	12.500	36.50	9.246	39.50	8.544	42.50	7.941	45.50	7.417	48.50	6.958	51.50	6.553	54.50	6.192
28.00	12.053	36.62	9.216	39.62	8.518	42.62	7.918	45.62	7.398	48.62	6.941	51.62	6.538	54.62	6.179
29.00	11.638	36.75	9.183	39.75	8.490	42.75	7.894	45.75	7.377	48.75	6.923	51.75	6.521	54.75	6.164
29.50	11.441	36.87	9.153	39.87	8.465	42.87	7.872	45.87	7.357	48.87	6.906	51.87	6.506	54.87	6.150
30.00	11.250	37.00	9.121	40.00	8.437	43.00	7.848	46.00	7.336	49.00	6.887	52.00	6.490	55.00	6.136
30.50	11.065	37.12	9.092	40.12	8.412	43.12	7.826	46.12	7.317	49.12	6.870	52.12	6.475	55.12	6.123
31.00	10.887	37.25	9.060	40.25	8.385	43.25	7.803	46.25	7.297	49.25	6.852	52.25	6.459	55.25	6.108
31.50	10.714	37.37	9.031	40.37	8.360	43.37	7.781	46.37	7.278	49.37	6.836	52.37	6.444	55.37	6.095
32.00	10.547	37.50	9.000	40.50	8.333	43.50	7.758	46.50	7.258	49.50	6.818	52.50	6.428	55.50	6.081
32.50	10.385	37.62	8.971	40.62	8.308	43.62	7.737	46.62	7.239	49.62	6.801	52.62	6.413	55.62	6.068
33.00	10.227	37.75	8.940	40.75	8.282	43.75	7.714	46.75	7.219	49.75	6.783	52.75	6.398	55.75	6.054
33.50	10.075	37.87	8.912	40.87	8.257	43.87	7.693	46.87	7.200	49.87	6.767	52.87	6.383	55.87	6.041
34.00	9.926	38.00	8.881	41.00	8.231	44.00	7.670	47.00	7.180	50.00	6.750	53.00	6.367	56.00	6.027
34.25	9.854	38.12	8.853	41.12	8.207	44.12	7.649	47.12	7.162	50.12	6.733	53.12	6.353	56.50	5.973
34.50	9.783	38.25	8.823	41.25	8.181	44.25	7.627	47.25	7.142	50.25	6.716	53.25	6.338	57.00	5.921
34.75	9.712	38.37	8.795	41.37	8.158	44.37	7.606	47.37	7.124	50.37	6.700	53.37	6.323	57.50	5.869
35.00	9.643	38.50	8.766	41.50	8.132	44.50	7.584	47.50	7.105	50.50	6.683	53.50	6.308	58.00	5.819
35.25	9.574	38.62	8.738	41.62	8.109	44.62	7.563	47.62	7.087	50.62	6.667	53.62	6.294	58.50	5.769
35.50	9.507	38.75	8.708	41.75	8.083	44.75	7.541	47.75	7.068	50.75	6.650	53.75	6.279	59.00	5.720
35.75	9.440	38.87	8.682	41.87	8.060	44.87	7.521	47.87	7.050	50.87	6.634	53.87	6.265	60.00	5.625

TABLE 13

VERTEX DISTANCE CONVERSION SCALE (mm)

SPECTACLE LENS	PLUS LENSES								MINUS LENSES							
POWER	8	9	10	11	12	13	14	15	8	9	10	11	12	13	14	15
4.00	4.12	4.12	4.12	4.12	4.25	4.25	4.25	4.25	3.87	3.87	3.87	3.87	3.87	3.75	3.75	3.75
4.50	4.62	4.75	4.75	4.75	4.75	4.75	4.75	4.87	4.37	4.37	4.25	4.25	4.25	4.25	4.25	4.25
5.00	5.25	5.25	5.25	5.25	5.25	5.37	5.37	5.37	4.75	4.75	4.75	4.75	4.75	4.75	4.62	4.62
5.50	5.75	5.75	5.75	5.87	5.87	5.87	6.00	6.00	5.25	5.25	5.25	5.12	5.12	5.12	5.12	5.12
6.00	6.25	6.37	6.37	6.37	6.50	6.50	6.50	6.62	5.75	5.62	5.62	5.62	5.62	5.50	5.50	5.50
6.50	6.87	6.87	7.00	7.00	7.00	7.12	7.12	7.25	6.12	6.12	6.12	6.00	6.00	6.00	6.00	5.87
7.00	7.37	7.50	7.50	7.62	7.62	7.75	7.75	7.75	6.62	6.62	6.50	6.50	6.50	6.37	6.37	6.37
7.50	8.00	8.00	8.12	8.12	8.25	8.25	8.37	8.50	7.12	7.00	7.00	6.87	6.87	6.87	6.75	6.75
8.00	8.50	8.62	8.75	8.75	8.87	8.87	9.00	9.12	7.50	7.50	7.37	7.37	7.25	7.25	7.25	7.25
8.50	9.12	9.25	9.25	9.37	9.50	9.50	9.62	9.75	8.00	7.87	7.87	7.75	7.75	7.62	7.62	7.50
9.00	9.75	9.75	9.87	10.00	10.12	10.25	10.37	10.37	8.37	8.37	8.25	8.25	8.12	8.00	8.00	8.00
9.50	10.25	10.37	10.50	10.62	10.75	10.87	11.00	11.12	8.87	8.75	8.62	8.62	8.50	8.50	8.37	8.37
10.00	10.87	11.00	11.12	11.25	11.37	11.50	11.62	11.75	9.25	9.12	9.12	9.00	8.87	8.87	8.75	8.75
10.50	11.50	11.62	11.75	11.87	12.00	12.12	12.25	12.50	9.62	9.62	9.50	9.37	9.37	9.25	9.12	9.12
11.00	12.00	12.25	12.37	12.50	12.75	12.87	13.00	13.12	10.12	10.00	9.87	9.75	9.75	9.62	9.50	9.50
11.50	12.62	12.87	13.00	13.12	13.37	13.50	13.75	13.87	10.50	10.37	10.37	10.25	10.12	10.00	9.87	9.87
12.00	13.25	13.50	13.62	13.87	14.00	14.25	14.50	14.62	11.00	10.87	10.75	10.62	10.50	10.37	10.25	10.12
12.50	13.87	14.12	14.25	14.50	14.75	15.00	15.25	15.37	11.37	11.25	11.12	11.00	10.87	10.75	10.62	10.50
13.00	14.50	14.75	15.00	15.25	15.50	15.62	16.00	16.12	11.75	11.62	11.50	11.37	11.25	11.12	11.00	10.87
13.50	15.12	15.37	15.62	15.87	16.12	16.37	16.62	16.87	12.25	12.00	11.87	11.75	11.62	11.50	11.37	11.25
14.00	15.75	16.00	16.25	16.50	16.75	17.12	17.50	17.75	12.62	12.50	12.25	12.12	12.00	11.87	11.75	11.50
14.50	16.50	16.75	17.00	17.25	17.50	17.87	18.25	18.50	13.00	12.75	12.62	12.50	12.37	12.25	12.00	11.87
15.00	17.00	17.37	17.75	18.00	18.25	18.62	19.00	19.37	13.37	13.25	13.00	12.87	12.75	12.50	12.37	12.25
15.50	17.75	18.00	18.25	18.75	19.00	19.37	19.75	20.25	13.75	13.62	13.50	13.25	13.00	12.87	12.75	12.62
16.00	18.25	18.75	19.00	19.37	19.75	20.25	20.50	21.00	14.25	14.00	13.75	13.62	13.50	13.25	13.00	12.87
16.50	19.00	19.37	19.75	20.25	20.50	21.00	21.50	21.87	14.50	14.37	14.12	14.00	13.75	13.62	13.50	13.25
17.00	19.75	20.25	20.50	21.00	21.50	22.00	22.25	22.87	15.00	14.75	14.50	14.25	14.12	14.00	13.75	13.50
17.50	20.50	20.75	21.25	21.75	22.25	22.75	23.25	23.75	15.37	15.12	14.87	14.75	14.50	14.25	14.00	13.87
18.00	21.00	21.50	22.00	22.50	23.00	23.50	24.00	24.62	15.75	15.50	15.25	15.00	14.75	14.62	14.37	14.12
18.50	21.75	22.25	22.75	23.25	23.75	24.50	25.00	25.62	16.12	15.87	15.62	15.37	15.12	14.87	14.75	14.50
19.00	22.50	23.00	23.50	24.00	24.75	25.25	26.00	26.50	16.50	16.25	16.00	15.75	15.50	15.25	15.00	14.75

TABLE 14

MJK SPHEROCYLINDRICAL VERTEX CHART

VERTEX DISTANCE = 13.00 mm | **CYLINDER INCREMENT = 0.25 DIOPTER** | **SPHERE INCREMENT = 0.125 DIOPTER**

SR	SRV	−0.25	−0.50	−0.75	−1.00	−1.25	−1.50	−1.75	−2.00	−2.25	−2.50	−2.75	−3.00
−3.00	−2.87	−0.25	−0.50	−0.75	−1.00	−1.25	−1.25	−1.50	−1.75	−2.00	−2.25	−2.50	−2.75
−3.25	−3.12	−0.25	−0.50	−0.75	−1.00	−1.25	−1.25	−1.50	−1.75	−2.00	−2.25	−2.50	−2.75
−3.50	−3.37	−0.25	−0.50	−0.75	−1.00	−1.25	−1.25	−1.50	−1.75	−2.00	−2.25	−2.50	−2.75
−3.75	−3.62	−0.25	−0.50	−0.75	−1.00	−1.00	−1.25	−1.50	−1.75	−2.00	−2.25	−2.50	−2.75
−4.00	−3.75	−0.25	−0.50	−0.75	−1.00	−1.00	−1.25	−1.50	−1.75	−2.00	−2.25	−2.50	−2.50
−4.25	−4.00	−0.25	−0.50	−0.75	−1.00	−1.00	−1.25	−1.50	−1.75	−2.00	−2.25	−2.50	−2.50
−4.50	−4.25	−0.25	−0.50	−0.75	−1.00	−1.00	−1.25	−1.50	−1.75	−2.00	−2.25	−2.25	−2.50
−4.75	−4.50	−0.25	−0.50	−0.75	−1.00	−1.00	−1.25	−1.50	−1.75	−2.00	−2.25	−2.25	−2.50
−5.00	−4.75	−0.25	−0.50	−0.75	−0.75	−1.00	−1.25	−1.50	−1.75	−2.00	−2.25	−2.25	−2.50
−5.25	−4.87	−0.25	−0.50	−0.75	−0.75	−1.00	−1.25	−1.50	−1.75	−2.00	−2.25	−2.25	−2.50
−5.50	−5.12	−0.25	−0.50	−0.75	−0.75	−1.00	−1.25	−1.50	−1.75	−2.00	−2.00	−2.25	−2.50
−5.75	−5.37	−0.25	−0.50	−0.75	−0.75	−1.00	−1.25	−1.50	−1.75	−2.00	−2.00	−2.25	−2.50
−6.00	−5.62	−0.25	−0.50	−0.75	−0.75	−1.00	−1.25	−1.50	−1.75	−2.00	−2.00	−2.25	−2.50
−6.25	−5.75	−0.25	−0.50	−0.75	−0.75	−1.00	−1.25	−1.50	−1.75	−1.75	−2.00	−2.25	−2.50
−6.50	−6.00	−0.25	−0.50	−0.75	−0.75	−1.00	−1.25	−1.50	−1.75	−1.75	−2.00	−2.25	−2.50
−6.75	−6.25	−0.25	−0.50	−0.75	−0.75	−1.00	−1.25	−1.50	−1.75	−1.75	−2.00	−2.25	−2.50
−7.00	−6.37	−0.25	−0.50	−0.50	−0.75	−1.00	−1.25	−1.50	−1.75	−1.75	−2.00	−2.25	−2.50
−7.25	−6.62	−0.25	−0.50	−0.50	−0.75	−1.00	−1.25	−1.50	−1.75	−1.75	−2.00	−2.25	−2.50
−7.50	−6.87	−0.25	−0.50	−0.50	−0.75	−1.00	−1.25	−1.50	−1.50	−1.75	−2.00	−2.25	−2.50
−7.75	−7.00	−0.25	−0.50	−0.50	−0.75	−1.00	−1.25	−1.50	−1.50	−1.75	−2.00	−2.25	−2.50
−8.00	−7.25	−0.25	−0.50	−0.50	−0.75	−1.00	−1.25	−1.50	−1.50	−1.75	−2.00	−2.25	−2.50
−8.25	−7.50	−0.25	−0.50	−0.50	−0.75	−1.00	−1.25	−1.50	−1.50	−1.75	−2.00	−2.25	−2.25
−8.50	−7.62	−0.25	−0.50	−0.50	−0.75	−1.00	−1.25	−1.50	−1.50	−1.75	−2.00	−2.25	−2.25
−8.75	−7.87	−0.25	−0.50	−0.50	−0.75	−1.00	−1.25	−1.50	−1.50	−1.75	−2.00	−2.25	−2.25
−9.00	−8.00	−0.25	−0.50	−0.50	−0.75	−1.00	−1.25	−1.25	−1.50	−1.75	−2.00	−2.25	−2.25
−9.25	−8.25	−0.25	−0.50	−0.50	−0.75	−1.00	−1.25	−1.25	−1.50	−1.75	−2.00	−2.00	−2.25
−9.50	−8.50	−0.25	−0.50	−0.50	−0.75	−1.00	−1.25	−1.25	−1.50	−1.75	−2.00	−2.00	−2.25
−9.75	−8.62	−0.25	−0.50	−0.50	−0.75	−1.00	−1.25	−1.25	−1.50	−1.75	−2.00	−2.00	−2.25
−10.00	−8.87	−0.25	−0.50	−0.50	−0.75	−1.00	−1.25	−1.25	−1.50	−1.75	−2.00	−2.00	−2.25
−10.25	−9.00	−0.25	−0.50	−0.50	−0.75	−1.00	−1.25	−1.25	−1.50	−1.75	−2.00	−2.00	−2.25
−10.50	−9.25	−0.25	−0.50	−0.50	−0.75	−1.00	−1.25	−1.25	−1.50	−1.75	−2.00	−2.00	−2.25
−10.75	−9.37	−0.25	−0.50	−0.50	−0.75	−1.00	−1.25	−1.25	−1.50	−1.75	−2.25	−2.00	−2.25
+4.00	+4.25	−0.25	−0.50	−0.75	−1.00	−1.25	−1.75	−2.00	−2.25	−2.50	−2.75	−3 00	−3.25
+4.25	+4.50	−0.25	−0.50	−0.75	−1.00	−1.50	−1.75	−2.00	−2.25	−2.50	−2.75	−3.00	−3.25
+4.50	+4.75	−0.25	−0.50	−0.75	−1.00	−1.50	−1.75	−2.00	−2.25	−2.50	−2.75	−3.00	−3.25
+4.75	+5.12	−0.25	−0.50	−0.75	−1.00	−1.50	−1.75	−2.00	−2.25	−2.50	−2.75	−3.00	−3.25
+5.00	+5.37	−0.25	−0.50	−0.75	−1.00	−1.50	−1.75	−2.00	−2.25	−2.50	−2.75	−3.00	−3.25
+5.25	+5.62	−0.25	−0.50	−0.75	−1.00	−1.50	−1.75	−2.00	−2.25	−2.50	−2.75	−3.00	−3.25
+5.50	+5.87	−0.25	−0.50	−0.75	−1.00	−1.50	−1.75	−2.00	−2.25	−2.50	−2.75	−3.00	−3.25
+5.75	+6.25	−0.25	−0.50	−0.75	−1.00	−1.50	−1.75	−2.00	−2.25	−2.50	−2.75	−3.00	−3.25
+6.00	+6.50	−0.25	−0.50	−0.75	−1.00	−1.50	−1.75	−2.00	−2.25	−2.50	−2.75	−3.00	−3.50
+6.25	+6.75	−0.25	−0.50	−1.00	−1.00	−1.50	−1.75	−2.00	−2.25	−2.50	−2.75	−3.25	−3.50
+6.50	+7.12	−0.25	−0.50	−1.00	−1.00	−1.50	−1.75	−2.00	−2.25	−2.50	−3.00	−3.25	−3.50
+6.75	+7.37	−0.25	−0.50	−1.00	−1.00	−1.50	−1.75	−2.00	−2.25	−2.50	−3.00	−3.25	−3.50
+7.00	+7.75	−0.25	−0.50	−1.00	−1.00	−1.50	−1.75	−2.00	−2.25	−2.75	−3.00	−3.25	−3.50
+7.25	+8 00	−0.25	−0.50	−1.00	−1.00	−1.50	−1.75	−2.00	−2.25	−2.75	−3.00	−3.25	−3.50
+7.50	+8.25	−0.25	−0.50	−1.00	−1.00	−1.50	−1.75	−2.00	−2.50	−2.75	−3.00	−3.25	−3.50
+7.75	+8.62	−0.25	−0.50	−1.00	−1.00	−1.50	−1.75	−2.00	−2.50	−2.75	−3.00	−3 25	−3.50
+8.00	+8.87	−0.25	−0.50	−1.00	−1.00	−1.50	−1.75	−2.25	−2.50	−2.75	−3.00	−3.25	−3.50
+8.25	+9.25	−0.25	−0.50	−1.00	−1.00	−1.50	−1.75	−2.25	−2.50	−2.75	−3.00	−3.25	−3.50
+8.50	+9 25	−0.25	−0.75	−1.00	−1.25	−1.50	−1.75	−2.25	−2.50	−2.75	−3.00	−3.25	−3.75
+8.75	+9.87	−0.25	−0.75	−1.00	−1.25	−1.50	−1.75	−2.25	−2.50	−2.75	−3.00	−3.25	−3.75
+9.00	+10.25	−0.25	−0.75	−1.00	−1.25	−1.50	−2.00	−2.25	−2.50	−2.75	−3.00	−3.50	−3.75
+9.25	+10.50	−0.25	−0.75	−1.00	−1.25	−1.50	−2.00	−2.25	−2.50	−2.75	−3.00	−3.50	−3.75
+9.50	+10.87	−0.25	−0.75	−1.00	−1.25	−1.50	−2.00	−2.25	−2.50	−2.75	−3.25	−3.50	−3.75
+9.75	+11.12	−0.25	−0.75	−1.00	−1.25	−1.50	−2.00	−2.25	−2.50	−2.75	−3.25	−3.50	−3.75
+10.00	+11.50	−0.25	−0.75	−1.00	−1.25	−1.50	−2.00	−2.25	−2.50	−3.00	−3.25	−3.50	−3.75
+10.25	+11.87	−0.25	−0.75	−1.00	−1.25	−1.75	−2.00	−2.25	−2.50	−3.00	−3.25	−3.50	−3.75
+10 50	+12.12	−0.25	−0.75	−1.00	−1.25	−1.75	−2.00	−2.25	−2.50	−3.00	−3 25	−3.50	−3.75
+10.75	+12.50	−0.25	−0.75	−1.00	−1.25	−1.75	−2.00	−2.25	−2.50	−3.00	−3.25	−3.50	−4.00
+11.00	+12.87	−0.25	−0.75	−1.00	−1.25	−1.75	−2.00	−2.25	−2.75	−3.00	−3.25	−3.50	−4.00
+11.25	+13.12	−0.25	−0.75	−1.00	−1.25	−1.75	−2.00	−2.25	−2.75	−3.00	−3.25	−3.50	−4.00
+11.50	+13.50	−0.25	−0.75	−1.00	−1.25	−1.75	−2.00	−2.25	−2.75	−3.00	−3.25	−3.75	−4.00
+11.75	+13.87	−0.25	−0.75	−1.00	−1.25	−1.75	−2.00	−2.25	−2.75	−3.00	−3.25	−3.75	−4.00

Example: Spectacle refraction (SR) at 13 mm = −5.75 − 2.50 × 180.
Matching up −5.75 on the left, gives effective spherical power (SRV) of −5.37.
Following underlined values to the right and reading in the −2.50 cylinder column gives a cylinder value of −2.00.

Corneal plane refraction = −5.37 − 2.00 × 180.

Legend: In this chart of spherocylindrical corneal plane refractions, the spherical value is calculated and rounded off to the nearest 0.12 diopter, while the cylinder value is rounded off to the nearest 0.25 diopter.

8. SPORTS AND RECREATIONAL LENSES

As public concern mounts over the number of sports-related ocular injuries, the importance of protective eyewear has gained wider recognition. The National Society for the Prevention of Blindness reports that some 33,808 sports- and recreation-related eye injuries required emergency room treatment in 1987 alone. Statistics such as this, plus adoption of protective eyewear by such prominent athletes as Kareem Abdul Jabbar and Eric Dickerson, have done much to promote greater acceptance of protective eyewear among younger athletes.

Special eyewear is now available for use not only in sports such as squash, racquetball, and tennis, but also in basketball, baseball, soccer, football, and hockey. This eyewear replaces traditional spectacle lenses, ordinary plastic lenses, and open or "lens-less" eyeguards, none of which provide adequate protection. Four types are available.

- Standard frames fitted with 2-mm polycarbonate lenses — adequate for athletes participating in noncontact sports such as track and field
- Sports frames with 3-mm polycarbonate lenses — best for higher-risk sports such as baseball, basketball, and soccer
- A molded, polycarbonate lens/frame combination — available with a corrective prescription, or, for contact lens wearers and others who do not ordinarily wear spectacles, without one
- Face masks attached to a helmet — suitable for use in the highest-risk sports, such as hockey, football, and lacrosse

Available products and their sources are listed in **Table 15**. Note that most sports glasses are made for adults and are too large for small children, or even older children with a narrow interpupillary distance. For the little ones, smaller-sized sports goggles trade-named "Rec-Specs, Jr" are available from Liberty Optical. If even these are too large, the child should be fitted with a sturdy frame and polycarbonate lenses 3 mm thick at the center. For suppliers, see **Table 16.**

Adapted from Jeffers JB. An ongoing tragedy: pediatric sports-related eye injuries. *Semin Ophthalmol.* 1990;5(No. 4):216-223.

TABLE 15

PROTECTIVE SPORTS EYEWEAR

MODEL	PRESCRIPTION CAPABILITY	NAME AND ADDRESS
Rec-Specs, Jr*	Yes	Liberty Optical
Pro-Guard	Yes	380 Verona Ave
All-Pro	Yes	Newark, NJ 07104
		800-879-9992
Essex	Yes	LST Leader Sports
Troy	No	PO Box 591
New Yorker	No	60 Lakeshore Rd
Vision Plus (Football)	No	Essex, NY
		800-847-2001
Action Eyes "Thor-Style"	Yes	Viking Sports
		5355 Sierra Rd
		San Jose, CA 95132
		800-535-3300
Regent	No	Ektelon
Arbitor	No	8929 Aero Dr
Interceptor	Yes	San Diego, CA 92123
		800-854-2958
Sports Specs	No	Herslof Optical
		12000 W Carmen Ave
		Milwaukee, WI 53225
		800-558-7073
Face Guard (Baseball)	No	Face Guard Incorporated
		PO Box 8425
		Roanoke, VA 24014
		800-336-9683

Rec-Specs, Jr are designed to fit younger children. They come in a variety of neon colors to make them more attractive to children.

TABLE 16

ADDRESSES FOR PEDIATRIC SAFETY EYEWEAR

American Optical Safety Division
14 Mechanic Street
Southbridge, MA 01550
800-982-2828

Titmus Company
PO Box 191
Petersburg, VA 23804
800-446-1802

SECTION 5

VISION STANDARDS AND LOW VISION

1. VISION STANDARDS

TABLE 1

VISION STANDARDS FOR PILOTS

	WITHOUT RX[1]	REQUIRING RX[1] CORRECTED TO	NEAR VISION WITH/ WITHOUT RX	PHORIAS[2]	FIELDS	COLOR	PATHOLOGY
1st class	20/20	20/100 to 20/20	20/40 (J_3)	6 D eso/exo 1 Δ hyper	Normal	Normal	4
2nd class	20/20	20/100 to 20/20	20/40 (J_3)	6 D eso/exo 1 Δ hyper	Normal	3	5
3rd class	20/50	To 20/30	20/60 (J_6)	. . .	. . .	3	5

1. Each eye.
2. If exceeded, further evaluation required to determine bifoveal fixation and adequate vergence phoria relationship.
3. Able to distinguish aviation signal red, aviation signal green, and white.
4. No acute or chronic pathologic condition of either eye of adnexa that might interfere with its proper function, might progress to that degree, or be aggravated by flying.
5. No serious pathology.

Note: By amendment regulations (12/21/76) correction may be by spectacles or contact lenses.

TABLE 2

VISION STANDARDS FOR ADMISSION TO SERVICE ACADEMIES

US Coast Guard Academy	Minimum uncorrected 20/200 each eye; correctable to 20/20 each eye; refractive error not more than ±5.50 D any meridian; astigmatism not over 3.00 D; anisometropia not exceeding 3.50 D; full visual fields; normal color vision; no chronic, disfiguring, disabling, ocular pathology.
US Merchant Marine Academy	Minimum uncorrected 20/100 each eye; correctable to 20/20 each eye; refractive error as for Coast Guard Academy; color vision normal by Farnsworth lantern test or pseudoisochromatic; plates; certain pathologies may disqualify.
US Naval Academy	Uncorrected vision 20/20 each eye; limited waivers if correctable to 20/20 each eye and to refraction standards, Coast Guard Academy; color vision normal–no waivers; no chronic, disfiguring, disabling ocular pathology.
US Military Academy	Distance vision correctable to 20/20 each eye; refractive error as for Coast Guard Academy; able to distinguish vivid red and green; ET less than 15 prism diopters; XT less than 10 prism diopters; hypertropia less than 2 prism diopters; certain pathologies may disqualify.
US Air Force Academy	*Pilot:* Uncorrected vision 20/20 or better each eye, far and near; refractive error hyperopia no greater than +1.75 D and nearsightedness less than plano in any one meridian; the astigmatic error must not exceed 0.75 D. *Navigator:* Uncorrected vision 20/70 or better correctable with ordinary glasses to 20/20 each eye; near acuity 20/20 or better each eye, uncorrected; hyperopia not greater than +3.00 D and myopia not greater than –1.50 D any meridian; astigmatism not to exceed 2.00 D. *Commission:* Distance acuity correctable 20/40 one eye and 20/70 other, or 20/30 one eye and 20/100 other; near acuity correctable to 20/20 (J_1) one eye and 20/30 (J_2) in other; refractive error of equivalent sphere not more than ±8.00 D; no chronic, disfiguring, disabling ocular pathology.

Based on information as of 17 May, 1983, Medical Examination Review Board, Department of Defense.

TABLE 3

VISION STANDARDS FOR COMMERCIAL DRIVERS

	VISUAL ACUITY	VISUAL FIELD				
	BINOC	MONOC	BINOC	COLOR	OTHER	RETEST
Alabama	20/70	No	No	No	No	No
Alaska	20/40	No	No	No	No	Periodic
Arizona	20/40	No	No	No	No	Periodic
Arkansas	20/50	NS	NS	NS	NS	NS
California	20/40	70, 70	NS	R,G,A	NS	Periodic
Colorado	20/40	Yes	Yes	Yes	ST	Periodic
Connecticut	20/40	Yes	Yes	Yes	ST	No
Delaware	20/40	No	No	No	No	Periodic
Florida	20/70	No	No	No	No	Periodic
Georgia	20/60	140, 140	140	No	No	Periodic
Hawaii	20/40	70, 70	140	R,G,A	ST, EC	Periodic
Idaho	20/40	NS	NS	NS	NS	Periodic
Illinois	20/40	70, 70	140	NS	NS	Periodic
Indiana	20/50	No	No	No	NS	Periodic
Iowa	20/70	No	No	No	NS	Periodic
Kansas	20/40	NS	NS	NS	NS	Periodic
Kentucky	20/45, PV	No	No	No	No	No
Louisiana	20/40	No	No	No	No	Periodic
Maine	20/40	NS	NS	NS	NS	No
Maryland	20/40	140, 140	140	No	No	Periodic
Massachusetts	20/40	90, 90	120	Yes	No	Periodic
Michigan	20/40	70, 70	140	NS	NS	Periodic
Minnesota	20/40	NS	NS	NS	NS	Periodic
Mississippi	20/40	90, 90	180	No	ST	No
Missouri	20/40	55, 55	No	No	No	Periodic
Montana	20/40	75, 75	No	Yes	ST	Periodic
Nebraska	20/40	70, 70	140	Yes	No	Periodic
Nevada	20/40	No	No	No	No	Periodic
New Hampshire	20/40	NS	NS	NS	NS	Periodic
New Jersey	20/40	70, 70	No	R,G,A	No	NS
New Mexico	20/40	NS	NS	NS	NS	Periodic
New York	20/40	NS	NS	NS	NS	Periodic
North Carolina	20/50	No	70	Yes	No	Periodic
North Dakota	20/40	70, 70	140	No	No	Periodic
Ohio	20/40	70, 70	No	No	No	Periodic
Oklahoma	20/40	No	No	No	No	No
Oregon	20/40	No	110	No	No	No
Pennsylvania	20/40	No	140	No	No	No
Rhode Island	20/40	60, 60	120	Yes	No	Periodic
South Carolina	PV	NS	NS	NS	NS	Periodic
South Dakota	20/40	No	No	No	No	Periodic
Tennessee	20/40	No	No	No	No	No
Texas	20/50	No	No	No	No	Periodic
Utah	20/40	NS	NS	Yes	ST	Periodic
Vermont	20/40	NS	NS	NS	NS	No
Virginia	20/40	100, 100	100	No	NS	Periodic
Washington	20/40	No	140	R,G,A	No	Periodic
West Virginia	20/40	No	No	No	No	No
Wisconsin	20/40	70, 70	140	No	No	Periodic
Wyoming	20/40	No	No	No	No	Periodic

Key: Visual acuity is expressed in Snellen notation; visual field is given in degrees along the horizontal meridian; color abbreviations: R = red, G = green, A = amber; abbreviations for other conditions: EC = eye coordination; ST = stereopsis (absence of); NS = standard not specified; No = no standard; PV = default to private vehicle standard.

Source: US Dept of Transportation. *Visual Disorders and Commercial Drivers.* Washington, DC: Federal Highway Administration, Office of Motor Carriers; Nov 1991. US Dept of Transportation publication FHWA-MC-92-003, HCS-10/1-92(200)E.

2. LOW-VISION AIDS

Under federal regulation, a patient is considered legally blind when the best vision attained in the better eye is 20/200 or less, or when, whatever the acuity achieved, the field of vision of the better eye is 20° or less. While most states have adopted these standards, individual variations may exist at the local level.

Patients whose vision is reduced or inadequate for their visual tasks — those whose best corrected vision ranges from 20/50 downward toward the 20/200 level — can frequently be aided by the same techniques and devices used for the legally blind and visually rehabilitated. These modalities include rehabilitation training programs and optical and nonoptical aids. They often can help restore independence and mobility, allowing the patient to remain productive.

For those patients considered partially sighted rather than partially blind, increased vision is obtained by magnification or approximation. For distance, this may be accomplished by telescopic devices. Although difficult to use while moving about, these instruments may be quite effective for distinguishing a street sign or the number of a house or bus. They are also useful aids in the theater or classroom and at sporting events.

Telescopic devices can be obtained in magnifications of 2.2, 2.5, 3.0, 3.5, 4.0, 6.0, 8.0, and 10× from suppliers such as Vision, Keeler, Nikon, Selsi, Walters, and Zeiss. Some are fixed focus; others may be refocused for viewing closer material. Telescopes fitted with reading cap lenses permit reading at greater distances than high-plus aids. A familiar example of this system is the surgical loupe.

Because the field diminishes as the power increases, the magnification of telescopic devices should be kept to the minimum needed to secure desired acuity. Differences in design and construction of these devices may cause slight variations in the fields produced at a given magnification. A representative sample may be drawn from the devices produced by Designs for Vision:

MAGNIFICATION	FIELD AT 20 FEET
2.2 standard	12°
2.2 wide Angle	17°
3.0 standard	8°
3.0 wide angle	12°
4.0 standard	6°

Near vision can be augmented by higher adds, high-plus "Micro" lenses (American Optical, Lucerne Optical), binocular loupes, and handheld or stand magnifiers. The higher plus values permit approximation to increase the angle subtended with little or no demand on accommodation. The add to obtain J_5 can be estimated by the inverse of the best distance vision obtained. For example, if best distance vision is 20/200, the add is 200/20, or 10 D.

Greater detail can be obtained through increased add power or supplementary magnifiers. If the patient will not read at extremely close range, lower adds may be used in combination with magnifiers. Required magnification at desired working distance can also be provided by a telemicroscope system modified with a reading cap or objective lens, as in a surgical loupe.

When binocular function is present, prism base-in may be required in the near prescription (about 1 prism diopter per diopter of add). Plastic-lens, half-eye spectacles of 6, 8, or 10 D with incorporated prism are available from American Optical and Lucerne Optical. Handheld magnifiers ranging from 23 to 83 are available from Bausch & Lomb, Coburn, Coil, Eschenbach, McLeod, and Selsi. Once again, the higher powers have reduced fields of view. Patients with physical infirmities can use stand magnifiers that rest on the material and remain in focus as they are moved across the page.

Nonoptical aids include reading masks, large-print publications, heavily ruled stationery, check-writing guides, large playing cards, and easy-to-thread needles. Also available are fixed-power opaque projection magnifiers (Nesbit Co) and closed-circuit television devices with variable magnification.

Television permits a greater range of magnification and can, when polarity is reversed, provide a white-on-black image instead of the usual black-on-white. This effect, for many, is an additional aid. Products are available from Telesensory Systems and Visualtek. Advances in electronics have also made possible talking clocks, calculators, and many other business machines whose "voices" open the way to gainful employment for the visually impaired.

A *Catalogue of Optical Aids* is available from the New York Association for the Blind, 111 East 59th Street, New York, NY 10022. Available from the American Foundation for the Blind, 15 West 16th Street, New York, NY 10011, are Aid for the 80's, *Products for People with Visual Handicaps*, and a *Catalogue of Publications,* all of which can further help the visually impaired. The Talking Books Program can be joined by applying to the National Library Science for the Blind and Physically Handicapped, Library of Congress, Washington, DC 20542.

For those with clouded vision, absorptive lenses provide glare protection and can help improve acuity. Neutral gray lenses with 5% to 15% transmission are specifically recommended for achromatopes, who may also require the protection of wide side shield frames. Albinotic patients are aided by brown tints with 75% transmission indoors and 25% outdoors. Retinitis pigmentosa patients generally require daytime outdoor protection with the darker sunglass tints. Many are aided in night vision by the Kalichrome lenses (Bausch & Lomb) and the Hazemaster line (American Optical).

SECTION 6

EVALUATION OF PERMANENT VISUAL IMPAIRMENT

The purpose of this section is to provide criteria and a method for evaluating permanent impairments of the visual system and relating them to permanent impairment of the whole person. The visual system consists of the eyes, ocular adnexa, and visual pathways.

Visual impairment occurs in the presence of a deviation from normal in one or more of the functions of the eye, which include (1) corrected visual acuity for near and far objects; (2) visual field perception; and (3) ocular motility with diplopia. Evaluation of visual impairment is based on evaluation of the three functions. Although not all of the functions are equally important, vision is imperfect without coordination of all three. Other ocular functions and disturbances are considered to the extent that they affect one or more of the three functions. Impairment percents representing the functions are *combined* (Combined Values Chart, p.70).

If an ocular or adnexal disturbance or deformity interferes with visual function and is not reflected in diminished visual acuity, decreased visual fields, or ocular motility with diplopia, the significance of the disturbance or deformity should be evaluated by the examining physician. In that situation, the physician may *combine* an additional 5% to 10% impairment with the impaired visual function of the involved eye. Abnormalities that might result in such impairments include media opacities, corneal or lens opacities, and abnormalities resulting in such symptoms as epiphora, photophobia, or metamorphopsia.

Permanent deformities of the orbit, such as scars or cosmetic defects that do not alter ocular function, also may be considered to be factors causing whole-person impairments as high as 10%. If facial disfigurement due to scarring above the upper lip is evaluated by means of *the Guides to the Evaluation of Permanent Impariment* on the ear, nose, throat, and related structures, then any overlapping impairment percentage due to ocular scarring should be subtracted from the greater value.

Equipment

The following equipment is necessary to test the functions of the visual system.

1. *Visual Acuity Test Charts*: For distance vision tests, the Snellen test chart with nonserif block letters or numbers, the illiterate E chart, or Landolt's brokenring chart are acceptable. For near vision, charts with print similar to that of the Snellen chart, with Revised Jaeger Standard print, or with American point-type notation for use at 35 cm (14 in) are acceptable. The 10 equally difficult block letters (D, K, R, H, V, C, N, Z, S, and O) of Louise L. Sloan are recommended for testing distance vision. Each letter subtends a visual angle of 5 minutes and a stroke width of 1 minute.

2. *Visual Field Testing:* The standard for testing visual fields is the traditional stimulus III-4e of the Goldmann perimeter. Other acceptable perimeters and stimuli are listed in **Table 1.** The tangent screen may be used for diplopia testing.

3. *Refraction Equipment:* The necessary equipment consists of a phoropter or a combination of hand-held lenses and a retinoscope.

TABLE 1

STIMULI EQUIVALENT TO THE GOLDMANN KINETIC STIMULUS

	Phakic	Aphakic
Goldmann (kinetic)	III-4E	IV-4e
ARC perimeter (kinetic)	3 mm white at radius 330 mm	6 mm white at radius 330 mm
Allergan-Humphrey (static, size 3)	10 dB	6 dB
Octopus (static, size 3)	7 dB	3 dB

Preparation for Medical Evaluation

Before using the information in this section, the reader should become familiar with Chapters 1 and 2 and the Glossary of *the Guides to the Evaluation of Permament Impairment*, which discuss the purpose of the Guides and the situations in which they are useful and also provide basic definitions. Chapters 1 and 2 discuss the methods for examining patients and preparing reports. A medical evaluation report should include information such as the following.

A. Medical Evaluation

- History of medical condition
- Results of most recent clinical evaluation
- Assessment of current clinical status and state ment of further medical plans
- Diagnosis

B. Analysis of Findings

- Impact of medical condition on life activities
- Explanation for concluding that the condition is stable and unlikely to change during the next year
- Explanation for concluding that the individual is or is not likely to suffer further impairment by engaging in ordinary activities
- Explanation for concluding that accommodations or restrictions are or are not warranted

C. Comparison of Analysis with Impairment Criteria

- Description of clinical findings and how these findings relate to specific criteria
- Explanation of each impairment estimate
- Summary of all impairment estimates
- Overall estimate of whole-person impairment

CENTRAL VISUAL ACUITY

Test chart illumination of at least 5 foot-candles is recommended to attain a distinct contrast of 0.85 or greater and a comfortable luminance of approximately 85 ± 5 candelas per square meter. The chart or reflecting surface should not be dirty or discolored. The far test distance simulates infinity at 6 m (20 ft) or at no less than 4 m (13 ft 1 in). The near test distance should be fixed at 35 cm (14 in) in keeping with the Revised Jaeger Standard. Adequate and comfortable illumination must be diffused onto the test card at a level about three times greater than that of usual room illumination. **Table 2** shows standards for distance and near visual acuity.

There are no universally accepted standards for contrast and glare sensitivity testing and glare disability testing. Thus, the results of such testing are not incorporated in visual tests of central visual acuity. However, such testing, if it is done with generally accepted methods, may be the basis for an additional impairment of visual function of the involved eye as high as 10%.

Central vision should be measured and recorded for distance and for near objects, without correction and with best corrected conventional spectacle refraction. If a patient is well adapted to contact lenses and wishes to wear them, best corrected vision with contact lenses is acceptable as the basis for estimating impairment. In certain ocular conditions, particularly in the presence of corneal abnormalities, contact lens-corrected vision may be better than that which can be obtained with spectacle correction. If the patient does not already wear contact lenses, it is not necessary to fit a contact lens to determine best corrected visual acuity.

Visual acuity for distance should be recorded in the Snellen notation, using a fraction in which the numerator is the test distance in feet or meters and the denominator is the distance at which the smallest letter discriminated by the patient would subtend 5 minutes of arc and at which an eye with 20/20 vision would see that letter. The fraction notation is one of convenience that does not indicate percentage of visual acuity. A similar Snellen notation using centimeters or inches, or a comparable Revised Jaeger Standard or American point type notation, may be used in designating near visual acuity.

The values shown in **Table 2** for distance and near visual acuity and loss were used to develop **Table 3**. **Table 3** combines both types of loss to derive an overall estimate of loss of central vision in an eye. Using **Table 3**, the examiner identifies the Snellen rating for near vision along the top row and the Snellen rating for distance along the first column. Reading down from the former and across from the latter, the examiner locates two impairment values for loss of central vision where the column and row cross. It can be seen that each impairment percentage for loss of central vision is the mean of the impairment percentages for the losses of distance acuity and near visual acuity. **Tables 2** and **3** were developed in 1955 by the Council on Industrial Health of the American Medical Association.

TABLE 2

VISUAL ACUITY NOTATIONS WITH CORRESPONDING PERCENTAGES OF LOSS OF CENTRAL VISION

FOR DISTANCE

	SNELLEN NOTATIONS		
ENGLISH	METRIC 6	METRIC 4	% LOSS
20/15	6/5	4/3	0
20/20	6/6	4/4	0
20/25	6/7.5	4/5	5
20/30	6/10	4/6	10
20/40	6/12	4/8	15
20/50	6/15	4/10	25
20/60	6/20	4/12	35
20/70	6/22	4/14	40
20/80	6/24	4/16	45
20/100	6/30	4/20	50
20/125	6/38	4/25	60
20/150	6/50	4/30	70
20/200	6/60	4/40	80
20/300	6/90	4/60	85
20/400	6/120	4/80	90
20/800	6/240	4/160	95

FOR NEAR

NEAR SNELLEN		REVISED JAEGER	AMERICAN	
INCHES	CENTIMETERS	STANDARD	POINT-TYPE	% LOSS
14/14	35/35	1	3	0
14/18	35/45	2	4	0
14/21	35/53	3	5	5
14/24	35/60	4	6	7
14/28	35/70	5	7	10
14/35	35/88	6	8	50
14/40	35/100	7	9	55
14/45	35/113	8	10	60
14/60	35/150	9	11	80
14/70	35/175	10	12	85
14/80	35/200	11	13	87
14/88	35/220	12	14	90
14/112	35/280	13	21	95
14/140	35/350	14	23	98

Monocular aphakia or monocular pseudophakia is considered to be an additional central vision impairment. If either is present, the remaining central vision is decreased by 50%, as shown by **Table 3.** With monocular pseudophakia, despite a normal Snellen acuity, there is more light scattering and a greater likelihood of glare, diminished contrast sensitivity, and spherical aberration than with a normal phakic eye. Also, capsular opacification, lens decentralization with visualization of the lens edge or positioning hole, or pupillary abnormalities may occur, and there is total loss of accomodation. For these reasons an initial 50% impairment in the central visual acuity of the pseuduophakic eye is allowed, to which 50% of the observed impairment for loss of central vision is added.

Determining the Loss of Central Vision in One Eye
First, measure and record the best central visual acuity for distance and the best acuity for near vision, with and without conventional corrective spectacles or contact lenses.

Then consult **Table 3** to derive the overall loss, combining the values for best corrected near and distance acuities. Allow, if indicated, for the additional loss of central vision that results from monocular aphakia or pseudophakia.

Example: A 55-year-old man's Snellen rating for distance vision of the left eye was 20/30, and the rating for near vision of the same eye was 14/24. The man's native lens was present. **Table 3** indicates that the loss of central vision of the eye was 9%.

VISUAL FIELDS

While central visual acuity represents the ability to discern fine details, visual field acuity represents visual ability over a wider breadth of view while the subject is looking straight ahead. There are two elements to the visual field evaluation. One is the peripheral-most location at which a standard object

TABLE 3

LOSS IN % OF CENTRAL VISION* IN A SINGLE EYE.

SNELLEN RATING FOR DISTANCE IN FEET	APPROXIMATE SNELLEN RATING FOR NEAR IN INCHES													
	14/14	14/18	14/21	14/24	14/28	14/35	14/40	14/45	14/60	14/70	14/80	14/88	14/112	14/140
20/15	0	0	3	4	5	25	27	30	40	43	44	45	48	49
	50	50	52	52	53	63	64	65	70	72	72	73	74	75
20/20	0	0	3	4	5	25	27	30	40	43	44	46	48	49
	50	50	52	52	53	63	64	65	70	72	72	73	74	75
20/25	3	3	5	6	8	28	30	33	43	45	46	48	50	52
	52	52	53	53	54	64	65	67	72	73	73	74	75	76
20/30	5	5	8	9	10	30	32	35	45	48	49	50	53	54
	53	53	54	54	55	65	66	68	73	74	74	75	76	77
20/40	8	8	10	11	13	33	35	38	48	50	51	53	55	57
	54	54	55	56	57	67	68	69	74	75	76	77	78	79
20/50	13	13	15	16	18	38	40	43	53	55	56	58	60	62
	57	57	58	58	59	69	70	72	77	78	78	79	80	81
20/60	16	16	18	20	22	41	44	46	56	59	60	61	64	65
	58	58	59	60	61	70	72	73	78	79	80	81	82	83
20/70	18	18	21	22	23	43	46	48	58	61	62	63	66	67
	59	59	61	61	62	72	73	74	79	81	81	82	83	84
20/80	20	20	23	24	25	45	47	50	60	63	64	65	68	69
	60	60	62	62	63	73	74	75	80	82	82	83	84	85
20/100	25	25	28	29	30	50	52	55	65	68	69	70	73	74
	63	63	64	64	65	75	76	78	83	84	84	85	87	87
20/125	30	30	33	34	35	55	57	60	70	73	74	75	78	79
	65	65	67	67	68	78	79	80	85	87	87	88	89	90
20/150	34	34	37	38	39	59	61	64	74	77	78	79	82	83
	67	67	68	69	70	80	81	82	87	88	89	90	91	92
20/200	40	40	43	44	45	65	67	70	80	83	84	85	88	89
	70	70	72	72	73	83	84	85	90	91	92	93	94	95
20/300	43	43	45	46	48	68	70	73	83	85	86	88	90	92
	72	72	73	73	74	84	85	87	91	93	93	94	95	96
20/400	45	45	48	49	50	70	72	75	85	88	89	90	93	94
	73	73	74	74	75	85	86	88	93	94	94	95	97	97
20/800	48	48	50	51	53	73	75	78	88	90	91	93	95	97
	74	74	75	76	77	87	88	89	94	95	96	97	98	99

*Upper number shows % loss of central vision without allowance for monocular aphakia or monocular pseudophakia; lower number shows % loss of central vision with allowance for monocular aphakia or monocular pseudophakia.

can be detected. The other is the quality of visual functioning at every point within the field of view.

For the purpose of evaluating impairment in a standard fashion, a patient's visual field is evaluated as the ability to see a standard stimulus, either in terms of the peripheral-most extent along eight meridians at which the stimulus is seen (method 1) or in terms of the proportion of a predefined region in which the standard stimulus is or is not visible (method 2).

With either method, tests that have been performed for medical diagnosis may be used for calculation of impairment or to determine that a certain level of impairment has been exceeded. Sometimes, however, the available test results are not adequate for this purpose, so a specific examination must be done to allow determination of impairment. **Figure 1** shows a type of chart that is used to measure visual fields.

The traditional standard stimulus is the III-4e kinetic stimulus of the Goldmann perimeter. The IV-4e stimulus should be used in aphakic patients without a lens implant or contact lens. The equivalent stimuli with other instruments are given in **Table 1**.

Determining Loss of Monocular Visual Fields

In method 1 of measuring the visual field, the peripheral-most extent over which the static stimulus is seen is noted in each of eight principal meridians. The normal extent of these meridians is given in **Table 4**; the total extent summed over eight meridians

TABLE 4

NORMAL VISUAL FIELDS FOR EIGHT PRINCIPAL MERIDIANS.

DIRECTION OF VISION	DEGREES OF FIELD
Temporally	85
Down temporally	85
Direct down	65
Down nasally	50
Nasally	60
Up nasally	55
Direct up	45
Up temporally	55
Total	500

Figure 1. Example of Perimetric Charts Used to Plot Extent or Outline of Visual Field Along Eight Principal Meridians Separated by 45° Intervals.

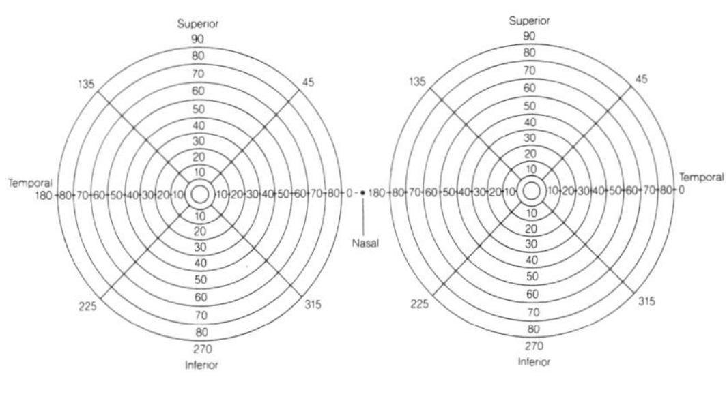

is 500. To calculate the percentage of retained vision, one adds the extent of the visual field along each of the eight meridians, considering the maximum normal values for the meridians given in **Table 4**, then divides by 5 to determine the percentage of visual field perception that remains. One must subtract the percentage of visual field remaining from 100% to obtain the percentage of visual field lost. **Table 5** tabulates the losses of monocular visual fields calculated by this method.

If the boundary of the visual field coincides with a principal meridian, as in hemianopia or nasal step, the value used for that meridian is the midpoint. Thus, in a hemianopic patient in whom the vertical meridian is split by the III-4e isopter from the point of fixation (0°) up to 40°, that meridian is given a value of 20°. In the case of a nasal step extending from 30° to 60° with the standard stimulus, a value of 45° is used for the nasal meridian.

If a meridian passes through a scotoma, the width of the scotoma is subtracted from the maximum number of degrees for that meridian. The visual field loss in each eye is increased by 5% for an inferior quadrant loss and by 10% for an inferior hemianopic loss, because major loss of a visual field below has more of a functional consequence than an equivalent field loss above. The increase of 5% or 10% is *added* to the percentage representing the visual field loss.

In method 2, an Esterman grid is used (**Figs. 2A** and **2B**,). The extent over which the standard stimulus is seen or not seen in an ordinary monocular field test is transferred onto the Esterman 100 unit monocular grid. A simple count of the number of dots seen within the field among the 100 dots that are in the grid gives the percentage of retained vision. A count of the number of dots *not* seen gives the percentage lost. The Esterman grid is available from the American Academy of Ophthalmology, 655 Beech St., P.O. Box 7424, San Francisco, CA 94120-7424.

When it is available, a binocular field test performed with both eyes open and the chin in the middle of the instrument is preferred if method 2 is to be used, except for patients with one eye or those with a strabismic deviation of one eye (heterotropia). The binocular field result is determined by using the Esterman 120-unit binocular grid, and the dot count is multiplied by 5/6 to obtain the percentage of retained or lost field.

Some automated machines can perform a test of one or two eyes with a method corresponding to method 2, presenting the standard stimulus at the 100 or 120 prescribed locations and recording the result.

If a medical test of visual fields is already available, it may or may not be valid for determining visual impairment. Kinetic visual field tests should not be used if the standard stimulus was not among those plotted. An exception may occur if a stimulus stronger than the standard was plotted and the field is quite restricted. The loss is gauged by calculating the percentage of loss with the stronger stimulus; then it is certain that the percentage loss with the standard stimulus would be greater.

Another way of using a previously determined diagnostic field occurs if it covers only part of the maximum visual field, for example, only the central 30°. Methods 1 and 2 will yield the desired percentage calculation only if the patient can visualize the standard stimulus within the tested region. Thus, if the 10-decibel (dB) stimulus of the Allergan-Humphrey instrument is seen only inside 15° along all eight meridians but is not seen outside 15°, in considering the 20° or 30° field one may calculate that the retained vision is 24% (15° x 8/5). However, if the 10-dB stimulus is seen out to the edge of the 30° field along each meridian and for an unknown extent beyond, one cannot calculate the percentage of retained vision or visual loss. In such an instance, one can document the loss only if the visual field examination covers a larger field.

If an automated central field examination is normal, it is acceptable as documentation that the entire field is normal, if the ocular history and examination do not suggest lesions that would affect the outer extent of the field.

Figure 2A.–Esterman 120-unit *Binocular* Scoring Grid* for Use with Both Eyes Open.

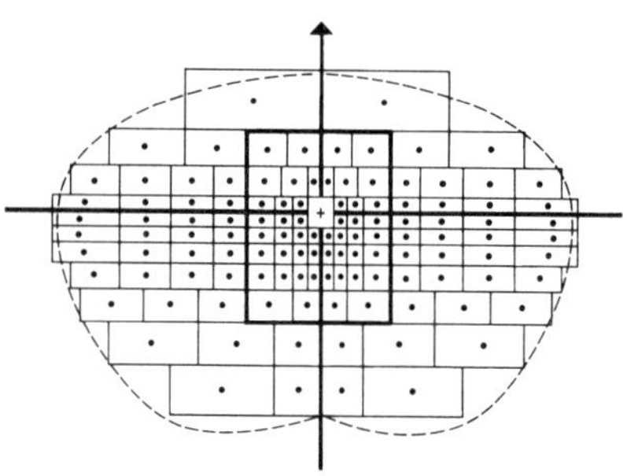

Figure 2B.–Esterman 100-unit *Monocular* Scoring Grid* for Arc or Bowl Perimeter or Similar Automated Instrument Providing Full Monocular Field Analysis.

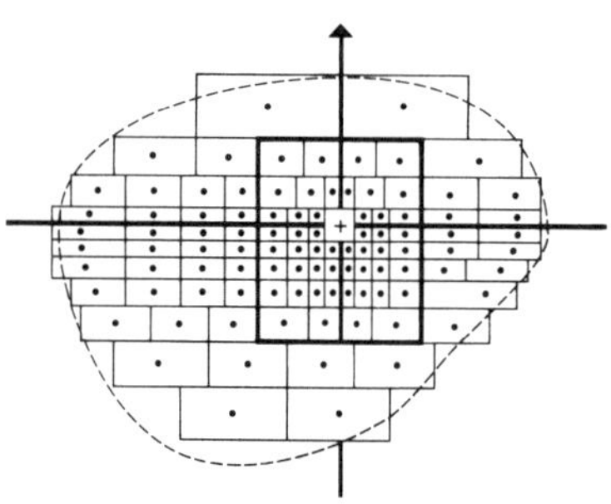

Examples of determining visual field impairments follow.

Example 1: Determine the visual field impairment and percentage of retained visual field in Field 1, right eye (below) using method 1.

Direction of vision	Degrees of field	Comments
Temporally	77	
Down temporally	84	
Direct down	55	65° maximum from table,minus 10° of scotoma between 15° and 25°
Down nasally	50	Not 55°, because maximum from table is 50°
Nasally	37	Midway between 22° and 52°
Up nasally	15	
Direct up	10	
Up temporally	33	40° peripheral extent, minus 7° excluded by isopter between 10° and 17°
Total	361	361 divided by 5 = 72

Thus, the retained visual field is 72%, and the impairment is 28%.

Field 1

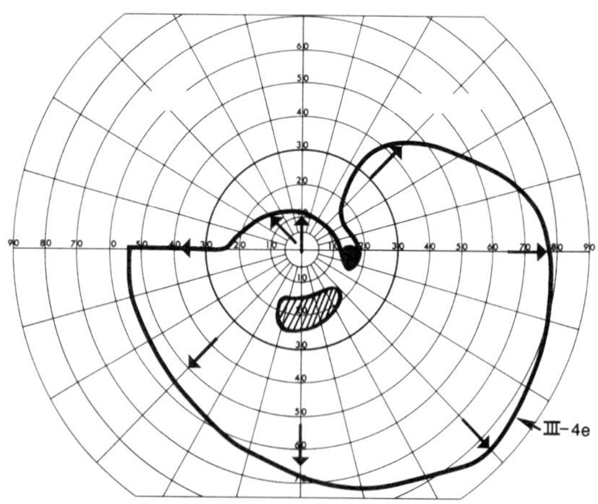

*Grids may be obtained from the American Academy of Ophthalmology, 655 Beech St., San Francisco, CA 94120

Example 2: Determine the percentage of field loss in *Field 2*, left eye (below) using method 2.

Solution: Twenty-seven of the dots are excluded by the standard isopter. This is considered to be a 27% visual field loss, with 73% of the visual field retained.

Example 3: Calculate the visual field using method 1 and the diagnostic results shown in Field 3, right eye (below).

A line is drawn around the location where visibility is better than 10 dB, the standard stimulus for the Humphrey Visual Field Analyzer. Although the field may extend slightly beyond the 30° edge of the tested region, it is obvious that the field is quite restricted. The eight meridians are summed as follows.

Direction of vision	Degree of field	Comments
Temporally	30	
Down temporally	5	
Direct down	3	Midpoint between 6 and 0°
Down nasally	0	
Nasally	8	Midpoint between 15 and 0°
Up nasally	15	
Direct up	17.5	
Up temporally	20	
Total	98.5	98.5 divided by 5 = 19.7, or about 20%

Thus, the patient retains 20% of the visual field and has an 80% loss.

Field 2

Temporal **Nasal**

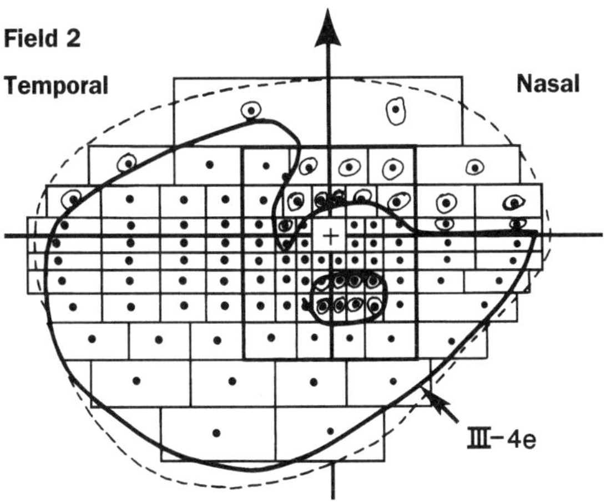

Field 3

Nasal **Temporal**

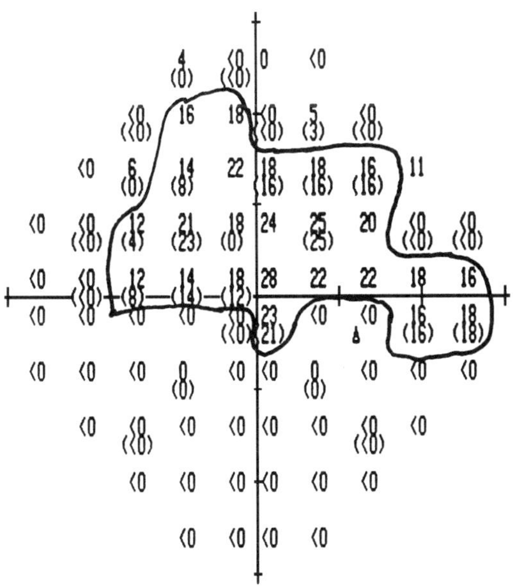

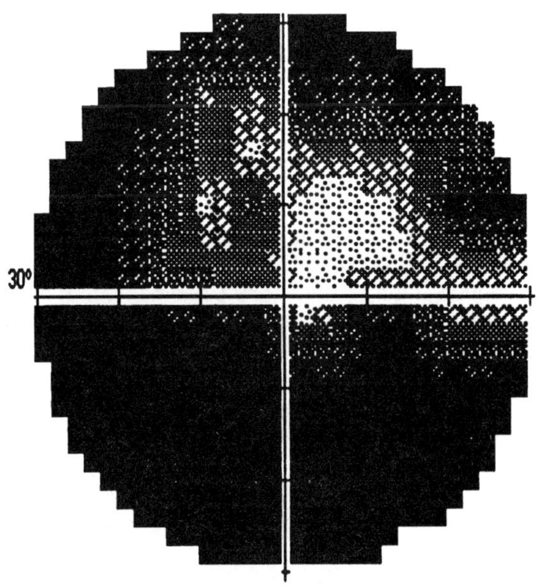

TABLE 5

LOSS OF MONOSCULAR VISUAL FIELD

TOTAL DEGREES LOST	TOTAL DEGREES RETAINED	% OF LOSS
0	500	0
5	495	1
10	490	2
15	485	3
20	480	4
25	475	5
30	470	6
35	465	7
40	460	8
45	455	9
50	450	10
55	445	11
60	440	12
65	435	13
70	430	14
75	425	15
80	420	16
85	415	17
90	410	18
95	405	19
100	400	20
105	395	21
110	390	22
115	385	23
120	380	24
125	375	25
130	370	26
135	365	27
140	360	28
145	355	29
150	350	30
155	345	31
160	340	32
165	335	33
170	330	34
175	325	35
180	320	36
185	315	37
190	310	38
195	305	39
200	300	40
205	295	41
210	290	42
215	285	43
220	280	44
225	275	45
230	270	46
235	265	47
240	260	48
245	255	49
250	250	50
255	245	51
260	240	52
265	235	53
270	230	54
275	225	55
280	220	56
285	215	57
290	210	58
295	205	59
300	200	60
305	195	61
310	190	62
315	185	63
320	180	64
325	175	65
330	170	66
335	165	67
340	160	68
345	155	69
350	150	70
355	145	71
360	140	72
365	135	73
370	130	74
375	125	75
380	120	76
385	115	77
390	110	78
395	105	79
400	100	80
405	95	81
410	90	82
415	85	83
420	80	84
425	75	85
430	70	86
435	65	87
440	60	88
445	55	89
450	50	90
455	45	91
460	40	92
465	35	93
470	30	94
475	25	95
480	20	96
485	15	97
490	10	98
495	5	99
500	0	100

*Or more.

ABNORMAL OCULAR MOTILITY AND BINOCULAR DIPLOPIA

Unless a patient has diplopia within 30° of the center of fixation, the diplopia rarely causes significant visual impairment. An exception is diplopia on looking downward. The extent of diplopia in the various directions of gaze is determined on an arc perimeter at 33 cm or with a bowl perimeter. A tangent screen also is acceptable for evaluating the central 30°. Examination is made in each of the eight major meridians by using a small test light or the projected light of approximately Goldmann III-4e without adding colored lenses or correcting prisms.

To determine the impairment of ocular motility, the patient is seated with both eyes open and the chin resting in the chin rest and centered so that the eyes are equidistant from the sides of the central fixation target.

The presence of diplopia is then plotted along the eight meridians of a suitable visual field chart (**Fig. 1**). The impairment percentage for loss of ocular motility due to diplopia in the meridian of maximum impairment, according to **Fig. 3**, is *combined* with any other visual impairment (Combined Values Chart, p. 70).

Example 1: Diplopia within the central 20° is estimated to be a 100% impairment of ocular motility (**Fig. 3**). This is equivalent to the total loss of vision of one eye, which is estimated to be a 25% impairment of the visual system and a 24% whole-person impairment (**Table 6**).

Figure 3. Percentage Loss of Ocular Motility of One Eye in Diplopia Fields.

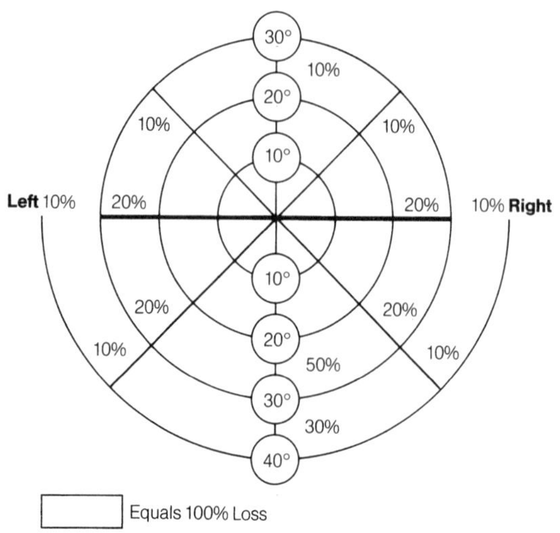

Example 2: Diplopia on looking horizontally off center from 20° to 30° is equivalent to 20% loss of ocular motility. Diplopia of the same eye when looking diagonally from 30° to 40° is equivalent to 10% loss of ocular motility. The impairments from diplopia are added, and the total loss of ocular motility is 30%.

STEPS IN DETERMINING IMPAIRMENT OF THE VISUAL SYSTEM AND OF THE WHOLE PERSON

Step 1: Determine and record the percentage loss of central vision for each eye separately, combining the losses of near and distance vision.

Step 2: Determine and record the percentage loss of visual field for each eye separately (monocular) or for both eyes together (binocular).

Step 3: Determine and record the percentage loss of ocular motility.

Procedure with Monocular Visual Fields Test

If the percentage loss of visual field is calculated for each eye separately (monocular), *combine* (Combined Values Chart, p. 70) the percentage loss of central vision with the percentage loss of visual field in each eye and record the values.

Example 1:
Right Eye
Loss of central vision
(both near and distance) 56%
Loss of visual field 32%
56% *combined* with 32%
(Combined Values) 70%
Thus, the estimated impairment of the right eye is 70%.

Left Eye
Loss of central vision
(both near and distance) 46%
Loss of visual field 32%
46% *combined* with 32%
(Combined Values) 63%
Estimated impairment of the left eye is 63%.

Again using the Combined Values, *combine* the percentage for impairment of ocular motility with the combined value for central vision and visual field in the eye manifesting the greater impairment, the right eye in example 1. Disregard the loss of ocular motility in the other eye.

TABLE 6

IMPAIRMENT OF THE VISUAL SYSTEM AS IT RELATES TO IMPAIRMENT OF THE WHOLE PERSON

% IMPAIRMENT OF		% IMPAIRMENT OF		% IMPAIRMENT OF		% IMPAIRMENT OF		% IMPAIRMENT OF		% IMPAIRMENT OF	
VISUAL SYSTEM	WHOLE PERSON	VISUAL SYSTEM	WHOLE PERSON	VISUAL SYSTEM	WHOLE PERSON	VISUAL SYSTEM	WHOLE PERSON	VISUAL SYSTEM	WHOLE PERSON	VISUAL SYSTEM	WHOLE PERSON
0	0	15	14	30	28	45	42	60	57	75	71
1	1	16	15	31	29	46	43	61	58	76	72
2	2	17	16	32	30	47	44	62	59	77	73
3	3	18	17	33	31	48	45	63	59	78	74
4	4	19	18	34	32	49	46	64	60	79	75
5	5	20	19	35	33	50	47	65	61	80	76
6	6	21	20	36	34	51	48	66	62	81	76
7	7	22	21	37	35	52	49	67	63	82	77
8	8	23	22	38	36	53	50	68	64	83	78
9	8	24	23	39	37	54	51	69	65	84	79
10	9	25	24	40	38	55	52	70	66	85	80
11	10	26	25	41	39	56	53	71	67	86	81
12	11	27	25	42	40	57	54	72	68	87	82
13	12	28	26	43	41	58	55	73	69	88	83
14	13	29	27	44	42	59	56	74	70	89	84
										90-100	85

	% IMPAIRMENT VISUAL SYSTEM	% IMPAIRMENT WHOLE PERSON
Total loss of vision one eye	25	24
Total loss of vision both eyes	100	85

Example 2:
In the patient described above, the eye with the greater motility loss has a 25% motility impairment.

Right Eye
Impairment of central vision and visual field 70%
Loss of ocular motility 25%
70% *combined* with 25%
(Combined Values Chart) 78%

The examiner may *combine* as much as a 10% impairment for an ocular abnormality or dysfunction that he or she believes is not adequately reflected in the visual acuity, visual fields, or diplopia testing (Combined Values Chart). In the above example, an impairment of 78% combined with a 10% impairment would result in a visual impairment of the right eye of 80%.

Step 4: After determining the level of impairment of each eye, use **Table 7** to determine visual system impairment. In the above example, consider- ing impairments of 80% and 63%, impairment of the visual system is seen from **Table 7** to be 67%.

Step 5: Consult **Table 6** to ascertain the impairment of the whole person that is contributed by impairment of the visual system. A 67% impairment of the patient's visual system, as shown in the example above, is equivalent to a 63% impairment of the whole person (**Table 6**).

Procedure with Binocular Esterman Field Test
If the percentage loss of visual fields is determined for both eyes together by means of the Esterman binocular grid, consult **Table 7** to ascertain the impairment of the visual system due to loss of central vision.

Example 3:

Right Eye
Loss of central vision for both near and
distance is 56%

Left Eye
Loss of central vision for both near and
distance is 46%
From **Table 7** it is seen that impairment due to
the loss of central vision of both eyes is 49%

Using the Combined Values Chart, *combine* the impairment due to loss of central vision with the impairment due to binocular visual field loss.

Binocular visual field testing is not recommended when loss of ocular motility is present.

With the patient in example 3:
Impairment due to loss of central vision of
both eyes is 49%
Impairment due to binocular visual field loss
is determined to be 20%
Combine the central vision and visual field losses
(Combined Values Chart); the impairment
of the visual system is 59%

Consult **Table 6** to ascertain the impairment of the whole person that is contributed by the visual system.

In example 3, the 59% visual system impairment is equivalent to a 56% whole-person impairment (**Table 6**).

OTHER CONDITIONS

Up to an additional 10% impairment may be *combined* with the whole-person impairment related to the visual system for such conditions as permanent deformities of the orbit, scars, and other cosmetic deformities that do not otherwise alter ocular function. *Combine* the estimates by means of the Combined Values Chart.

Example:
Impairment due to loss of central vision
of both eyes 49%
Impairment due to binocular visual field loss . .20%
Impairment of visual system
(Combined Values Chart) 59%
Impairment of whole person related to visual
system (**Table 6**) 56%
10% impairment for orbital scar and
deformity 10%
Whole-person impairment
(Combined Values Chart) 60%

REFERENCES
1. Sloan LL. New test charts for the measurement of visual acuity. *Am J Ophthalmol.* 1959;48:808-813.
2. Report of Working Group 39, Committee on Vision, National Academy of Sciences. Recommended standard procedures for the clinical measurement and specification of visual acuity. *Adv Ophthalmol.* 1980;41:103-143.
3. Esterman B. Grid for scoring visual field, II perimeter. *Arch Ophthalmol.* 1968;79:400-406.
4. Keeney AH, Duerson HL Jr. Collated near-vision test card. *Am J Ophthalmol.* 1958;46:592-594.
5. Keeney AH. *Ocular Examination: Basis and Technique.* 2nd ed. St Louis, Mo: CV Mosby Co; 1976.
6. Newell FW. *Ophthalmology: Principles and Concepts.* 7th ed. St Louis, Mo: CV Mosby Co; 1992.
7. Esterman B. Functional scoring of the binocular visual field. *Ophthalmology.* 1982;89:1226-1234.
8. Esterman B, Blance E, Wallach M, Bonelli A. Computerized scoring of the functional field: preliminary report. Doc *Ophthalmol Proc Ser.* 1985;42:333-339.
9. Anderson DR. *Perimetry: With and Without Automation.* 2nd ed. St Louis, Mo: CV Mosby Co; 1987.
10. American Academy of Ophthalmology. Contrast sensitivity and glare testing in the evaluation of anterior segment disease. *Ophthalmology.* 1990;97:1233-1237.
11. Frisen L. *Clinical Tests of Vision.* New York, NY: Raven Press; 1990.

TABLE 7

VISUAL SYSTEM

The values in this table are based on the following formula:

$$\frac{3 \times \text{impairment value of better eye} + \text{impairment value of worse eye}}{4} = \text{impairment of visual system}$$

The guides to the table are percentage impairment values for each eye. The percentage for the worse eye is read at the side of the table. The percentage for the better eye is read at the bottom of the table. At the intersection of the column for the worse eye and the column for the better eye is the impairment of visual system value.

For example, when there is 60% impairment of one eye and 30% impairment of the other eye, read down the side of the table until you come to the larger value (60%). Then follow across the row until it is intersected by the column headed by 30% at the bottom of the page. At the intersection of these two columns is printed the number 38. This number (38) represents the percentage impairment of the visual system when there is 60% impairment of one eye and 30% impairment of the other eye.

If bilateral aphakia is present and corrected central vision has been used in evaluation, impairment of the visual system is weighted by an additional 25% decrease in the value of the remaining corrected vision. For example, a 38% impairment (62% remaining) would be increased to 38% + (25%) (62%) = 54%.

% Impairment Worse Eye	0	1	2	3	4	5	6	7	8	9	10	11	12	13	14	15	16	17	18	19	20	21	22	23	24	25	26	27	28	29	30	31	32	33	34	35	36	37	38	39	40	41	42	43	44	45	46	47	48	49
0	0																																																	
1	0	1																																																
2	1	1	2																																															
3	1	2	2	3																																														
4	1	2	3	3	4																																													
5	1	2	3	4	4	5																																												
6	2	2	3	4	5	5	6																																											
7	2	3	3	4	5	6	6	7																																										
8	2	3	4	4	5	6	7	7	8																																									
9	2	3	4	5	5	6	7	8	8	9																																								
10	3	3	4	5	6	6	7	8	9	9	10																																							
11	3	4	4	5	6	7	7	8	9	10	10	11																																						
12	3	4	5	5	6	7	8	8	9	10	11	11	12																																					
13	3	4	5	6	6	7	8	9	9	10	11	12	12	13																																				
14	4	4	5	6	7	7	8	9	10	10	11	12	13	13	14																																			
15	4	5	5	6	7	8	8	9	10	11	11	12	13	14	14	15																																		
16	4	5	6	6	7	8	9	9	10	11	12	12	13	14	15	15	16																																	
17	4	5	6	7	7	8	9	10	10	11	12	13	13	14	15	16	16	17																																
18	5	5	6	7	8	8	9	10	11	11	12	13	14	14	15	16	17	17	18																															
19	5	6	6	7	8	9	9	10	11	12	12	13	14	15	15	16	17	18	18	19																														
20	5	6	7	7	8	9	10	10	11	12	13	13	14	15	16	16	17	18	19	19	20																													
21	5	6	7	8	8	9	10	11	11	12	13	14	14	15	16	17	17	18	19	20	20	21																												
22	6	6	7	8	9	9	10	11	12	12	13	14	15	15	16	17	18	18	19	20	21	21	22																											
23	6	7	7	8	9	10	10	11	12	13	13	14	15	16	16	17	18	19	19	20	21	22	22	23																										
24	6	7	8	8	9	10	11	11	12	13	14	14	15	16	17	17	18	19	20	20	21	22	23	23	24																									
25	6	7	8	9	9	10	11	12	12	13	14	15	15	16	17	18	18	19	20	21	21	22	23	24	24	25																								
26	7	7	8	9	10	10	11	12	13	13	14	15	16	16	17	18	19	19	20	21	22	22	23	24	25	25	26																							
27	7	8	8	9	10	11	11	12	13	14	14	15	16	17	17	18	19	20	20	21	22	23	23	24	25	26	26	27																						
28	7	8	9	9	10	11	12	12	13	14	15	15	16	17	18	18	19	20	21	21	22	23	24	24	25	26	27	27	28																					
29	7	8	9	10	10	11	12	13	13	14	15	16	16	17	18	19	19	20	21	22	22	23	24	25	25	26	27	28	28	29																				
30	8	8	9	10	11	11	12	13	14	14	15	16	17	17	18	19	20	20	21	22	23	23	24	25	26	26	27	28	29	29	30																			
31	8	9	9	10	11	12	12	13	14	15	15	16	17	18	18	19	20	21	21	22	23	24	24	25	26	27	27	28	29	30	30	31																		
32	8	9	10	10	11	12	13	13	14	15	16	16	17	18	19	19	20	21	22	22	23	24	25	25	26	27	28	28	29	30	31	31	32																	
33	8	9	10	11	11	12	13	14	14	15	16	17	17	18	19	20	20	21	22	23	23	24	25	26	26	27	28	29	29	30	31	32	32	33																
34	9	9	10	11	12	12	13	14	15	15	16	17	18	18	19	20	21	21	22	23	24	24	25	26	27	27	28	29	30	30	31	32	33	33	34															
35	9	10	10	11	12	13	13	14	15	16	16	17	18	19	19	20	21	22	22	23	24	25	25	26	27	28	28	29	30	31	31	32	33	34	34	35														
36	9	10	11	11	12	13	14	14	15	16	17	17	18	19	20	20	21	22	23	23	24	25	26	26	27	28	29	29	30	31	32	32	33	34	35	35	36													
37	9	10	11	12	12	13	14	15	15	16	17	18	18	19	20	21	21	22	23	24	24	25	26	27	27	28	29	30	30	31	32	33	33	34	35	36	36	37												
38	10	10	11	12	13	13	14	15	16	16	17	18	19	19	20	21	22	22	23	24	25	25	26	27	28	28	29	30	31	31	32	33	34	34	35	36	37	37	38											
39	10	11	11	12	13	14	14	15	16	17	17	18	19	20	20	21	22	23	23	24	25	26	26	27	28	29	29	30	31	32	32	33	34	35	35	36	37	38	38	39										
40	10	11	12	12	13	14	15	15	16	17	18	18	19	20	21	21	22	23	24	24	25	26	27	27	28	29	30	30	31	32	33	33	34	35	36	36	37	38	39	39	40									
41	10	11	12	13	13	14	15	16	16	17	18	19	19	20	21	22	22	23	24	25	25	26	27	28	28	29	30	31	31	32	33	34	34	35	36	37	37	38	39	40	40	41								
42	11	11	12	13	14	14	15	16	17	17	18	19	20	20	21	22	23	23	24	25	26	26	27	28	29	29	30	31	32	32	33	34	35	35	36	37	38	38	39	40	41	41	42							
43	11	12	12	13	14	15	15	16	17	18	18	19	20	21	21	22	23	24	24	25	26	27	27	28	29	30	30	31	32	33	33	34	35	36	36	37	38	39	39	40	41	42	42	43						
44	11	12	13	13	14	15	16	16	17	18	19	19	20	21	22	22	23	24	25	25	26	27	28	28	29	30	31	31	32	33	34	34	35	36	37	37	38	39	40	40	41	42	43	43	44					
45	11	12	13	14	14	15	16	17	17	18	19	20	20	21	22	23	23	24	25	26	26	27	28	29	29	30	31	32	32	33	34	35	35	36	37	38	38	39	40	41	41	42	43	44	44	45				
46	12	12	13	14	15	15	16	17	18	18	19	20	21	21	22	23	24	24	25	26	27	27	28	29	30	30	31	32	33	33	34	35	36	36	37	38	39	39	40	41	42	42	43	44	45	45	46			
47	12	13	13	14	15	16	16	17	18	19	19	20	21	22	22	23	24	25	25	26	27	28	28	29	30	31	31	32	33	34	34	35	36	37	37	38	39	40	40	41	42	43	43	44	45	46	46	47		
48	12	13	14	14	15	16	17	17	18	19	20	20	21	22	23	23	24	25	26	26	27	28	29	29	30	31	32	32	33	34	35	35	36	37	38	38	39	40	41	41	42	43	44	44	45	46	47	47	48	
49	12	13	14	15	15	16	17	18	18	19	20	21	21	22	23	24	24	25	26	27	27	28	29	30	30	31	32	33	33	34	35	36	36	37	38	39	39	40	41	42	42	43	44	45	45	46	47	48	48	49

% Impairment Better Eye

% Impairment Better Eye (columns) / % Impairment Worse Eye (rows)

	0	1	2	3	4	5	6	7	8	9	10	11	12	13	14	15	16	17	18	19	20	21	22	23	24	25	26	27	28	29	30	31	32	33	34	35	36	37	38	39	40	41	42	43	44	45	46	47	48	49	
50	13	13	14	15	16	16	17	18	19	19	20	21	22	22	23	24	25	25	26	27	28	28	29	30	31	31	32	33	34	34	35	36	37	37	38	39	40	40	41	42	43	43	44	45	46	46	47	48	49	49	50
51	13	14	14	15	16	17	17	18	19	20	20	21	22	23	23	24	25	26	26	27	28	29	29	30	31	32	32	33	34	35	35	36	37	38	38	39	40	41	41	42	43	44	44	45	46	47	47	48	49	50	51
52	13	14	15	15	16	17	18	18	19	20	21	21	22	23	24	24	25	26	27	27	28	29	30	30	31	32	33	33	34	35	36	36	37	38	39	39	40	41	42	42	43	44	45	45	46	47	48	48	49	50	52
53	13	14	15	16	16	17	18	19	19	20	21	22	22	23	24	25	25	26	27	28	28	29	30	31	31	32	33	34	34	35	36	37	37	38	39	40	40	41	42	43	43	44	45	46	46	47	48	49	49	50	53
54	14	14	15	16	17	17	18	19	20	20	21	22	23	23	24	25	26	26	27	28	29	29	30	31	32	32	33	34	35	35	36	37	38	38	39	40	41	41	42	43	44	44	45	46	47	47	48	49	50	50	54
55	14	15	15	16	17	18	18	19	20	21	21	22	23	24	24	25	26	27	27	28	29	30	30	31	32	33	33	34	35	36	36	37	38	39	39	40	41	42	42	43	44	45	45	46	47	48	48	49	50	51	55
56	14	15	16	16	17	18	19	19	20	21	22	22	23	24	25	25	26	27	28	28	29	30	31	31	32	33	34	34	35	36	37	37	38	39	40	40	41	42	43	43	44	45	46	46	47	48	49	49	50	51	56
57	14	15	16	17	17	18	19	20	20	21	22	23	23	24	25	26	26	27	28	29	29	30	31	32	32	33	34	35	35	36	37	38	38	39	40	41	41	42	43	44	44	45	46	47	47	48	49	50	50	51	57
58	15	15	16	17	18	18	19	20	21	21	22	23	24	24	25	26	27	27	28	29	30	30	31	32	33	33	34	35	36	36	37	38	39	39	40	41	42	42	43	44	45	45	46	47	48	48	49	50	51	51	58
59	15	16	16	17	18	19	19	20	21	22	22	23	24	25	25	26	27	28	28	29	30	31	31	32	33	34	34	35	36	37	37	38	39	40	40	41	42	43	43	44	45	46	46	47	48	49	49	50	51	52	59
60	15	16	17	17	18	19	20	20	21	22	23	23	24	25	26	26	27	28	29	29	30	31	32	32	33	34	35	35	36	37	38	38	39	40	41	41	42	43	44	44	45	46	47	47	48	49	50	50	51	52	60
61	15	16	17	18	18	19	20	21	21	22	23	24	24	25	26	27	27	28	29	30	30	31	32	33	33	34	35	36	36	37	38	39	39	40	41	42	42	43	44	45	45	46	47	48	48	49	50	51	51	52	61
62	16	16	17	18	19	19	20	21	22	22	23	24	25	25	26	27	28	28	29	30	31	31	32	33	34	34	35	36	37	37	38	39	40	40	41	42	43	43	44	45	46	46	47	48	49	49	50	51	52	52	62
63	16	17	17	18	19	20	20	21	22	23	23	24	25	26	26	27	28	29	29	30	31	32	32	33	34	35	35	36	37	38	38	39	40	41	41	42	43	44	44	45	46	47	47	48	49	50	50	51	52	53	63
64	16	17	18	18	19	20	21	21	22	23	24	24	25	26	27	27	28	29	30	30	31	32	33	33	34	35	36	36	37	38	39	39	40	41	42	42	43	44	45	45	46	47	48	48	49	50	51	51	52	53	64
65	16	17	18	19	19	20	21	22	22	23	24	25	25	26	27	28	28	29	30	31	31	32	33	34	34	35	36	37	37	38	39	40	40	41	42	43	43	44	45	46	46	47	48	49	49	50	51	52	52	53	65
66	17	17	18	19	20	20	21	22	23	23	24	25	26	26	27	28	29	29	30	31	32	32	33	34	35	35	36	37	38	38	39	40	41	41	42	43	44	44	45	46	47	47	48	49	50	50	51	52	53	53	66
67	17	18	18	19	20	21	21	22	23	24	24	25	26	27	27	28	29	30	30	31	32	33	33	34	35	36	36	37	38	39	39	40	41	42	42	43	44	45	45	46	47	48	48	49	50	51	51	52	53	54	67
68	17	18	19	19	20	21	22	22	23	24	25	25	26	27	28	28	29	30	31	31	32	33	34	34	35	36	37	37	38	39	40	40	41	42	43	43	44	45	46	46	47	48	49	49	50	51	52	52	53	54	68
69	17	18	19	20	20	21	22	23	23	24	25	26	26	27	28	29	29	30	31	32	32	33	34	35	35	36	37	38	38	39	40	41	41	42	43	44	44	45	46	47	47	48	49	50	50	51	52	53	53	54	69
70	18	18	19	20	21	21	22	23	24	24	25	26	27	27	28	29	30	30	31	32	33	33	34	35	36	36	37	38	39	39	40	41	42	42	43	44	45	45	46	47	48	48	49	50	51	51	52	53	54	54	70
71	18	19	19	20	21	22	22	23	24	25	25	26	27	28	28	29	30	31	31	32	33	34	34	35	36	37	37	38	39	40	40	41	42	43	43	44	45	46	46	47	48	49	49	50	51	52	52	53	54	55	71
72	18	19	20	20	21	22	23	23	24	25	26	26	27	28	29	29	30	31	32	32	33	34	35	35	36	37	38	38	39	40	41	41	42	43	44	44	45	46	47	47	48	49	50	50	51	52	53	53	54	55	72
73	18	19	20	21	21	22	23	24	24	25	26	27	27	28	29	30	30	31	32	33	33	34	35	36	36	37	38	39	39	40	41	42	42	43	44	45	45	46	47	48	48	49	50	51	51	52	53	54	54	55	73
74	19	19	20	21	22	22	23	24	25	25	26	27	28	28	29	30	31	31	32	33	34	34	35	36	37	37	38	39	40	40	41	42	43	43	44	45	46	46	47	48	49	49	50	51	52	52	53	54	55	55	74
75	19	20	20	21	22	23	23	24	25	26	26	27	28	29	29	30	31	32	32	33	34	35	35	36	37	38	38	39	40	41	41	42	43	44	44	45	46	47	47	48	49	50	50	51	52	53	53	54	55	56	75
76	19	20	21	21	22	23	24	24	25	26	27	27	28	29	30	30	31	32	33	33	34	35	36	36	37	38	39	39	40	41	42	42	43	44	45	45	46	47	48	48	49	50	51	51	52	53	54	54	55	56	76
77	19	20	21	22	22	23	24	25	25	26	27	28	28	29	30	31	31	32	33	34	34	35	36	37	37	38	39	40	40	41	42	43	43	44	45	46	46	47	48	49	49	50	51	52	52	53	54	55	55	56	77
78	20	20	21	22	23	23	24	25	26	26	27	28	29	29	30	31	32	32	33	34	35	35	36	37	38	38	39	40	41	41	42	43	44	44	45	46	47	47	48	49	50	50	51	52	53	53	54	55	56	56	78
79	20	21	21	22	23	24	24	25	26	27	27	28	29	30	30	31	32	33	33	34	35	36	36	37	38	39	39	40	41	42	42	43	44	45	45	46	47	48	48	49	50	51	51	52	53	54	54	55	56	57	79
80	20	21	22	22	23	24	25	25	26	27	28	28	29	30	31	31	32	33	34	34	35	36	37	37	38	39	40	40	41	42	43	43	44	45	46	46	47	48	49	49	50	51	52	52	53	54	55	55	56	57	80
81	20	21	22	23	23	24	25	26	26	27	28	29	29	30	31	32	32	33	34	35	35	36	37	38	38	39	40	41	41	42	43	44	44	45	46	47	47	48	49	50	50	51	52	53	53	54	55	56	56	57	81
82	21	21	22	23	24	24	25	26	27	27	28	29	30	30	31	32	33	33	34	35	36	36	37	38	39	39	40	41	42	42	43	44	45	45	46	47	48	48	49	50	51	51	52	53	54	54	55	56	57	57	82
83	21	22	22	23	24	25	25	26	27	28	28	29	30	31	31	32	33	34	34	35	36	37	37	38	39	40	40	41	42	43	43	44	45	46	46	47	48	49	49	50	51	52	52	53	54	55	55	56	57	58	83
84	21	22	23	23	24	25	26	26	27	28	29	29	30	31	32	32	33	34	35	35	36	37	38	38	39	40	41	41	42	43	44	44	45	46	47	47	48	49	50	50	51	52	53	53	54	55	56	56	57	58	84
85	21	22	23	24	24	25	26	27	27	28	29	30	30	31	32	33	33	34	35	36	36	37	38	39	39	40	41	42	42	43	44	45	45	46	47	48	48	49	50	51	51	52	53	54	54	55	56	57	57	58	85
86	22	22	23	24	25	25	26	27	28	28	29	30	31	31	32	33	34	34	35	36	37	37	38	39	40	40	41	42	43	43	44	45	46	46	47	48	49	49	50	51	52	52	53	54	55	55	56	57	58	58	86
87	22	23	23	24	25	26	26	27	28	29	29	30	31	32	32	33	34	35	35	36	37	38	38	39	40	41	41	42	43	44	44	45	46	47	47	48	49	50	50	51	52	53	53	54	55	56	56	57	58	59	87
88	22	23	24	24	25	26	27	27	28	29	30	30	31	32	33	33	34	35	36	36	37	38	39	39	40	41	42	42	43	44	45	45	46	47	48	48	49	50	51	51	52	53	54	54	55	56	57	57	58	59	88
89	22	23	24	25	25	26	27	28	28	29	30	31	31	32	33	34	34	35	36	37	37	38	39	40	40	41	42	43	43	44	45	46	46	47	48	49	49	50	51	52	52	53	54	55	55	56	57	58	58	59	89
90	23	23	24	25	26	26	27	28	29	29	30	31	32	32	33	34	35	35	36	37	38	38	39	40	41	41	42	43	44	44	45	46	47	47	48	49	50	50	51	52	53	53	54	55	56	56	57	58	59	59	90
91	23	24	24	25	26	27	27	28	29	30	30	31	32	33	33	34	35	36	36	37	38	39	39	40	41	42	42	43	44	45	45	46	47	48	48	49	50	51	51	52	53	54	54	55	56	57	57	58	59	60	91
92	23	24	25	25	26	27	28	28	29	30	31	31	32	33	34	34	35	36	37	37	38	39	40	40	41	42	43	43	44	45	46	46	47	48	49	49	50	51	52	52	53	54	55	55	56	57	58	58	59	60	92
93	23	24	25	26	26	27	28	29	29	30	31	32	32	33	34	35	35	36	37	38	38	39	40	41	41	42	43	44	44	45	46	47	47	48	49	50	50	51	52	53	53	54	55	56	56	57	58	59	59	60	93
94	24	24	25	26	27	27	28	29	30	30	31	32	33	33	34	35	36	36	37	38	39	39	40	41	42	42	43	44	45	45	46	47	48	48	49	50	51	51	52	53	54	54	55	56	57	57	58	59	60	60	94
95	24	25	25	26	27	28	28	29	30	31	31	32	33	34	34	35	36	37	37	38	39	40	40	41	42	43	43	44	45	46	46	47	48	49	49	50	51	52	52	53	54	55	55	56	57	58	58	59	60	61	95
96	24	25	26	26	27	28	29	29	30	31	32	32	33	34	35	35	36	37	38	38	39	40	41	41	42	43	44	44	45	46	47	47	48	49	50	50	51	52	53	53	54	55	56	56	57	58	59	59	60	61	96
97	24	25	26	27	27	28	29	30	30	31	32	33	33	34	35	36	36	37	38	39	39	40	41	42	42	43	44	45	45	46	47	48	48	49	50	51	51	52	53	54	54	55	56	57	57	58	59	60	60	61	97
98	25	25	26	27	28	28	29	30	31	31	32	33	34	34	35	36	37	37	38	39	40	40	41	42	43	43	44	45	46	46	47	48	49	49	50	51	52	52	53	54	55	55	56	57	58	58	59	60	61	61	98
99	25	26	26	27	28	29	29	30	31	32	32	33	34	35	35	36	37	38	38	39	40	41	41	42	43	44	44	45	46	47	47	48	49	50	50	51	52	53	53	54	55	56	56	57	58	59	59	60	61	62	99
100	25	26	27	27	28	29	30	30	31	32	33	33	34	35	36	36	37	38	39	39	40	41	42	42	43	44	45	45	46	47	48	48	49	50	51	51	52	53	54	54	55	56	57	57	58	59	60	60	61	62	100
	0	1	2	3	4	5	6	7	8	9	10	11	12	13	14	15	16	17	18	19	20	21	22	23	24	25	26	27	28	29	30	31	32	33	34	35	36	37	38	39	40	41	42	43	44	45	46	47	48	49	

% Impairment Better Eye

% Impairment Worse Eye	50	51	52	53	54	55	56	57	58	59	60	61	62	63	64	65	66	67	68	69	70	71	72	73	74	75	76	77	78	79	80	81	82	83	84	85	86	87	88	89	90	91	92	93	94	95	96	97	98	99	100
50	50
51	50	51
52	51	51	52
53	51	52	52	53
54	51	52	53	53	54
55	51	52	53	54	54	55
56	52	52	53	54	55	55	56
57	52	53	53	54	55	56	56	57
58	52	53	54	54	55	56	57	57	58
59	52	53	54	55	55	56	57	58	58	59
60	53	53	54	55	56	56	57	58	59	59	60
61	53	54	54	55	56	57	57	58	59	60	60	61
62	53	54	55	55	56	57	58	58	59	60	61	61	62
63	53	54	55	56	56	57	58	59	59	60	61	62	62	63
64	54	54	55	56	57	57	58	59	60	60	61	62	63	63	64
65	54	55	55	56	57	58	58	59	60	61	61	62	63	64	64	65
66	54	55	56	56	57	58	59	59	60	61	62	62	63	64	65	65	66
67	54	55	56	57	57	58	59	60	60	61	62	63	63	64	65	66	66	67
68	55	55	56	57	58	58	59	60	61	61	62	63	64	64	65	66	67	67	68
69	55	56	56	57	58	59	59	60	61	62	62	63	64	65	65	66	67	68	68	69
70	55	56	57	57	58	59	60	60	61	62	63	63	64	65	66	66	67	68	69	69	70
71	55	56	57	58	58	59	60	61	61	62	63	64	64	65	66	67	67	68	69	70	70	71
72	56	56	57	58	59	59	60	61	62	62	63	64	65	65	66	67	68	68	69	70	71	71	72
73	56	57	57	58	59	60	60	61	62	63	63	64	65	66	66	67	68	69	69	70	71	72	72	73
74	56	57	58	58	59	60	61	61	62	63	64	64	65	66	67	67	68	69	70	70	71	72	73	73	74
75	56	57	58	59	59	60	61	62	62	63	64	65	65	66	67	68	68	69	70	71	71	72	73	74	74	75
76	57	57	58	59	60	60	61	62	63	63	64	65	66	66	67	68	69	69	70	71	72	72	73	74	75	75	76
77	57	58	58	59	60	61	61	62	63	64	64	65	66	67	67	68	69	70	70	71	72	73	73	74	75	76	76	77
78	57	58	59	59	60	61	62	62	63	64	65	65	66	67	68	68	69	70	71	71	72	73	74	74	75	76	77	77	78
79	57	58	59	60	60	61	62	63	63	64	65	66	66	67	68	69	69	70	71	72	72	73	74	75	75	76	77	78	78	79
80	58	58	59	60	61	61	62	63	64	64	65	66	67	67	68	69	70	70	71	72	73	73	74	75	76	76	77	78	79	79	80
81	58	59	59	60	61	62	62	63	64	65	65	66	67	68	68	69	70	71	71	72	73	74	74	75	76	77	77	78	79	80	80	81
82	58	59	60	60	61	62	63	63	64	65	66	66	67	68	69	69	70	71	72	72	73	74	75	75	76	77	78	78	79	80	81	81	82
83	58	59	60	61	61	62	63	64	64	65	66	67	67	68	69	70	70	71	72	73	73	74	75	76	76	77	78	79	79	80	81	82	82	83
84	59	59	60	61	62	62	63	64	65	65	66	67	68	68	69	70	71	71	72	73	74	74	75	76	77	77	78	79	80	80	81	82	83	83	84
85	59	60	60	61	62	63	63	64	65	66	66	67	68	69	69	70	71	72	72	73	74	75	75	76	77	78	78	79	80	81	81	82	83	84	84	85
86	59	60	61	61	62	63	64	64	65	66	67	67	68	69	70	70	71	72	73	73	74	75	76	76	77	78	79	79	80	81	82	82	83	84	85	85	86
87	59	60	61	62	62	63	64	65	65	66	67	68	68	69	70	71	71	72	73	74	74	75	76	77	77	78	79	80	80	81	82	83	83	84	85	86	86	87
88	60	60	61	62	63	63	64	65	66	66	67	68	69	69	70	71	72	72	73	74	75	75	76	77	78	78	79	80	81	81	82	83	84	84	85	86	87	87	88
89	60	61	61	62	63	64	64	65	66	67	67	68	69	70	70	71	72	73	73	74	75	76	76	77	78	79	79	80	81	82	82	83	84	85	85	86	87	88	88	89
90	60	61	62	62	63	64	65	65	66	67	68	68	69	70	71	71	72	73	74	74	75	76	77	77	78	79	80	80	81	82	83	83	84	85	86	86	87	88	89	89	90
91	60	61	62	63	63	64	65	66	66	67	68	69	69	70	71	72	72	73	74	75	75	76	77	78	78	79	80	81	81	82	83	84	84	85	86	87	87	88	89	90	90	91
92	61	61	62	63	64	64	65	66	67	67	68	69	70	70	71	72	73	73	74	75	76	76	77	78	79	79	80	81	82	82	83	84	85	85	86	87	88	88	89	90	91	91	92
93	61	62	62	63	64	65	65	66	67	68	68	69	70	71	71	72	73	74	74	75	76	77	77	78	79	80	80	81	82	83	83	84	85	86	86	87	88	89	89	90	91	92	92	93
94	61	62	63	63	64	65	66	66	67	68	69	69	70	71	72	72	73	74	75	75	76	77	78	78	79	80	81	81	82	83	84	84	85	86	87	87	88	89	90	90	91	92	93	93	94
95	61	62	63	64	64	65	66	67	67	68	69	70	70	71	72	73	73	74	75	76	76	77	78	79	79	80	81	82	82	83	84	85	85	86	87	88	88	89	90	91	91	92	93	94	94	95
96	62	62	63	64	65	65	66	67	68	68	69	70	71	71	72	73	74	74	75	76	77	77	78	79	80	80	81	82	83	83	84	85	86	86	87	88	89	89	90	91	92	92	93	94	95	95	96
97	62	63	63	64	65	66	66	67	68	69	69	70	71	72	72	73	74	75	75	76	77	78	78	79	80	81	81	82	83	84	84	85	86	87	87	88	89	90	90	91	92	93	93	94	95	96	96	97
98	62	63	64	64	65	66	67	67	68	69	70	70	71	72	73	73	74	75	76	76	77	78	79	79	80	81	82	82	83	84	85	85	86	87	88	88	89	90	91	91	92	93	94	94	95	96	97	97	98
99	62	63	64	65	65	66	67	68	68	69	70	71	71	72	73	74	74	75	76	77	77	78	79	80	80	81	82	83	83	84	85	86	86	87	88	89	89	90	91	92	92	93	94	95	95	96	97	98	98	99
100	63	63	64	65	66	66	67	68	69	69	70	71	72	72	73	74	75	75	76	77	78	78	79	80	81	81	82	83	84	84	85	86	87	87	88	89	90	90	91	92	93	93	94	95	96	96	97	98	99	99	100

% Impairment Better Eye

TABLE 8

COMBINED VALUES CHART

The values are derived from the formula A + B (1 – A) = combined value of A and B, where A and B are the decimal equivalents of the impairment ratings. In the chart all values are expressed as percents. To combine any two impairment values, locate the larger of the values on the side of the chart and read along that row until you come to the column indicated by the smaller value at the bottom of the chart. At the intersection of the row and the column is the combined value.

For example, to combine 35% and 20% read down the side of the chart until you come to the larger value, 35%. Then read across the 35% row until you come to the column indicated by 20% at the bottom of the chart. At the intersection of the row and column is the number 48. Therefore, 35% combined with 20% is 48%. Due to the construction of this chart, the larger impairment value must be identified at the side of the chart.

If three or more impairment values are to be combined, select any two and find their combined values as above. Then use that value and the third value to locate the combined value of all. This process can be repeated indefinitely, the final value in each instance being the combination of all the previous values. In each step of this process the larger impairment value must be identified at the side of the chart.

1	2																																																
2	3	4																																															
3	4	5	6																																														
4	5	6	7	8																																													
5	6	7	8	9	10																																												
6	7	8	9	10	11	12																																											
7	8	9	10	11	12	13	14																																										
8	9	10	11	12	13	14	14	15																																									
9	10	11	12	13	14	14	15	16	17																																								
10	11	12	13	14	15	15	16	17	18	19																																							
11	12	13	14	15	15	16	17	18	19	20	21																																						
12	13	14	15	16	16	17	18	19	20	21	22	23																																					
13	14	15	16	16	17	18	19	20	21	22	23	23	24																																				
14	15	16	17	17	18	19	20	21	22	23	23	24	25	26																																			
15	16	17	18	18	19	20	21	22	23	24	24	25	26	27	28																																		
16	17	18	19	19	20	21	22	23	24	24	25	26	27	28	29	29																																	
17	18	19	19	20	21	22	23	24	24	25	26	27	28	29	29	30	31																																
18	19	20	20	21	22	23	24	25	25	26	27	28	29	29	30	31	32	33																															
19	20	21	21	22	23	24	25	25	26	27	28	29	30	30	31	32	33	34	34																														
20	21	22	22	23	24	25	26	26	27	28	29	30	30	31	32	33	34	34	35	36																													
21	22	23	23	24	25	26	27	27	28	29	30	30	31	32	33	34	34	35	36	37	38																												
22	23	24	24	25	26	27	27	28	29	30	31	31	32	33	34	34	35	36	37	38	38	39																											
23	24	25	25	26	27	28	28	29	30	31	31	32	33	34	35	35	36	37	38	38	39	40	41																										
24	25	26	26	27	28	29	29	30	31	32	32	33	34	35	35	36	37	38	38	39	40	41	41	42																									
25	26	27	27	28	29	30	30	31	32	33	33	34	35	36	36	37	38	39	39	40	41	42	42	43	44																								
26	27	27	28	29	30	30	31	32	33	33	34	35	36	36	37	38	39	39	40	41	42	42	43	44	45	45																							
27	28	28	29	30	31	31	32	33	34	34	35	36	36	37	38	39	39	40	41	42	42	43	44	45	45	46	47																						
28	29	29	30	31	32	32	33	34	34	35	36	37	37	38	39	40	40	41	42	42	43	44	45	45	46	47	47	48																					
29	30	30	31	32	33	33	34	35	35	36	37	38	38	39	40	40	41	42	42	43	44	45	45	46	47	47	48	49	50																				
30	31	31	32	33	34	34	35	36	36	37	38	38	39	40	41	41	42	43	43	44	45	45	46	47	48	48	49	50	50	51																			
31	32	32	33	34	34	35	36	37	37	38	39	39	40	41	41	42	43	43	44	45	45	46	47	48	48	49	50	50	51	52	52																		
32	33	33	34	35	35	36	37	37	38	39	39	40	41	42	42	43	44	44	45	46	46	47	48	48	49	50	50	51	52	52	53	54																	
33	34	34	35	36	36	37	38	38	39	40	40	41	42	42	43	44	44	45	46	46	47	48	48	49	50	50	51	52	52	53	54	54	55																
34	35	35	36	37	37	38	39	39	40	41	41	42	43	43	44	45	45	46	47	47	48	49	49	50	51	51	52	52	53	54	54	55	56	56															
35	36	36	37	38	38	39	40	40	41	42	42	43	43	44	45	45	46	47	47	48	49	49	50	51	51	52	53	53	54	55	55	56	56	57	58														
36	37	37	38	39	39	40	40	41	42	42	43	44	44	45	46	46	47	48	48	49	49	50	51	51	52	53	53	54	55	55	56	56	57	58	58	59													
37	38	38	39	40	40	41	41	42	43	43	44	45	45	46	46	47	48	48	49	50	50	51	51	52	53	53	54	55	55	56	57	57	58	58	59	60	60												
38	39	39	40	40	41	42	42	43	44	44	45	45	46	47	47	48	49	49	50	50	51	52	52	53	54	54	55	55	56	57	57	58	58	59	60	60	61	62											
39	40	40	41	41	42	43	43	44	44	45	46	46	47	48	48	49	49	50	51	51	52	52	53	54	54	55	55	56	57	57	58	59	59	60	60	61	62	62	63										
40	41	41	42	42	43	44	44	45	45	46	47	47	48	48	49	50	50	51	51	52	53	53	54	54	55	56	56	57	57	58	59	59	60	60	61	62	62	63	63	64									
41	42	42	43	43	44	45	45	46	46	47	47	48	49	49	50	50	51	52	52	53	53	54	55	55	56	56	57	58	58	59	59	60	60	61	62	62	63	63	64	65	65								
42	43	43	44	44	45	45	46	47	47	48	48	49	50	50	51	51	52	52	53	54	54	55	55	56	57	57	58	58	59	59	60	61	61	62	62	63	63	64	65	65	66	66							
43	44	44	45	45	46	46	47	48	48	49	49	50	50	51	52	52	53	53	54	54	55	56	56	57	57	58	58	59	60	60	61	61	62	62	63	64	64	65	65	66	66	67	68						
44	45	45	46	46	47	47	48	48	49	50	50	51	51	52	52	53	54	54	55	55	56	56	57	57	58	59	59	60	60	61	61	62	62	63	64	64	65	65	66	66	67	68	68	69					
45	46	46	47	47	48	48	49	49	50	51	51	52	52	53	53	54	54	55	55	56	57	57	58	58	59	59	60	60	61	62	62	63	63	64	64	65	65	66	66	67	68	68	69	69	70				
46	47	47	48	48	49	49	50	50	51	51	52	52	53	54	54	55	55	56	56	57	57	58	58	59	60	60	61	61	62	62	63	63	64	64	65	65	66	67	67	68	68	69	69	70	70	71			
47	48	48	49	49	50	50	51	51	52	52	53	53	54	54	55	55	56	57	57	58	58	59	59	60	60	61	61	62	62	63	63	64	64	65	66	66	67	67	68	68	69	69	70	70	71	71	72		
48	49	49	50	50	51	51	52	52	53	53	54	54	55	55	56	56	57	57	58	58	59	59	60	60	61	62	62	63	63	64	64	65	65	66	66	67	67	68	68	69	69	70	70	71	71	72	72	73	
49	50	50	51	51	52	52	53	53	54	54	55	55	56	56	57	57	58	58	59	59	60	60	61	61	62	62	63	63	64	64	65	65	66	66	67	67	68	68	69	69	70	70	71	71	72	72	73	73	74	
50	51	51	52	52	53	53	54	54	55	55	56	56	57	57	58	58	59	59	60	60	61	61	62	62	63	63	64	64	65	65	66	66	67	67	68	68	69	69	70	70	71	71	72	72	73	73	74	74	75	75
	1	**2**	**3**	**4**	**5**	**6**	**7**	**8**	**9**	**10**	**11**	**12**	**13**	**14**	**15**	**16**	**17**	**18**	**19**	**20**	**21**	**22**	**23**	**24**	**25**	**26**	**27**	**28**	**29**	**30**	**31**	**32**	**33**	**34**	**35**	**36**	**37**	**38**	**39**	**40**	**41**	**42**	**43**	**44**	**45**	**46**	**47**	**48**	**49**	**50**

COMBINED VALUES CHART (CONTINUED)

	1	2	3	4	5	6	7	8	9	10	11	12	13	14	15	16	17	18	19	20	21	22	23	24	25
51	51	52	52	53	53	54	54	55	55	56	56	57	57	58	58	59	59	60	60	61	61	62	62	63	63
52	52	53	53	54	54	55	55	56	56	57	57	58	58	59	59	60	60	61	61	62	62	63	63	64	64
53	53	54	54	55	55	56	56	57	57	58	58	59	59	60	60	61	61	61	62	62	63	63	64	64	65
54	54	55	55	56	56	57	57	58	58	59	59	59	60	60	61	61	62	62	63	63	64	64	65	65	66
55	55	56	56	57	57	58	58	59	59	60	60	60	61	61	62	62	63	63	64	64	64	65	65	66	66
56	56	57	57	58	58	59	59	60	60	60	61	61	62	62	63	63	63	64	64	65	65	66	66	67	67
57	57	58	58	59	59	60	60	60	61	61	62	62	63	63	63	64	64	65	65	66	66	66	67	67	68
58	58	59	59	60	60	61	61	61	62	62	63	63	63	64	64	65	65	66	66	66	67	67	68	68	68
59	59	60	60	61	61	61	62	62	63	63	64	64	64	65	65	66	66	66	67	67	68	68	68	69	69
60	60	61	61	62	62	62	63	63	64	64	64	65	65	66	66	66	67	67	68	68	68	69	69	70	70
61	61	62	62	63	63	63	64	64	65	65	65	66	66	66	67	67	68	68	68	69	69	70	70	70	71
62	62	63	63	64	64	64	65	65	65	66	66	67	67	67	68	68	68	69	69	70	70	70	71	71	72
63	63	64	64	64	65	65	66	66	66	67	67	67	68	68	69	69	69	70	70	70	71	71	72	72	72
64	64	65	65	65	66	66	67	67	67	68	68	68	69	69	69	70	70	70	71	71	72	72	72	73	73
65	65	66	66	66	67	67	67	68	68	69	69	69	70	70	70	71	71	71	72	72	72	73	73	73	74
66	66	67	67	67	68	68	68	69	69	69	70	70	70	71	71	71	72	72	72	73	73	73	74	74	75
67	67	68	68	68	69	69	69	70	70	70	71	71	71	72	72	72	73	73	73	74	74	74	75	75	75
68	68	69	69	69	70	70	70	71	71	71	72	72	72	72	73	73	73	74	74	74	75	75	75	76	76
69	69	70	70	70	71	71	71	71	72	72	72	73	73	73	74	74	74	75	75	75	76	76	76	76	77
70	70	71	71	71	72	72	72	72	73	73	73	74	74	74	75	75	75	75	76	76	76	77	77	77	78
71	71	72	72	72	72	73	73	73	74	74	74	74	75	75	75	76	76	76	77	77	77	77	78	78	78
72	72	73	73	73	73	74	74	74	75	75	75	75	76	76	76	76	77	77	77	78	78	78	78	79	79
73	73	74	74	74	74	75	75	75	75	76	76	76	77	77	77	77	78	78	78	78	79	79	79	79	80
74	74	75	75	75	75	76	76	76	76	77	77	77	77	78	78	78	78	79	79	79	79	80	80	80	81
75	75	76	76	76	76	77	77	77	77	78	78	78	78	79	79	79	79	80	80	80	80	81	81	81	81
76	76	76	77	77	77	77	78	78	78	78	79	79	79	79	80	80	80	80	81	81	81	81	82	82	82
77	77	77	78	78	78	78	79	79	79	79	80	80	80	80	80	81	81	81	81	82	82	82	82	83	83
78	78	78	79	79	79	79	80	80	80	80	80	81	81	81	81	82	82	82	82	82	83	83	83	83	84
79	79	79	80	80	80	80	80	81	81	81	81	82	82	82	82	82	83	83	83	83	83	84	84	84	84
80	80	80	81	81	81	81	81	82	82	82	82	82	83	83	83	83	83	84	84	84	84	84	85	85	85
81	81	81	82	82	82	82	82	83	83	83	83	83	83	84	84	84	84	84	85	85	85	85	85	86	86
82	82	82	83	83	83	83	83	83	84	84	84	84	84	85	85	85	85	85	85	86	86	86	86	86	87
83	83	83	84	84	84	84	84	84	85	85	85	85	85	85	86	86	86	86	86	86	87	87	87	87	87
84	84	84	84	85	85	85	85	85	85	86	86	86	86	86	86	87	87	87	87	87	87	88	88	88	88
85	85	85	85	86	86	86	86	86	86	87	87	87	87	87	87	87	88	88	88	88	88	88	88	89	89
86	86	86	86	87	87	87	87	87	87	87	88	88	88	88	88	88	88	89	89	89	89	89	89	89	90
87	87	87	87	88	88	88	88	88	88	88	88	89	89	89	89	89	89	89	89	90	90	90	90	90	90
88	88	88	88	88	89	89	89	89	89	89	89	89	90	90	90	90	90	90	90	90	91	91	91	91	91
89	89	89	89	89	90	90	90	90	90	90	90	90	90	91	91	91	91	91	91	91	91	91	92	92	92
90	90	90	90	90	91	91	91	91	91	91	91	91	91	91	92	92	92	92	92	92	92	92	92	92	93
91	91	91	91	91	91	92	92	92	92	92	92	92	92	92	92	92	93	93	93	93	93	93	93	93	93
92	92	92	92	92	92	92	93	93	93	93	93	93	93	93	93	93	93	93	94	94	94	94	94	94	94
93	93	93	93	93	93	93	93	94	94	94	94	94	94	94	94	94	94	94	94	94	94	95	95	95	95
94	94	94	94	94	94	94	94	94	95	95	95	95	95	95	95	95	95	95	95	95	95	95	95	95	96
95	95	95	95	95	95	95	95	95	95	96	96	96	96	96	96	96	96	96	96	96	96	96	96	96	96
96	96	96	96	96	96	96	96	96	96	96	96	96	97	97	97	97	97	97	97	97	97	97	97	97	97
97	97	97	97	97	97	97	97	97	97	97	97	97	97	97	97	97	98	98	98	98	98	98	98	98	98
98	98	98	98	98	98	98	98	98	98	98	98	98	98	98	98	98	98	98	98	98	98	98	98	98	99
99	99	99	99	99	99	99	99	99	99	99	99	99	99	99	99	99	99	99	99	99	99	99	99	99	99
	1	2	3	4	5	6	7	8	9	10	11	12	13	14	15	16	17	18	19	20	21	22	23	24	25

	26	27	28	29	30	31	32	33	34	35	36	37	38	39	40	41	42	43	44	45	46	47	48	49	50
51	64	64	65	65	66	66	67	67	68	68	69	69	70	70	71	71	72	72	73	73	74	74	75	75	76
52	64	65	65	66	66	67	67	68	68	69	69	70	70	71	71	72	72	73	73	74	74	75	75	76	76
53	65	66	66	67	67	68	68	69	69	69	70	70	71	71	72	72	73	73	74	74	75	75	76	76	77
54	66	66	67	67	68	68	69	69	70	70	71	71	71	72	72	73	73	74	74	75	75	76	76	77	77
55	67	67	68	68	69	69	69	70	70	71	71	72	72	73	73	73	74	74	75	75	76	76	77	77	78
56	67	68	68	69	69	70	70	71	71	71	72	72	73	73	74	74	74	75	75	76	76	77	77	78	78
57	68	69	69	69	70	70	71	71	72	72	72	73	73	74	74	75	75	75	76	76	77	77	78	78	79
58	69	69	70	70	71	71	71	72	72	73	73	74	74	74	75	75	76	76	76	77	77	78	78	79	79
59	70	70	70	71	71	72	72	73	73	73	74	74	75	75	75	76	76	77	77	77	78	78	79	79	80
60	70	71	71	72	72	72	73	73	74	74	74	75	75	76	76	76	77	77	78	78	78	79	79	80	80
61	71	72	72	72	73	73	73	74	74	75	75	75	76	76	77	77	77	78	78	79	79	79	80	80	81
62	72	72	73	73	73	74	74	75	75	75	76	76	76	77	77	78	78	78	79	79	79	80	80	81	81
63	73	73	73	74	74	74	75	75	76	76	76	77	77	77	78	78	79	79	79	80	80	80	81	81	82
64	73	74	74	74	75	75	76	76	76	77	77	77	78	78	78	79	79	79	80	80	81	81	81	82	82
65	74	74	75	75	76	76	76	77	77	77	78	78	78	79	79	79	80	80	80	81	81	81	82	82	83
66	75	75	76	76	76	77	77	77	78	78	78	79	79	79	80	80	80	81	81	81	82	82	82	83	83
67	76	76	76	77	77	77	78	78	78	79	79	79	80	80	80	81	81	81	82	82	82	83	83	83	84
68	76	77	77	77	78	78	78	79	79	79	80	80	80	80	81	81	81	82	82	82	83	83	83	84	84
69	77	77	78	78	78	79	79	79	80	80	80	80	81	81	81	82	82	82	83	83	83	84	84	84	85
70	78	78	78	79	79	79	80	80	80	81	81	81	81	82	82	82	83	83	83	84	84	84	84	85	85
71	79	79	79	79	80	80	80	81	81	81	81	82	82	82	83	83	83	83	84	84	84	85	85	85	86
72	79	80	80	80	80	81	81	81	82	82	82	82	83	83	83	83	84	84	84	85	85	85	85	86	86
73	80	80	81	81	81	81	82	82	82	82	83	83	83	84	84	84	84	85	85	85	85	86	86	86	87
74	81	81	81	82	82	82	82	83	83	83	83	84	84	84	84	85	85	85	85	86	86	86	86	87	87
75	82	82	82	82	83	83	83	83	84	84	84	84	85	85	85	85	86	86	86	86	87	87	87	87	88
76	82	82	83	83	83	83	84	84	84	84	85	85	85	85	86	86	86	86	87	87	87	87	88	88	88
77	83	83	83	84	84	84	84	85	85	85	85	86	86	86	86	86	87	87	87	87	88	88	88	88	89
78	84	84	84	84	85	85	85	85	85	86	86	86	86	87	87	87	87	87	88	88	88	88	89	89	89
79	84	85	85	85	85	86	86	86	86	86	87	87	87	87	87	88	88	88	88	88	89	89	89	89	90
80	85	85	86	86	86	86	86	87	87	87	87	87	88	88	88	88	88	89	89	89	89	89	90	90	90
81	86	86	86	87	87	87	87	87	87	88	88	88	88	88	89	89	89	89	89	90	90	90	90	90	91
82	87	87	87	87	87	88	88	88	88	88	88	89	89	89	89	89	90	90	90	90	90	90	91	91	91
83	87	88	88	88	88	88	88	89	89	89	89	89	89	90	90	90	90	90	90	91	91	91	91	91	92
84	88	88	88	89	89	89	89	89	89	90	90	90	90	90	90	91	91	91	91	91	91	92	92	92	92
85	89	89	89	89	90	90	90	90	90	90	90	91	91	91	91	91	91	91	92	92	92	92	92	92	93
86	90	90	90	90	90	90	90	91	91	91	91	91	91	91	92	92	92	92	92	92	92	93	93	93	93
87	90	91	91	91	91	91	91	91	91	92	92	92	92	92	92	92	92	93	93	93	93	93	93	93	94
88	91	91	91	91	92	92	92	92	92	92	92	92	93	93	93	93	93	93	93	93	94	94	94	94	94
89	92	92	92	92	92	92	93	93	93	93	93	93	93	93	93	94	94	94	94	94	94	94	94	94	95
90	93	93	93	93	93	93	93	93	93	94	94	94	94	94	94	94	94	94	94	95	95	95	95	95	95
91	93	93	94	94	94	94	94	94	94	94	94	94	94	95	95	95	95	95	95	95	95	95	95	95	96
92	94	94	94	94	94	94	95	95	95	95	95	95	95	95	95	95	95	95	96	96	96	96	96	96	96
93	95	95	95	95	95	95	95	95	95	95	96	96	96	96	96	96	96	96	96	96	96	96	96	96	97
94	96	96	96	96	96	96	96	96	96	96	96	96	96	96	96	96	97	97	97	97	97	97	97	97	97
95	96	96	96	96	96	97	97	97	97	97	97	97	97	97	97	97	97	97	97	97	97	97	97	97	98
96	97	97	97	97	97	97	97	97	97	97	97	97	98	98	98	98	98	98	98	98	98	98	98	98	98
97	98	98	98	98	98	98	98	98	98	98	98	98	98	98	98	98	98	98	98	98	98	98	98	98	99
98	99	99	99	99	99	99	99	99	99	99	99	99	99	99	99	99	99	99	99	99	99	99	99	99	99
99	99	99	99	99	99	99	99	99	99	99	99	99	99	99	99	99	99	99	99	99	99	99	99	99	100
	26	27	28	29	30	31	32	33	34	35	36	37	38	39	40	41	42	43	44	45	46	47	48	49	50

COMBINED VALUES CHART (CONTINUED)

51	76
52	76	77
53	77	77	78
54	77	78	78	79
55	78	78	79	79	80
56	78	79	79	80	80	81
57	79	79	80	80	81	81	82
58	79	80	80	81	81	82	82	82
59	80	80	81	81	82	82	82	83	83
60	80	81	81	82	82	82	83	83	84	84
61	81	81	82	82	82	83	83	84	84	84	85
62	81	82	82	83	83	83	84	84	84	85	85	86
63	82	82	83	83	83	84	84	84	85	85	86	86	86
64	82	83	83	83	84	84	85	85	85	86	86	86	87	87
65	83	83	84	84	84	85	85	85	86	86	86	87	87	87	88
66	83	84	84	84	85	85	85	86	86	86	87	87	87	88	88	88
67	84	84	84	85	85	85	86	86	86	87	87	87	88	88	88	88	89
68	84	85	85	85	86	86	86	87	87	87	88	88	88	88	89	89	89	90
69	85	85	85	86	86	86	87	87	87	88	88	88	89	89	89	89	90	90	90
70	85	86	86	86	87	87	87	87	88	88	88	89	89	89	90	90	90	90	91	91
71	86	86	86	87	87	87	88	88	88	88	89	89	89	90	90	90	90	91	91	91	92
72	86	87	87	87	87	88	88	88	89	89	89	89	90	90	90	93	91	91	91	92	92	92
73	87	87	87	88	88	88	88	89	89	89	89	90	90	90	91	91	91	91	92	92	92	92	93
74	87	88	88	88	88	89	89	89	89	90	90	90	90	91	91	91	91	92	92	92	92	93	93	93
75	88	88	88	89	89	89	89	90	90	90	90	91	91	91	91	92	92	92	92	93	93	93	93	94	94
76	88	88	89	89	89	89	90	90	90	90	91	91	91	91	92	92	92	92	93	93	93	93	94	94	94	94
77	89	89	89	89	90	90	90	90	91	91	91	91	91	92	92	92	92	93	93	93	93	94	94	94	94	94	95
78	89	89	90	90	90	90	91	91	91	91	91	92	92	92	92	93	93	93	93	93	94	94	94	94	95	95	95	95
79	90	90	90	90	91	91	91	91	91	92	92	92	92	92	93	93	93	93	93	94	94	94	94	95	95	95	95	95	96
80	90	90	91	91	91	91	91	92	92	92	92	92	93	93	93	93	93	94	94	94	94	94	95	95	95	95	95	96	96	96
81	91	91	91	91	91	92	92	92	92	92	93	93	93	93	93	94	94	94	94	94	94	95	95	95	95	95	96	96	96	96	96
82	91	91	92	92	92	92	92	92	93	93	93	93	93	94	94	94	94	94	94	95	95	95	95	95	96	96	96	96	96	96	97	97
83	92	92	92	92	92	93	93	93	93	93	93	94	94	94	94	94	94	95	95	95	95	95	95	96	96	96	96	96	96	97	97	97	97
84	92	92	92	93	93	93	93	93	93	94	94	94	94	94	94	95	95	95	95	95	95	96	96	96	96	96	96	96	97	97	97	97	97	97
85	93	93	93	93	93	93	94	94	94	94	94	94	94	95	95	95	95	95	95	96	96	96	96	96	96	96	97	97	97	97	97	97	97	98	98
86	93	93	93	94	94	94	94	94	94	94	95	95	95	95	95	95	95	96	96	96	96	96	96	96	97	97	97	97	97	97	97	97	98	98	98	98
87	94	94	94	94	94	94	94	95	95	95	95	95	95	95	95	96	96	96	96	96	96	96	96	97	97	97	97	97	97	97	98	98	98	98	98	98	98
88	94	94	94	94	95	95	95	95	95	95	95	95	95	96	96	96	96	96	96	96	97	97	97	97	97	97	97	97	97	98	98	98	98	98	98	98	98	99
89	95	95	95	95	95	95	95	95	95	96	96	96	96	96	96	96	96	96	97	97	97	97	97	97	97	97	97	98	98	98	98	98	98	98	98	98	99	99	99
90	95	95	95	95	96	96	96	96	96	96	96	96	96	96	97	97	97	97	97	97	97	97	97	97	98	98	98	98	98	98	98	98	98	98	99	99	99	99	99	99
91	96	96	96	96	96	96	96	96	96	96	96	97	97	97	97	97	97	97	97	97	97	97	98	98	98	98	98	98	98	98	98	98	98	99	99	99	99	99	99	99	99
92	96	96	96	96	96	96	97	97	97	97	97	97	97	97	97	97	97	97	98	98	98	98	98	98	98	98	98	98	98	98	98	99	99	99	99	99	99	99	99	99	99	99
93	97	97	97	97	97	97	97	97	97	97	97	97	97	97	98	98	98	98	98	98	98	98	98	98	98	98	98	98	99	99	99	99	99	99	99	99	99	99	99	99	99	99	100
94	97	97	97	97	97	97	97	97	98	98	98	98	98	98	98	98	98	98	98	98	98	98	98	98	99	99	99	99	99	99	99	99	99	99	99	99	99	99	99	99	99	100	100	100
95	98	98	98	98	98	98	98	98	98	98	98	98	98	98	98	98	98	98	98	99	99	99	99	99	99	99	99	99	99	99	99	99	99	99	99	99	99	99	99	100	100	100	100	100	100
96	98	98	98	98	98	98	98	98	98	98	98	98	99	99	99	99	99	99	99	99	99	99	99	99	99	99	99	99	99	99	99	99	99	99	99	99	99	100	100	100	100	100	100	100	100	100
97	99	99	99	99	99	99	99	99	99	99	99	99	99	99	99	99	99	99	99	99	99	99	99	99	99	99	99	99	99	99	99	99	99	100	100	100	100	100	100	100	100	100	100	100	100	100	100
98	99	99	99	99	99	99	99	99	99	99	99	99	99	99	99	99	99	99	99	99	99	99	99	99	100	100	100	100	100	100	100	100	100	100	100	100	100	100	100	100	100	100	100	100	100	100	100	100
99	100	100	100	100	100	100	100	100	100	100	100	100	100	100	100	100	100	100	100	100	100	100	100	100	100	100	100	100	100	100	100	100	100	100	100	100	100	100	100	100	100	100	100	100	100	100	100	100	100
	51	**52**	**53**	**54**	**55**	**56**	**57**	**58**	**59**	**60**	**61**	**62**	**63**	**64**	**65**	**66**	**67**	**68**	**69**	**70**	**71**	**72**	**73**	**74**	**75**	**76**	**77**	**78**	**79**	**80**	**81**	**82**	**83**	**84**	**85**	**86**	**87**	**88**	**89**	**90**	**91**	**92**	**93**	**94**	**95**	**96**	**97**	**98**	**99**

SECTION 7

PRODUCT IDENTIFICATION GUIDE

To aid in quick identification, manufacturers participating in this section have furnished full-color photographs of selected ophthalmic products. Capsules and tablets are shown in actual size. Tubes, bottles, boxes, and other types of packaging appear in reduced size to fit available space.

For more information on any of the products in this section, please turn to the Pharmaceutical Product Information section, or check directly with the manufacturer. The page number of each product's text entry appears above its photograph.

While every effort has been made to guarantee faithful reproduction of the products in this section, changes in size, color, and design are always a possibility. Be sure to confirm a product's identity with the manufacturer or your pharmacist.

For your convenience, reporductions of the Rosenbaum Vision Screener and a Color Vision Screening Chart can be found at the end of the section.

MANUFACTURERS INDEX

PRODUCT INDEX

AKORN, INC.

P. 203
(Also Available in Ampuls)

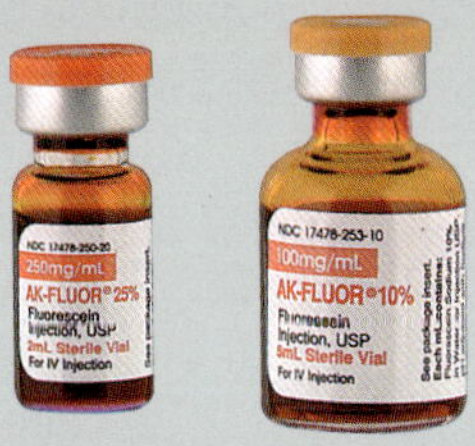

25% 2 mL 10% 5 mL

AK-Fluor®
(fluorescein injection U.S.P.)

ALLERGAN, INC.

P. 244

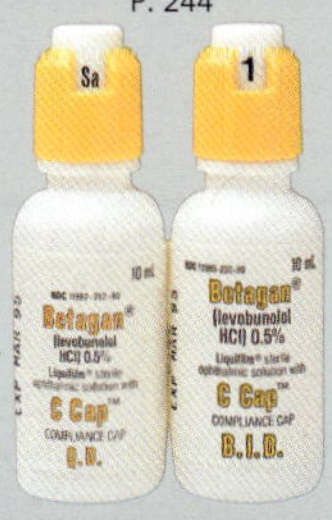

Betagan® Liquifilm® Sterile Ophthalmic Solution
With C Cap® Compliance Cap Q.D. and B.I.D.
(levobunolol HCl) 0.5%

P. 255

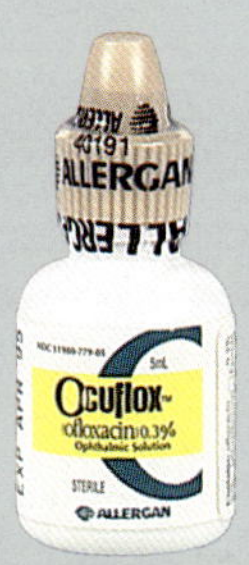

5 mL

Ocuflox™
(ofloxacin ophthalmic solution) 0.3%

P. 263

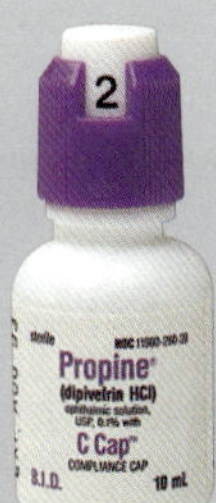

Propine®
Ophthalmic Solution, USP, 0.1%
With C Cap® Compliance B.I.D.
(dipivefrin HCl)

BAUSCH & LOMB

Personal Products Division
P. 265

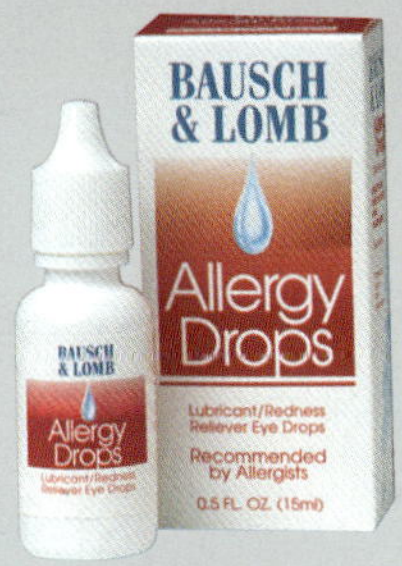

0.5 fl. oz.

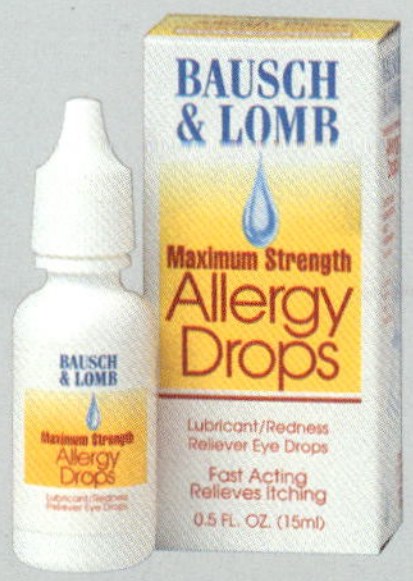

0.5 fl. oz.

Bausch & Lomb® Allergy Drops
Regular & Maximum Strength
Lubricant/Redness Reliever Eye Drops

Bausch & Lomb
P. 265

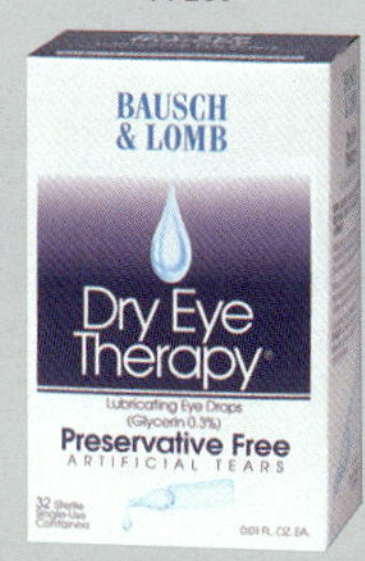

32 Sterile Single-Use Containers
0.01 fl. oz.

Dry Eye Therapy®
Lubricating Eye Drops
Preservative-Free Artificial Tears

P. 266

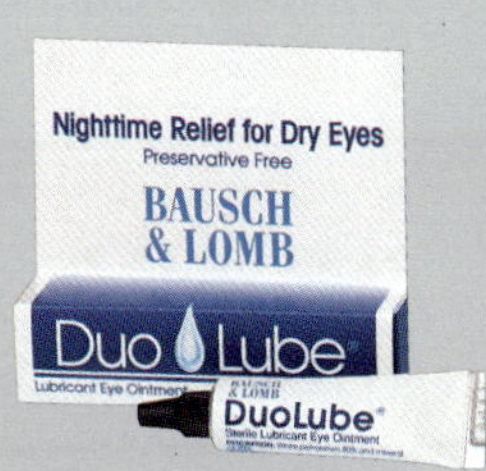

1/8 oz.

Duolube®
Lubricant Eye Ointment Preservative-Free
Nighttime Relief for Dry Eyes

P. 266

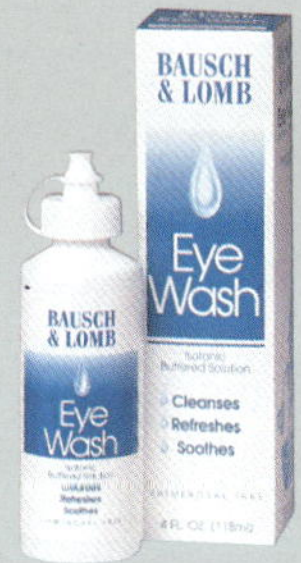

4 fl. oz.

Bausch & Lomb® Eye Wash
Cleanses, Refreshes and
Soothes Irritated Eyes

P. 266

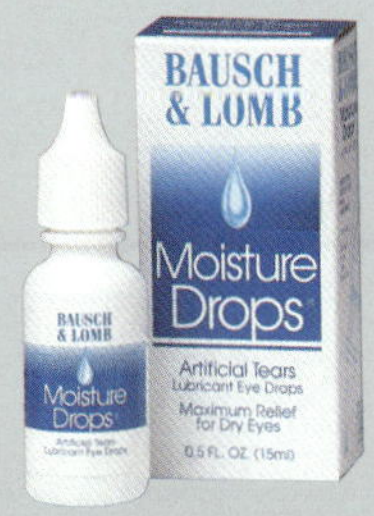

0.5 and 1.0 fl. oz. sizes

Moisture Drops® Artificial Tears
Lubricant Eye Drops
Soothing Relief for Dry Eyes

BAUSCH & LOMB

Pharmaceutical Division
P. 267

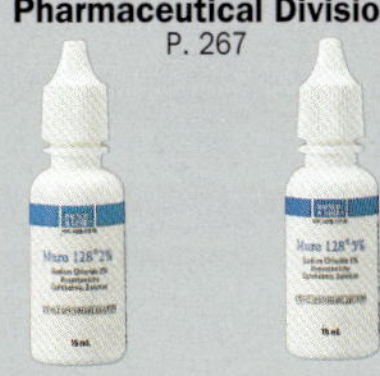

2% 15 mL 5% 15 mL

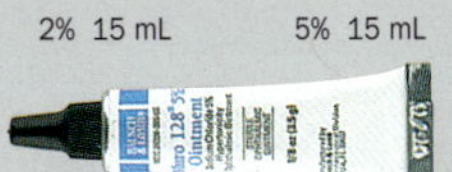

5% Ointment 3.5 g

Muro 128®
Hypertonicity Solutions & Ointment
(sodium chloride 2%, 5%)

P. 268

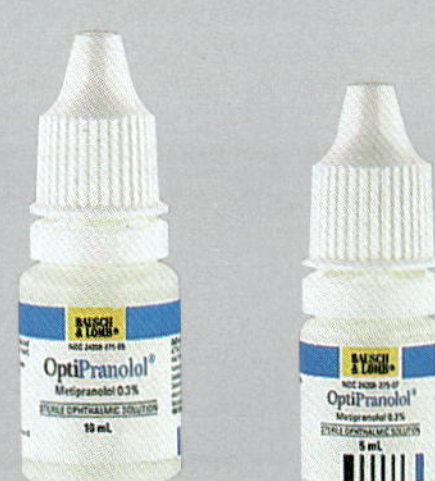

10 mL 5 mL

OptiPranolol®
Sterile Ophthalmic Solution
(metipranolol .3%)

BURROUGHS WELLCOME

P. 271

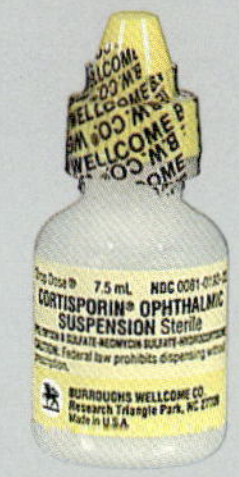

Plastic Drop Dose® dispenser bottle 7.5 mL

Cortisporin® Ophthalmic Suspension Sterile
(neomycin and polymyxin B sulfates,
hydrocortisone)

P. 270

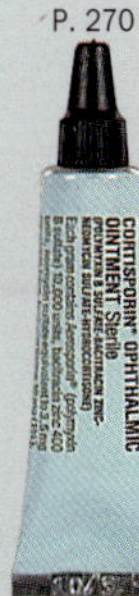

1/8 oz. (3.5 g) tube with ophthalmic tip

Cortisporin® Ophthalmic Ointment Sterile
(polysporin B sulfate, bacitracin zinc,
neomycin sulfate, hydrocortisone)

P. 272

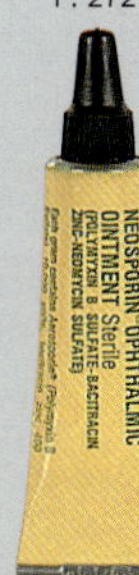

1/8 oz. (3.5 g) tube with ophthalmic tip

Neosporin® Ophthalmic Ointment Sterile
(polymyxin B sulfate, bacitracin zinc,
neomycin sulfate)

P. 273

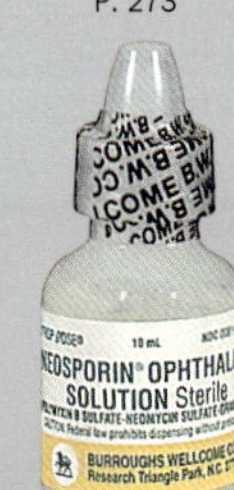

10 mL
Plastic Drop Dose® dispenser bottle

Neosporin® Ophthalmic Solution Sterile
(neomycin and polymyxin B sulfates,
bacitracin zinc)

Burroughs Wellcome
P. 274

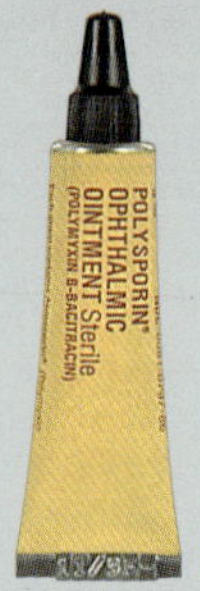

1/8 oz. tube with ophthalmic tip

Polysporin® Ophthalmic Ointment Sterile
(polymyxin B, bacitracin)

P. 274

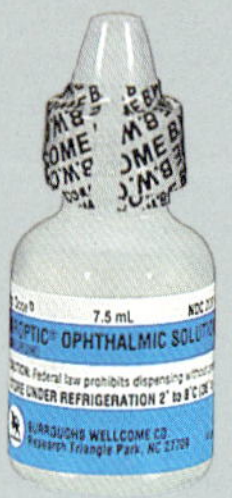

7.5 mL
Plastic Drop Dose® dispenser bottle

Viroptic® Ophthalmic Solution
1% Sterile
(trifluridine)

CIBA VISION

Ophthalmics
P. 277

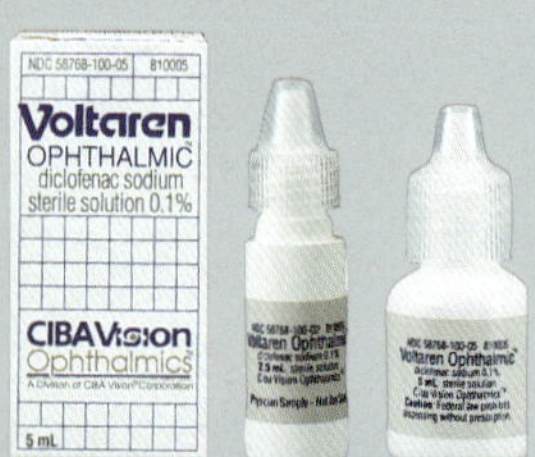

2.5 mL 5 mL

Voltaren Ophthalmic®
(diclofenac sodium sterile ophthalmic solution 0.1%)

IOLAB

P. 283

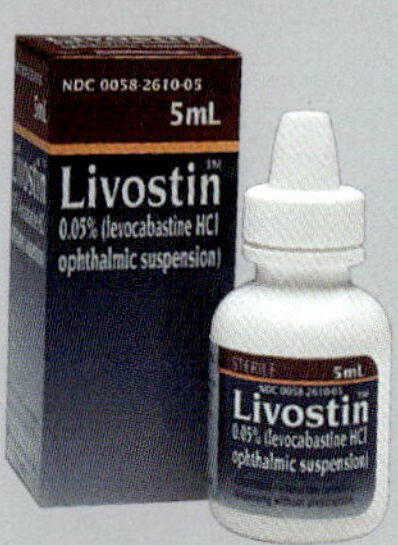

5 mL Ophthalmic Suspension

Livostin™
(levocabastine HCl)

IOLAB
P. 284

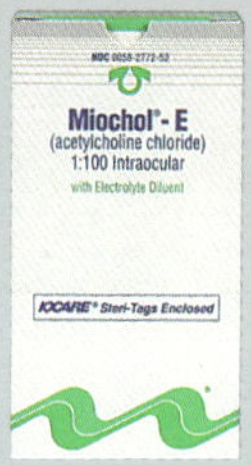

Pack contains: Miochol-E 2 mL univial, IOCARE Steri-Tags (sterile syringe labels for drug identification)

Miochol®-E 1:100 Intraocular with Electrolyte Diluent
(acetycholine chloride)

P. 284

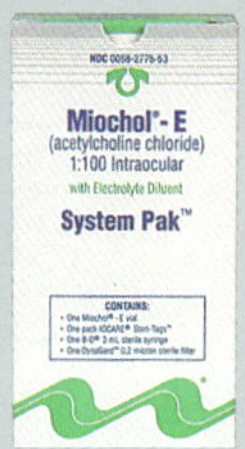

Pack contains: Miochol-E 2 mL univial, IOCARE Steri-Tags sterile labels, B-D 3 mL sterile syringe, DynaGard 0.2 micron sterile filter

Miochol®-E 1:100 Intraocular with Electrolyte Diluent System Pak™
(acetylcholine chloride intraocular)

P. 284

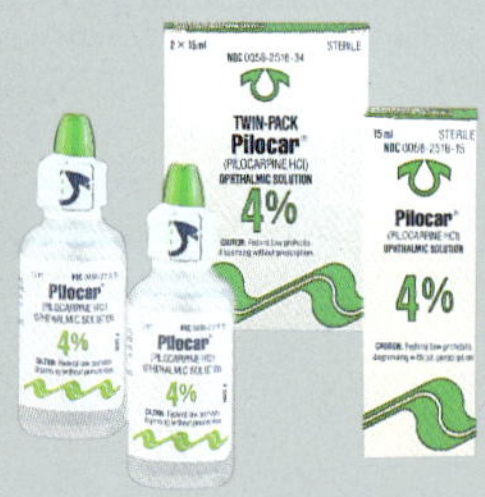

Available in 6 strengths:
1/2%, 1%, 2%, 3%, 4%, 6%
Twin Packs (2x15 mL) & Singles (15 mL)

Pilocar® Ophthalmic Solution
(pilocarpine HCl)

MERCK & CO., INC.

P. 290

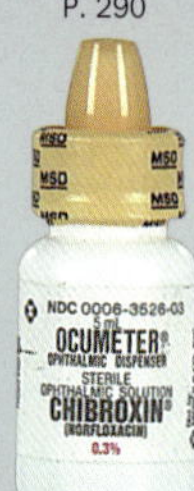

3526* 5 mL 0.3%

Chibroxin®
Sterile Ophthalmic Solution
OCUMETER® Ophthalmic Dispenser
(norfloxacin)

Merck & Co., Inc.
P. 291

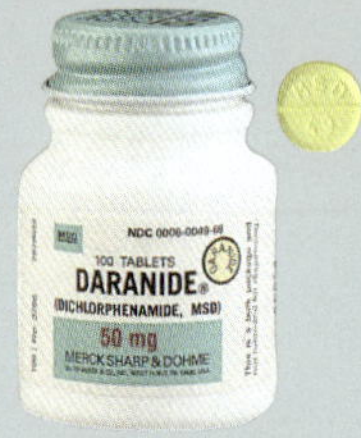

3256* 50 mg Bottle of 100

Daranide®
(dichlorphenamide)

P. 292

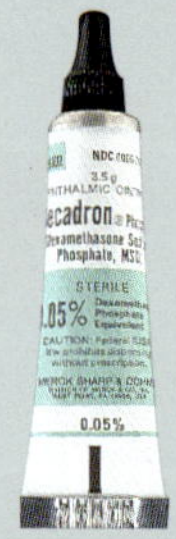

7615* 3.5-g tube 0.05%

Decadron® Phosphate
Sterile Ophthalmic Ointment
(dexamethasone sodium phosphate)

P. 293

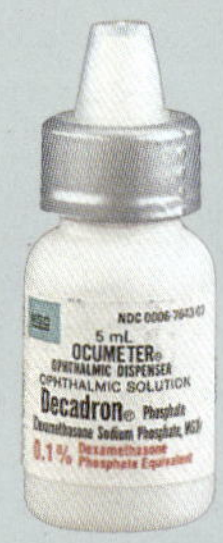

7643* 5 mL 0.1%

Decadron® Phosphate
Sterile Ophthalmic Solution
OCUMETER® Ophthalmic Dispenser
(dexamethasone sodium phosphate)

P. 294

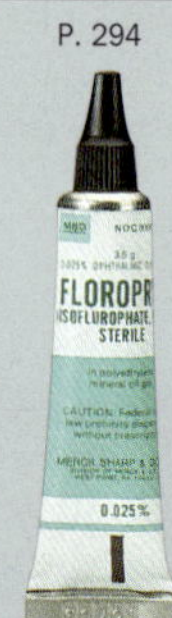

7742* 3.5-g tube 0.025%

Floropryl®
Sterile Ophthalmic Ointment
(isoflurophate)

Merck & Co., Inc.
P. 295

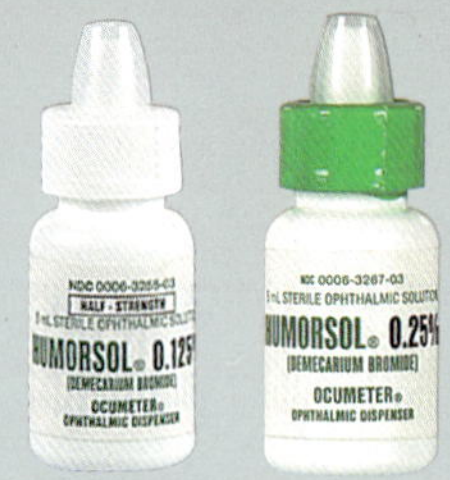

3255* 5 mL 0.125%　**3267*** 5 mL 0.25%

Humorsol®
Sterile Ophthalmic Solution
OCUMETER® Ophthalmic Dispenser
(demecarium bromide)

P. 297

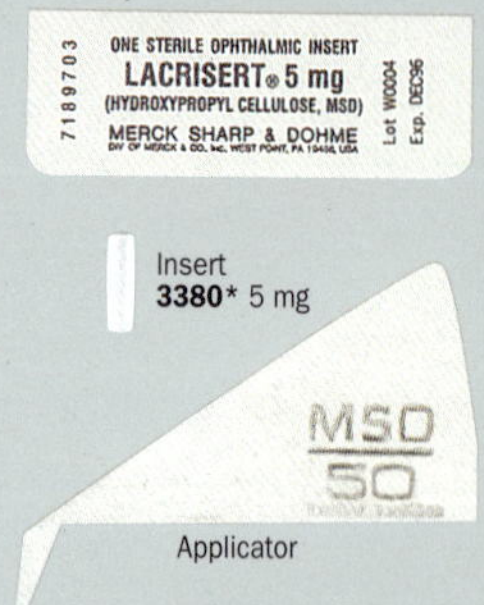

Insert
3380* 5 mg

Applicator

Lacrisert®
Sterile Ophthalmic Insert
(hydroxypropyl cellulose)

P. 298

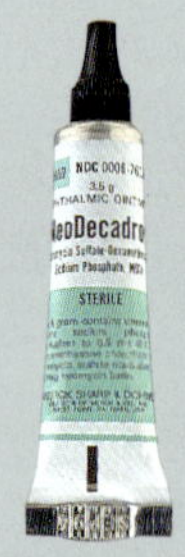

7617* 3.5-g tube 0.05%

NeoDecadron®
Sterile Ophthalmic Ointment
(neomycin sulfate-dexamethasone sodium phosphate)

P. 299

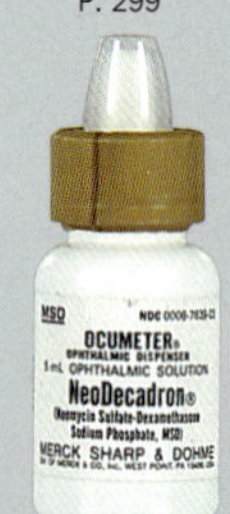

7639* 5 mL

NeoDecadron®
Sterile Ophthalmic Solution
OCUMETER® Ophthalmic Dispenser
(neomycin sulfate-dexamethasone sodium phosphate)

*Manufacturer's identification code

P. 299

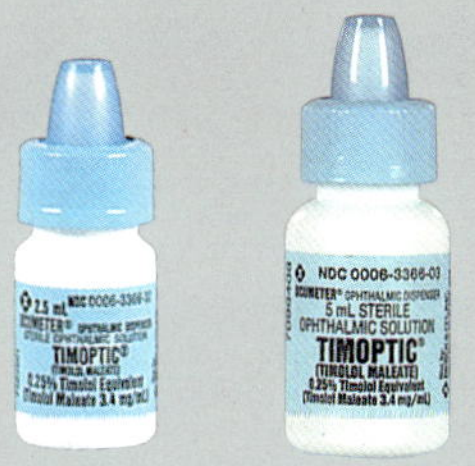

2.5 mL 5 mL

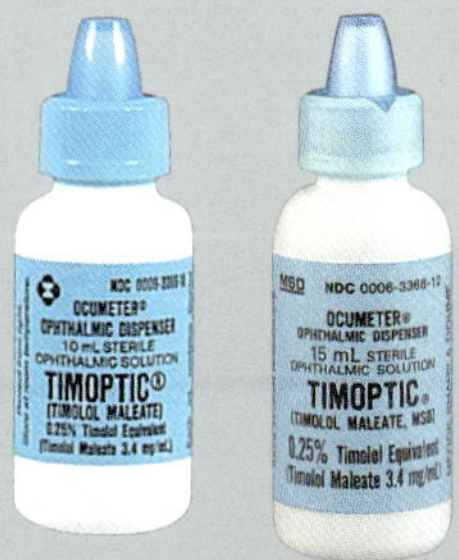

10 mL 15 mL
3366* 0.25% timolol equivalent

Timoptic®
Sterile Ophthalmic Solution
OCUMETER® Ophthalmic Dispenser
(timolol maleate)

P. 299

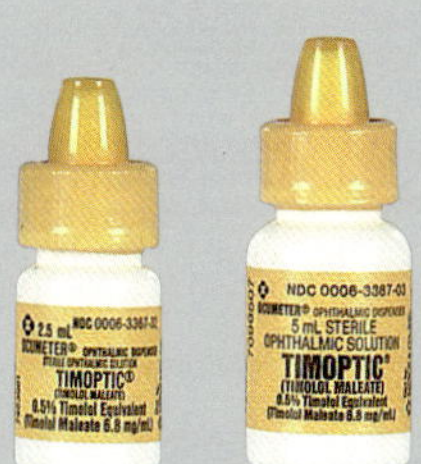

2.5 mL 5 mL

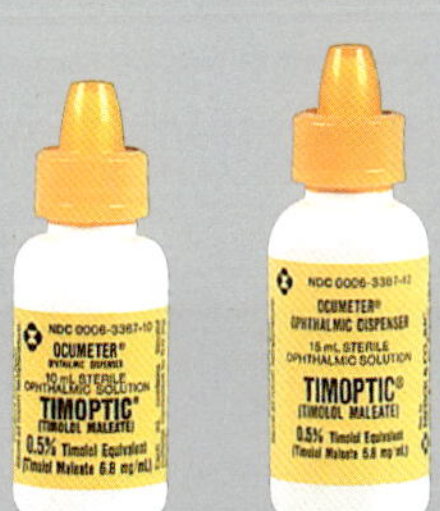

10 mL 15 mL
3367* 0.5% timolol equivalent

Timoptic®
Sterile Ophthalmic Solution
OCUMETER® Ophthalmic Dispenser
(timolol maleate)

Merck & Co., Inc.
P. 302

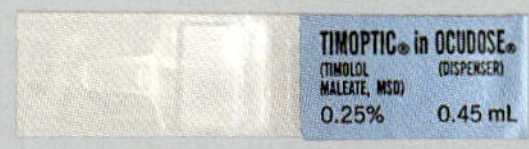

3542* 0.45 mL
0.25% timolol equivalent

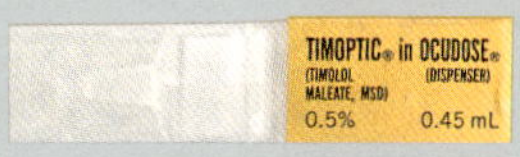

3543* 0.45 mL
0.5% timolol equivalent

Timoptic®
Preservative-Free
Sterile Ophthalmic Solution
in OCUDOSE® Dispenser
(timolol maleate)

P. 305

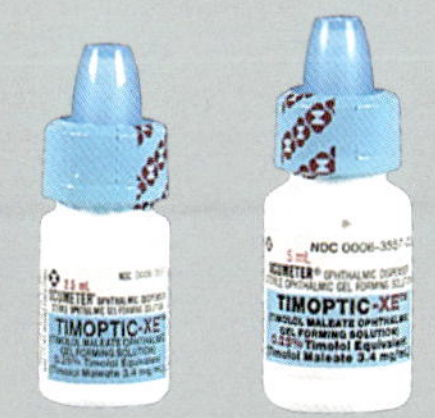

2.5 mL 5 mL
3557* 0.25% timolol equivalent

Timoptic-XE™
Sterile Ophthalmic Gel Forming Solution
OCUMETER® Ophthalmic Dispenser
(timolol maleate ophthalmic
gel forming solution)

P. 305

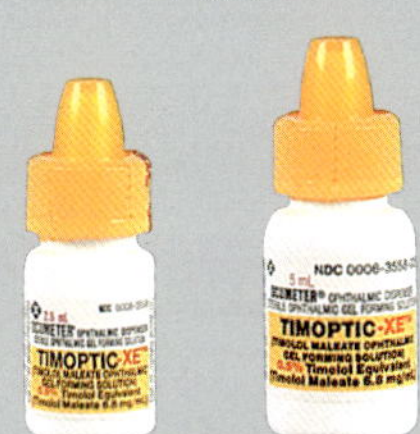

2.5 mL 5 mL

3558* 0.5% timolol equivalent

Timoptic-XE™
Sterile Ophthalmic Gel Forming Solution
OCUMETER® Ophthalmic Dispenser
(timolol maleate ophthalmic
gel forming solution)

OTSUKA AMERICA
Pharmaceutical, Inc.
P. 308

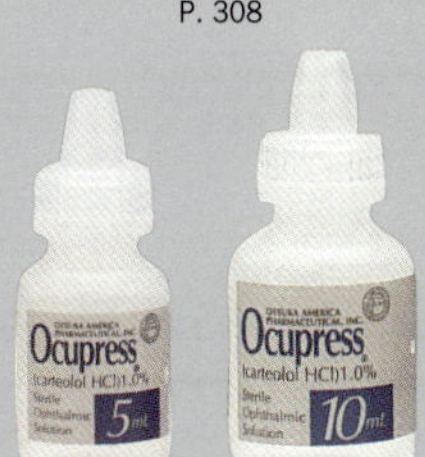

5 mL 10 mL

Ocupress®
(carteolol HCl) 1%

PARKE-DAVIS
P. 311

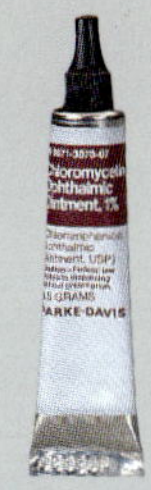

3.5 grams

Chloromycetin®
Ophthalmic Ointment 1%
Preservative Free (chloramphenicol
ophthalmic ointment, USP)

P. 311

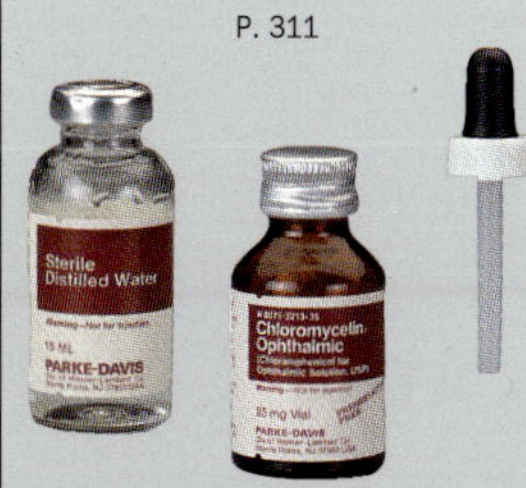

Distilled Water | 25 mg Sterile Powder | Dropper

Chloromycetin® Ophthalmic
Preservative Free
(chloramphenicol for ophthalmic
solution, USP)

P. 310

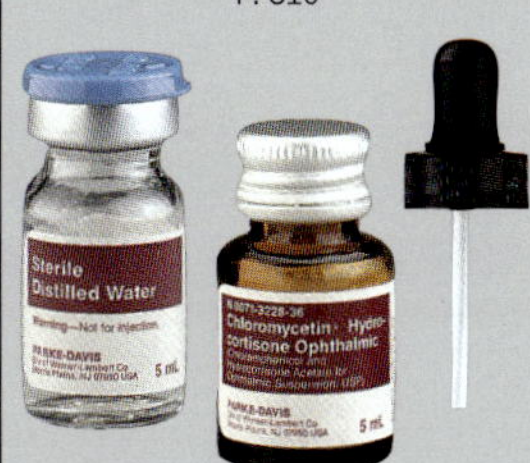

Distilled Water | 5 mL Sterile Powder | Dropper

Chloromycetin® Hydrocortisone Ophthalmic
(chloramphenicol and hydrocortisone
acetate for suspension, USP)

P. 312

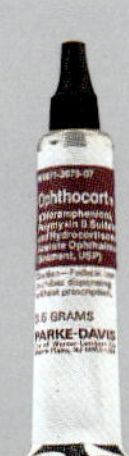

3.5 grams

Ophthocort®
Preservative Free
(chloramphenicol, polymyxin
B sulfate, and hydrocortisone
acetate ophthalmic ointment, USP)

P. 313

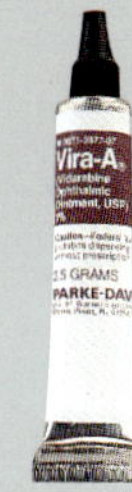

3.5 grams

Vira-A®
Ophthalmic Ointment 3%
Preservative Free
(vidarabine ophthalmic ointment,USP)

PFIZER
Consumer Health Care
P. 314

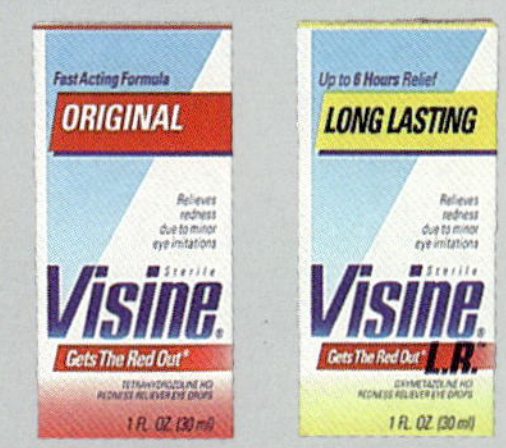

Original Formula | Long Lasting Relief

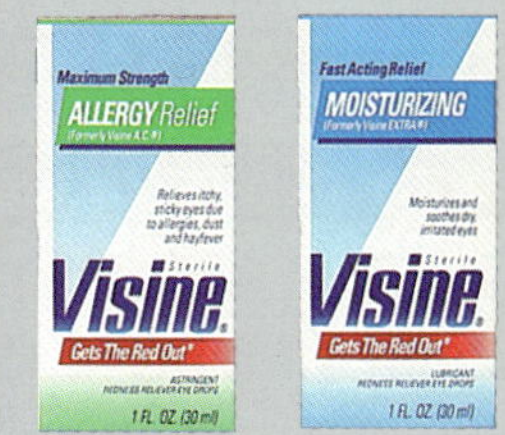

Allergy Relief | Moisturizing Relief

Visine®
Redness Reliever Eye Drops

PHARMAVITE
P. 317

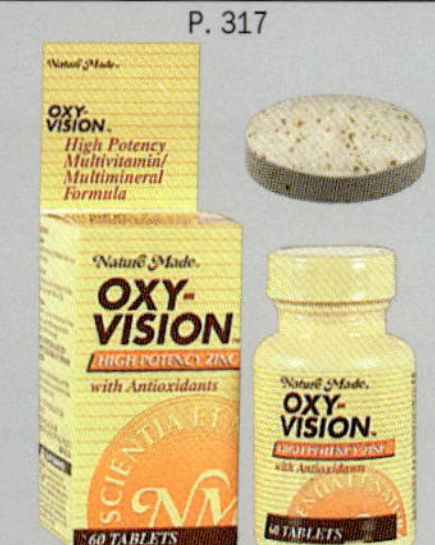

60 Tablets
Multivitamin/Multimineral Formula

Nature Made® Oxy-Vision™
High Potency Zinc with Antioxidants

*Manufacturer's identification code

ROCHE

P. 317

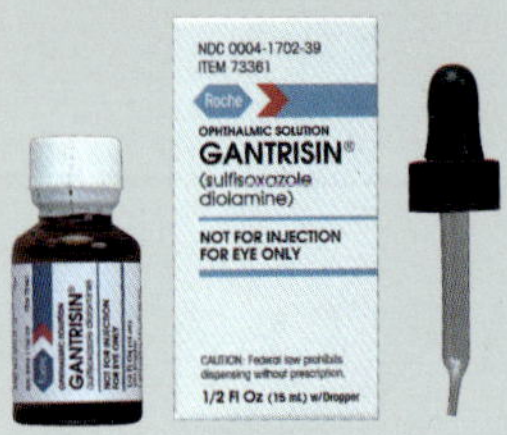

4% (40 mg/mL)

Gantrisin®
Ophthalmic Solution
(sulfisoxazole diolamine)

STORZ OPHTHALMICS

P. 319

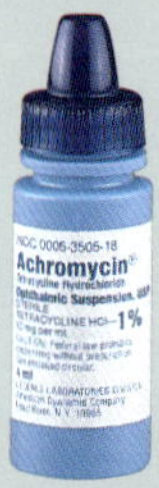

Achromycin®
Ophthalmic Suspension 1.0%
(tetracycline HCl)

P. 320

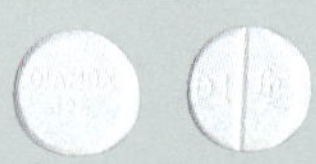

D1** 125 mg

D2** 250 mg

Diamox® Tablets

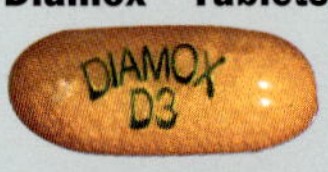

D3** 500 mg

Diamox® Sequels®
(acetazolamide)

P. 323

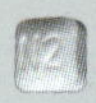

N2** 25 mg

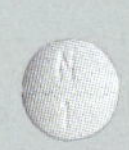

N1** 50 mg

Neptazane®
(methazolamide)

Storz Ophthalmics

P. 324

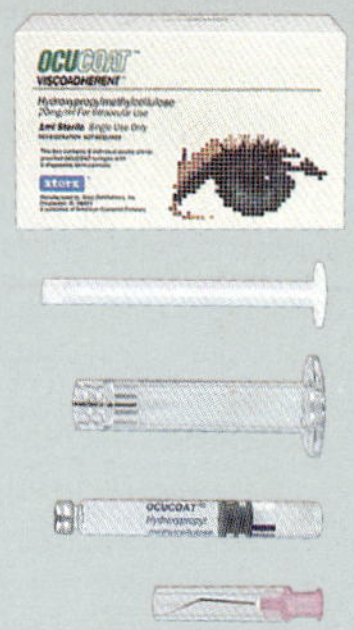

OcuCoat™
(2% hydroxypropylmethylcellulose)

P. 324

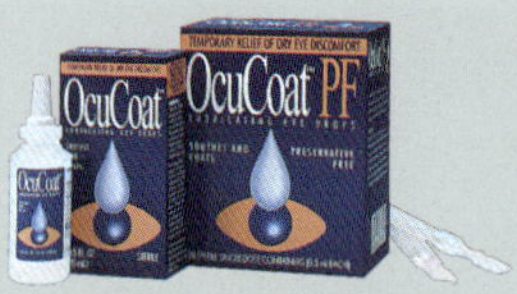

15 mL bottle

28 single-dose containers (.5 mL each)

OcuCoat™ and OcuCoat™ PF
Lubricating Eye Drops

P. 325

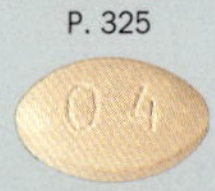

04**

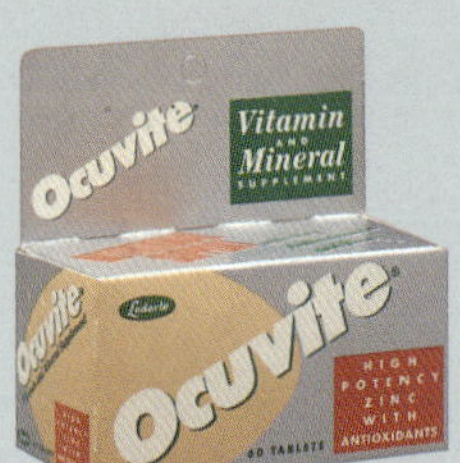

Ocuvite®
Vitamin and Mineral Supplement

WYETH-AYERST

P. 327

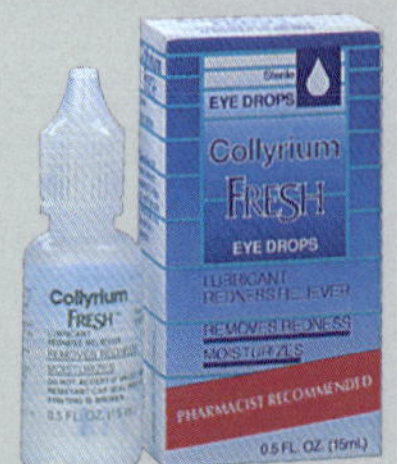

1/2 fl. oz. (15 mL)

Collyrium Fresh™
Eye drops with tetrahydrozoline HCl plus glycerin

Wyeth-Ayerst

P. 326

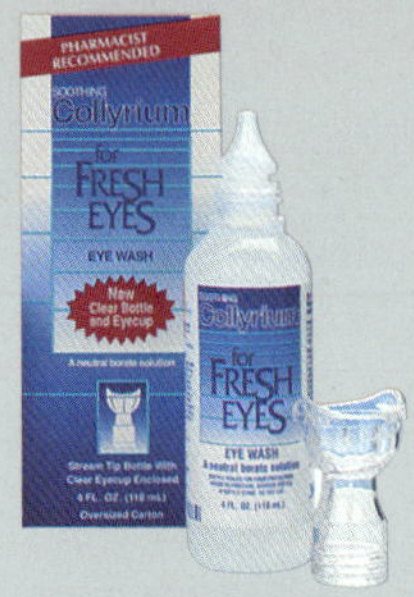

Lotion 4 fl. oz. (118 mL)
with separate eyecup bottle cap

Collyrium for Fresh Eyes
Eye Wash

P. 327

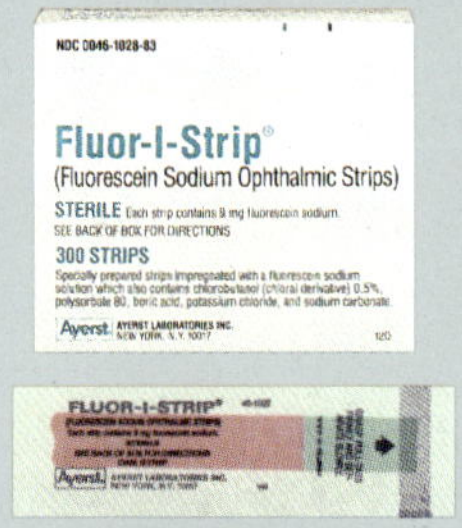

Box of 300 strips
Each strip contains
9 mg fluorescein sodium

Fluor-I-Strip®
(fluorescein sodium ophthalmic strips)

P. 327

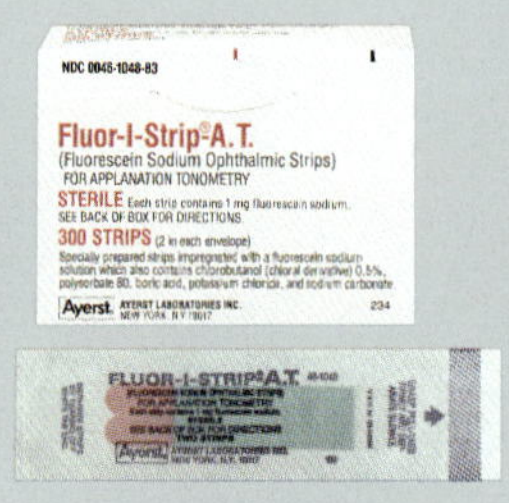

Box of 300 strips
Each strip contains
1 mg fluorescein sodium

Fluor-I-Strip®-A.T.
For Applanation Tonometry
(fluorescein sodium ophthalmic strips)

P. 327

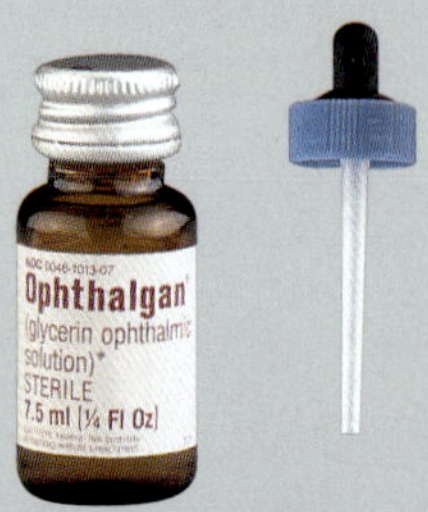

7.5 mL (1/4 fl. oz.)

Ophthalgan®
Sterile
(glycerin ophthalmic solution)

Wyeth-Ayerst

P. 328

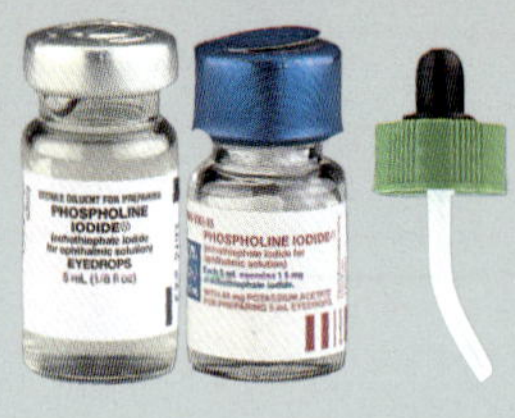

Sterile diluent | 0.03% (1/32%) sterile powder | 1.5 mg/ 5 mL

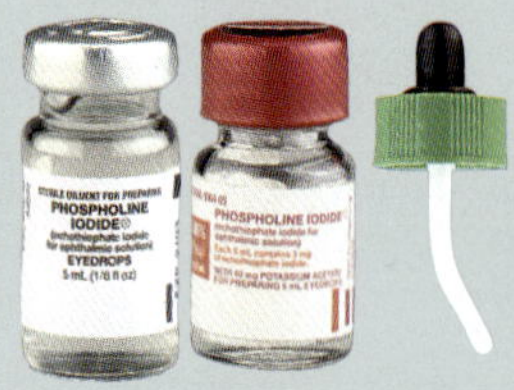

Sterile diluent | 0.06% (1/16%) sterile powder | 3 mg/ 5 mL

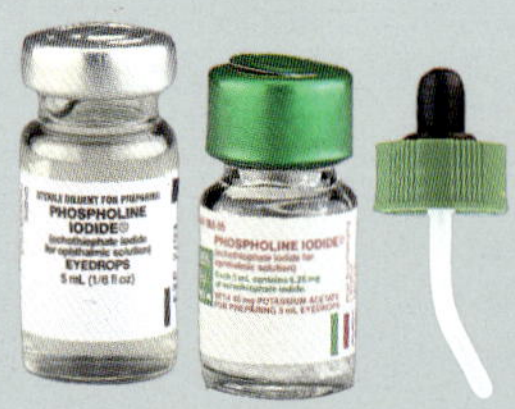

Sterile diluent | 0.125% (1/8%) sterile powder | 6.25 mg/ 5 mL

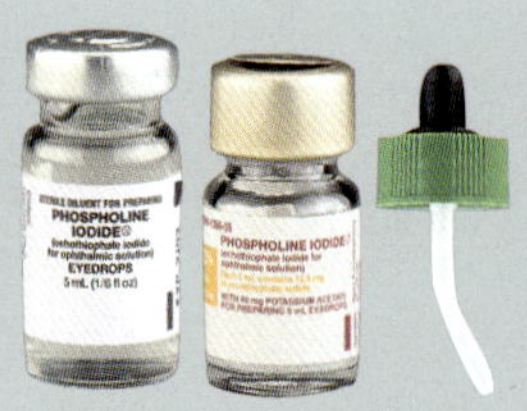

Sterile diluent | 0.25% (1/4%) sterile powder | 12.5 mg/ 5 mL

Phospholine Iodide®
(echothiophate iodide for ophthalmic solution)

While every effort has been made to reproduce products faithfully, this section is to be considered a Quick–Reference identification aid.

For more detailed information on products illustrated in this section, consult the Product Information Section or manufacturers may be contacted directly.

**Ledermark identification code

ROSENBAUM VISION SCREENER

95			=			distance equivalent $\frac{20}{800}$
874			ACCOMMODATION TEST			$\frac{20}{400}$
			Point	Jaeger		
2843			26	16		$\frac{20}{200}$
638	E Ш Ǝ	X O O	14	10		$\frac{20}{100}$
8 7 4 5	Ǝ m Ш	O X O	10	7		$\frac{20}{70}$
6 3 9 2 5	m E Ǝ	X O X	8	5		$\frac{20}{50}$
4 2 8 3 6 5	Ш E m	O X O	6	3		$\frac{20}{40}$
3 7 4 2 5 8	Ǝ Ш Ǝ	X X O	5	2		$\frac{20}{30}$
9 3 7 8 2 6	Ш m E	X O O	4	1		$\frac{20}{25}$
4 2 8 7 3 9	E Ш m	O O X	3	1+		$\frac{20}{20}$

Chart is held in good light 14 inches from eye. Record vision for each eye separately with and without glasses. Presbyopic patients should read through bifocal segment. Check myopes with glasses only.

DESIGN COURTESY OF J.G. ROSENBAUM, M.D. FACS, CLEVELAND, OHIO

PUPIL GAUGE (mm.)

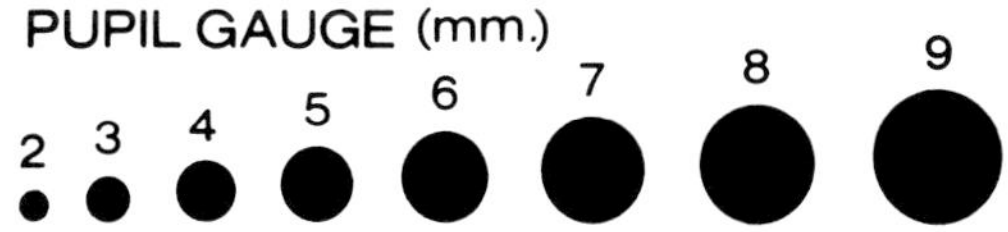

COLOR VISION SCREENING CHART

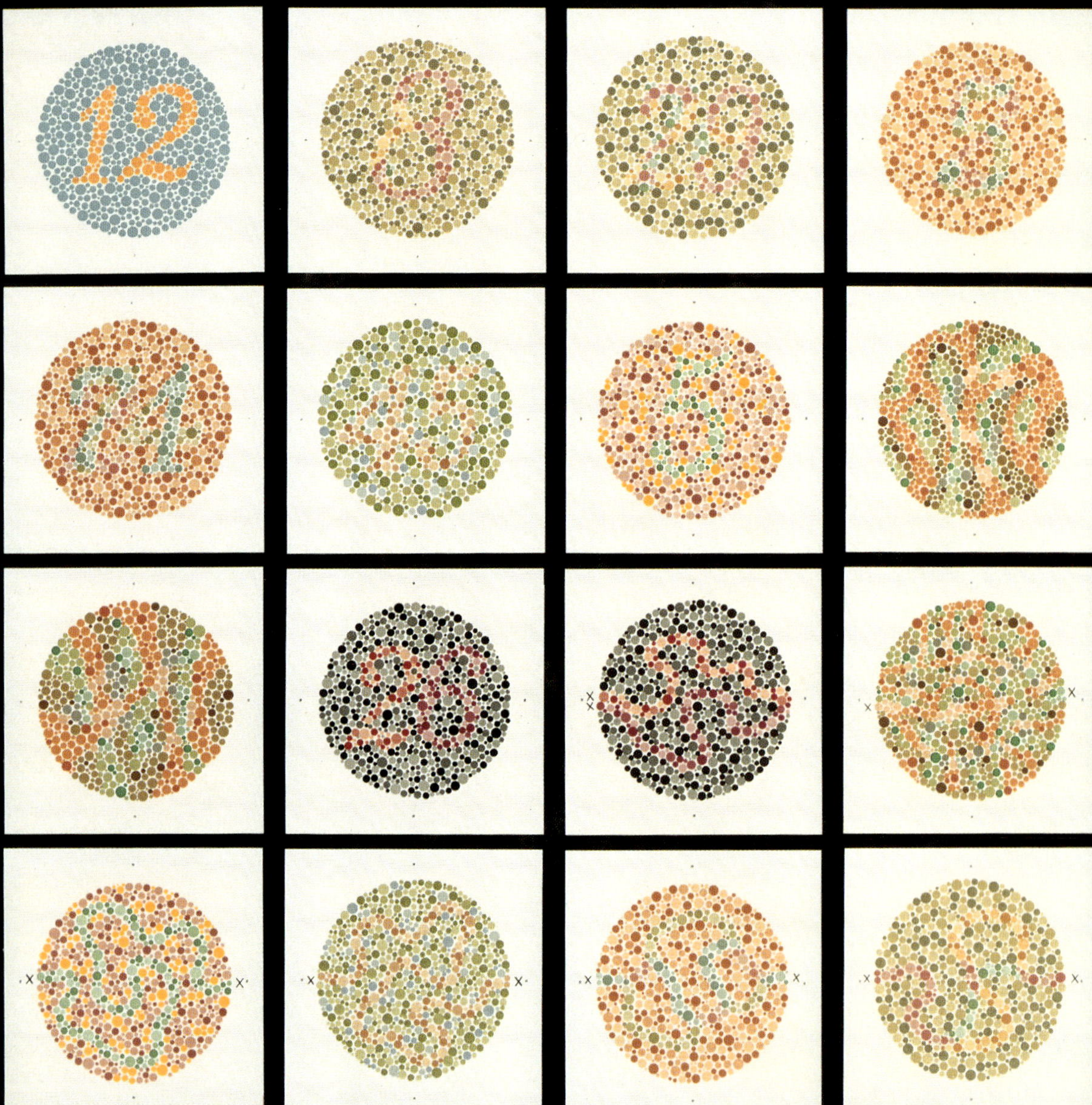

NO.	NORMAL EYE	COLOR BLIND EYE
1	12	12
2	8	3
3	29	70
4	5	2
5	74	21
6	45	NOTHING
7	5	NOTHING
8	NOTHING	5

NO.	NORMAL EYE	COLOR BLIND EYE
9	NOTHING	45
10	26	2 OR 6
11	2 LINES X TO X	LINE X TO X
12	NOTHING	LINE X TO X
13	LINE X TO X	NOTHING
14	LINE X TO X	NOTHING
15	LINE X TO X	NOTHING
16	LINE X TO X	LINE X TO X

Reprinted with permission of Robert S. Rosner, M.D., Cleveland, OH

COVER ANSWERS BEFORE TESTING PATIENT

SECTION 8

PHARMACEUTICAL PRODUCT INFORMATION

This book is made possible through the courtesy of the manufacturers whose products appear in this and the following sections. The information concerning each product has been prepared by the manufacturer, and edited and approved by the manufacturer's medical department, medical director, or medical counsel.

For those products that have official package circulars, the descriptions in *Physicians' Desk Reference For Ophthalmology* must be in full compliance with Food and Drug Administration regulations pertaining to the labeling of prescription drugs. In presenting the following material, the publisher is not necessarily advocating the use of any product listed.

Akorn, Inc.
100 AKORN DRIVE
ABITA SPRINGS, LA 70420

NDC 17478 PRODUCT

-286- **AKBETA™** ℞
Levobunolol HCl 0.25%, sterile ophthalmic solution.
5mL: -10
10mL: -11

-287- **AKBETA™** ℞
Levobunolol HCl 0.5%, sterile ophthalmic solution.
5mL: -10
10mL: -11
15mL: -12

-281- **AK-CHLOR™** ℞
Chloramphenicol, 0.5%, sterile ophthalmic solution.
7.5mL: -09
15mL: -12

-280-35 **AK-CHLOR™ OINTMENT** ℞
Chloramphenicol 1.0%, sterile ophthalmic ointment.
3.5gm

-275-10 **AK-CIDE®** ℞
Sulfacetamide Sodium 100mg, Prednisolone Acetate 5mg, sterile ophthalmic suspension.
5mL

-276-35 **AK-CIDE® OINTMENT** ℞
Sulfacetamide Sodium 10%, Prednisolone Acetate 0.5%, sterile ophthalmic ointment.
3.5gm

-216-12 **AK-CON™** ℞
Naphazoline HCl 0.1%, sterile ophthalmic solution.
15mL

-215-12 **AK-CON-A™** ℞
Naphazoline HCl 0.025%, Pheniramine Maleate 0.3%, sterile ophthalmic solution.
15mL

-279-10 **AK-DEX®** ℞
Dexamethasone Sodium Phosphate 0.1%, sterile ophthalmic solution.
5mL

-278-35 **AK-DEX® OINTMENT** ℞
Dexamethasone Sodium Phosphate 0.05%, sterile ophthalmic ointment.
3.5gm

-200- **AK-DILATE™ 2.5%** ℞
Phenylephrine HCl, sterile ophthalmic solution.
2mL: -20
15mL: -12

-205-10 **AK-DILATE™ 10%** ℞
Phenylephrine HCl, sterile ophthalmic solution.
5mL

-254-10 **AK-FLUOR® 10% GLASS AMPUL** ℞
Fluorescein injection, USP, sterile aqueous ophthalmic solution.
5mL

-251-20 **AK-FLUOR® 25% GLASS AMPUL** ℞
Fluorescein injection, USP, sterile aqueous ophthalmic solution.
2mL

-253-10 **AK-FLUOR® 10% SINGLE DOSE VIAL** ℞
Fluorescein injection, USP, sterile aqueous ophthalmic solution.
5mL

-250-20 **AK-FLUOR® 25% SINGLE DOSE VIAL** ℞
Fluorescein injection, USP, sterile aqueous ophthalmic solution.
2mL

-621-12 **AK-NaCl™ 5%**
Sodium Chloride 5%, sterile hypertonic ophthalmic solution.
15mL

-620-35 **AK-NaCl™ 5% OINTMENT**
(Preservative Free) Sodium Chloride 5%, sterile ophthalmic ointment.
3.5gm

-220-12 **AK-NEFRIN™**
Phenylephrine HCl 0.12%, sterile ophthalmic solution.
15mL

-277-10 **AK-NEO-DEX™** ℞
Neomycin Sulfate, Dexamethasone Sodium Phosphate, sterile ophthalmic solution.
5mL

-100- **AK-PENTOLATE™ 1%** ℞
Cyclopentolate HCl, sterile ophthalmic solution.
2mL: -20
15mL: -10

-238-35 **AK-POLY-BAC™ OINTMENT** ℞
(Preservative-Free) Polymyxin B Sulfate, Bacitracin Zinc, sterile ophthalmic ointment.
3.5gm

-218-10 **AK-PRED™ 0.125%** ℞
Prednisolone Sodium Phosphate 0.125%, sterile ophthalmic solution.
5mL

-219- **AK-PRED™ 1%** ℞
Prednisolone Sodium Phosphate 1%, sterile ophthalmic solution.
5mL: -10
10mL -11
15mL: -12

-269- **AK-RINSE™** ℞
Irrigating solution.
4fl.oz.: -18
1fl.oz.: -30

-790- **AK-SPORE®** ℞
Polymyxin B, Neomycin, Gramicidin, sterile opthalmic solution.
2mL: -20
10mL: -11

-235-35 **AK-SPORE® OINTMENT** ℞
(Preservative-Free) Polymyxin B, Neomycin, Bacitracin, sterile ophthalmic ointment.
3.5gm

-231-09 **AK-SPORE® HC** ℞
Neomycin Sulfate, Polymyxin B Sulfate, Hydrocortisone, sterile ophthalmic suspension.
7.5mL

-232-35 **AK-SPORE® HC OINTMENT** ℞
(Preservative-Free) Polymyxin B, Bacitracin, Neomycin, Hydrocortisone, sterile ophthalmic ointment.
3.5gm

-237-11 **AK-SPORE® HC OTIC SOLUTION** ℞
Polymyxin B, Neomycin, Hydrocortisone, sterile otic solution.
10mL

-236-11 **AK-SPORE® HC OTIC SUSPENSION** ℞
Polymyxin B, Neomycin, Hydrocortisone, sterile otic suspension.
10mL

Continued on next page

Akorn—Cont.

-221- **AK-SULF®** ℞
Sulfacetamide Sodium
10%, sterile ophthalmic
solution.
2mL: -20
15mL: -12

-227-35 **AK-SULF® OINTMENT** ℞
Sulfacetamide Sodium
10%, sterile ophthalmic
ointment.
3.5gm

-245-12 **AK-T-CAINE™** ℞
Tetracaine HCl 0.5%,
sterile ophthalmic solution.
15mL

-240- **AK-TAINE®** ℞
Proparacaine HCl, 0.5%,
sterile ophthalmic solution.
2mL: -20
15mL: -12

-230-35 **AKTETRA™** ℞
Oxytetracycline HCl,
Polymyxin B Sulfate,
sterile ophthalmic
ointment.
3.5gm

-290-10 **AKTOB™** ℞
Tobramycin 0.3%,
sterile ophthalmic
solution.
5mL

-233-35 **AK-TRACIN™ OINTMENT** ℞
(Preservative-Free)
Bacitracin, sterile
ophthalmic ointment.
3.5gm

-239-10 **AK-TROL®** ℞
Dexamethasone 0.1%,
Neomycin Sulfate,
Polymyxin B Sulfate,
sterile ophthalmic
suspension.
5mL

-240-35 **AK-TROL® OINTMENT** ℞
Dexamethasone 0.1%,
Neomycin Sulfate,
Polymyxin B Sulfate,
sterile ophthalmic ointment.
3.5gm

-223-12 **AKARPINE™ 1%** ℞
Pilocarpine HCl,
sterile ophthalmic solution.
15mL

-224-12 **AKARPINE™ 2%** ℞
Pilocarpine HCl,
sterile ophthalmic solution.
15mL

-226-12 **AKARPINE™ 4%** ℞
Pilocarpine HCl,
sterile ophthalmic solution.
15mL

-920- **AKORN BALANCED SALT SOLUTION** ℞
(Preservative-Free)
Sterile surgical solution.
18mL: -19
500mL: -90

-060-12 **AKWA TEARS®**
Polyvinyl Alcohol,
ocular lubricant solution.
15mL

-062-35 **AKWA TEARS® OINTMENT**
(Preservative Free)
White Petrolatum,
Mineral Oil, Lanolin
Derivatives, sterile
ophthalmic ointment.
3.5gm

-214- **ATROPINE CARE™ 1%** ℞
Atropine Sulfate 1%,
sterile ophthalmic solution.
2mL: -20
5mL: -10
15mL: -12

-610-12 **EYE-SINE™**
Tetrahydrozoline HCl
.05%, sterile
ophthalmic solution.
½ oz.

-311-10 **FLUORACAINE®** ℞
Fluorescein Sodium
0.25%, Proparacaine HCl
0.5%, sterile
ophthalmic solution.
5mL

-400-01 **FLUORETS™**
Fluorescein Sodium 1mg,
sterile ophthalmic strips.
100/box

-283- **GENTAK®** ℞
Gentamicin Sulfate,
sterile ophthalmic solution.
5mL: -10
15mL: -12

-284-35 **GENTAK® OINTMENT** ℞
Gentamicin Sulfate,
sterile ophthalmic
ointment.
3.5gm

-525-01 **GLAUCTABS™** ℞
Methazolamide tablets
USP 25mg.
100/btl.

-550-01 **GLAUCTABS™** ℞
Methazolamide tablets
USP 50mg.
100/btl.

-070-12 **GONAK™**
Hydroxypropyl Methyl-
cellulose 2.5%, sterile
ophthalmic solution.
15mL

-820-06 **LID WIPES-SPF™**
Sterile, Preservative-Free. Hypo-allergenic,
isotonic eye-lid
cleansing pad, for
sensitive eyes.
30/box

-805-60 **OCUCAPS ANTIOXIDANTS**
Vitamin
and mineral supplement.
60/btl.

-810-100 **PALMITATE-A**
15,000 IU Vitamin A.
100/btl.

-815-01 **PALMITATE-A 5000**
5,000 IU Vitamin A.
100/btl.

57217-9521-1 **ROSETS™**
1.3mg Rose Bengal,
individually wrapped,
sterile ophthalmic strips.
100/box

-116- **SULSTER™** ℞
Sulfacetamide Sodium
10%, Prednisolone
Sodium Phosphate .25%,
sterile ophthalmic
solution.
5mL: -10
10mL: -11

-401-01 **SNO STRIPS™**
Sterile, individually
wrapped, tear flow
test strips.
100/box

-061-12 **TEARS RENEWED®**
Dexitran 70,
Hydroxypropyl Methyl-
cellulose 2906,
sterile ophthalmic solution.
15mL

-063-35 **TEARS RENEWED® OINTMENT**
(Preservative and Lanolin Free)
White petrolatum and
light mineral oil,
sterile ophthalmic ointment.
3.5gm

-101-12 **TROPICACYL® 0.5%** ℞
Tropicamide, sterile
ophthalmic solution.
15mL

-102- **TROPICACYL® 1%** ℞
Tropicamide, sterile
ophthalmic solution.
2mL: -20
15mL: -12

AK-CIDE® ℞
brand of prednisolone acetate, USP and sulfacetamide sodium, USP
Ophthalmic Suspension–Sterile
Ophthalmic Ointment–Sterile

Description: AK-CIDE Ophthalmic **Suspension** is a steroid/anti-infective sterile preparation having a pH range of 7.0 to 7.4. Each mL contains: 5 mg prednisolone acetate, USP; 100 mg sulfacetamide sodium, USP; sodium phosphate dibasic, sodium phosphate monobasic, tyloxapol, sodium thiosulfate, edetate disodium, and purified water; 5 mg phenylethyl alcohol and 0.25 mg benzalkonium chloride as preservatives.
AK-CIDE Ophthalmic **Ointment** is a steroid/anti-infective sterile preparation containing in each gram: 5 mg prednisolone acetate, USP and 100 mg sulfacetamide sodium, USP; 0.5 mg methylparaben and 0.1 mg propylparaben as preservatives, in a bland, unctuous base of mineral oil and white petrolatum.
The empirical formula for prednisolone acetate, a 1-unsaturated analog of hydrocortisone acetate, is $C_{23}H_{30}O_6$. The molecular weight is 402.49. Chemically it is 11β,17,21-trihydroxypregna-1,4-diene-3,20-dione 21-acetate, with the following structural formula:

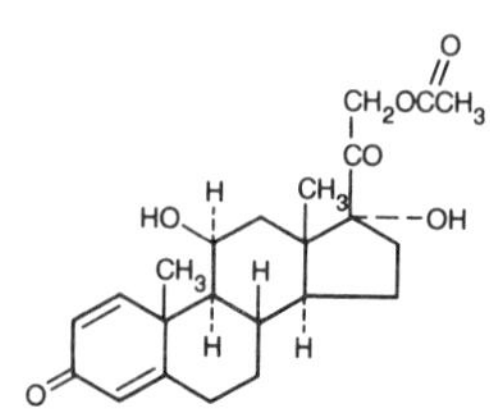

Prednisolone acetate is a nearly odorless, white to practically white, crystalline powder. It is slightly soluble in acetone, alcohol, and chloroform, and practically insoluble in water.
Sulfacetamide sodium, $C_8H_9N_2NaO_3S \cdot H_2O$, is a sulfonamide antibacterial agent with a molecular weight of 254.24. Chemically it is *N*-[4-amino-phenyl)sulfonyl]-, acetamide, monosodium salt, monohydrate, with the following structural formula:

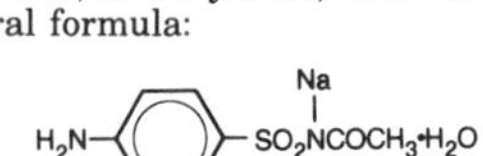

Sulfacetamide sodium is an odorless, white, crystalline powder. It is freely soluble in water, sparingly soluble in alcohol, and practically insoluble in benzene, chloroform, and ether.

Clinical Pharmacology: Corticosteroids suppress the inflammatory response to a variety of agents, and they probably delay or slow healing. Since corticosteroids may inhibit the body's defense mechanism against infection, a concomitant antimicrobial drug may be used when this inhibition is considered to be clinically significant in a particular case.
The anti-infective component in the combination is included to provide action against specific organisms susceptible to it.
When a decision is made to administer both a corticoid and an antimicrobial, the administration of such drugs in combination has the advantages of greater patient compliance and convenience and added assurance that the appropriate dosage of both drugs is administered. There is also assured compatibility of ingredients when both types of drug are in the same formulation and, particularly, that the correct volume of drug is delivered and retained.
The relative potency of corticosteroids depends on the molecular structure, concentration, and release from the vehicle.
Indications and Usage: AK-CIDE Ophthalmic **Suspension** or **Ointment** is indicated for steroid-responsive inflammatory ocular conditions for which a corticosteroid is indicated and where bacterial infection or a risk of bacterial ocular infection exists.
Ocular steroids are indicated in inflammatory conditions of the palpebral and bulbar conjunctivae, cornea, and anterior segment of the globe where the inherent risk of steroid use in certain infective conjunctivitides is accepted to obtain a diminution in edema and inflammation. They are also indicated in chronic anterior uveitis and corneal injury from chemical, radiation, or thermal burns, or penetration of foreign bodies.
The use of a combination drug with an anti-infective component is indicated where the risk of infection is high or where there is an expectation that potentially dangerous numbers of bacteria will be present in the eye.
The particular anti-infective drug in this product is active against the following common bacterial eye pathogens: *Pseudomonas* species, *Hemophilus influenzae, Klebsiella* species, *Staphylococcus aureus, Streptococcus pneumoniae, Streptococcus* (Viridans group), *Escherichia coli,* and *Enterobacter* species.
This product does not provide adequate coverage against: *Neisseria* species and *Serratia marcescens.*
Contraindications: AK-CIDE is contraindicated in epithelial herpes simplex keratitis (dendritic keratitis), vaccinia, varicella, and many other viral diseases of the cornea or conjunctiva; mycobacterial infection of the eye; and fungal diseases of ocular structures. AK-CIDE is contraindicated in individuals with known or suspected hypersensitivity to any of the ingredients of the preparation, or to other sulfonamides, or other corticosteroids. (Hypersensitivity to the antibacterial component occurs at a higher rate than for other components.) The use of these combinations is always contraindicated after uncomplicated removal of a corneal foreign body.
Warnings: Prolonged use may result in glaucoma, with damage to the optic nerve, defects in visual acuity and fields of vision, and in posterior subcapsular cataract formation. Prolonged use may suppress the host response and thus increase the hazard of secondary ocular infections. In those diseases causing thinning of the cornea or sclera, perforations have been known to occur with the use of topical steroids. In acute purulent conditions of the eye, steroids may mask infection or enhance existing infection. If these products are used for ten days or longer, intraocular pressure should be routinely monitored even though this may be difficult in children and uncooperative patients.
Employment of steroid medication in the treatment of herpes simplex requires great caution. A significant percentage of staphylococcal isolates are completely resistant to sulfonamides.
Precautions: The initial prescription and renewal of the medication order beyond 20 mL of AK-CIDE Ophthalmic **Suspension** or beyond 8 g of the **Ointment** should be made by a physician only after examination of the patient with the aid of magnification, such as slitlamp biomicroscopy and where appropriate, fluorescein staining.
The possibility of fungal infections of the cornea should be considered after prolonged steroid dosing.
Sensitization may recur when a sulfonamide is readministered irrespective of the route of administration, and cross-sensitivity among different sulfonamides may occur. (See **Adverse Reactions.**) Cross-allergenicity among corticosteroids has been demonstrated. If signs of hypersensitivity or other untoward reactions occur, discontinue use of the preparation.
Adverse Reactions: Adverse reactions have occurred which can be attributed to the steroid component, the anti-infective component, or the combination. Exact incidence figures are not available since no denominator of treated patients is available.
Reactions occurring most often from the presence of the anti-infective ingredient are allergic sensitizations. Instances of Stevens-Johnson syndrome and systemic lupus erythematosus (in one case producing a fatal outcome) have been reported following the use of ophthalmic sulfonamide-containing preparations.
The reactions due to the steroid component in decreasing order of frequency are: elevaton of intraocular pressure (IOP) with possible development of glaucoma, and infrequent optic nerve damage; posterior subcapsular cataract formation; and delayed wound healing.
Corticosteroid-containing preparations can also cause acute anterior uveitis or perforation of the globe. Mydriasis, loss of accommodation, and ptosis have occasionally been reported following local use of corticosteroids.
Secondary Infection: The development of secondary infection has occurred after use of combinations containing steroids and antimicrobials. Fungal infections of the cornea are particularly prone to develop coincidentally with long-term applications of the steroid. The possibility of fungal invasion must be considered in any persistent corneal ulceration where steroid treatment has been used.
Secondary bacterial ocular infection following suppression of host responses also occurs.
Dosage and Administration: AK-CIDE Ophthalmic **Suspension:** Two or three drops should be instilled into the conjunctival sac every one to two hours during the day and at bedtime until a favorable response is obtained.
AK-CIDE Ophthalmic **Ointment:** A thin film should be applied three or four times daily and once at bedtime until a favorable response is obtained.
The initial prescription of AK-CIDE Ophthalmic should *not* be more than 20 mL of the **Suspension** or 8 g of the **Ointment** and the prescription should not be refilled without further evaluation as outlined in **Precautions.**
Dosage should be adjusted according to the specific needs of the patient. AK-CIDE Ophthalmic **Suspension** or **Ointment** dosage may be reduced, but care should be taken not to discontinue therapy prematurely. In chronic conditions, withdrawal of treatment should be carried out by gradually decreasing the frequency of application.
How Supplied: AK-CIDE Ophthalmic **Suspension,** 5 mL dropper bottle; box of one; NDC 17478-275-10. **Store between 2° and 25°C (36° and 77°F). Clumping may occur on long standing at high temperatures. Shake well before using. Protect from light.**
AK-CIDE Ophthalmic **Ointment,** 3.5 g applicator tube; box of one; NDC 17478-276-35. **Store between 2° and 30°C (36° and 86°F).**

Manufactured by Schering Corporation,
Kenilworth, NJ 07033
for Akorn, Inc., Abita Springs, LA 70420.

AK–FLUOR® ℞

Fluorescein Injection, USP
10% & 25% Sterile Solution

Description: AK-FLUOR® (Fluorescein Injection, USP) is a sterile solution in Water for Injection, of Fluorescein prepared with the aid of Sodium Hydroxide. Hydrochloric Acid and/or Sodium Hydroxide may be used to adjust pH (8.0–9.8). AK-FLUOR® is used intravenously as a diagnostic aid. The active ingredient exists as a sodium salt of fluorescein and is represented by the chemical structure:

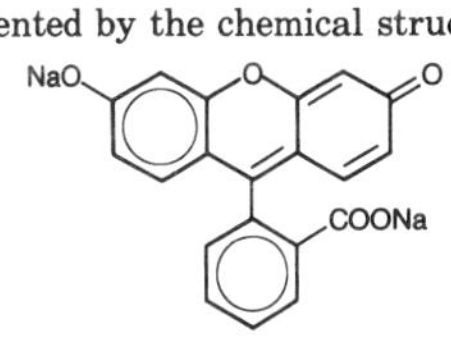

Established Name:
Fluorescein Sodium
Chemical Name:
Spiro[isobenzofuran-1(3H),9′-[9H]xanthene]-3-one, 3′6′-dihydroxy, disodium salt
Clinical Pharmacology: The yellowish-green fluorescence of the product demarcates the vascular area under observation, distinguishing it from adjacent areas.
Indications and Usage: Indicated in diagnostic fluorescein angiography or angioscopy of the fundus and of the iris vasculature.
Contraindications: Contraindicated in those persons who have shown hypersensitivity to any component of this preparation.
Warnings: Care must be taken to avoid extravasation during injection as the high pH of fluorescein solution can result in severe local tissue damage. The following complications resulting from extravasation of fluorescein have been noted to occur: sloughing of the skin, superficial phlebitis, subcutaneous granuloma, and toxic neuritis along the median curve in the antecubital area. Complications resulting from extravasation can cause severe pain in the arm for up to several hours. When significant extravasation occurs, the injection should be discontinued and conservative measures to treat damaged tissues and to relieve pain should be implemented.
Precautions: Caution is to be exercised in patients with a history of allergy or bronchial asthma. An emergency tray including such items as 0.1% epinephrine for intravenous or intramuscular use; an antihistamine, soluble steroid, and aminophylline for intravenous use; oxygen should always be available in the event of possible reaction to fluorescein injection.[1]
Pediatric Use: Safety and effectiveness in children have not been established.
Carcinogenesis, Mutagenesis, Impairment of Fertility: There have been no long-term studies done using fluorescein in animals to evaluate carcinogenic potential.
Use in Pregnancy: Avoid angiography on patients who are pregnant, especially those in first trimester. There have been no reports of fetal complications for fluorescein injection during pregnancy.
Nursing Mothers: It is not known whether this drug is excreted in human milk. Because many drugs are excreted in human milk, cau-

Continued on next page

Akorn—Cont.

tion should be exercised when AK-FLUOR® (Fluorescein Injection, USP) is administered to a nursing woman.

Patient Warning: Skin will attain a temporary yellowish discoloration. Urine attains a bright yellow color. Discoloration of the skin fades in 6 to 12 hours; urine fluorescence in 24 to 36 hours.

Adverse Reactions: Nausea, vomiting, headache, gastrointestinal distress, syncope, vomiting, hypotension, and other symptoms and signs of hypersensitivity have occurred. Cardiac arrest, basilar artery ischemia, severe shock, convulsions, and thrombophlebitis at the injection site and rare cases of death have been reported.

Extravasation of the solution at the injection site causes intense pain at the site and a dull aching pain in the injected arm. (SEE WARNINGS.) Generalized hives and itching, bronchospasm and anaphylaxis have been reported. A strong taste may develop after injection.

The most common reaction is nausea.

Dosage and Administration: Inject the contents of the ampul or vial rapidly into the antecubital vein, *after taking precautions to avoid extravasation.* A syringe, filled with fluorescein, is attached to transparent tubing and a 25 gauge scalp vein needle for injection. Insert the needle and draw the patient's blood to the hub of the syringe so that a *small* air bubble separates the patient's blood in the tubing from the fluorescein. With the room lights on, slowly inject the blood back into the vein while watching the skin over the needle tip. If the needle has extravasated, the patient's blood will be seen to bulge the skin and the injection should be stopped before any fluorescein is injected. When assured that extravasation has not occurred, the room light may be turned off and the fluorescein injection completed. Luminescence appears in the retina and choroidal vessels in 9 to 14 seconds and can be observed by standard viewing equipment. If potential allergy is suspected, an intradermal skin test may be performed prior to intravenous administration, i.e., 0.05 mL injected intradermally to be evaluated 30 to 60 minutes following injection. For children, the dose is calculated on the basis of 35 mg for each ten pounds of body weight.

Parenteral drug products should be inspected visually for particulate matter and discoloration, whenever solution and container permit.

How Supplied:

AK-FLUOR®, 10% (Fluorescein Injection, USP—Sterile) 100 mg/mL

NDC 17478-253-10 12 × 5mL Single Dose Vials

NDC 17478-254-10 25 × 5mL Ampuls

AK-FLUOR®, 25% (Fluorescein Injection, USP—Sterile) 250 mg/mL

NDC 17478-250-20 12 × 2mL Single Dose Vials

NDC 17478-251-20 12 × 2mL Ampuls

Storage: Store at 15°–30°C (59°–86°F); protect from freezing.

Reference:

1. Schatz, Burton, Yannuzzi, Rabb. Interpretation of Fundus Fluorescein Angiography, p. 38, C.V. Mosby Co., St. Louis, Mo., 1978.

Caution: Federal (USA) law prohibits dispensing without prescription.

Akorn
Abita Springs, LA 70420

Shown in Product Identification Guide, page 103

AK-PRED ℞

(prednisolone sodium phosphate)
Sterile Ophthalmic Solution

Description: AK-PRED is a water soluble form of the synthetic anti-inflammatory steroid prednisolone.

Available in two strengths as follows:

Contents:

Each ml contains:

	Ak-Pred 0.125%	Ak-Pred-1%
Prednisolone Sodium Phosphate	0.125%	1.0%
(Equivalent to Prednisolone)	0.1%	0.8%
Benzalkonium Chloride (Preservative)	0.01%	0.01%

In an isotonic, phosphate buffered saline solution containing Sodium Bisulfite, Sodium Edetate and Hydroxypropyl Methylcellulose.

Actions: This drug causes inhibition of inflammatory response to inciting agents of mechanical, chemical, or immunological nature. No generally accepted explanation of this steroid property has been advanced.

Indications: For the treatment of: Steroid responsive inflammatory conditions of the palpebral and bulbar conjuctiva, cornea and anterior segment of the globe, such as allergic conjunctivitis, acne rosacea, superficial punctate keratitis, herpes zoster keratitis, iritis, cyclitis, selected infective conjunctivitis when the inherent hazard of steroid use is accepted to obtain an advisable diminution in edema and inflammation: corneal injury from chemical, radiation, or thermal burns, or penetration of foreign bodies.

Contraindications:

1. Acute superficial herpes simplex keratitis
2. Fungal diseases of ocular structures
3. Vaccinia, varicella and most other viral diseases of the cornea and conjunctiva
4. Tuberculosis of the eye
5. Hypersensitivity to a component of this medication.

Warnings:

1. Steroid medication in the treatment of herpes simplex keratitis involving the stroma requires great caution; frequent slit-lamp microscopy is mandatory.
2. Prolonged use may result in glaucoma, damage to the optic nerve, defect in visual acuity and fields of vision, posterior subcapsular cataract formation, or may aid in the establishment of secondary ocular infections from pathogens liberated from ocular tissues.
3. In those diseases causing thinning of the cornea or sclera, perforation has been known to occur with the use of topical steroids.
4. Acute purulent untreated infection of the eye may be masked or activity enhanced by presence of steroid medication.
5. Usage in pregnancy: Safety of intensive or protracted use of topical steroids during pregnancy has not been established.

Precautions: As fungal infections of the cornea are particularly prone to develop coincidentally with long-term steroid applications, fungus invasion must be suspected in any persistent corneal ulceration where a steroid has been used or is in use.

Introacular pressure should be checked frequently.

The use of AK-PRED should be discontinued if improvement in the condition being treated does not occur within several days.

Care should be exercised to avoid contamination of the material during its use.

Store in a cool place. Protect from light.

Adverse Reactions: Glaucoma with optic nerve damage, visual acuity and field defects, posterior subcapsular cataract formation, secondary ocular infections from pathogens liberated from ocular tissues, perforation of the globe.

Dosage: Initially, 1 or 2 drops placed in the conjunctival sac every hour until improvement occurs. Thereafter, gradually reduce to 1 or 2 drops every 3 or 4 hours.

Supply:

0.125%—5 mL NDC 17478-218-10
1%—5 mL NDC 17478-219-10
1%—15 mL NDC 17478-219-12

AK-SPORE ℞

(neomycin sulfate-polymyxin B sulfate-gramicidin) Sterile Ophthalmic Solution
(neomycin sulfate-polymyxin B sulfate-bacitracin zinc) Sterile Ophthalmic Ointment

Description: Solution—AK-SPORE Solution is a sterile aqueous solution formulated for ophthalmic use in the treatment of superficial external ocular infections. Each ml contains Polymyxin B Sulfate 10,000 units, Neomycin Sulfate (equivalent to 1.75 mg Neomycin base), Gramicidin 0.025 mg. The vehicle contains Alcohol 0.5%, Thimerosal (preservative) 0.001%, Propylene glycol, Polyoxyethylene-polyoxypropylene compound, Sodium chloride and Purified Water.

Ointment—AK-SPORE ointment is a sterile antimicrobial ointment formulated for ophthalmic use to contain bacitracin zinc, neomycin sulfate, and polymyxin B sulfate in a special white petrolatum-mineral oil base. Each gram contains 400 units of bacitracin, 3.5 milligrams of neomycin, and 10,000 units of Polymyxin B. Contains no preservatives.

Clinical Pharmacology: The anti-infective components in AK-SPORE Solution and Ointment are included to provide action against specific organisms susceptible to them. Neomycin Sulfate is considered effective against a wide range of gram-negative and gram-positive organisms, including many strains of **Proteus, Klebsiella, Staphylococcus aureus, Escherichia coli,** and **Haemophilus influenzae.** Polymyxin B Sulfate's effectiveness is sharply restricted to gram-negative bacteria, including many strains of **Escherichia coli, Haemophilus influenzae,** and **Pseudomonas aeruginosa.** Gramicidin is effective against gram-positive organisms including **Pneumococci, Staphylococci, Streptococci, Diphtheria bacilli,** and certain **anaerobic bacilli.**

Bacitracin is bactericidal for a variety of gram-positive and gram-negative organisms. It interferes with bacterial cell wall synthesis by inhibition of the regeneration of phospholipid receptors involved in peptidoglycan synthesis.

Indications and Usage: This product is indicated in the short-term treatment of superficial external ocular infections. The particular anti-infective drug(s) in this product are active against the following common bacterial eye pathogens:

Staphylococcus aureus
Streptococci, including **Streptococcus pneumoniae**
Escherichia coli
Haemophilus influenzae
Klebsiella/Enterobacter species
Nelsseria species
Pseudomonas aeruginosa

The product does not provide adequate coverage against:

Serratia marcescens

Contraindications: This product is contraindicated in those persons who have shown sensitivity to any of its components.

Warnings: Neomycin sulfate may cause cutaneous sensitization. A precise incidence of hypersensitivity reactions (primarily skin rash) due to topical neomycin is now known. The ophthalmic manifestations of sensitization to neomycin are usually itching, reddening and edema of the conjunctiva and eyelid. It may be manifest simply as a failure to heal. During long-term use of neomycin-containing products, periodic examination for such signs is advisable, and the patient should be told to discontinue the product if they are observed. These symptoms subside quickly on withdrawing the medication. Neomycin-containing applications should be avoided for the patient thereafter.

Precautions: General: As with other antibiotic preparations, prolonged use may result in overgrowth of nonsusceptible organisms including fungi. Appropriate measures should be taken if this occurs.

Culture and susceptibility testing should be performed during treatment.

Allergic cross-reactions may occur which could prevent the use of any or all of the following antibiotics for the treatment of future infections; kanamycin, paromomycin, streptomycin, and possibly gentamicin.

Information for Patients: If redness, irritation, swelling or pain persists or increases, discontinue use and contact your physician.

Avoid contaminating the applicator tip with material from the eye, fingers, or other source. This caution is necessary if the sterility of the solution is to be preserved.

Adverse Reactions: The most frequent adverse reactions are localized hypersensitivity, including itching, swelling, and conjunctival erythema. Local irritation on instillation has also been reported. Exact incidence figures are not available since no denominator of treated patients is available.

Dosage and Administration: The suggested dosage is one or two drops in the affected eye, two to four times daily or more frequently, as required. In acute infection, initiate therapy with one or two drops every 15 to 30 minutes, reducing the frequency of instillation gradually as the infection is controlled. The patient should be instructed to avoid contaminating the applicator tip with material from an infected eye or other source. This is best done by preventing the tip from touching the eyelid or surrounding area. This caution is necessary in order to keep the sterile solution as free from contaminating organisms as possible. Apply the ointment every 3 or 4 hours for 7 to 10 days, depending on the severity of the infection.

How Supplied:

2 mL NDC 17478-790-20
10 mL NDC 17478-790-11
3.5 gm (1/8oz.) NDC 17478-235-35

AK-TROL ℞

(neomycin sulfate–polymyxin B sulfate–dexamethasone 0.1%)
Sterile Ophthalmic Suspension
Sterile Ophthalmic Ointment

Description: AK-Trol Ophthalmic Ointment and Suspension are anti-infective steroid combinations in a sterile suspension form and sterile ointment form for topical application.

Contents: Each ml of the suspension and each gram of the ointment contains:

Neomycin Sulfate ... Equivalent to 3.5 mg Neomycin base
Polymyxin B Sulfate 10,000 units
Dexamethasone 0.1%

In a solution containing Benzalkonium Chloride 0.01% (preservative) with Polysorbate 20, Sodium Chloride, Hydroxpropyl Methylcellulose, Hydrochloric Acid and/or Sodium Hydroxide to adjust the pH and Purified Water or in an ointment base containing Methylparaben 0.05%, Propylparaben 0.01% (as preservatives) with White Petrolatum, Anhydrous Liquid Lanolin and Mineral Oil as inactive ingredients.

Clinical Pharmacology: Corticoids suppress the inflammatory response to a variety of agents and they probably delay or slow healing. Since corticoids may inhibit the body's defense mechanism against infection, a concomitant antimicrobial drug may be used when this inhibition is considered to be clinically significant in a particular case.

The anti-infective component in the combination is included to provide action against specific organisms susceptible to it. Neomycin Sulfate and Polymyxin B Sulfate are considered active against the following microrganisms:

Staphylococcus aureus
Escherichia coli
Haemophilus influenzae
Klebsiella/Enterobacter species
Neisseria species
Pseudomonas aeruginosa

When a decision to administer both a corticoid and an antimicrobial is made, the administration of such drugs in combination has the advantage of greater patient compliance and convenience, with the added assurance that the appropriate dosage of both drugs is administered, plus assured compatibility of ingredients when both types of drug are in the same formulation and, particularly, that the correct volume of drug is delivered and retained.

The relative potency of corticosteroids depends on the molecular structure, concentration, and release from the vehicle.

Indications and Usage: For steroid-responsive inflammatory ocular conditions for which a corticosteroid is indicated and where bacterial infection or a risk of bacterial ocular infection exists.

Ocular steroids are indicated in inflammatory conditions of the palpebral and bulbar conjunctiva, cornea, and anterior segment of the globe where the inherent risk of steroid use in certain infective conjunctivitides is accepted to obtain a diminution in edema and inflammation. They are also indicated in chronic anterior uveitis and corneal injury from chemical, radiation or thermal burns, or penetration of foreign bodies.

The use of a combination drug with an anti-infective component is indicated where the risk of infection is high or where there is an expectation that potentially dangerous numbers of bacteria will be present in the eye.

The particular anti-infective drugs in this product are active against the following common bacterial eye pathogens:

Staphylococcus aureus
Escherichia coli
Haemophilus influenzae
Klebsiella/Enterobacter species
Neisseria species
Pseudomonas aerugenosa

The product does not provide adequate coverage against:

Serratia marcescens
Streptococci, including *Streptococcus pneumoniae*

Contraindications: Epithelial herpes simplex keratitis (dendritic keratitis), vaccinia, varicella and many other viral diseases of the cornea and conjunctiva. Mycobacterial infection of the eye. Fungal diseases of ocular structures. Hypersensitivity to a component of the medication. (Hypersensitivity to the antibiotic component occurs at a higher rate than for other components.)

The use of these combinations is always contraindicated after uncomplicated removal of a corneal foreign body.

Warnings: Prolonged use may result in glaucoma, with damage to the optic nerve, defects in visual acuity and fields of vision, and posterior subcapsular cataract formation. Prolonged use may suppress the host response and thus increase the hazard of secondary ocular infections. In those diseases causing thinning of the cornea of sclera, perforations have been known to occur with the use of topical steroids. In acute purulent conditions of the eye, steroids may mask infection or enhance existing infection. If these products are used for 10 days or longer, intraocular pressure should be routinely monitored even though it may be difficult in children and uncooperative patients.

Employment of steroid medication in the treatment of herpes simplex requires great caution. Neomycin Sulfate cause cutaneous sensitization. A precise incidence of hypersensitivity reactions (primarily skin rash) due to topical neomycin is not known.

Precautions: The initial prescription and renewal of the medication beyond 20 milliliters should be made by a physician only after examination of the patient with the aid of magnification, such as slit lamp biomicroscopy and where appropriate, flourescein staining. The possibility of persistent fungal infections of the cornea should be considered after prolonged steroid dosing.

Adverse Reactions: Adverse reactions have occurred with steroid/anti-infective combination drugs which can be attributed to the steroid component, the anti-infective component, or the combination. Exact incidence figures are not available since no denominator of treated patients is available. Reactions occurring most often from the presence of the anti-infective ingredients are allergic sensitizations. The reactions due to the steroid component in decreasing order of frequency are; elevation of intraocular pressure (OP) with possible development of glaucoma and infrequent optic nerve damage; posterior subcapsular cataract formation; and delayed wound healing.

Secondary Infection:

The development of secondary infection has occurred after use of combinations containing steroids and antimicrobials. Fungal infections of the cornea are particularly prone to develop coincidentally with long-term applications of steroids. The possibility of fungal invasion must be considered in any persistent corneal ulceration where steroid treatment has been used. Secondary bacterial ocular infection following suppression of host responses also occurs.

Dosage and Administration: AK-Trol Ophthalmic Suspension: One to two drops topically in the conjunctival sac(s). In severe disease, drops may be used hourly, being tapered to discontinuation as the inflammation subsides. In mild disease, drops may be used up to four to six times daily. Not more than 20 milliliters should be prescribed initially and the prescription should not be refilled without further evaluation as outlined in PRECAUTIONS above.

SHAKE WELL BEFORE USING.

AK-Trol Ophthalmic Ointment: Apply a small amount into the conjunctival sac(s) up to three or four times daily. Not more than 8 grams should be prescribed initially and the prescription should not be refilled without further evaluation as outlined in PRECAUTIONS above.

How Supplied: Ophthalmic Suspension is supplied in 5 ml (plastic drop container). Ointment is supplied in 3.5 gram (1/8oz.) ophthalmic tube.

5 mL NDC 17478-239-10
3.5 gm NDC 17478-240-35

AKTETRA ℞

oxytetracycline HCl with
POLYMYXIN B SULFATE
OPHTHALMIC OINTMENT
STERILE

Description: Each gram of sterile ointment contains oxytetracycline HCl equivalent to

Continued on next page

Akorn—Cont.

5 mg oxytetracycline, 10,000 units of polymyxin B sulfate, white petrolatum, and liquid petrolatum.

Actions: AKTETRA is a widely used antibiotic with clinically proved activity against gram-positive and gram-negative bacteria, rickettsiae, spirochetes, large viruses, and certain protozoa.

Polymyxin B Sulfate, one of a group of related antibiotics derived from *Bacillus polymyxa,* is rapidly bactericidal. This action is exclusively against gram-negative organisms. It is particularly effective against *Pseudomonas aeruginosa (B. pyocyaneus),* and Koch-Weeks bacillus, frequently found in local infections of the eye.

There is thus made available a particularly effective antimicrobial combination of the broad-spectrum antibiotic AKTETRA as well as polymyxin B sulfate against primarily causative or secondarily infecting organisms.

Indications: The sterile preparation, AKTETRA with Polymyxin B Sulfate Ophthalmic Ointment, is indicated for the treatment of superficial ocular infections involving the conjunctiva and/or cornea caused by AKTETRA with Polymyxin B Sulfate-susceptible organisms.

It may be administered topically alone, or as an adjunct to systemic therapy.

It is effective in infections caused by susceptible strains of staphylococci, streptococci, pneumococci, *Hemophilus influenzae, Pseudomonas aeruginosa,* Koch-Weeks bacillus, and *Proteus.*

Contraindications: This drug is contraindicated in individuals who have shown hypersensitivity to any of its components.

Precautions: As with all antibiotic preparations, use of this drug may result in overgrowth of nonsusceptible organisms, including fungi. If superinfection occurs, the antibiotic should be discontinued and appropriate specific therapy should be instituted.

Adverse Reactions: AKTETRA with Polymyxin B Sulfate Ophthalmic Ointment is well tolerated by the epithelial membranes and other tissues of the eye. Allergic or inflammatory reactions due to individual hypersensitivity are rare.

Dosage and Administration: Approximately ½ inch of the ointment is squeezed from the tube onto the lower lid of the affected eye two to four times daily.

The patient should be instructed to avoid contamination of the tip of the tube when applying the ointment.

How Supplied: AKTETRA with Polymyxin B Sulfate Ophthalmic Ointment is supplied in ⅓ oz. (3.5 g) tubes (NDC 17478-230-35).

FLUORACAINE® ℞

Fluorescein Sodium and Proparacaine Hydrochloride Ophthalmic Solution, USP Sterile

Description: Fluoracaine® (Fluorescein Sodium and Proparacaine Hydrochloride Ophthalmic Solution USP) is a sterile ophthalmic solution combining the disclosing action of Fluorescein with the anesthetic action of Proparacaine Hydrochloride. The active ingredients are represented by the structures:

[See structures at top of next column.]

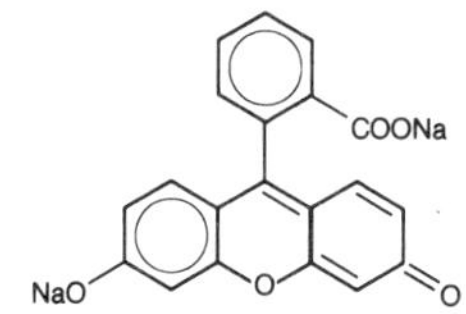

Established name: Fluorescein Sodium

Chemical name: Spiro[isobenzofuran-1(3H), 9'-[9H]xanthene]-3-one, 3'6'-dihydroxy, disodium salt

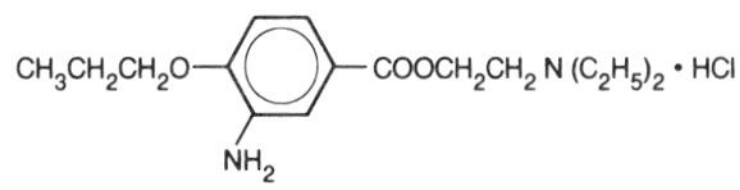

Established name: Proparacaine Hydrochloride

Chemical name: Benzoic acid, 3-amino-4-propoxy-, 2-(diethyl-amino)ethylester, monohydrochloride

Each mL contains: Actives: Proparacaine Hydrochloride 0.5%, Fluorescein Sodium 0.25%. **Preservative:** Thimerosal 0.01%. **Inactives:** Povidone, Glycerine, Boric Acid, Polysorbate 80, Sodium Hydroxide and/or Hydrochloric Acid (to adjust pH), Purified Water USP.

Clinical Pharmacology: Fluoracaine® is the combination of a disclosing agent with a rapidly acting anesthetic agent of short duration.

Indications and Usage: For procedures requiring a disclosing agent in combination with an anesthetic agent such as tonometry, gonioscopy, removal of corneal foreign bodies and other short corneal or conjunctival procedures.

Contraindications: Known hypersensitivity to any component of this product.

Warnings: Prolonged use of a topical ocular anesthetic is not recommended. It may produce permanent corneal opacification with accompanying visual loss.

Precautions: Fluoracaine® (Fluorescein Sodium and Proparacaine Hydrochloride Ophthalmic Solution, USP) should be used cautiously and sparingly in patients with known allergies, cardiac disease, or hyperthyroidism. The long-term toxicity is unknown; prolonged use may possibly delay wound healing. Although exceedingly rare with ophthalmic application of local anesthetics, systemic toxicity (manifested by central nervous system stimulation followed by depression) may occur. Protection of the eye from irritating chemicals, foreign bodies and rubbing during the period of anesthesia is very important. Tonometers soaked in sterilizing or detergent solutions should be thoroughly rinsed with sterile distilled water prior to use. Patients should be advised to avoid touching the eye until the anesthesia has worn off.

Use in Pregnancy: Pregnancy Category C. Animal reproduction studies have not been conducted with Fluoracaine®. It is also not known whether Fluoracaine® can cause fetal harm when administered to a pregnant woman or can affect reproduction capacity. Fluoracaine® should be given to a pregnant woman only if clearly needed.

Nursing Mothers: It is not known whether this drug is excreted in human milk. Because many drugs are excreted in human milk, caution should be exercised when Fluoracaine® is administered to a nursing woman.

Pediatric Use: Safety and effectiveness in children have not been established.

Adverse Reactions: Occasional temporary stinging, burning, and conjunctival redness have been reported after use of ocular anesthetics, as well as a rare, severe, immediate-type, apparently hyperallergic corneal reaction, with acute, intense and diffuse epithelial keratitis, a gray, ground glass appearance, sloughing of large areas of necrotic epithelium corneal filaments and sometimes, iritis with descemetitis.

Allergic contact dermatitis with drying and fissuring of the fingertips has been reported.

Dosage and Administration: Removal of foreign bodies and sutures, and for tonometry: 1 to 2 drops (in single installations) in each eye before operating.

Deep ophthalmic anesthesia: 1 drop in each eye every 5 to 10 minutes for 5–7 doses.

NOTE: The use of an eye patch is recommended.

How Supplied: Fluoracaine® is supplied as 5mL contained in a pastic bottle with dropper tip (NDC 17478-310-10) or 5 mL contained in a glass bottle with a separate sterile dropper applicator (NDC 17478-311-10).

Storage: Refrigerate at 2°–8°C (35°–46°F) before and after opening. Protect from light.

Caution: Federal (USA) law prohibits dispensing without prescription.

Akorn
Abita Springs, LA 70420

GENTAK® ℞

brand of gentamicin sulfate
Ophthalmic Solution, USP –Sterile
Ophthalmic Ointment, USP –Sterile
Each mL or gram contains gentamicin sulfate, USP equivalent to 3.0 mg gentamicin.

Description: Gentamicin sulfate is a water-soluble antibiotic of the aminoglycoside group. Gentamicin Sulfate **Ophthalmic Solution** is a sterile, aqueous solution buffered to approximately pH 7 for ophthalmic use. Each mL contains gentamicin sulfate, USP (equivalent to 3.0 mg gentamicin), disodium phosphate, monosodium phosphate, sodium chloride, and benazalkonium chloride (0.1 mg) as a preservative.

Gentamicin Sulfate **Ophthalmic Ointment** is a sterile ointment, each gram containing gentamicin sulfate, USP (equivalent to 3.0 mg gentamicin) in a base of white petrolatum, with methylparaben (0.5 mg) and propylparaben (0.1 mg) as preservatives.

Gentamicin is obtained from cultures of *Micromonospora purpurea.* It is a mixture of the sulfate salts of gentamicin C_1, C_2, and C_{1A}. All three components appear to have similar antimicrobial activities. Gentamicin sulfate occurs as a white powder and is soluble in water and insoluble in alcohol. The structure is as follows:

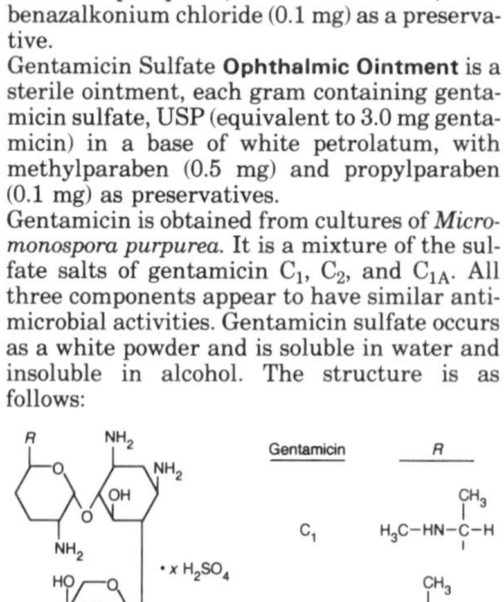

Clinical Pharmacology: Microbiology: Gentamicin sulfate is active *in vitro* against many strains of the following microorganisms: *Staphylococcus aureus, Staphylococcus epidermidis, Streptococcus pyogenes, Streptococcus pneumoniae, Enterobacter aerogenes, Escherichia coli, Haemophilus influenzae, Klebsiella pneumoniae, Neisseria gonorrhoeae, Pseudomonas aeruginosa,* and *Serratia marcescens.*

Indications and Usage: GENTAK **Sterile Ophthalmic Solution** and **Ointment** are indi-

cated in the topical treatment of ocular bacterial infections, including conjunctivitis, keratitis, keratoconjunctivitis, corneal ulcers, blepharitis, blepharoconjunctivitis, acute meibomianitis, and dacryocystitis caused by susceptible strains of the following microorganisms:
Staphylococcus aureus, Staphylococcus epidermidis, Streptococcus pyogenes, Streptococcus pneumoniae, Enterobacter aerogenes, Escherichia coli, Haemophilus influenzae, Klebsiella pneumoniae, Neisseria gonorrhoeae, Pseudomonas aeruginosa, and *Serratia marcescens*.

Contraindications: GENTAK **Ophthalmic Solution** and **Ointment** are contraindicated in patients with known hypersensitivity to any of the components.

Warnings: NOT FOR INJECTION INTO THE EYE. GENTAK **Ophthalmic Solution** and **Ointment** are not for injection. They should never be injected subconjunctivally, nor should they be directly introduced into the anterior chamber of the eye.

Precautions: General: Prolonged use of topical antibiotics may give rise to overgrowth of nonsusceptible organisms including fungi. Baceterial resistance to gentamicin may also develop. If purulent discharge, inflammation or pain becomes aggravated, the patient should discontinue use of the medication and consult a physician.
If irritation or hypersensitivity to any component of the drug develops, the patient should discontinue use of this preparation, and appropriate therapy should be instituted.
Ophthalmic ointments may retard corneal healing.

Information for Patients: To avoid contamination, do not touch tip of container to the eye, eyelid, or any surface.

Carcinogenesis, Mutagenesis, Impairment of Fertility: There are no published carcinogenicity or impairment of fertility studies on gentamicin. Aminoglycoside antibiotics have been found to be non-mutagenic.

Pregnancy: Pregnancy Category C. Gentamicin has been shown to depress body weights, kidney weights, and median glomerular counts in newborn rats when administered systemically to pregnant rats in daily doses approximately 500 times the maximum recommended ophthalmic human dose. There are no adequate and well-controlled studies in pregnant women. Gentamicin should be used during pregnancy only if the potential benefit justifies the potential risk to the fetus.

Adverse Reactions: Bacterial and fungal corneal ulcers have developed during treatment with gentamicin ophthalmic preparations.
The most frequently reported adverse reactions are ocular burning and irritation upon drug instillation, non-specific conjunctivitis, conjunctival epithelial defects, and conjunctival hyperemia.
Other adverse reactions which have occurred rarely are allergic reactions, thrombocytopenic purpura, and hallucinations.

Dosage and Administration: GENTAK **Ophthalmic Solution:** Instill one or two drops into the affected eye every four hours. In severe infections, dosage may be increased to as much as two drops once every hour.
GENTAK **Ophthalmic Ointment:** Apply a small amount (about ½ inch) to the affected eye two to three times a day.

How Supplied: GENTAK Ophthalmic Solution–Sterile, 5-mL plastic dropper bottle, box of one (NDC-17478-283-10).
GENTAK Ophthalmic Ointment–Sterile, 3.5 g tube, box of one (NDC-17478-284-35).
Store GENTAK Ophthalmic Ointment and Solution between 3° and 30°C (36° and 86°F).
Manufactured by Schering Corporation,
Kenilworth, NJ 07033
for Akorn, Inc., Abita Springs, LA 70420.
11/93

17924702

GLAUCTABS ℞
Methazolamide Tablets USP
25 mg and 50 mg

Description: Methazolamide, a sulfonamide derivative, is a white crystalline powder, weakly acidic, slightly soluble in water, alcohol and acetone. The chemical name for methazolamide is: N-[5-(aminosulfonyl)-3-methyl-1,3,4-thiadiazol-2(3H)-ylidene]-acetamide and it has the following structural formula:

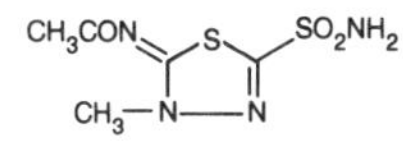

$C_5H_8N_4O_3S_2$ 236.26

Each tablet, for oral administration, contains 25 mg or 50 mg methazolamide. In addition, each tablet contains the following inactive ingredients: colloidal silicon dioxide, croscarmellose sodium, dibasic calcium phosphate dihydrate, magnesium stearate (powder), and microcrystalline cellulose.

Clinical Pharmacology: Methazolamide is a potent inhibitor of carbonic anhydrase.
Methazolamide is well absorbed from the gastrointestinal tract. Peak plasma concentrations are observed 1 to 2 hours after dosing. In a multiple-dose, pharmacokinetic study, administration of methazolamide 25 mg bid, 50 mg bid, and 100 mg bid demonstrated a linear relationship between plasma methazolamide levels and methazolamide dose. Peak plasma concentrations (C_{max}) for the 25 mg, 50 mg and 100 mg bid regimens were 2.5 mcg/mL, 5.1 mcg/mL, and 10.7 mcg/mL, respectively. The area under the plasma concentration-time curves (AUC) was 1130 mcg.min/mL, 2571 mcg.min/mL, and 5418 mcg.min/mL for the 25 mg, 50 mg, and 100 mg dosage regimens, respectively.
Methazolamide is distributed throughout the body including the plasma, cerebrospinal fluid, aqueous humor of the eye, red blood cells, bile and extra-cellular fluid. The mean apparent volume of distribution (V_{area}/F) ranges from 17 L to 23 L. Approximately 55% is bound to plasma proteins. The steady-state methazolamide red blood cell: plasma ratio varies with dose and was found to be 27:1, 16:1, and 10:1 following the administration of methazolamide 25 mg bid, 50 mg bid, and 100 mg bid, respectively.
The mean steady-state plasma elimination half-life for methazolamide is approximately 14 hours. At steady state approximately 25% of the dose is recovered unchanged in the urine over the dosing interval. Renal clearance accounts for 20% to 25% of the total clearance of drug. After repeated bid-tid dosing, methazolamide accumulates to steady-state concentrations in 7 days.
Methazolamide's inhibitory action on carbonic anhydrase decreases the secretion of aqueous humor and results in a decrease in intraocular pressure. The onset of the decrease in intraocular pressure generally occurs within 2 to 4 hours, has a peak effect in 6 to 8 hours and a total duration of 10 to 18 hours.
Methazolamide is a sulfonamide derivative; however, it does not have any clinically significant antimicrobial properties. Although methazolamide achieves a high concentration in the cerebrospinal fluid, it is not considered an effective anticonvulsant.
Methazolamide has a weak and transient diuretic effect, therefore use results in an increase in urinary volume, with excretion of sodium, potassium, and chloride. The drug should not be used as a diuretic. Inhibition of renal bicarbonate reabsorption produces an alkaline urine. Plasma bicarbonate decreases, and a relative, transient metabolic acidosis may occur due to a disequilibrium in carbon dioxide transport in the red cell. Urinary citrate excretion is decreased by approximately 40% after doses of 100 mg every 8 hours. Uric acid output has been shown to decrease 36% in the first 24 hour period.

Indications and Usage: Glauctabs are indicated in the treatment of ocular conditions where lowering intraocular pressure is likely to be of therapeutic benefit, such as chronic open-angle glaucoma, secondary glaucoma, and preoperatively in acute angle-closure glaucoma where lowering the intraocular pressure is desired before surgery.

Contraindications: Methazolamide therapy is contraindicated in situations in which sodium and/or potassium serum levels are depressed, in cases of marked kidney or liver disease or dysfunction, in adrenal gland failure, and in hyperchloremic acidosis. In patients with cirrhosis, use may precipitate the development of hepatic encephalopathy.
Long-term administration of methazolamide is contraindicated in patients with angle-closure glaucoma, since organic closure of the angle may occur in spite of lowered intraocular pressure.

Warnings: Fatalities have occurred, although rarely, due to severe reactions to sulfonamides including Stevens-Johnson syndrome, toxic epidermal necrolysis, fulminant hepatic necrosis, agranulocytosis, aplastic anemia, and other blood dyscrasias. Hypersensitivity reactions may recur when a sulfonamide is readministered, irrespective of the route of administration.
If hypersensitivity or other serious reactions occur, the use of this drug should be discontinued.
Caution is advised for patients receiving high-dose aspirin and methazolamide concomitantly, as anorexia, tachypnea, lethargy, coma, and death have been reported with concomitant use of high-dose aspirin and carbonic anhydrase inhibitors.

Precautions: General: Potassium excretion is increased initially upon administration of methazolamide and in patients with cirrhosis or hepatic insufficiency could precipitate a hepatic coma.
In patients with pulmonary obstruction or emphysema, where alveolar ventilation may be impaired, methazolamide should be used with caution because it may precipitate or aggravate acidosis.
Information for Patients: Adverse reactions common to all sulfonamide derivatives may occur: anaphylaxis, fever, rash (including erythema multiforme, Stevens-Johnson syndrome, toxic epidermal necrolysis), crystalluria, renal calculus, bone marrow depression, thrombocytopenic purpura, hemolytic anemia, leukopenia, pancytopenia, and agranulocytosis. Precaution is advised for early detection of such reactions, and the drug should be discontinued and appropriate therapy instituted.
Caution is advised for patients receiving high-dose aspirin and methazolamide concomitantly.
Laboratory Tests: To monitor for hematologic reactions common to all sulfonamides, it is recommended that a baseline CBC and platelet count be obtained on patients prior to initiating methazolamide therapy and at regular intervals during therapy. If significant changes occur, early discontinuance and institution of appropriate therapy are important. Periodic monitoring of serum electrolytes is also recommended.

Continued on next page

Akorn—Cont.

Drug Interactions: Methazolamide should be used with caution in patients on steroid therapy because of the potential for developing hypokalemia.
Caution is advised for patients receiving high-dose aspirin and methazolamide concomitantly, as anorexia, tachypnea, lethargy, coma and death have been reported with concomitant use of high-dose aspirin and carbonic anhydrase inhibitors (see WARNINGS).
Carcinogenesis, Mutagenesis, Impairment of Fertility: Long-term studies in animals to evaluate the carcinogenic potential of methazolamide and its effect on fertility have not been conducted. Methazolamide was not mutagenic in the Ames bacterial test.
Pregnancy: *Teratogenic effects.* Pregnancy Category C. Methazolamide has been shown to be teratogenic (skeletal anomalies) in rats when given in doses approximately 40 times the human dose. There are no adequate and well controlled studies in pregnant women. Methazolamide should be used during pregnancy only if the potential benefit justifies the potential risk to the fetus.
Nursing Mothers: It is not known whether this drug is excreted in human milk. Because many drugs are excreted in human milk and because of the potential for serious adverse reactions in nursing infants from methazolamide, a decision should be made whether to discontinue nursing or to discontinue the drug, taking into account the importance of the drug to the mother.
Pediatric Use: The safety and effectiveness of methazolamide in children have not been established.
Adverse Reactions: Adverse reactions, occurring most often early in therapy, include paresthesias, particularly a "tingling" feeling in the extremities; hearing dysfunction or tinnitus; fatigue; malaise; loss of appetite; taste alteration; gastrointestinal disturbances such as nausea, vomiting, and diarrhea; polyuria; and occasional instances of drowsiness and confusion.
Metabolic acidosis and electrolyte imbalance may occur.
Transient myopia has been reported. This condition invariably subsides upon diminution or discontinuance of the medication.
Other occasional adverse reactions include urticaria, melena, hematuria, glycosuria, hepatic insufficiency, flaccid paralysis, photosensitivity, convulsions, and, rarely, crystalluria and renal calculi. Also see PRECAUTIONS: Information for Patients for possible reactions common to sulfonamide derivatives. Fatalities have occurred, although rarely, due to severe reactions to sulfonamides including Stevens-Johnson syndrome, toxic epidermal necrolysis, fulminant hepatic necrosis, agranulocytosis, aplastic anemia, and other blood dyscrasias (see WARNINGS).
Overdosage: No data are available regarding methazolamide overdosage in humans as no cases of acute poisoning with this drug have been reported. Animal data suggest that even a high dose of methazolamide is nontoxic. No specific antidote is known. Treatment should be symptomatic and supportive.
Electrolyte imbalance, development of an acidotic state, and central nervous system effects might be expected to occur. Serum electrolyte levels (particularly potassium) and blood pH levels should be monitored.
Supportive measures may be required to restore electrolyte and pH balance.
Dosage and Administration: The effective therapeutic dose administered varies from 50 mg to 100 mg two or three times daily. The drug may be used concomitantly with miotic and osmotic agents.
How Supplied: Glauctabs (Methazolamide Tablets USP), 25 mg, are round, white tablets, debossed "EFF" on one side and "21" on the other side and are supplied in bottles of 100, NDC 17478-525-01.
Glauctabs (Methazolamide Tablets USP), 50 mg, are round, white, scored tablets debossed "EFF" on one side and "20" on the other side and are supplied in bottles of 100, NDC #17478-550-01.
Store at controlled room temperature, 15°–30°C (50°–86°F).
Dispense in a tight container as defined in the USP, with a child-resistant closure (as required).
CAUTION: Federal law prohibits dispensing without prescription.

Manufactured by:
MIKART, INC.
Atlanta, GA 30318
Marketed by:
AKORN, INC.
Abita Springs, LA 70420

Code 617B00 & 628B00 Rev. 05/94

LID WIPES-SPF™ OTC

Description: Lid Wipes-SPF™ are sterile, preservative-free, individually packaged, pre-soaked cleansing pads. Lid Wipes-SPF™ are isotonic, non-ionic, pH-adjusted and hypo-allergenic. Lid Wipes-SPF™ are specially formulated to be non-irritating.
Ingredients: PEG-200 Glyceryl Monotallowate, PEG-80 Glyceryl Monococate, Laureth-23, Cocoamido Propyl Amine Oxide, Sodium Chloride, Glycerin, Sodium Phosphate Monobasic, Sodium Hydroxide and/or Phosphoric Acid (to adjust pH) and Purified Water.
Use: For use when daily, long-term hygiene of the eyelid margins is indicated.
Directions: Gently cleanse skin and eyelid margins with the pre-moistened pad to remove oils, debris, crusted matter and cosmetics. Rinse with warm water and dry. Ready to use, do not dilute.
How Supplied: Lid Wipes-SPF™ is available as 30 individually packaged, pre-soaked cleansing pads in a convenient dispenser box.
NDC 17478-820-06 Box of 30.

OCUCAPS® Antioxidants OTC
Vitamin and Mineral Supplement

Description: Each OcuCaps® caplet contains: [see table below]
Indications: OcuCaps® is formulated as an antioxidant vitamin & mineral supplement. OcuCaps® is a nutritional supplement to the diets of people who may have or be at risk of deficiencies of the ingredients found in OcuCaps®.
Recommended Intake: Adults should take one caplet once or twice daily, as directed by a physician.
How Supplied: White, coated caplets.
NDC 17478-805-60 Bottle of 60
Store at controlled room temperature, keep tightly closed.
[See table below.]

OCUCAPS®

Ingredient	Source	Amount	% US RDA
Vitamin A	Beta Carotene	5000 IU	100%
Vitamin C	Ascorbic Acid	400mg	667%
Vitamin E	dL-Alpha-Tocopheryl Acetate	200 IU	667%
Zinc	Zinc Ascorbate	40mg	267%
L-Glutathione		5mg	***
Sodium Pyruvate		3mg	***
Copper	Copper Ascorbate	2mg	100%
Selenium	L-Selenomethionine	40mcg	***

*** US RDA not established.

TEARS RENEWED OINTMENT OTC
Preservative Free and Lanolin-Free
Sterile Ophthalmic Lubricating Ointment

Description: An ocular emollient containing white petrolatum and light mineral oil. Contains no preservatives and no lanolin.
Indications: For use as a lubricant or protectant to prevent further irritation or to relieve dryness of the eye.
Directions: Pull down lower lid of the affected eye and apply a small amount (1/4 inch) of ointment to the inside of the eyelid.
How Supplied: 3.5 gm (1/8 oz.) ophthalmic tube with applicator tip. NDC 17478-063-35

Alcon Laboratories, Inc.
and its affiliates
CORPORATE HEADQUARTERS:
6201 SOUTH FREEWAY
FORT WORTH, TX 76134

ADSORBONAC® 2% and 5% OTC
(Sodium Chloride Ophthalmic Solution)
Hypertonicity Eye Drops

Ingredients: Each mL contains: **Active:** Sodium chloride 2% or 5%. **Preservative:** Thimerosal 0.004%, added. **Inactive:** ADSORBOBASE® polymers (Povidone, PEG-90M, Hydroxyethyl Cellulose and Poloxamer 188), Edetate Disodium, Dibasic Sodium Phosphate, Hydrochloric Acid and/or Sodium Hydroxide to adjust pH, Purified Water.
Indications:

FDA APPROVED USE
For the temporary relief of corneal edema.

Warnings: This product contains thimerosal 0.004% added as a preservative. Do not use this product if you are sensitive to thimerosal or any other ingredient containing mercury. Do not use this product except under the advice and supervision of a doctor. If you experience eye pain, changes in vision, continued redness or irritation of the eye, or if the condition worsens or persists, consult a doctor. This product may cause temporary burning and irritation on being instilled into the eye. If solution changes color or becomes cloudy, do not use. To avoid contamination, do not touch tip of container to any surface. Replace cap after using. Keep this and all drugs out of the reach of children. In case of accidental ingestion, seek professional assistance or contact a Poison Control Center immediately.
Directions: Instill 1 or 2 drops in the affected eye(s) every 3 or 4 hours, or as directed by a doctor.
How Supplied: 15mL sterile control dropper dispensers—2% and 5% strengths.
2% NDC 0998-0504-15
5% NDC 0998-0505-15
Storage: PROTECT FROM LIGHT—STORE CONTAINER IN ORIGINAL CARTON AT 8°–27°C (46°–80°F).

ADSORBOTEAR® OTC
Artificial Tear

Ingredients: hydroxyethylcellulose 0.4% and ADSORBOBASE® (povidone 1.67% with water soluble polymers) in a buffered, isotonic solution. Preservatives: thimerosal 0.004%, edetate disodium 0.1%.
Indications: ADSORBOTEAR® is a sterile, tear-like lubricant which provides temporary relief for dry conditions of the eyes when the natural tear production is deficient.
FOR TOPICAL EYE USE ONLY.
Warnings: This product contains thimerosal 0.004% as a preservative. Do not use this product if you are sensitive to thimerosal or any other ingredient containing mercury.
If you experience eye pain, changes in vision, continued redness or irritation of the eye, or if the condition worsens or persists for more than 72 hours, discontinue use and consult a physician.
To avoid contamination, do not touch tip of container to any surface. Replace cap after using. If solution changes color or becomes cloudy, do not use. Keep this and all drugs out of the reach of children. In case of accidental ingestion, seek professional assistance or contact a Poison Control Center immediately.
Directions: Apply one or two drops of ADSORBOTEAR® to the eye(s) three times a day or as needed.
How Supplied: 15mL sterile control dropper dispensers.
NDC 0998-0410-15
Storage: PROTECT FROM LIGHT. STORE CONTAINER IN ORIGINAL CARTON AT 8°–27°C (46°–80°F).
TAMPER RESISTANT: Do not use if cap band marked **Alcon** is damaged or missing. For added protection, carton end-panels are sealed.

ALCAINE® ℞
(proparacaine hydrochloride Ophthalmic Solution, USP) 0.5%

Description: ALCAINE® (Proparacaine Hydrochloride) is a topical anesthetic prepared as a sterile aqueous ophthalmic solution. The active ingredient is represented by the chemical structure:

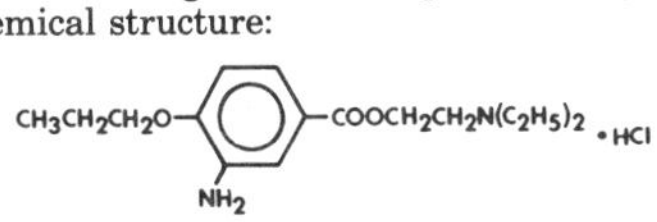

Established name:
Proparacaine Hydrochloride

Chemical name:
Benzoic acid, 3-amino-4-propoxy-, 2-(diethylamino) ethyl ester, monohydrochloride.

Each mL contains: Active: Proparacaine Hydrochloride 0.5% (5mg). Preservative: Benzalkonium Chloride 0.01%. Inactive: Glycerin, Hydrochloric Acid and/or Sodium Hydroxide (to adjust pH), Purified Water.
Clinical Pharmacology: ALCAINE Solution is a rapid acting local anesthetic suitable for ophthalmic use. The onset of anesthesia usually begins within 30 seconds and persists for 15 minutes or longer.
The main site of anesthetic action is the nerve cell membrane where proparacaine interferes with the large transient increase in the membrane permeability to sodium ions that is normally produced by a slight depolarization of the membrane. As the anesthetic action progressively develops in a nerve, the threshold for electrical stimulation gradually increases and the safety factor for conduction decreases; when this action is sufficiently well developed, block of conduction is produced.
The exact mechanism whereby proparacaine and other local anesthetics influence the permeability of the cell membrane is unknown; however, several studies indicate that local anesthetics may limit sodium ion permeability through the lipid layer of the nerve cell membrane. This limitation prevents the fundamental change necessary for the generation of the action potential.
Indications and Usage: ALCAINE Solution is indicated for topical anesthesia in ophthalmic practice. Representative ophthalmic procedures in which the preparation provides good local anesthesia include measurement of intraocular pressure (tonometry), removal of foreign bodies and sutures from the cornea, conjunctival scraping in diagnosis and gonioscopic examination; it is also indicated for use as a topical anesthetic prior to surgical operations such as cataract extraction.
Contraindications: This preparation is contraindicated in patients with known hypersensitivity to any component of the solution. This product should never be prescribed for the patient's own use.
Warnings: For topical ophthalmic use only. Prolonged use of a topical ocular anesthetic may produce permanent corneal opacification with accompanying loss of vision.
Precautions:
General. Proparacaine hydrochloride should be used cautiously and sparingly in patients with known allergies, cardiac disease, or hyperthyroidism. The long-term toxicity of proparacaine is unknown; prolonged use may possibly delay wound healing. Although exceedingly rare with ophthalmic application of local anesthetics, it should be borne in mind that systemic toxicity (manifested by central nervous system stimulation followed by depression) may occur.
Protection of the eye from irritating chemicals, foreign bodies and rubbing during the period of anesthesia is very important. Tonometers soaked in sterilizing or detergent solutions should be thoroughly rinsed with sterile distilled water prior to use. Patients should be advised to avoid touching the eye until the anesthesia has worn off. Do not touch dropper tip to any surface as this may contaminate the solution.
Carcinogenesis, Mutagenesis, Impairment of Fertility. Long-term studies in animals have not been performed to evaluate carcinogenic potential, mutagenicity, or possible impairment of fertility in males or females.
Pregnancy Category C. Animal reproduction studies have not been conducted with ALCAINE Solution. It is also not known whether proparacaine hydrochloride can cause fetal harm when administered to a pregnant woman or can affect reproduction capacity. Proparacaine hydrochloride should be administered to a pregnant woman only if clearly needed.
Nursing Mothers. It is not known whether this drug is excreted in human milk. Because many drugs are excreted in human milk, caution should be exercised when proparacaine hydrochloride is administered to a nursing woman.
Pediatric Use. Controlled clinical studies have not been performed with ALCAINE Solution to establish safety and effectiveness in children; however, the literature cites the use of proparacaine hydrochloride as a topical ophthalmic anesthetic agent in children.
Adverse Reactions: Pupillary dilation or cycloplegic effects have rarely been observed with proparacaine hydrochloride. The drug appears to be safe for use in patients sensitive to other local anesthetics, but local or systemic sensitivity occasionally occurs. Instillation of proparacaine in the eye at recommended concentration and dosage usually produces little or no initial irritation, stinging, burning, conjunctival redness, lacrimation or increased winking. However, some local irritation and stinging may occur several hours after the instillation.
Rarely, a severe, immediate-type, apparently hyperallergic corneal reaction may occur which includes acute, intense and diffuse epithelial keratitis; a gray, ground-glass appearance; sloughing of large areas of necrotic epithelium; corneal filaments and, sometimes, iritis with descemetitis.
Allergic contact dermatitis with drying and fissuring of the fingertips has been reported. Softening and erosion of the corneal epithelium and conjunctival congestion and hemorrhage have been reported.
Dosage and Administration:
Deep anesthesia as in cataract extraction:
Instill 1 drop every 5 to 10 minutes for 5 to 7 doses.
Removal of sutures:
Instill 1 or 2 drops 2 or 3 minutes before removal of stitches.
Removal of foreign bodies:
Instill 1 or 2 drops prior to operating.
Tonometry:
Instill 1 or 2 drops immediately before measurement.
How Supplied: ALCAINE (Proparacaine Hydrochloride Ophthalmic Solution, USP) 0.5% is supplied in 15 mL DROP-TAINER® dispensers.
NDC 0998-0016-15
Storage: Store at 8°–24°C (46°–75°F) before opening. Store at 2°–8°C (35°–46°F) after opening to retard discoloration of solution. Do not use a discolored solution.
Caution: Federal (USA) law prohibits dispensing without prescription.

ALOMIDE® 0.1% ℞
(Lodoxamide Tromethamine Ophthalmic Solution)

Description: ALOMIDE® is a sterile ophthalmic solution containing the mast cell stabilizer lodoxamide tromethamine for topical administration to the eyes. Lodoxamide tromethamine is a white, crystalline, water-soluble powder with a molecular weight of 553.91. The chemical structure is presented below:

Structural Formula:

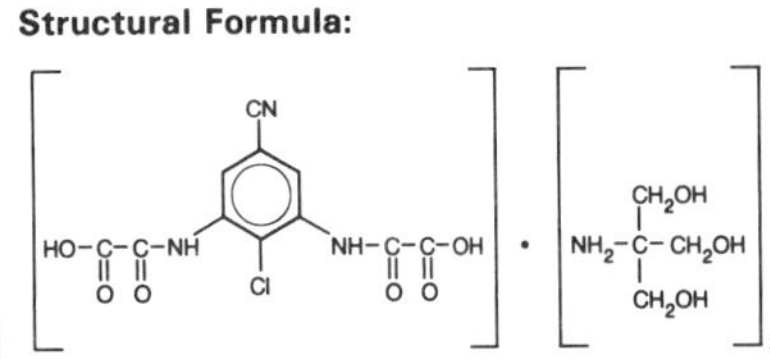

Chemical Name:
N,N′-(2-chloro-5-cyano-m-phenylene)dioxamic acid tromethamine salt
Empirical Formula: $C_{19}H_{28}O_{12}N_5Cl$
Each mL of ALOMIDE® Ophthalmic Solution contains: Active: 1.78 mg lodoxamide tromethamine equivalent to 1 mg lodoxamide. **Preservative:** benzalkonium chloride 0.007%. **Inactive:** mannitol, hydroxypropyl methylcellulose 2910, sodium citrate, citric acid, edetate disodium, tyloxapol, hydrochloric acid and/or sodium hydroxide (adjust pH), and purified water.
Clinical Pharmacology: Lodoxamide tromethamine is a mast cell stabilizer that inhibits the *in vivo* Type 1 immediate hypersensitivity reaction. Lodoxamide therapy inhibits the increases in cutaneous vascular permeability that are associated with reagin or IgE and antigen-mediated reactions.
In vitro studies have demonstrated the ability of lodoxamide to stabilize rodent mast cells and

Continued on next page

Alcon—Cont.

prevent antigen-stimulated release of histamine. In addition, lodoxamide prevents the release of other mast cell inflammatory mediators (i.e., SRS-A, slow-reacting substances of anaphylaxis, also known as the peptidoleukotrienes) and inhibits eosinophil chemotaxis. Although lodoxamide's precise mechanism of action is unknown, the drug has been reported to prevent calcium influx into mast cells upon antigen stimulation.
Lodoxamide has no intrinsic vasoconstrictor, antihistaminic, cyclooxygenase inhibition, or other anti-inflammatory activity.
The disposition of ^{14}C-lodoxamide was studied in six healthy adult volunteers receiving a 3 mg (50 μCi) oral dose of lodoxamide. Urinary excretion was the major route of elimination. The elimination half-life of ^{14}C-lodoxamide was 8.5 hours in urine. In a study conducted in twelve healthy adult volunteers, topical administration of ALOMIDE® 0.1% (Lodoxamide Tromethamine Ophthalmic Solution), one drop in each eye four times per day for ten days, did not result in any measurable lodoxamide plasma levels at a detection limit of 2.5 ng/mL.

Indications and Usage: ALOMIDE® Ophthalmic Solution 0.1% is indicated in the treatment of the ocular disorders referred to by the terms vernal keratoconjunctivitis, vernal conjunctivitis, and vernal keratitis.

Contraindications: Hypersensitivity to any component of this product.

Warnings: Not for injection. As with all ophthalmic preparations containing benzalkonium chloride, patients should be instructed not to wear soft contact lenses during treatment with ALOMIDE® Ophthalmic Solution.

Precautions: **General:** Patients may experience a transient burning or stinging upon instillation of ALOMIDE® Ophthalmic Solution. Should these symptoms persist, the patient should be advised to contact the prescribing physician.

Carcinogenesis, Mutagenesis, Impairment of Fertility:
A long-term study with lodoxamide tromethamine in rats (two-year oral administration) showed no neoplastic or tumorigenic effects at doses 100 mg/kg/day (more than 5000 times the proposed human clinical dose). No evidence of mutagenicity or genetic damage was seen in the Ames *Salmonella* Assay, Chromosomal Aberration in CHO Cells Assay, or Mouse Forward Lymphoma Assay. In the BALB/c-3T3 Cells Transformation Assay, some increase in the number of transformed foci was seen at high concentrations (greater than 4000 μg/mL). No evidence of impairment of reproductive function was shown in laboratory animal studies.

Pregnancy: Pregnancy Category B. Reproduction studies with lodoxamide tromethamine administered orally to rats and rabbits in doses of 100 mg/kg/day (more than 5000 times the proposed human clinical dose) produced no evidence of developmental toxicity. There are, however, no adequate and well-controlled studies in pregnant women. Because animal reproduction studies are not always predictive of human response, ALOMIDE® 0.1% (Lodoxamide Tromethamine Ophthalmic Solution) should be used during pregnancy only if clearly needed.

Nursing Mothers: It is not known whether lodoxamide tromethamine is excreted in human milk. Because many drugs are excreted in human milk, caution should be exercised when ALOMIDE® Ophthalmic Solution 0.1% is administered to nursing women.

Pediatric Use: Safety and effectiveness in children younger than 2 years of age have not been established.

Adverse Reactions: During clinical studies of ALOMIDE® Ophthalmic Solution 0.1%, the most frequently reported ocular adverse experiences were transient burning, stinging, or discomfort upon instillation, which occurred in approximately 15% of the subjects. Other ocular events occurring in 1 to 5% of the subjects included ocular itching/pruritus, blurred vision, dry eye, tearing/discharge hyperemia, crystalline deposits, and foreign body sensation. Events that occurred in less than 1% of the subjects included corneal erosion/ulcer, scales on lid/lash, eye pain, ocular edema/swelling, ocular warming sensation, ocular fatigue, chemosis, corneal abrasion, anterior chamber cells, keratopathy/keratitis, blepharitis, allergy, sticky sensation, and epitheliopathy.
Nonocular events reported were headache (1.5%) and (at less than 1%) heat sensation, dizziness, somnolence, nausea, stomach discomfort, sneezing, dry nose, and rash.

Overdosage: There have been no reports of ALOMIDE® 0.1% (Lodoxamide Tromethamine Ophthalmic Solution) overdose following topical ocular application. Accidental overdose of an oral preparation of 120 to 180 mg of lodoxamide resulted in a temporary sensation of warmth, profuse sweating, diarrhea, lightheadedness, and a feeling of stomach distension; no permanent adverse effects were observed. Side effects reported following systemic oral administration of 0.1 mg to 10.0 mg of lodoxamide include a feeling of warmth or flushing, headache, dizziness, fatigue, sweating, nausea, loose stools, and urinary frequency/urgency. The physician may consider emesis in the event of accidental ingestion.

Dosage and Administration: The dose for adults and children greater than two years of age is one to two drops in each affected eye four times daily for up to 3 months.

How Supplied: ALOMIDE® Ophthalmic Solution 0.1% is supplied as follows: 10 mL in plastic ophthalmic DROP-TAINER® dispenser.

10 mL: **NDC** 0065-0345-10

Storage:
Store at 15°C–27°C (59°F–80°F).

Caution: Federal (USA) law prohibits dispensing without prescription.

BETOPTIC® ℞

(betaxolol hydrochloride)
0.5% as base
Sterile Ophthalmic Solution

Description: BETOPTIC® Sterile Ophthalmic Solution contains betaxolol hydrochloride, a cardioselective beta-adrenergic receptor blocking agent, in a sterile isotonic solution. Betaxolol hydrochloride is a white, crystalline powder, soluble in water, with a molecular weight of 343.89. The chemical structure is presented below:

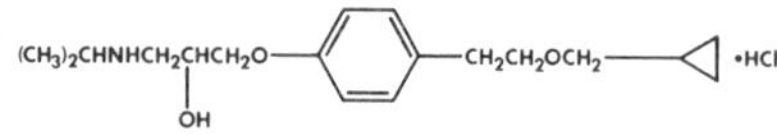

Empirical Formula:
$C_{18}H_{29}NO_3 \cdot HCl$
Chemical Name:
(±)-1-[p-[2-(Cyclopropylmethoxy)ethyl] phenoxy]-3-(isopropylamino)-2-propanol hydrochloride.

Each mL of BETOPTIC Ophthalmic Solution (0.5%) contains: Active: 5.6 mg betaxolol hydrochloride equivalent to betaxolol base 5 mg. Preservative: Benzalkonium Chloride 0.01%. Inactives: Edetate Disodium, Sodium Chloride, Hydrochloric Acid and/or Sodium Hydroxide (to adjust pH), and Purified Water.

Clinical Pharmacology: Betaxolol HCl, a cardioselective (beta-1-adrenergic) receptor blocking agent, does not have significant membrane-stabilizing (local anesthetic) activity and is devoid of intrinsic sympathomimetic action. Orally administered beta-adrenergic blocking agents reduce cardiac output in healthy subjects and patients with heart disease. In patients with severe impairment of myocardial function, beta-adrenergic receptor antagonists may inhibit the sympathetic stimulatory effect necessary to maintain adequate cardiac function.
When instilled in the eye, BETOPTIC Ophthalmic Solution has the action of reducing elevated as well as normal intraocular pressure, whether or not accompanied by glaucoma. Ophthalmic betaxolol has minimal effect on pulmonary and cardiovascular parameters.
Ophthalmic betaxolol (one drop in each eye) was compared to timolol and placebo in a three-way crossover study challenging nine patients with reactive airway disease who were selected on the basis of having at least a 15% reduction in the forced expiratory volume in one second (FEV_1) after administration of ophthalmic timolol. Betaxolol HCl had no significant effect on pulmonary function as measured by FEV_1, Forced Vital Capacity (FVC) and FEV_1/VC. Additionally, the action of isoproterenol, a beta stimulant, administered at the end of the study was not inhibited by ophthalmic betaxolol. In contrast, ophthalmic timolol significantly decreased these pulmonary functions.
[See table below.]
No evidence of cardiovascular beta-adrenergic blockade during exercise was observed with betaxolol in a double-masked, three-way crossover study in 24 normal subjects comparing ophthalmic betaxolol, timolol and placebo for effect on blood pressure and heart rate. Mean arterial blood pressure was not affected by any treatment; however, ophthalmic timolol pro-

FEV_1 —Percent Change from Baseline[1]

	Means		
	Betaxolol 1.0%[a]	Timolol 0.5%	Placebo
Baseline	1.6	1.4	1.4
60 Minutes	2.3	−25.7*	5.8
120 Minutes	1.6	−27.4*	7.5
240 Minutes	−6.4	−26.9*	6.9
Isoproterenol[b]	36.1	−12.4*	42.8

[1] Schoene, R. B. *et al.*, Am. J. Ophthal. 97:86, 1984.
[a] Twice the clinical concentration.
[b] Inhaled at 240 minutes; measurement at 270 minutes.
*Timolol statistically different from betaxolol and placebo ($p < 0.05$).

duced a significant decrease in the mean heart rate.

[See table at top right.]

Clinical Studies: Optic nerve head damage and visual field loss are the result of a sustained elevated intraocular pressure and poor ocular perfusion. BETOPTIC Ophthalmic Solution has the action of reducing elevated as well as normal intraocular pressure, and the mechanism of ocular hypotensive action appears to be a reduction of aqueous production as demonstrated by tonography and aqueous fluorophotometry. The onset of action with BETOPTIC Ophthalmic Solution can generally be noted within 30 minutes and the maximal effect can usually be detected 2 hours after topical administration. A single dose provides a 12-hour reduction in intraocular pressure. Clinical observation of glaucoma patients treated with BETOPTIC Ophthalmic Solution for up to three years shows that the intraocular pressure lowering effect is well maintained. Clinical studies show that topical BETOPTIC Ophthalmic Solution reduces mean intraocular pressure 25% from baseline. In trials using 22 mmHg as a generally accepted index of intraocular pressure control, BETOPTIC Ophthalmic Solution was effective in more than 94% of the population studied, of which 73% were treated with the beta blocker alone. In controlled, double-masked studies, the magnitude and duration of the ocular hypotensive effect of BETOPTIC Ophthalmic Solution and ophthalmic timolol solution were clinically equivalent.

BETOPTIC Ophthalmic Solution has also been used successfully in glaucoma patients who have undergone a laser trabeculoplasty and have needed additional long-term ocular hypotensive therapy.

BETOPTIC Ophthalmic Solution has been well-tolerated in glaucoma patients wearing hard or soft contact lenses and in aphakic patients.

BETOPTIC Ophthalmic Solution does not produce miosis or accommodative spasm which are frequently seen with miotic agents. The blurred vision and night blindness often associated with standard miotic therapy are not associated with BETOPTIC Ophthalmic Solution. Thus, patients with central lenticular opacities avoid the visual impairment caused by a constricted pupil.

Indications and Usage: BETOPTIC Ophthalmic Solution has been shown to be effective in lowering intraocular pressure and is indicated in the treatment of ocular hypertension and chronic open-angle glaucoma. It may be used alone or in combination with other anti-glaucoma drugs.

In clinical studies BETOPTIC® was safely used to lower intraocular pressure in 47 patients with both glaucoma and reactive airway disease who were followed for a mean period of 15 months. However, caution should be used in treating patients with severe reactive airway disease or a history of asthma.

Contraindications: Hypersensitivity to any component of this product. BETOPTIC Ophthalmic Solution is contraindicated in patients with sinus bradycardia, greater than a first degree atrioventricular block, cardiogenic shock, or patients with overt cardiac failure.

Warning: Topically applied beta-adrenergic blocking agents may be absorbed systemically. The same adverse reactions found with systemic administration of beta-adrenergic blocking agents may occur with topical administration. For example, severe respiratory reactions and cardiac reactions, including death due to bronchospasm in patients with asthma, and rarely death in association with cardiac failure, have been reported with topical application of beta-adrenergic blocking agents.

BETOPTIC Ophthalmic Solution has been shown to have a minor effect on heart rate and blood pressure in clinical studies. Caution should be used in treating patients with a history of cardiac failure or heart block. Treatment with BETOPTIC Ophthalmic Solution should be discontinued at the first signs of cardiac failure.

Mean Heart Rates[1]

Bruce Stress Exercise Test Minutes	TREATMENT Betaxolol 1%[a]	Timolol 0.5%	Placebo
0	79.2	79.3	81.2
2	130.2	126.0	130.4
4	133.4	128.0*	134.3
6	136.4	129.2*	137.9
8	139.8	131.8*	139.4
10	140.8	131.8*	141.3

[1] Atkins, J. M. *et al.*, Am. J. Oph. 99:173–175, Feb., 1985.
[a] Twice the clinical concentration.
*Mean pulse rate significantly lower for timolol than betaxolol or placebo ($p < 0.05$).

Precautions:

General: Information for Patients. Do not touch dropper tip to any surface as this may contaminate the solution.

Diabetes Mellitus. Beta-adrenergic blocking agents should be administered with caution in patients subject to spontaneous hypoglycemia or to diabetic patients (especially those with labile diabetes) who are receiving insulin or oral hypoglycemic agents. Beta-adrenergic receptor blocking agents may mask the signs and symptoms of acute hypoglycemia.

Thyrotoxicosis. Beta-adrenergic blocking agents may mask certain clinical signs (e.g., tachycardia) of hyperthyroidism. Patients suspected of developing thyrotoxicosis should be managed carefully to avoid abrupt withdrawal of beta-adrenergic blocking agents, which might precipitate a thyroid storm.

Muscle Weakness. Beta-adrenergic blockade has been reported to potentiate muscle weakness consistent with certain myasthenic symptoms (e.g., diplopia, ptosis, and generalized weakness).

Major Surgery. Consideration should be given to the gradual withdrawal of beta-adrenergic blocking agents prior to general anesthesia because of the reduced ability of the heart to respond to beta-adrenergically mediated sympathetic reflex stimuli.

Pulmonary. Caution should be exercised in the treatment of glaucoma patients with excessive restriction of pulmonary function. There have been reports of asthmatic attacks and pulmonary distress during betaxolol treatment. Although rechallenges of some such patients with ophthalmic betaxolol has not adversely affected pulmonary function test results, the possibility of adverse pulmonary effects in patients sensitive to beta blockers cannot be ruled out.

Risk from Anaphylactic Reaction: While taking beta-blockers, patients with a history of atopy or a history of severe anaphylactic reaction to a variety of allergens may be more reactive to repeated accidental, diagnostic, or therapeutic challenge with such allergens. Such patients may be unresponsive to the usual doses of epinephrine used to treat anaphylactic reactions.

Drug Interactions: Patients who are receiving a beta-adrenergic blocking agent orally and BETOPTIC Ophthalmic Solution should be observed for a potential additive effect either on the intraocular pressure or on the known systemic effects of beta blockade.

Close observation of the patient is recommended when a beta blocker is administered to patients receiving catecholamine-depleting drugs such as reserpine, because of possible additive effects and the production of hypotension and/or bradycardia.

Betaxolol is an adrenergic blocking agent; therefore, caution should be exercised in patients using concomitant adrenergic psychotropic drugs.

Ocular: In patients with angle-closure glaucoma, the immediate treatment objective is to reopen the angle by constriction of the pupil with a miotic agent. Betaxolol has little or no effect on the pupil. When BETOPTIC Ophthalmic Solution is used to reduce elevated intraocular pressure in angle-closure glaucoma, it should be used with a miotic and not alone.

Carcinogenesis, Mutagenesis, Impairment of Fertility: Lifetime studies with betaxolol HCl have been completed in mice at oral doses of 6, 20 or 60 mg/kg/day and in rats at 3, 12 or 48 mg/kg/day; betaxolol HCl demonstrated no carcinogenic effect. Higher dose levels were not tested.

In a variety of *in vitro* and *in vivo* bacterial and mammalian cell assays, betaxolol HCl was nonmutagenic.

Pregnancy: Pregnancy Category C. Reproduction, teratology, and peri- and postnatal studies have been conducted with orally administered betaxolol HCl in rats and rabbits. There was evidence of drug related postimplantation loss in rabbits and rats at dose levels above 12 mg/kg and 128 mg/kg, respectively. Betaxolol HCl was not shown to be teratogenic, however, and there were no other adverse effects on reproduction at subtoxic dose levels. There are no adequate and well-controlled studies in pregnant women. BETOPTIC Ophthalmic Solution should be used during pregnancy only if the potential benefit justifies the potential risk to the fetus.

Nursing Mothers: It is not known whether betaxolol HCl is excreted in human milk. Because many drugs are excreted in human milk, caution should be exercised when BETOPTIC Ophthalmic Solution is administered to nursing women.

Pediatric Use: Safety and effectiveness in children have not been established.

Adverse Reactions: The following adverse reactions have been reported in clinical trials with BETOPTIC Ophthalmic Solution.

Ocular: Discomfort of short duration was experienced by one in four patients, but none discontinued therapy; occasional tearing has been reported. Rare instances of decreased corneal sensitivity, erythema, itching sensation, corneal punctate staining, keratitis, ani-

Continued on next page

Alcon—Cont.

socoria, edema, and photophobia have been reported.

Additional medical events reported with other formulations of betaxolol include blurred vision, foreign body sensation, dryness of the eyes, inflammation, discharge, ocular pain, decreased visual acuity, and crusty lashes.

Systemic: Systemic reactions following administration of BETOPTIC Ophthalmic Solution 0.5% or BETOPTIC S Ophthalmic Suspension 0.25% have been rarely reported. These include:

Cardiovascular: Bradycardia, heart block and congestive failure.

Pulmonary: Pulmonary distress characterized by dyspnea, bronchospasm, thickened bronchial secretions, asthma and respiratory failure.

Central Nervous System: Insomnia, dizziness, vertigo, headaches, depression, lethargy, and increase in signs and symptoms of myasthenia gravis.

Other: Hives, toxic epidermal necrolysis, hair loss and glossitis.

Overdosage: No information is available on overdosage of humans. The oral LD_{50} of the drug ranged from 350–920 mg/kg in mice and 860–1050 mg/kg in rats. The symptoms which might be expected with an overdose of a systemically administered beta-1-adrenergic receptor blocker agent are bradycardia, hypotension and acute cardiac failure. A topical overdose of BETOPTIC Ophthalmic Solution may be flushed from the eye(s) with warm tap water.

Dosage and Administration: The recommended dose is one to two drops of BETOPTIC Ophthalmic Solution in the affected eye(s) twice daily. In some patients, the intraocular pressure lowering responses to BETOPTIC Ophthalmic Solution may require a few weeks to stabilize. As with any new medication, careful monitoring of patients is advised.

If the intraocular pressure of the patient is not adequately controlled on this regimen, concomitant therapy with pilocarpine and other miotics, and/or epinephrine and/or carbonic anhydrase inhibitors can be instituted.

How Supplied: BETOPTIC Ophthalmic Solution is a sterile, isotonic, aqueous solution of betaxolol hydrochloride. Supplied as follows: 2.5, 5, 10 and 15 mL in plastic ophthalmic DROP-TAINER® dispensers.

2.5 mL: **NDC** 0065-0245-20
5 mL: **NDC** 0065-0245-05
10 mL: **NDC** 0065-0245-10
15 mL: **NDC** 0065-0245-15

Storage: Store at room temperature.

Caution: Federal (USA) law prohibits dispensing without prescription.

U.S. Patents Nos. 4,252,984; 4,311,708; 4,342,783

BETOPTIC® S ℞

(betaxolol HCl)
0.25% as base
Sterile Ophthalmic Suspension

Description: BETOPTIC S Ophthalmic Suspension 0.25% contains betaxolol hydrochloride, a cardioselective beta-adrenergic receptor blocking agent, in a sterile resin suspension formulation. Betaxolol hydrochloride is a white, crystalline powder, with a molecular weight of 343.89. The chemical structure is presented below:

[See structure at top of next column.]

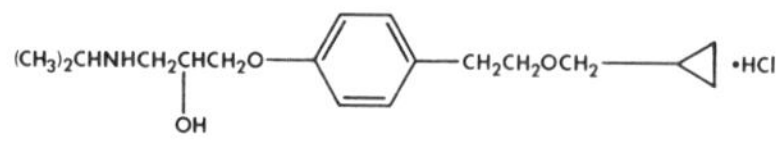

Empirical Formula:
$C_{18}H_{29}NO_3 \cdot HCl$

Chemical Name:
(±)-1-[p-[2-(cyclopropylmethoxy)ethyl] phenoxy]-3-(isopropylamino)-2-propanol hydrochloride.

Each mL of BETOPTIC S Ophthalmic Suspension contains: Active: betaxolol HCl 2.8 mg equivalent to 2.5 mg of betaxolol base. Preservative: benzalkonium chloride 0.01%. Inactive: Mannitol, Poly(Styrene-Divinyl Benzene) sulfonic acid, Carbomer 934P, edetate disodium, hydrochloric acid or sodium hydroxide (to adjust pH) and purified water.

Clinical Pharmacology: Betaxolol HCl, a cardioselective (beta-1-adrenergic) receptor blocking agent, does not have significant membrane-stabilizing (local anesthetic) activity and is devoid of intrinsic sympathomimetic action. Orally administered beta-adrenergic blocking agents reduce cardiac output in healthy subjects and patients with heart disease. In patients with severe impairment of myocardial function, beta-adrenergic receptor antagonists may inhibit the sympathetic stimulatory effect necessary to maintain adequate cardiac function.

When instilled in the eye, BETOPTIC S Ophthalmic Suspension 0.25% has the action of reducing elevated intraocular pressure, whether or not accompanied by glaucoma. Ophthalmic betaxolol has minimal effect on pulmonary and cardiovascular parameters.

Elevated IOP presents a major risk factor in glaucomatous field loss. The higher the level of IOP, the greater the likelihood of optic nerve damage and visual field loss. Betaxolol has the action of reducing elevated as well as normal intraocular pressure and the mechanism of ocular hypotensive action appears to be a reduction of aqueous production as demonstrated by tonography and aqueous fluorophotometry. The onset of action with betaxolol can generally be noted within 30 minutes and the maximal effect can usually be detected 2 hours after topical administration. A single dose provides a 12-hour reduction in intraocular pressure.

In controlled, double-masked studies, the magnitude and duration of the ocular hypotensive effect of BETOPTIC S Ophthalmic Suspension 0.25% and BETOPTIC Ophthalmic Solution 0.5% were clinically equivalent. BETOPTIC S Suspension was significantly more comfortable than BETOPTIC Solution.

Ophthalmic betaxolol solution at 1% (one drop in each eye) was compared to placebo in a crossover study challenging nine patients with reactive airway disease. Betaxolol HCl had no significant effect on pulmonary function as measured by FEV_1, Forced Vital Capacity (FVC), FEV_1/FVC and was not significantly different from placebo. The action of isoproterenol, a beta stimulant, administered at the end of the study was not inhibited by ophthalmic betaxolol.

No evidence of cardiovascular beta adrenergic-blockade during exercise was observed with betaxolol in a double-masked, crossover study in 24 normal subjects comparing ophthalmic betaxolol and placebo for effects on blood pressure and heart rate.

Indications and Usage: BETOPTIC S Ophthalmic Suspension 0.25% has been shown to be effective in lowering intraocular pressure and may be used in patients with chronic open-angle glaucoma and ocular hypertension. It may be used alone or in combination with other intraocular pressure lowering medications.

Contraindications: Hypersensitivity to any component of this product. BETOPTIC S Ophthalmic Suspension 0.25% is contraindicated in patients with sinus bradycardia, greater than a first degree atrioventricular block, cardiogenic shock, or patients with overt cardiac failure.

Warning: Topically applied beta-adrenergic blocking agents may be absorbed systemically. The same adverse reactions found with systemic administration of beta-adrenergic blocking agents may occur with topical administration. For example, severe respiratory reactions and cardiac reactions, including death due to bronchospasm in patients with asthma, and rarely death in association with cardiac failure, have been reported with topical application of beta-adrenergic blocking agents.

BETOPTIC S Ophthalmic Suspension 0.25% has been shown to have a minor effect on heart rate and blood pressure in clinical studies. Caution should be used in treating patients with a history of cardiac failure or heart block. Treatment with BETOPTIC S Ophthalmic Suspension 0.25% should be discontinued at the first signs of cardiac failure.

Precautions:

General:

Diabetes Mellitus. Beta-adrenergic blocking agents should be administered with caution in patients subject to spontaneous hypoglycemia or to diabetic patients (especially those with labile diabetes) who are receiving insulin or oral hypoglycemic agents. Beta-adrenergic receptor blocking agents may mask the signs and symptoms of acute hypoglycemia.

Thyrotoxicosis. Beta-adrenergic blocking agents may mask certain clinical signs (e.g., tachycardia) of hyperthyroidism. Patients suspected of developing thyrotoxicosis should be managed carefully to avoid abrupt withdrawal of beta-adrenergic blocking agents, which might precipitate a thyroid storm.

Muscle Weakness. Beta-adrenergic blockade has been reported to potentiate muscle weakness consistent with certain myasthenic symptoms (e.g., diplopia, ptosis and generalized weakness).

Major Surgery. Consideration should be given to the gradual withdrawal of beta-adrenergic blocking agents prior to general anesthesia because of the reduced ability of the heart to respond to beta-adrenergically mediated sympathetic reflex stimuli.

Pulmonary. Caution should be exercised in the treatment of glaucoma patients with excessive restriction of pulmonary function. There have been reports of asthmatic attacks and pulmonary distress during betaxolol treatment. Although rechallenges of some such patients with ophthalmic betaxolol has not adversely affected pulmonary function test results, the possibility of adverse pulmonary effects in patients sensitive to beta blockers cannot be ruled out.

Information for Patients: Do not touch dropper tip to any surface, as this may contaminate the contents. Do not use with contact lenses in eyes.

Drug Interactions: Patients who are receiving a beta-adrenergic blocking agent orally and BETOPTIC S Ophthalmic Suspension 0.25% should be observed for a potential additive effect either on the intraocular pressure or on the known systemic effects of beta blockade.

Close observation of the patient is recommended when a beta blocker is administered to patients receiving catecholamine-depleting drugs such as reserpine, because of possible additive effects and the production of hypotension and/or bradycardia.

Betaxolol is an adrenergic blocking agent; therefore, caution should be exercised in patients using concomitant adrenergic psychotropic drugs.

Risk from anaphylactic reaction: While taking beta-blockers, patients with a history of atopy or a history of severe anaphylactic reaction to a variety of allergens may be more reactive to repeated accidental, diagnostic, or therapeutic challenge with such allergens. Such patients may be unresponsive to the usual doses of epinephrine used to treat anaphylactic reactions.
Ocular: In patients with angle-closure glaucoma, the immediate treatment objective is to reopen the angle by constriction of the pupil with a miotic agent. Betaxolol has little or no effect on the pupil. When BETOPTIC S Ophthalmic Suspension 0.25% is used to reduce elevated intraocular pressure in angle-closure glaucoma, it should be used with a miotic and not alone.
Carcinogenesis, Mutagenesis, Impairment of Fertility: Lifetime studies with betaxolol HCl have been completed in mice at oral doses of 6, 20 or 60 mg/kg/day and in rats at 3, 12 or 48 mg/kg/day; betaxolol HCl demonstrated no carcinogenic effect. Higher dose levels were not tested.
In a variety of *in vitro* and *in vivo* bacterial and mammalian cell assays, betaxolol HCl was nonmutagenic.
Pregnancy:
Pregnancy Category C. Reproduction, teratology, and peri- and postnatal studies have been conducted with orally administered betaxolol HCl in rats and rabbits. There was evidence of drug related postimplantation loss in rabbits and rats at dose levels above 12 mg/kg and 128 mg/kg, respectively. Betaxolol HCl was not shown to be teratogenic, however, and there were no other adverse effects on reproduction at subtoxic dose levels. There are no adequate and well-controlled studies in pregnant women. BETOPTIC S should be used during pregnancy only if the potential benefit justifies the potential risk to the fetus.
Nursing Mothers: It is not known whether betaxolol HCl is excreted in human milk. Because many drugs are excreted in human milk, caution should be exercised when BETOPTIC S Ophthalmic Suspension 0.25% is administered to nursing women.
Pediatric Use: Safety and effectiveness in children have not been established.
Adverse Reactions:
Ocular: In clinical trials, the most frequent event associated with the use of BETOPTIC S Ophthalmic Suspension 0.25% has been transient ocular discomfort. The following other conditions have been reported in small numbers of patients: blurred vision, corneal punctate keratitis, foreign body sensation, photophobia, tearing, itching, dryness of eyes, erythema, inflammation, discharge, ocular pain, decreased visual acuity and crusty lashes.
Additional medical events reported with other formulations of betaxolol include allergic reactions, decreased corneal sensitivity, corneal punctate staining which may appear in dendritic formations, edema and anisocoria.
Systemic: Systemic reactions following administration of BETOPTIC S Ophthalmic Suspension 0.25% or BETOPTIC Ophthalmic Solution 0.5% have been rarely reported. These include:
Cardiovascular: Bradycardia, heart block and congestive failure.
Pulmonary: Pulmonary distress characterized by dyspnea, bronchospasm, thickened bronchial secretions, asthma and respiratory failure.
Central Nervous System: Insomnia, dizziness, vertigo, headaches, depression, lethargy, and increase in signs and symptoms of myasthenia gravis.
Other: Hives, toxic epidermal necrolysis, hair loss, and glossitis.
Overdosage: No information is available on overdosage of humans. The oral LD50 of the drug ranged from 350–920 mg/kg in mice and 860–1050 mg/kg in rats. The symptoms which might be expected with an overdose of a systemically administered beta-1-adrenergic receptor blocking agent are bradycardia, hypotension and acute cardiac failure.
A topical overdose of BETOPTIC S Ophthalmic Suspension 0.25% may be flushed from the eye(s) with warm tap water.
Dosage and Administration: The recommended dose is one to two drops of BETOPTIC S Ophthalmic Suspension 0.25% in the affected eye(s) twice daily. In some patients, the intraocular pressure lowering responses to BETOPTIC S may require a few weeks to stabilize. As with any new medication, careful monitoring of patients is advised.
If the intraocular pressure of the patient is not adequately controlled on this regimen, concomitant therapy with pilocarpine and other miotics, and/or epinephrine and/or carbonic anhydrase inhibitors can be instituted.
How Supplied: BETOPTIC S Ophthalmic Suspension 0.25% is supplied as follows: 2.5, 5, 10 and 15 mL in plastic ophthalmic DROP-TAINER® dispensers.

2.5 mL: **NDC** 0065-0246-20
5.0 mL: **NDC** 0065-0246-05
10.0 mL: **NDC** 0065-0246-10
15.0 mL: **NDC** 0065-0246-15

Storage: Store upright at room temperature. Shake well before using.
Caution: Federal (USA) Law Prohibits Dispensing Without a Prescription.
U.S. Patents Nos. 4,252,984; 4,311,708; 4,342,783; 4,911,920.

BION® TEARS — OTC
Lubricant Eye Drops

Dry Eye
Dry eye refers to a condition in which people produce too few tears or tears that lack some important components. The result is an unstable tear film that cannot spread evenly over the surface of the eye causing dry spots to form. These dry spots can lead to discomfort, blurred vision and potential corneal infection. Dry eye occurs in varying degrees of severity ranging from symptoms of mild, intermittent burning, scratchiness and foreign-body sensation to a severe lack of tear secretion accompanied by ocular surface disease called Keratoconjunctivitis Sicca (KCS).
Causes of Dry Eye
Aging. Dry eye commonly affects older adults. As a general rule, tear production diminishes with age. At age 65, for example, people produce about 60% fewer tears than at age 18.
Systemic Disease. Dry eye is often associated with other conditions such as arthritis, allergies, lupus, Sjögren's Syndrome and some skin disorders.
Environment. Adverse environmental conditions such as dry air, smog, smoke and wind can aggravate the condition.
Medication. Tranquilizers, diuretics, cold medications containing antihistamines, birth control pills, and some medications used to control blood pressure or treat digestive disorders can cause or aggravate dry eye.
Treatment of Dry Eye
Treatment of dry eye is generally done through the use of tear substitutes. BION® TEARS are specially designed to be physiologically compatible with the surface of the eye and to treat dry eye symptoms by replacing needed tear components.
BION® TEARS advanced formula contains:
The unique DUASORB® polymeric system combines with natural tears to soothe sensitive dry spots.
A special lubricating vehicle designed to match the electrolyte balance of sodium, potassium, calcium, magnesium, zinc and bicarbonate found in natural tears.
No preservatives or decongestants that may cause irritation or limit use. BION® TEARS may be used as often as necessary to provide relief.
BION® TEARS special formula requires special packaging. Airtight foil pouches are used to maintain the delicate balance of ingredients until the product is ready for use in the eye. **To ensure optimal effectiveness once the pouch is opened, the containers inside the pouch must be used within four days (96 hours).**
PLEASE READ THESE WARNINGS PRIOR TO USING BION® TEARS LUBRICANT EYE DROPS AND KEEP THIS INSERT FOR FUTURE REFERENCE.
Warnings: If you experience eye pain, changes in vision, continued redness or irritation of the eye, or if the condition worsens or persists for more than 72 hours, discontinue use and consult a doctor.
If solution changes color or becomes cloudy, do not use.
To avoid contamination, do not touch tip of container to any surface. Do not reuse. Open opened, discard. Keep this and all drugs out of the reach of children. In case of accidental ingestion, seek professional assistance or contact a Poison Control Center immediately.
How Supplied: BION® TEARS Lubricant Eye Drops are supplied in boxes of 28 0.015 fl. oz. single-use containers.
Product Code 0065-0419-28

CILOXAN® — ℞
(Ciprofloxacin HCl)
0.3% as base
Sterile Ophthalmic Solution

Description: CILOXAN® (Ciprofloxacin HCl) Ophthalmic Solution is a synthetic, sterile, multiple dose, antimicrobial for topical ophthalmic use. Ciprofloxacin is a fluoroquinolone antibacterial active against a broad spectrum of gram-positive and gram-negative ocular pathogens. It is available as the monohydrochloride monohydrate salt of 1-cyclopropyl-6-fluoro-1,4-dihydro-4-oxo-7- (1-piperazinyl)-3-quinoline-carboxylic acid. It is a faint to light yellow crystalline powder with a molecular weight of 385.8. Its empirical formula is $C_{17}H_{18}FN_3O_3 \cdot HCl \cdot H_2O$ and its chemical structure is as follows:

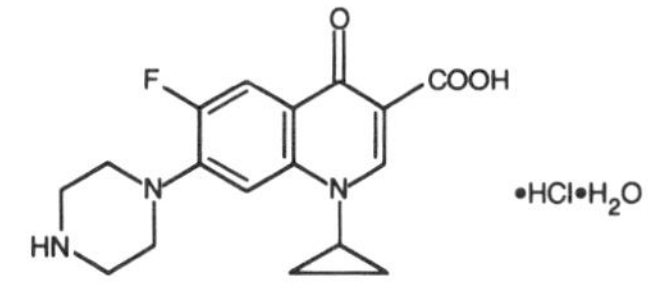

Ciprofloxacin differs from other quinolones in that it has a fluorine atom at the 6-position, a piperazine moiety at the 7-position, and a cyclopropyl ring at the 1-position.
Each mL of CILOXAN Ophthalmic Solution contains: Active: Ciprofloxacin HCl 3.5 mg equivalent to 3 mg base. Preservative: Benzalkonium Chloride 0.006%. Inactive: Sodium Acetate, Acetic Acid, Mannitol 4.6%, Edetate Disodium 0.05%, Hydrochloric Acid and/or Sodium Hydroxide (to adjust pH) and Purified Water. The pH is approximately 4.5 and the osmolality is approximately 300 mOsm.
Clinical Pharmacology:
Systemic Absorption: A systemic absorbtion study was performed in which CILOXAN Ophthalmic Solution was administered in each eye every two hours while awake for two days followed by every four hours while awake for an additional 5 days. The maximum reported plasma concentration of ciprofloxacin was less than 5 ng/mL. The mean concentration was usually less than 2.5 ng/mL.

Continued on next page

Alcon—Cont.

Microbiology: Ciprofloxacin has *in vitro* activity against a wide range of gram-negative and gram-positive organisms. The bactericidal action of ciprofloxacin results from interference with the enzyme DNA gyrase which is needed for the synthesis of bacterial DNA.

Ciprofloxacin has been shown to be active against most strains of the following organisms both *in vitro* and in clinical infections. (See *Indications and Usage* section).

Gram-Positive:
Staphylococcus aureus (including methicillin-susceptible and methicillin-resistant strains)
Staphylococcus epidermidis
Streptococcus pneumoniae
Streptococcus (Viridans Group)

Gram-Negative:
Pseudomonas aeruginosa
Serratia marcescens

Ciprofloxacin has been shown to be active *in vitro* against most strains of the following organisms, however, *the clinical significance of these data is unknown:*

Gram-Positive:
Enterococcus faecalis (Many strains are only moderately susceptible)
Staphylococcus haemolyticus
Staphylococcus hominis
Staphylococcus saprophyticus
Streptococcus pyogenes

Gram-Negative:
Acinetobacter calcoaceticus subsp. anitratus
Aeromonas caviae
Aeromonas hydrophila
Brucella melitensis
Campylobacter coli
Campylobacter jujuni
Citrobacter diversus
Citrobacter freundii
Edwardsiella tarda
Enterobacter aerogenes
Enterobacter cloacae
Escherichia coli
Haemophilus ducreyi
Haemophilus influenzae
Haemophilus parainfluenzae
Klebsiella pneumoniae
Klebsiella oxytoca
Legionella pneumophila
Moraxella (Branhamella) catarrhalis
Morganella morganii
Neisseria gonorrhoeae
Neisseria meningitidis
Pasteurella multocida
Proteus mirabilis
Proteus vulgaris
Providencia rettgeri
Providencia stuartii
Salmonella enteritidis
Salmonella typhi
Shigella sonneii
Shigella flexneri
Vibrio cholerae
Vibrio parahaemolyticus
Vibrio vulnificus
Yersinia enterocolitica

Other Organisms: *Chlamydia trachomatis* (only moderately susceptible) and *Mycobacterium tuberculosis* (only moderately susceptible).

Most strains of *Pseudomonas cepacia* and some strains of *Pseudomonas maltophilia* are resistant to ciprofloxacin as are most anaerobic bacteria, including *Bacteroides fragilis* and *Clostridium difficile.*

The minimal bactericidal concentration (MBC) generally does not exceed the minimal inhibitory concentration (MIC) by more than a factor of 2. Resistance to ciprofloxacin *in vitro* usually develops slowly (multiple-step mutation).

Ciprofloxacin does not cross-react with other antimicrobial agents such as beta-lactams or aminoglycosides; therefore, organisms resistant to these drugs may be susceptible to ciprofloxacin.

Clinical Studies:
Following therapy with CILOXAN Ophthalmic Solution, 76% of the patients with corneal ulcers and positive bacterial cultures were clinically cured and complete re-epithelialization occurred in about 92% of the ulcers.

In 3 and 7 day multicenter clinical trials, 52% of the patients with conjunctivitis and positive conjunctival cultures were clinically cured and 70–80% had all causative pathogens eradicated by the end of treatment.

Indications and Usage: CILOXAN Ophthalmic Solution is indicated for the treatment of infections caused by susceptible strains of the designated microorganisms in the conditions listed below:

Corneal Ulcers: *Pseudomonas aeruginosa*
*Serratia marcescens**
Staphylococcus aureus
Staphylococcus epidermidis
Streptococcus pneumoniae
Streptococcus (Viridans Group)*

Conjunctivitis: *Staphylococcus aureus*
Staphylococcus epidermidis
*Streptococcus pneumoniae**

*Efficacy for this organism was studied in fewer than 10 infections.

Contraindications: A history of hypersensitivity to ciprofloxacin or any other component of the medication is a contraindication to its use. A history of hypersensitivity to other quinolones may also contraindicate the use of ciprofloxacin.

Warnings: NOT FOR INJECTION INTO THE EYE.

Serious and occasionally fatal hypersensitivity (anaphylactic) reactions, some following the first dose, have been reported in patients receiving systemic quinolone therapy. Some reactions were accompanied by cardiovascular collapse, loss of consciousness, tingling, pharyngeal or facial edema, dyspnea, urticaria, and itching. Only a few patients had a history of hypersensitivity reactions. Serious anaphylactic reactions require immediate emergency treatment with epinephrine and other resuscitation measures, including oxygen, intravenous fluids, intravenous antihistamines, corticosteroids, pressor amines and airway management, as clinically indicated.

Precautions:

General: As with other antibacterial preparations, prolonged use of ciprofloxacin may result in overgrowth of nonsusceptible organisms, including fungi. If superinfection occurs, appropriate therapy should be initiated. Whenever clinical judgment dictates, the patient should be examined with the aid of magnification, such as slit lamp biomicroscopy and, where appropriate, fluorescein staining.

Ciprofloxacin should be discontinued at the first appearance of a skin rash or any other sign of hypersensitivity reaction.

In clinical studies of patients with bacterial corneal ulcer, a white crystalline precipitate located in the superficial portion of the corneal defect was observed in 35 (16.6%) of 210 patients. The onset of the precipitate was within 24 hours to 7 days after starting therapy. In one patient, the precipitate was immediately irrigated out upon its appearance. In 17 patients, resolution of the precipitate was seen in 1 to 8 days (seven within the first 24–72 hours); in five patients, resolution was noted in 10–13 days. In nine patients, exact resolution days were unavailable; however, at follow-up examinations, 18–44 days after onset of the event, complete resolution of the precipitate was noted. In three patients, outcome information was unavailable. The precipitate did not preclude continued use of ciprofloxacin, nor did it adversely affect the clinical course of the ulcer or visual outcome. (SEE ADVERSE REACTIONS).

Drug Interactions: Specific drug interaction studies have not been conducted with ophthalmic ciprofloxacin. However, the systemic administration of some quinolones has been shown to elevate plasma concentrations of theophylline, interfere with the metabolism of caffeine, enhance the effects of the oral anticoagulant, warfarin, and its derivatives and have been associated with transient elevations in serum creatinine in patients receiving cyclosporine concomitantly.

Carcinogenesis, Mutagenesis, Impairment of Fertility: Eight *in vitro* mutagenicity tests have been conducted with ciprofloxacin and the test results are listed below:
Salmonella/Microsome Test (Negative)
E. coli DNA Repair Assay (Negative)
Mouse Lymphoma Cell Forward Mutation Assay (Positive)
Chinese Hamster V_{79} Cell HGPRT Test (Negative)
Syrian Hamster Embryo Cell Transformation Assay (Negative)
Saccharomyces cerevisiae Point Mutation Assay (Negative)
Saccharomyces cerevisiae Mitotic Crossover and Gene Conversion Assay (Negative)
Rat Hepatocyte DNA Repair Assay (Positive)

Thus, two of the eight tests were positive, but the results of the following three *in vivo* test systems gave negative results:
Rat Hepatocyte DNA Repair Assay
Micronucleus Test (Mice)
Dominant Lethal Test (Mice)

Long term carcinogenicity studies in mice and rats have been completed. After daily oral dosing for up to two years, there is no evidence that ciprofloxacin had any carcinogenic or tumorigenic effects in these species.

Pregnancy—Pregnancy Category C: Reproduction studies have been performed in rats and mice at doses up to six times the usual daily human oral dose and have revealed no evidence of impaired fertility or harm to the fetus due to ciprofloxacin. In rabbits, as with most antimicrobial agents, ciprofloxacin (30 and 100 mg/kg orally) produced gastrointestinal disturbances resulting in maternal weight loss and an increased incidence of abortion. No teratogenicity was observed at either dose. After intravenous administration, at doses up to 20 mg/kg, no maternal toxicity was produced and no embryotoxicity or teratogenicity was observed. There are no adequate and well controlled studies in pregnant women. CILOXAN Ophthalmic Solution should be used during pregnancy only if the potential benefit justifies the potential risk to the fetus.

Nursing Mothers: It is not known whether topically applied ciprofloxacin is excreted in human milk; however, it is known that orally administered ciprofloxacin is excreted in the milk of lactating rats and oral ciprofloxacin has been reported in human breast milk after a single 500 mg dose. Caution should be exercised when CILOXAN Ophthalmic Solution is administered to a nursing mother.

Pediatric Use: Safety and effectiveness in children below the age of 12 have not been established.

Although ciprofloxacin and other quinolones cause arthropathy in immature animals after oral administration, topical ocular administration of ciprofloxacin to immature animals did not cause any arthropathy and there is no evidence that the ophthalmic dosage form has any effect on the weight bearing joints.

Adverse Reactions: The most frequently reported drug related adverse reaction was local burning or discomfort. In corneal ulcer studies with frequent administration of the drug, white crystalline precipitates were seen in approximately 17% of patients (SEE PRECAUTIONS). Other reactions occurring in less than

10% of patients included lid margin crusting, crystals/scales, foreign body sensation, itching, conjunctival hyperemia and a bad taste following instillation. Additional events occurring in less than 1% of patients included corneal staining, keratopathy/keratitis, allergic reactions, lid edema, tearing, photophobia, corneal infiltrates, nausea and decreased vision.

Overdosage: A topical overdose of CILOXAN Ophthalmic Solution may be flushed from the eye(s) with warm tap water.

Dosage and Administration: The recommended dosage regimen for the treatment of **corneal ulcers** is: Two drops into the affected eye every 15 minutes for the first six hours and then two drops into the affected eye every 30 minutes for the remainder of the first day. On the second day, instill two drops in the affected eye hourly. On the third through the fourteenth day, place two drops in the affected eye every four hours. Treatment may be continued after 14 days if corneal re-epithelialization has not occurred.

The recommended dosage regimen for the treatment of **bacterial conjunctivitis** is: One or two drops instilled into the conjunctival sac(s) every two hours while awake for two days and one or two drops every four hours while awake for the next five days.

How Supplied: As a sterile ophthalmic solution: 2.5 mL and 5 mL in plastic DROP-TAINER® dispensers.

2.5 mL—NDC 0065-0656-25
5 mL —NDC 0065-0656-05

Storage: Store at 2° to 30°C (36° to 86°F). Protect from light.

Animal Pharmacology: Ciprofloxacin and related drugs have been shown to cause arthropathy in immature animals of most species tested following oral administration. However, a one-month topical ocular study using immature Beagle dogs did not demonstrate any articular lesions.

Caution: Federal (USA) law prohibits dispensing without prescription.

U.S. Patent No. 4,670,444

CYCLOGYL® ℞
(cyclopentolate hydrochloride ophthalmic solution, USP)

Description: CYCLOGYL® (cyclopentolate hydrochloride ophthalmic solution, USP) is an anticholinergic prepared as a sterile, borate buffered solution for topical ocular use. It is supplied in three strengths. The active ingredient is represented by the structural formula:

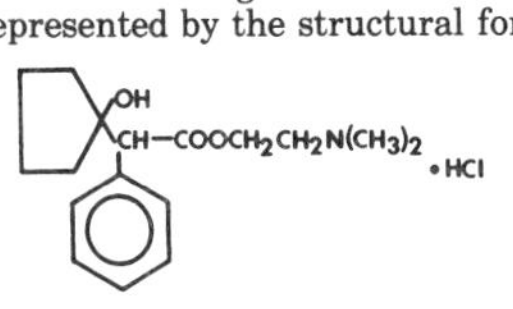

MW = 327.85 $C_{17}H_{25}NO_3 \cdot HCl$

Established name:
Cyclopentolate Hydrochloride

Chemical name:
2-(Dimethylamino)ethyl 1-hydroxy-α-phenylcyclopentaneacetate hydrochloride

Each mL contains: Active: Cyclopentolate Hydrochloride 0.5%, 1% or 2%. **Preservative:** Benzalkonium Chloride 0.01%. **Inactive:** Boric Acid, Edetate Disodium, Potassium Chloride (except 2% strength), Sodium Carbonate and/or Hydrochloric Acid (to adjust pH), Purified Water. The pH range is between 3.0 and 5.5.

Clinical Pharmacology: This anticholinergic preparation blocks the responses of the sphincter muscle of the iris and the accommodative muscle of the ciliary body to cholinergic stimulation, producing pupillary dilation (mydriasis) and paralysis of accommodation (cycloplegia). It acts rapidly, but has a shorter duration than atropine. Maximal cycloplegia occurs within 25 to 75 minutes after instillation. Complete recovery of accommodation usually takes 6 to 24 hours. Complete recovery from mydriasis in some individuals may require several days.

Indications and Usage: Cyclopentolate hydrochloride is used to produce mydriasis and cycloplegia.

Contraindications: Should not be used when narrow-angle glaucoma or anatomical narrow angles are present, or where there is hypersensitivity to any component of this preparation.

Warnings: For topical use only—not for injection. This preparation may cause CNS disturbances. This is especially true in younger age groups, but may occur at any age, especially with the stronger solutions. Premature and small infants are especially prone to CNS and cardiopulmonary side effects from systemic absorption of cyclopentolate. To minimize absorption, use only 1 drop of 0.5% CYCLOGYL solution per eye, followed by pressure applied over the nasolacrimal sac for two to three minutes. Observe infants closely for at least 30 minutes following instillation.

Precautions:

General: To avoid inducing angle closure glaucoma, an estimation of the depth of the angle of the anterior chamber should be made. The lacrimal sac should be compressed by digital pressure for two to three minutes after instillation to avoid excessive systemic absorption. Caution should be observed when considering use of this medication in the presence of Down's syndrome and in those predisposed to angle-closure glaucoma.

Information for Patients: Do not touch dropper tip to any surface as this may contaminate the solution. A transient burning sensation may occur upon instillation. Patients should be advised not to drive or engage in other hazardous activities while pupils are dilated. Patients may experience sensitivity to light and should protect eyes in bright illumination during dilation. Parents should be warned not to get this preparation in their child's mouth and to wash their own hands and the child's hands following administration.

Drug Interactions: Cyclopentolate may interfere with the anti-glaucoma action of carbachol or pilocarpine; also, concurrent use of these medications may antagonize the anti-glaucoma and miotic actions of ophthalmic cholinesterase inhibitors.

Carcinogenesis, Mutagenesis, and Impairment of Fertility: Studies in animals or humans have not been conducted to evaluate the potential of these effects.

Pregnancy Category C: Animal reproduction studies have not been conducted with cyclopentolate. It is also not known whether cyclopentolate can cause fetal harm when administered to a pregnant woman or can affect reproduction capacity. Cyclopentolate should be administered to a pregnant woman only if clearly needed.

Nursing Mothers: It is not known whether this drug is excreted in human milk. Because many drugs are excreted in human milk, caution should be exercised when cyclopentolate hydrochloride is administered to a nursing woman.

Pediatrics: Increased susceptibility to cyclopentolate has been reported in infants, young children, and in children with spastic paralysis or brain damage. Therefore, cyclopentolate should be used with great caution in these patients. Feeding intolerance may follow ophthalmic use of this product in neonates. It is recommended that feeding be withheld for four (4) hours after examination. Do not use in concentrations higher than 0.5% in small infants (see WARNINGS).

Geriatrics: In the elderly and others where increased intraocular pressure may be encountered, mydriatics and cycloplegics should be used cautiously.

Adverse Reactions:

Ocular: Increased intraocular pressure, burning, photophobia, blurred vision, irritation, hyperemia, conjunctivitis, blepharoconjunctivitis, punctate keratitis, synechiae.

Systemic: Use of cyclopentolate has been associated with psychotic reactions and behavioral disturbances, usually in children, especially with 2% concentration. These disturbances include ataxia, incoherent speech, restlessness, hallucinations, hyperactivity, seizures, disorientation as to time and place, and failure to recognize people. This drug produces reactions similar to those of other anticholinergic drugs, but the central nervous system manifestations as noted above are more common. Other toxic manifestations of anticholinergic drugs are skin rash, abdominal distention in infants, unusual drowsiness, tachycardia, hyperpyrexia, vasodilation, urinary retention, diminished gastrointestinal motility and decreased secretion in salivary and sweat glands, pharynx, bronchii and nasal passages. Severe manifestations of toxicity include coma, medullary paralysis and death.

Overdosage: Excessive dosage may produce exaggerated symptoms as noted in ADVERSE REACTIONS. When administration of the drug product is discontinued, the patient usually recovers spontaneously. In case of severe manifestations of toxicity the antidote of choice is physostigmine salicylate.

Pediatric Dose: As an antidote, slowly inject intravenously 0.5 mg physostigmine salicylate. If toxic symptoms persist and no cholinergic symptoms are produced, repeat at five minute intervals to a maximum cumulative dose of 2 mg.

Adolescent and Adult: As an antidote, slowly inject 2 mg physostigmine salicylate intravenously. A second dose of 1 to 2 mg may be given after 20 minutes if no reversal of toxic manifestations has occurred.[1,2,3]

Dosage and Administration: Adults: One or two drops of 0.5%, 1% or 2% solution in the eye which may be repeated in five to ten minutes if necessary. Complete recovery usually occurs in 24 hours. **Children:** One or two drops of 0.5%, 1% or 2% solution in the eye which may be repeated five to ten minutes later by a second application of 0.5% or 1% solution if necessary. **Small Infants:** A single instillation of one drop of 0.5% CYCLOGYL in the eye. To minimize absorption, apply pressure over the nasolacrimal sac for two to three minutes. Observe infant closely for at least 30 minutes following instillation. Individuals with heavily pigmented irides may require higher strengths.

How Supplied:
In multiple-dose plastic DROP-TAINER® dispensers:

0.5% CYCLOGYL
2mL NDC 0065-0395-02
5mL NDC 0065-0395-05
15mL NDC 0065-0395-15

1% CYCLOGYL
2mL NDC 0065-0396-02
5mL NDC 0065-0396-05
15mL NDC 0065-0396-15

2% CYCLOGYL
2mL NDC 0065-0397-02
5mL NDC 0065-0397-05
15mL NDC 0065-0397-15

Storage: Store at 8°–27°C (46°–80°F).

Caution: Federal (USA) law prohibits dispensing without prescription.

Continued on next page

Alcon—Cont.

References:
1. Rumack, B. H.: Anticholinergic Poisoning: Treatment with Physostigmine. **Pediatrics** 52(6):449–51, 1973.
2. Duvoisin, R. C. and Katz, R.: Reversal of Central Anticholinergic Syndromes in Man by Physostigmine, **J. Am. Med. Assn.** 206(9): 1963–65, 1968.
3. Grant, W. M.: **Toxicology of the Eye.** Second Edition, Volume 1. Springfield, Illinois, Charles C. Thomas: 1974.

CYCLOMYDRIL® ℞
(cyclopentolate hydrochloride, phenylephrine hydrochloride)
Sterile Ophthalmic Solution

Description: CYCLOMYDRIL® (Cyclopentolate Hydrochloride, Phenylephrine Hydrochloride) is a mydriatic prepared as a sterile topical ophthalmic solution. The active ingredients are represented by the chemical structures:

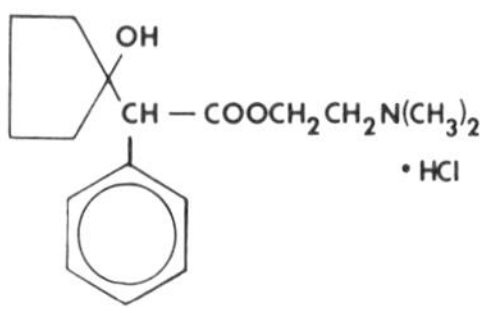

Established name:
Cyclopentolate Hydrochloride

Chemical name:
2-(Dimethylamino)ethyl 1-hydroxy-α-phenylcyclopentaneacetate hydrochloride

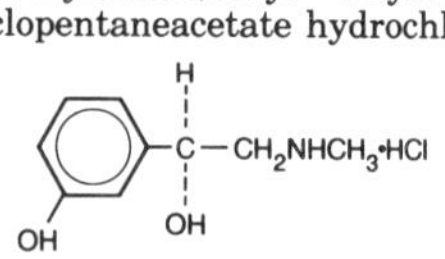

Established name:
Phenylephrine Hydrochloride

Chemical name:
3-hydroxy- α[(methylamino)-methyl]-, Benzenemethanol, hydrochloride (*R*)-.

Each mL contains: Active: Cyclopentolate Hydrochloride 0.2%, Phenylephrine Hydrochloride 1%. Preservative: Benzalkonium Chloride 0.01%. Inactive: Edetate Disodium, Boric Acid, Hydrochloric Acid and/or Sodium Carbonate (to adjust pH), Purified Water.

Clinical Pharmacology: Cyclopentolate Hydrochloride is an anticholinergic drug and Phenylephrine Hydrochloride is an adrenergic drug. This combination induces mydriasis that is considerably greater than that of either drug alone. The concentrations of Cyclopentolate Hydrochloride and of Phenylephrine Hydrochloride have been selected to induce safe and rapid mydriasis with little or no accompanying cycloplegia.

Indications and Usage: For the production of mydriasis.

Contraindications: Do not use in patients with narrow-angle glaucoma or with anatomically narrow angles or where there is hypersensitivity to any component of this preparation.

Warnings: Do not touch dropper tip to any surface, as this may contaminate the solution. For topical use only—not for injection. The use of this combination may have an adverse effect on individuals suffering from cardiovascular disease, hypertension, and hyperthyroidism; and it may cause CNS disturbances. Small infants are especially prone to CNS and cardiopulmonary side effects from systemic absorption of cyclopentolate.

Precautions: To avoid inducing angle closure glaucoma, an estimation of the depth of the angle of the anterior chamber should be made. The lacrimal sac should be compressed by digital pressure for two to three minutes after instillation to avoid excessive systemic absorption. The effect of long-term use of this preparation has not been established, therefore it should be restricted to short-term use.

Patient Warning: Patient should be advised not to drive or engage in other hazardous activities while pupils are dilated. Patient may experience sensitivity to light and should protect eyes in bright illumination during dilation. Parents should be warned not to get this preparation in their child's mouth and to wash their own hands and the child's hands following administration. Feeding intolerance may follow ophthalmic use of this product in neonates. It is recommended that feeding be withheld for four (4) hours after examination.

Adverse Reactions: Increased intraocular pressure. Use of Cyclopentolate has been associated with psychotic reactions and behavioral disturbances in children, especially with 2% concentration. These disturbances include ataxia, incoherent speech, restlessness, hallucinations, hyperactivity, seizures, disorientation as to time and place, and failure to recognize people. This drug produces reactions similar to those of other anticholinergic drugs; however, the central nervous system manifestations as noted above are more common. Other toxic manifestations of anticholinergic drugs are tachycardia, hyperpyrexia, vasodilation, urinary retention, diminished gastrointestinal motility and decreased secretion in salivary and sweat glands, pharynx, bronchii and nasal passages. Severe manifestations of toxicity include coma, medullary paralysis and death.

Overdosage: When administration of the drug product is discontinued, the patient usually recovers spontaneously. In case of severe manifestations of toxicity, the antidote of choice is physostigmine salicylate.

Pediatric Dose: As an antidote, slowly inject intravenously 0.5 mg of physostigmine salicylate. If toxic symptoms persist and no cholinergic symptoms are produced repeat at five minute intervals to a maximum dose of 2.0 mg.

Adolescent and Adult Dose: As an antidote, slowly inject intravenously 2.0 mg of physostigmine salicylate. A second dose of 1–2 mg may be given after 20 minutes if no reversal of toxic manifestations has occurred.[1,2,3]

Dosage and Administration: For funduscopy, instill one drop in each eye every five to ten minutes, not to exceed three times, to produce rapid mydriasis, permitting ready visual access to the fundus. Heavily pigmented irides may require larger doses. To minimize absorption in premature and small infants, apply pressure over the nasolacrimal sac for two to three minutes following instillation. Observe infants closely for at least 30 minutes.

How Supplied: 2 mL and 5 mL in plastic DROP-TAINER® dispensers.
2mL NDC 0065-0359-02
5mL NDC 0065-0359-05

Storage: Store at 46° to 80°F.

Caution: Federal (USA) law prohibits dispensing without prescription.

References:
1. Rumack, B. H.: Anticholinergic Poisoning: Treatment with Physostigmine. PEDIATRICS 52(6):449-51, 1973.
2. Duvoisin, R. C. and Katz, R.: Reversal of Central Anticholinergic Syndromes in Man by Physostigmine. J. AM. MED. ASSN. 206(9): 1963-65, 1968.
3. Grant, W. M.: *Toxicology of the Eye.* Second Edition, Volume 1. Springfield, Illinois. Charles C. Thomas: 1974.

DURATEARS NATURALE® OTC
Lubricant Eye Ointment

Description: A sterile bland, non-medicated unpreserved ointment.

Ingredients: Each gram contains: **Active:** White Petrolatum and Mineral Oil. **Inactive:** Anhydrous Liquid Lanolin.

Indications: For nighttime use as a lubricant to relieve dryness of the eye. FOR TOPICAL EYE USE ONLY.

Warnings: Remove contact lenses before using. If you experience eye pain, changes in vision, continued redness or irritation of the eye, or if the condition worsens or persists for more than 72 hours, discontinue use and consult a doctor.

To avoid contamination, do not touch tip of container to any surface. Replace cap after using. Keep this and all drugs out of the reach of children. In case of accidental ingestion, seek professional assistance or contact a Poison Control Center immediately.

Directions: Pull down the lower lid of the affected eye and apply a small amount (one-fourth inch) of ointment to the inside of the eyelid.

How Supplied: As a sterile ophthalmic ointment in 3.5 g tubes.
NDC 0065-0414-35

Storage: Store at 46°–80°F.

TAMPER RESISTANT: Prior to use, inspect the product container. If "skirt" on bottom of cap is visible, do not use. For added protection, carton end-panels are sealed.

⅛% ECONOPRED® ℞
1% ECONOPRED® PLUS ℞
(prednisolone acetate)
Ophthalmic Suspension

Description: ECONOPRED® and ECONOPRED® PLUS (Prednisolone Acetate) are adrenocortical steroid products prepared as sterile ophthalmic suspensions. The active ingredient is represented by the chemical structure:

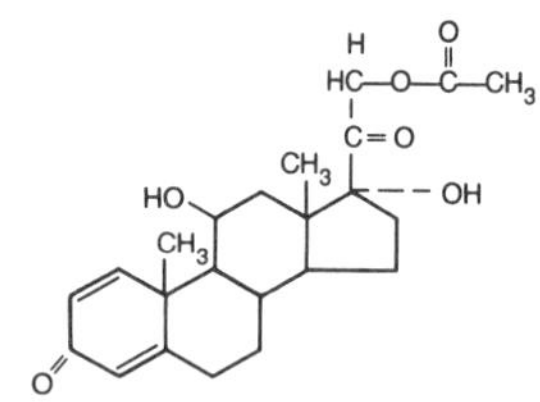

Established name:
Prednisolone Acetate

Chemical name:
Pregna-1,4-diene-3,20-dione, 21-(acetyloxy)-11,17-dihydroxy-,(11β)-.

Each mL contains: Active: Prednisolone Acetate 1.0% or 0.125%. Preservative: Benzalkonium Chloride 0.01%. Vehicle: Hydroxypropyl Methylcellulose. Inactive: Dried Sodium Phosphate, Polysorbate 80, Edetate Disodium, Glycerin, Citric Acid and/or Sodium Hydroxide (to adust pH), Purified Water.

Clinical Pharmacology: Corticosteroids inhibit the inflammatory response to a variety of inciting agents and probably delay or slow healing. They inhibit the edema, fibrin deposition, capillary dilation, leukocyte migration, capillary proliferation, fibroblast proliferation, deposition of collagen, and scar formation associated with inflammation.

There is no generally accepted explanation for the mechanism of action of ocular corticosteroids. However, corticosteroids are thought to act by the induction of phospholipase A_2 inhibi-

tory proteins, collectively called lipocortins. It is postulated that these proteins control the biosynthesis of potent mediators of inflammation such as prostaglandins and leukotrienes by inhibiting the release of their common precursor arachidonic acid. Arachidonic acid is released from membrane phospholipids by phospholipase A_2.
Corticosteroids are capable of producing a rise in intraocular pressure.
Indications and Usage: Steroid responsive inflammatory conditions of the palpebral and bulbar conjunctiva, cornea, and anterior segment of the globe such as allergic conjunctivitis, acne rosacea, superficial punctate keratitis, herpes zoster keratitis, iritis, cyclitis, selected infective conjunctivitides, when the inherent hazard of steroid use is accepted to obtain an advisable diminution in edema and inflammation; corneal injury from chemical, radiation, or thermal burns, or penetration of foreign bodies.
Contraindications: ECONOPRED and ECONOPRED Plus are contraindicated in most viral diseases of the cornea and conjunctiva including epithelial herpes simplex keratitis (dendritic keratitis), vaccinia, and varicella, and also in mycobacterial infection of the eye and fungal diseases of ocular structures. ECONOPRED and ECONOPRED Plus are also contraindicated in individuals with known or suspected hypersensitivity to any of the ingredients of this preparation and to other corticosteroids.
Warnings: Prolonged use of corticosteroids may result in glaucoma with damage to the optic nerve, defects in visual acuity and fields of vision, and in posterior subcapsular cataract formation. Prolonged use may also suppress the host immune response and thus increase the hazard of secondary ocular infections.
Various ocular diseases and long-term use of topical corticosteroids have been known to cause corneal and scleral thinning. Use of topical corticosteroids in the presence of thin corneal or scleral tissue may lead to perforation.
Acute purulent infections of the eye may be masked or activity enhanced by the presence of corticosteroid medication.
If this product is used for 10 days or longer, intraocular pressure should be routinely monitored even though it may be difficult in children and uncooperative patients. Steroids should be used with caution in the presence of glaucoma. Intraocular pressure should be checked frequently. The use of steroids after cataract surgery may delay healing and increase the incidence of bleb formation.
Use of ocular steroids may prolong the course and may exacerbate the severity of many viral infections of the eye (including herpes simplex). Employment of a corticosteroid medication in the treatment of patients with a history of herpes simplex requires great caution; frequent slit lamp microscopy is recommended.
Corticosteroids are not effective in mustard gas keratitis and Sjögren's keratoconjunctivitis.
Precautions: General: The initial prescription and renewal of the medication order should be made by a physician only after examination of the patient with the aid of magnification, such as slit lamp biomicroscopy and, where appropriate, fluorescein staining. If signs and symptoms fail to improve after two days, the patient should be re-evaluated.
As fungal infections of the cornea are particularly prone to develop coincidentally with long-term local corticosteroid applications, fungal invasion should be suspected in any persistent corneal ulceration where a corticosteroid has been used or is in use. Fungal cultures should be taken when appropriate.
If this product is used for 10 days or longer, intraocular pressure should be monitored (SEE WARNINGS).
Information for Patients: If inflammation or pain persists longer than 48 hours or becomes aggravated, the patient should be advised to discontinue use of the medication and consult a physician.
This product is sterile when packaged. To prevent contamination, care should be taken to avoid touching the bottle tip to eyelids or to any other surface. The use of this bottle by more than one person may spread infection. Keep bottle tightly closed when not in use. Keep out of the reach of children.
Carcinogenesis, Mutagenesis, Impairment of Fertility: No studies have been conducted in animals or in humans to evaluate the potential of these effects.
Pregnancy: Teratogenic effects. Pregnancy Category C. Prednisolone has been shown to be teratogenic in mice when given in doses 1–10 times the human dose. Dexamethasone, hydrocortisone and prednisolone were ocularly applied to both eyes of pregnant mice five times per day on days 10 through 13 of gestation. A significant increase in the incidence of cleft palate was observed in the fetuses of the treated mice. There are no adequate and well controlled studies in pregnant women. ECONOPRED® and ECONOPRED® Plus should be used during pregnancy only if the potential benefit justifies the potential risk to the fetus.
Nursing Mothers: It is not known whether topical administration of corticosteroids could result in sufficient systemic absorption to produce detectable quantities in human milk. Systemically administered corticosteroids appear in human milk and could suppress growth, interfere with endogenous corticosteroid production, or cause other untoward effects. Because of the potential for serious adverse reactions in nursing infants from prednisolone acetate, a decision should be made whether to discontinue nursing or to discontinue the drug, taking into account the importance of the drug to the mother.
Pediatric Use: Safety and effectiveness in children have not been established.
Adverse Reactions: Adverse reactions include, in decreasing order of frequency, elevation of intraocular pressure (IOP) with possible development of glaucoma and infrequent optic nerve damage, posterior subcapsular cataract formation, and delayed wound healing.
Although systemic effects are extremely uncommon, there have been rare occurrences of systemic hypercorticoidism after use of topical steroids.
Corticosteroid-containing preparations have also been reported to cause acute anterior uveitis and perforation of the globe. Keratitis, conjunctivitis, corneal ulcers, mydriasis, conjunctival hyperemia, loss of accommodation and ptosis have occasionally been reported following local use of corticosteroids.
The development of secondary ocular infection (bacterial, fungal and viral) has occurred. Fungal and viral infections of the cornea are particularly prone to develop coincidentally with long-term applications of steroid. The possibility of fungal invasion should be considered in any persistent corneal ulceration where steroid treatment has been used (SEE WARNINGS).
Dosage and Administration: SHAKE WELL BEFORE USING. Two drops topically in the eye(s) four times daily. In cases of bacterial infections, concomitant use of anti-infective agents is mandatory. Care should be taken not to discontinue therapy prematurely.
If signs and symptoms fail to improve after two days, the patient should be re-evaluated (see PRECAUTIONS).
The dosing of ECONOPRED and ECONOPRED Plus may be reduced, but care should be taken not to discontinue therapy prematurely. In chronic conditions, withdrawal of treatment should be carried out by gradually decreasing the frequency of applications.
How Supplied: 5mL and 10mL in plastic DROP-TAINER® dispensers.
1/8% ECONOPRED®:
5 mL NDC 0998-0635-05
10 mL NDC 0998-0635-10
1% ECONOPRED® Plus:
5 mL NDC 0998-0637-05
10 mL NDC 0998-0637-10
Storage: Store at 46°–75°F (8°–24°C) in an upright position.
Caution: Federal (USA) law prohibits dispensing without prescription.

EYE-STREAM® OTC
Sterile Eye Irrigating Solution

EYE-STREAM® is a sterile and stable irrigating solution that is specially designed and packaged for use in the eye(s). Formulated as a buffered salt solution, it closely approximates normal human tear fluid.
Ingredients: Each mL contains: **Tonicity Agents:** Sodium Chloride 0.64%, Potassium Chloride 0.075%, Calcium Chloride Dihydrate 0.048%, Magnesium Chloride Hexahydrate 0.03%. **Buffering Agents:** Sodium Acetate Trihydrate 0.39%, Sodium Citrate Dihydrate 0.17%. **pH Adjusters:** Sodium Hydroxide and/or Hydrochloric Acid. **Preservative:** Benzalkonium Chloride 0.013%. **Purified Water.** The pH of the solution is in the physiologic range.
Indications:

> FDA APPROVED USES
> For irrigating the eye to help relieve irritation, discomfort and burning by removing loose foreign material, air pollutants (smog or pollen), or chlorinated water.

Warnings: If you experience eye pain, changes in vision, continued redness or irritation of the eye, or if the condition worsens or persists, consult a doctor. Obtain immediate medical treatment for all open wounds in or near the eyes. If solution changes color or becomes cloudy, do not use. To avoid contamination, do not touch tip of container to any surface. Replace cap after using. Keep this and all drugs out of the reach of children. In case of accidental ingestion, seek professional assistance or contact a Poison Control Center immediately. Not to be used as a saline solution for rinsing and soaking soft contact lenses. NOT FOR INJECTION OR INTRAOCULAR SURGERY.
Directions: Flush the affected eye as needed, controlling the rate of flow of solution by pressure on the bottle. Please read this carton carefully and keep for future reference.
How Supplied: In 1 fluid ounce and 4 fluid ounce plastic squeeze bottles.
1 fl. oz: NDC 0065-0530-01
4 fl. oz.: NDC 0065-0530-04
Storage: Store at 8°–27°C (46°–80°F).

FLAREX® ℞
(fluorometholone acetate)
Sterile Ophthalmic Suspension

Description: FLAREX® (fluorometholone acetate) is a corticosteroid prepared as a sterile topical ophthalmic suspension. The active ingredient, fluorometholone acetate, is a white to creamy white powder with an empirical formula of $C_{24}H_{31}FO_5$ and a molecular weight of 418.5. Its chemical name is 9-fluoro-11β, 17-dihydroxy-6α-methylpregna-1, 4-diene-3, 20-dione 17-acetate. The chemical structure of Fluorometholone Acetate is presented below:
[See structure at top of next column.]

Continued on next page

Alcon—Cont.

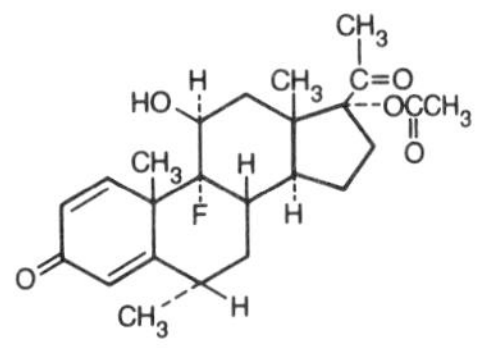

Each mL contains: Active: fluorometholone acetate 1 mg (0.1%). **Preservative:** benzalkonium chloride 0.01%. **Inactive:** sodium chloride, monobasic sodium phosphate, edetate disodium, hydroxyethyl cellulose, tyloxapol, hydrochloric acid and/or sodium hydroxide (to adjust pH), and purified water.

Clinical Pharmacology: Corticosteroids suppress the inflammatory response to inciting agents of mechanical, chemical or immunological nature. No generally accepted explanation of this steroid property has been advanced. Clinical studies demonstrate that Fluorometholone Acetate is significantly more efficacious than Fluorometholone for the treatment of external ocular inflammation.[1] Corticosteroids cause a rise in intraocular pressure in susceptible individuals. In a small study, FLAREX Ophthalmic Suspension demonstrated a significantly longer average time to produce a rise in intraocular pressure than did dexamethasone phosphate; however, the ultimate magnitude of the rise was equivalent for both drugs and in a small percentage of individuals a significant rise in intraocular pressure occurred within three days.[2]

Indications and Usage: FLAREX Ophthalmic Suspension is indicated for use in the treatment of steroid responsive inflammatory conditions of the palpebral and bulbar conjunctiva, cornea, and anterior segment of the eye.

Contraindications: Contraindicated in acute superficial herpes simplex keratitis, vaccinia, varicella, and most other viral diseases of cornea and conjunctiva; tuberculosis; fungal diseases; acute purulent untreated infections which, like other diseases caused by microorganisms, may be masked or enhanced by the presence of the steroid; and in those persons who have known hypersensitivity to any component of this preparation.

Warnings: Not for injection. Use in the treatment of herpes simplex infection requires great caution. Prolonged use may result in glaucoma, damage to the optic nerve, defects in visual acuity and visual field, cataract formation and/or may aid in the establishment of secondary ocular infections from pathogens due to suppression of host response. Acute purulent infections of the eye may be masked or exacerbated by presence of steroid medication. In those diseases causing thinning of the cornea or sclera, perforation has been known to occur with chronic use of topical steroids. It is advisable that the intraocular pressure be checked frequently.

Precautions:

General: Fungal infections of the cornea are particularly prone to develop coincidentally with long-term local steroid application. Fungus invasion must be considered in any persistent corneal ulceration where a steroid has been used or is in use.

Information for Patients: Do not touch dropper tip to any surface, as this may contaminate the suspension.

Carcinogenesis, mutagenesis, impairment of fertility: No studies have been conducted in animals or in humans to evaluate the possibility of these effects with fluorometholone.

Pregnancy: Pregnancy Category C. Fluorometholone has been shown to be embryocidal and teratogenic in rabbits when administered at low multiples of the human ocular dose. Fluorometholone was applied ocularly to rabbits daily on days 6–18 of gestation, and dose-related fetal loss and fetal abnormalities including cleft palate, deformed rib cage, anomalous limbs and neural abnormalities such as encephalocele, craniorachischisis, and spina bifida were observed. There are no adequate and well controlled studies of fluorometholone in pregnant women, and it is not known whether fluorometholone can cause fetal harm when administered to a pregnant woman. Fluorometholone should be used during pregnancy only if the potential benefit justifies the potential risk to the fetus.

Nursing Mothers: It is not known whether topical administration of corticosteroids could result in sufficient systemic absorption to produce detectable quantities in human milk. Systemically-administered corticosteroids appear in human milk and could suppress growth, interfere with endogenous corticosteroid production, or cause other untoward effects. Because of the potential for serious adverse reactions in nursing infants from fluorometholone, a decision should be made whether to discontinue nursing or to discontinue the drug.

Pediatric Use: Safety and effectiveness in children have not been established.

Adverse Reactions: Glaucoma with optic nerve damage, visual acuity and field defects, cataract formation, secondary ocular infection following suppression of host response, and perforation of the globe may occur.

Dosage and Administration: **Shake Well Before Using.** One to two drops instilled into the conjunctival sac(s) four times daily. During the initial 24 to 48 hours the dosage may be safely increased to two drops every two hours. If no improvement after two weeks, consult physician. Care should be taken not to discontinue therapy prematurely.

How Supplied: 2.5 mL, 5 mL and 10 mL in plastic DROP-TAINER® dispensers.

2.5 mL: **NDC** 0065-0096-25
5 mL: **NDC** 0065-0096-05
10 mL: **NDC** 0065-0096-10

Storage: Store upright between 2°–27°C (36°–80°F). Protect From Freezing.

References:

1. Leibowitz, H. M., et. al., Annals of Ophthalmology 1984; 16:1110.
2. Stewart, R.H., et al., Current Eye Research 1984; 3:835.

FLUORESCITE® INJECTION ℞
(fluorescein injection)
Sterile

Description: FLUORESCITE® Injection is a sterile aqueous solution in two strengths for use intravenously as a diagnostic aid. The active ingredient is represented by the chemical structure:

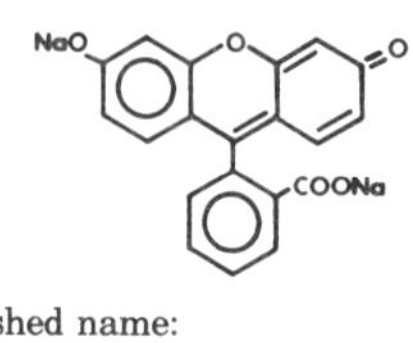

Established name:
Fluorescein Sodium
Chemical name:
Spiro[isobenzofuran-1(3*H*),9'-[9*H*] xanthene]-3-one, 3'6' dihydroxy, disodium salt.

The solution contains Fluorescein Sodium (equivalent to Fluorescein 10% or 25%), Sodium Hydroxide and/or Hydrochloric Acid (to adjust pH), and Water for Injection.

10% ampule
10% syringe
25% ampule

Clinical Pharmacology: The yellowish-green fluorescence of the drug demarcates the vascular area under observation, distinguishing it from adjacent areas.

Indications and Usage: Indicated in diagnostic fluorescein angiography or angioscopy of the fundus and of the iris vasculature.

Contraindications: Contraindicated in those persons who have shown hypersensitivity to any component of this preparation.

Warning: For ophthalmic use only—not for intrathecal injection. Care must be taken to avoid extravasation during injection as the high pH of fluorescein solution can result in severe local tissue damage. The following complications resulting from extravasation of fluorescein have been noted to occur: sloughing of the skin, superficial phlebitis, subcutaneous granuloma, and toxic neuritis along the median curve in the antecubital area. Complications resulting from extravasation can cause severe pain in the arm for up to several hours. When significant extravasation occurs, the injection should be discontinued and conservative measures to treat damaged tissue and to relieve pain should be implemented.

Precautions: General: Caution is to be exercised in patients with a history of allergy or bronchial asthma. An emergency tray including such items as 0.1% epinephrine for intravenous or intramuscular use; an antihistamine, soluble steroid, and aminophyllene for IV use; and oxygen should always be available in the event of possible reaction to fluorescein injection.[1]

Information for Patients: Skin will attain a temporary yellowish discoloration. Urine attains a bright yellow color. Discoloration of the skin fades in 6 to 12 hours; urine fluorescein in 24 to 36 hours.

Carcinogenesis, Mutagenesis, Impairment of Fertility: There have been no long-term studies done using fluorescein in animals to evaluate carcinogenic potential.

Use in Pregnancy: Avoid angiography on patients who are pregnant, especially those in first trimester. There have been no reports of fetal complications from fluorescein injection during pregnancy.

Nursing Mothers: Fluorescein has been demonstrated to be execreted in human milk. Caution should be exercised when fluorescein is administered to a nursing woman.

Adverse Reactions: Nausea and headache, gastrointestinal distress, syncope, vomiting, hypotension, and other symptoms and signs of hypersensitivity have occurred. Cardiac arrest, basilar artery ischemia, severe shock, convulsions, thrombophlebitis at the injection site and rare cases of death have been reported. Extravasation of the solution at the injection site causes intense pain at the site and a dull aching pain in the injected arm. (SEE WARNING.) Generalized hives and itching, bronchospasm and anaphylaxis have been reported. A strong taste may develop after injection.

Dosage and Administration: Parenteral drug products should be inspected visually for particulate matter and discoloration prior to administration, whenever solution and container permit. Inject the contents of the ampule or pre-filled syringe rapidly into the antecubital vein, *after taking precautions to avoid extravasation.* A syringe, filled with fluorescein, is attached to transparent tubing and a 25 gauge scalp vein needle for injection. Insert the needle and draw the patient's blood to the hub of the syringe so that a *small* air bubble separates the patient's blood in the tubing from the fluorescein. With the room lights on, slowly inject the blood back into the vein while watching the skin over the needle tip. If the needle has extravasated, the patient's blood will be seen to bulge the skin and the injection should be stopped before any fluorescein is injected. When assured that extravasation has not occurred, the room light may be turned off and the fluorescein injection completed. Luminescence appears in the retina and choroidal vessels in 9 to 14 seconds and can be observed by standard viewing equipment. If potential allergy is suspected, an intradermal skin test may be performed prior to intravenous administration, i.e., 0.05 mL injected intradermally to be evaluated 30 to 60 minutes following injection. For children, the dose is calculated on the basis of 35 mg for each ten pounds of body weight.

How Supplied: 5 mL of 10% in pre-filled syringe; 10% in 5 mL ampule and 25% in 2 mL ampule.

10% NDC 0065-0092-05
10% NDC 0065-0093-05 syringe
25% NDC 0065-0094-02

Storage: Store at 8°–27°C (46°–80°F).

Caution: Federal (USA) law prohibits dispensing without prescription.

REFERENCE:

1. Schatz, Burton, Yannuzzi, Rabb. Interpretation of Fundus Fluorescein Angiography, Page 38, C. V. Mosby Co., Saint Louis, 1978.

GLAUCON® ℞
(epinephrine)
Sterile Ophthalmic Solution

Description: GLAUCON® (epinephrine) is a sterile topical ophthalmic solution. The active ingredient is represented by the chemical structure:

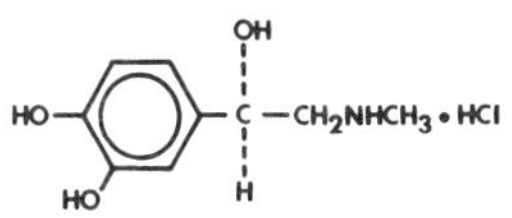

Established name:
Epinephrine Hydrochloride

Chemical name:
1,2-Benzenediol, 4-[1-hydroxy-2-(methylamino)ethyl]-, (*R*)-, monohydrochloride.

Each mL contains: Active: Epinephrine Hydrochloride equivalent to 1.0% or 2.0% Epinephrine base. **Preservative:** Benzalkonium Chloride 0.01%. **Inactive:** Sodium Metabisulfite, Edetate Disodium, Sodium Chloride in 1% solution only, Hydrochloric Acid, Sodium Hydroxide (to adjust pH), Purified Water.

Clinical Pharmacology: Lowers intraocular pressure by reducing the production of aqueous and increasing the facility of outflow.

Indications and Usage: For the control of simple (open angle) glaucoma. It may be used in combination with miotics, beta blockers, hyperosmotic agents, or carbonic anhydrase inhibitors when indicated.

Contraindications: Do not use in narrow or shallow angle (angle closure) glaucoma. Contraindicated in those persons who have shown hypersensitivity to any component of this preparation.

Warnings: For topical eye use only—not for injection. To avoid inducing angle closure glaucoma, an estimation of the depth of the angle of the anterior chamber should be made. Use with caution in individuals with history of hyperthyroidism, hypertension, organic cardiac disease and long-standing bronchial asthma. Maculopathy with associated decrease in visual acuity may occur in the aphakic eye; in this event, administration should be discontinued promptly. Do not use if solution is brown or contains a precipitate. Contains sodium metabisulfite, a sulfite that may cause allergic-type reactions including anaphylactic symptoms and life-threatening or less severe asthmatic episodes in certain susceptible people. The overall prevalence of sulfite sensitivity in the general population is unknown and probably low. Sulfite sensitivity is seen more frequently in asthmatic than in nonasthmatic people.

Precautions: General. Do not use this preparation while wearing soft contact lenses.

Information For Patients: Do not touch dropper tip to any surface, as this may contaminate the solution.

Carcinogenesis, Mutagenesis, Impairment of Fertility: There have been no long-term studies done using GLAUCON® (epinephrine) Ophthalmic Solution in animals to evaluate carcinogenic potential.

Pregnancy: Pregnancy Category C. Animal reproduction studies have not been conducted with epinephrine. It is also not known whether epinephrine can cause fetal harm when administered to a pregnant woman or can affect reproduction capacity. GLAUCON Ophthalmic Solution should be given to a pregnant woman only if clearly needed.

Nursing Mothers: It is not known whether these drugs are excreted in human milk. Because many drugs are excreted in human milk, caution should be exercised when epinephrine is administered to a nursing woman.

Adverse Reactions: Transient symptoms of stinging and burning may occur. Prolonged use may be associated with conjunctival or corneal pigmentation. Following prolonged administration, ocular irritation (hypersensitivity) may develop. Systemic side effects such as headache, palpitation, faintness, tachycardia, and extrasystoles may occur. Severe side effects such as hypertension and cardiac arrhythmia have been reported.

Dosage and Administration: Usual dosage is one drop topically in the eye(s) one or two times daily for the control of glaucoma.

How Supplied: 10 mL in 15 mL plastic DROP-TAINER® dispenser.

1% NDC 0998-0249-10
2% NDC 0998-0250-10

Storage: Store at 36° to 75°F (2° to 24° C).

Caution: Federal (USA) law prohibits dispensing without prescription.

GONIOSCOPIC PRISM SOLUTION ℞
Sterile prism solution

Description: A sterile buffered isotonic solution containing hydroxyethylcellulose, preserved with thimerosal 0.004% and edetate disodium 0.1%.

Indications and Usage: For professional use only. To be used in accordance with directions for bonding gonioscopic prisms to the eye. Refractive index approximately 1.35.

Warning: This product contains thimerosal. Do not use with patients allergic to thimerosal or any other ingredient containing mercury.

How Supplied: In 15mL (½ fl. oz.) plastic dispensers, NDC 0065-0259-15.

Storage: Store at room temperature.

IOPIDINE® ℞
(apraclonidine hydrochloride)
1% As Base
Sterile Ophthalmic Solution

Description: IOPIDINE® Ophthalmic Solution contains apraclonidine hydrochloride, an alpha adrenergic agonist, in a sterile isotonic solution for topical application to the eye. Apraclonidine hydrochloride is a white to off-white powder and is highly soluble in water. Its chemical name is 2-[(4-amino-2,6 dichlorophenyl) imino]imidazolidine monohydrochloride with an empirical formula of $C_9H_{11}Cl_3N_4$ and a molecular weight of 281.6. The chemical structure of apraclonidine hydrochloride is:

[See structure at top of next column.]

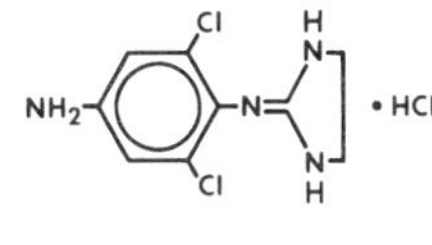

Each mL of IOPIDINE Ophthalmic Solution contains: Active: Apraclonidine hydrochloride 11.5 mg equivalent to apraclonidine base 10 mg. Preservative: Benzalkonium chloride 0.01%. Inactive: Sodium chloride, sodium acetate, sodium hydroxide and/or hydrochloric acid (pH 4.4–7.8) and purified water.

Clinical Pharmacology: Apraclonidine is a relatively selective, alpha adrenergic agonist and does not have significant membrane stabilizing (local anesthetic) activity. When instilled into the eye, IOPIDINE (apraclonidine hydrochloride) Ophthalmic Solution has the action of reducing intraocular pressure. Ophthalmic apraclonidine has minimal effect on cardiovascular parameters.

Optic nerve head damage and visual field loss may result from an acute elevation in intraocular pressure that can occur after argon or Nd:YAG laser surgical procedures. Elevated intraocular pressure, whether acute or chronic in duration, is a major risk factor in the pathogenesis of visual field loss. The higher the peak or spike of intraocular pressure, the greater the likelihood of visual field loss and optic nerve damage especially in patients with previously compromised optic nerves. The onset of action with IOPIDINE Ophthalmic Solution can usually be noted within one hour and the maximum intraocular pressure reduction usually occurs three to five hours after application of a single dose. The precise mechanism of the ocular hypotensive action of IOPIDINE Ophthalmic Solution is not completely established at this time. Aqueous fluorophotometry studies in man suggest that its predominant action may be related to a reduction of aqueous formation. Controlled clinical studies of patients requiring argon laser trabeculoplasty, argon laser iridotomy or Nd:YAG posterior capsulotomy showed that IOPIDINE Ophthalmic Solution controlled or prevented the postsurgical intraocular pressure rise typically observed in patients after undergoing those procedures. After surgery, the mean intraocular pressure was 1.2 to 4.0 mmHg below the corresponding presurgical baseline pressure before IOPIDINE Ophthalmic Solution treatment. With placebo treatment, postsurgical pressures were 2.5 to 8.4 mmHg higher than their corresponding presurgical baselines. Overall, only 2% of patients treated with IOPIDINE Ophthalmic Solution had severe intraocular pressure elevations (spike ≥ 10 mmHg) during the first three hours after laser surgery, whereas 22% of placebo-treated patients responded with severe pressure spikes (Table 1). Of the patients that experienced a pressure spike after surgery, the peak intraocular pressure was above 30 mmHg in most patients (Table 2) and was above 50 mmHg in seven placebo-treated patients and one IOPIDINE Ophthalmic Solution-treated patient.

[See tables on next page.]

Indications and Usage: IOPIDINE (apraclonidine hydrochloride) Ophthalmic Solution is indicated to control or prevent postsurgical elevations in intraocular pressure that occur in patients after argon laser trabeculoplasty, argon laser iridotomy or Nd:YAG posterior capsulotomy.

Contraindication: IOPIDINE® Ophthalmic Solution is contraindicated for patients receiving monoamine oxidase inhibitor therapy and for patients with hypersensitivity to any component of this medication or to clonidine.

Continued on next page

Alcon—Cont.

Precautions:

General: Since IOPIDINE Ophthalmic Solution is a potent depressor of intraocular pressure, patients who develop exaggerated reductions in intraocular pressure should be closely monitored.

Although the acute administration of two drops of IOPIDINE® Ophthalmic Solution has minimal effect on heart rate or blood pressure in clinical studies evaluating patients undergoing anterior segment laser surgery, the preclinical pharmacologic profile of this drug suggests that caution should be observed in treating patients with severe cardiovascular disease including hypertension.

The possibility of a vasovagal attack occurring during laser surgery should be considered and caution used in patients with history of such episodes.

Topical ocular administration of two drops of 0.5%, 1.0% and 1.5% IOPIDINE Ophthalmic Solution to New Zealand Albino rabbits three times daily for one month resulted in sporadic and transient instances of minimal corneal cloudiness in the 1.5% group only. No histopathological changes were noted in those eyes. No adverse ocular effects were observed in cynomolgus monkeys treated with two drops of 1.5% IOPIDINE Ophthalmic Solution applied three times daily for three months. No corneal changes were observed in 320 humans given at least one dose of 1.0% IOPIDINE Ophthalmic Solution.

Drug Interactions: Interactions with other agents have not been investigated.

Carcinogenesis, Mutagenesis, Impairment of Fertility: In a variety of *in vitro* cell assays, apraclonidine was nonmutagenic. Studies addressing carcinogenesis and the impairment of fertility have not been conducted.

Pregnancy: Pregnancy Category C: There are no adequate and well controlled studies of IOPIDINE Ophthalmic Solution in pregnant women. Animal reproduction studies have not been conducted with apraclonidine hydrochloride. This medication should be used in pregnancy only if the potential benefit to the mother justifies the potential risk to the fetus.

Nursing Mothers: It is not known if topically applied IOPIDINE Ophthalmic Solution is excreted in human milk. A decision should be considered to discontinue nursing temporarily for the one day on which IOPIDINE® Ophthalmic Solution is used.

Pediatric Use: Safety and effectiveness in children have not been established.

Adverse Reactions: The following adverse events were reported in association with the use of IOPIDINE Ophthalmic Solution in laser surgery: ocular injection (1.8%),upper lid elevation (1.3%), irregular heart rate (0.7%), ocular inflammation (0.45%), nasal decongestion (0.45%),conjunctival blanching (0.4%) and mydriasis (0.4%).

The following adverse events were observed in investigational studies dosing IOPIDINE Ophthalmic Solution once or twice daily for up to 28 days in nonlaser studies:

Ocular: Conjunctival blanching, upper lid elevation, mydriasis, burning, discomfort, foreign body sensation, dryness, itching, hypotony, blurred or dimmed vision, allergic response, conjunctival microhemorrhage.

Gastrointestinal: Abdominal pain, diarrhea, stomach discomfort, emesis.

Cardiovascular: Bradycardia, vasovagal attack, palpitations, orthostatic episode.

Central Nervous System: Insomnia, dream disturbances, irritability, decreased libido.

Other: Taste abnormalities, dry mouth, nasal burning or dryness, headache, head cold sensation, chest heaviness or burning, clammy or sweaty palms, body heat sensation, shortness of breath, increased pharyngeal secretion, extremity pain or numbness, fatigue, paresthesia, pruritus not associated with rash.

Overdosage: No information is available on overdosage in humans. The oral LD_{50} of the drug ranged from 3–8 mg/kg in mice and 38–107 mg/kg in rats. The intravenous LD_{50} of the drug ranged from 6–9 mg/kg in mice and 9–21 mg/kg in rats. LD_{50} values in these ranges are indicative of a drug with a high degree of toxicity.

Dosage and Administration: One drop of IOPIDINE Ophthalmic Solution should be instilled in the scheduled operative eye one hour before initiating anterior segment laser surgery and a second drop should be instilled to the same eye immediately upon completion of the laser surgical procedure. Use a separate container for each single-drop dose and discard each container after use.

How Supplied: IOPIDINE (apraclonidine hydrochloride) Ophthalmic Solution 1% as base is a sterile, isotonic, aqueous solution containing apraclonidine hydrochloride. Supplied as follows: 0.1 mL in plastic ophthalmic dispensers, packaged two per pouch. These dispensers are enclosed in a foil overwrap as an added barrier to evaporation.

0.1 mL: **NDC** 0065-0660-10

Storage: Store at room temperature: Protect from light.

U.S. Patent No. 4,517,199,5,212,196

Table 1
Incidence of Intraocular Pressure Spikes ≥ 10 mmHg

Study	Laser Procedure	P-Value	Treatment: Apraclonidine [a]N	(%)	Placebo [a]N	(%)
1	Trabeculoplasty	<0.05	0/40	(0%)	6/35	(17%)
2	Trabeculoplasty	=0.06	2/41	(5%)	8/42	(19%)
1	Iridotomy	<0.05	0/11	(0%)	4/10	(40%)
2	Iridotomy	=0.05	0/17	(0%)	4/19	(21%)
1	Nd:YAG Capsulotomy	<0.05	3/80	(4%)	19/83	(23%)
2	Nd:YAG Capsulotomy	<0.05	0/83	(0%)	22/81	(27%)

[a]N = Number Spikes/Number Eyes.

Table 2
Magnitude of Postsurgical Intraocular Pressure in Trabeculoplasty, Iridotomy and Nd:YAG Capsulotomy Patients With Severe Pressure Spikes ≥ 10 mmHg

Treatment	Total Spikes	Maximum Postsurgical Intraocular Pressure (mmHg): 20–29 mmHg	30–39 mmHg	40–49 mmHg	>50 mmHg
IOPIDINE	8	1	4	2	1
Placebo	78	16	47	8	7

IOPIDINE® 0.5% ℞
(Apraclonidine Ophthalmic Solution)
0.5% As Base

Description: IOPIDINE® 0.5% Ophthalmic Solution contains apraclonidine hydrochloride, an alpha adrenergic agonist, in a sterile isotonic solution for topical application to the eye. Apraclonidine hydrochloride is a white to off-white powder and is highly soluble in water. Its chemical name is 2-[(4-amino-2,6 dichlorophenyl) imino]imidazolidine monohydrochloride with an empirical formula of $C_9H_{11}Cl_3N_4$ and a molecular weight of 281.57. The chemical structure of apraclonidine hydrochloride is:

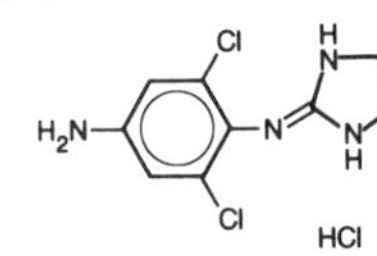

Each mL of IOPIDINE 0.5% Ophthalmic Solution contains: Active: apraclonidine hydrochloride 5.75 mg equivalent to apraclonidine base 5 mg; **Preservative:** benzalkonium chloride 0.01%. **Inactive:** sodium chloride, sodium acetate, sodium hydroxide and/or hydrochloric acid (pH 4.4–7.8) and purified water.

Clinical Pharmacology: Apraclonidine hydrochloride is a relatively selective alpha-2-adrenergic agonist. When instilled in the eye, IOPIDINE 0.5% Ophthalmic Solution, has the action of reducing elevated as well as normal, intraocular pressure (IOP), whether or not accompanied by glaucoma. Ophthalmic apraclonidine has minimal effect on cardiovascular parameters.

Elevated IOP presents a major risk factor in glaucomatous field loss. The higher the level of IOP the greater the likelihood of optic nerve damage and visual field loss. IOPIDINE 0.5% Ophthalmic Solution has the action of reducing IOP. The onset of action of apraclonidine can usually be noted within one hour, and maximum IOP reduction occurs about three hours after instillation. Aqueous fluorophotometry studies demonstrate that Apraclonidine's predominant mechanism of action is reduction of aqueous flow via stimulation of the alpha-adrenergic system,

Repeated dose-response and comparative studies (0.125% - 1.0% apraclonidine) demonstrate that 0.5% apraclonidine is at the top of the dose/response IOP reduction curve.

The clinical utility of IOPIDINE 0.5% Ophthalmic Solution is most apparent for those glaucoma patients on maximally tolerated medical therapy. Patients on maximally tolerated medical therapy with uncontrolled IOP and scheduled to undergo laser trabeculoplasty or trabeculectomy surgery were enrolled into a double masked, placebo-controlled, multi-center clinical trial to determine if IOPIDINE 0.5% Ophthalmic Solution, dosed three times daily (TID), could delay the need for surgery for up to three months.

All patients enrolled into this trial had advanced glaucoma and were undergoing maximally tolerated medical therapy, i.e., patients were using combinations of a topical beta blocker, sympathomimetics, parasympathomimetics and oral carbonic anhydrase inhibitors. Patients were considered to be treatment failures in this study if, in the opinion of the investigators, their IOP was uncontrolled by the masked study medication or there was evidence of further optic nerve damage or visual field loss, and surgery was indicated. Of 171 patients receiving masked medication, 84 were treated with IOPIDINE 0.5% Ophthalmic Solution and 87 were treated with placebo (Apraclonidine vehicle).

Apraclonidine treatment resulted in a significantly greater percentage of treatment successes compared to patients treated with placebo. In this placebo controlled maximum therapy trial, 14.3% of patients treated with IOPIDINE 0.5% Ophthalmic Solution were discontinued due to adverse events, primarily allergic like reactions (12.9%).

The IOP lowering efficacy of IOPIDINE 0.5% Ophthalmic Solution diminishes over time in some patients. This loss of effect, or tachyphylaxis, appears to be an individual occurrence with a variable time of onset and should be closely monitored.

An unpredictable decrease of IOP control in some patients and incidence of ocular allergic responses and systemic side effects may limit the utility of IOPIDINE 0.5% Ophthalmic Solution. However, patients on maximally tolerated medical therapy may still benefit from the additional IOP reduction provided by the short-term use of IOPIDINE 0.5% Ophthalmic Solution.

Topical use of IOPIDINE 0.5% Ophthalmic Solution leads to systemic absorption. Studies of IOPIDINE 0.5% Ophthalmic Solution dosed one drop three times a day in both eyes for 10 days in normal volunteers yielded mean peak and trough concentrations of 0.9 ng/mL and 0.5 ng/mL, respectively. The half-life of IOPIDINE® 0.5% (Apraclonidine Ophthalmic Solution) was calculated to be 8 hours.

IOPIDINE 0.5% Ophthalmic Solution, because of its alpha adrenergic activity, is a vasoconstrictor. Single dose ocular blood flow studies in monkeys, using the microsphere technique, demonstrated a reduced blood flow for the anterior segment; however, no reduction in blood flow was observed in the posterior segment of the eye after a topical dose of IOPIDINE 0.5% Ophthalmic Solution. Ocular blood flow studies have not been conducted in humans.

Indications and Usage: IOPIDINE 0.5% Ophthalmic Solution is indicated for short-term adjunctive therapy in patients on maximally tolerated medical therapy who require additional IOP reduction. Patients on maximally tolerated medical therapy who are treated with IOPIDINE 0.5% Ophthalmic Solution to delay surgery should have frequent followup examinations and treatment should be discontinued if the intraocular pressure rises significantly.

The addition of IOPIDINE 0.5% Ophthalmic Solution to patients already using two aqueous suppressing drugs (i.e., beta-blocker plus carbonic anhydrase inhibitor) as part of their maximally tolerated medical therapy may not provide additional benefit. This is because IOPIDINE 0.5% Ophthalmic Solution is an aqueous suppressing drug and the addition of a third aqueous suppressant may not significantly reduce IOP.

The IOP lowering efficacy of IOPIDINE 0.5% Ophthalmic Solution diminishes over time in some patients. This loss of effect, or tachyphylaxis, appears to be an individual occurrence with a variable time of onset and should be closely monitored. The benefit for most patients is less than one month.

Contraindications: IOPIDINE 0.5% Ophthalmic Solution is contraindicated in patients with hypersensitivity to Apraclonidine or any other component of this medication, as well as systemic clonidine. It is also contraindicated in patients receiving monoamine oxidase inhibitors (MAO inhibitors).

Warnings: Not for injection or oral ingestion. Topical ophthalmic use only.

Precautions: General: Glaucoma patients on maximally tolerated medical therapy who are treated with IOPIDINE 0.5% Ophthalmic Solution to delay surgery should have their visual fields monitored periodically.

Although the topical use of IOPIDINE 0.5% Ophthalmic Solution has not been studied in renal failure patients, structurally related clonidine undergoes a significant increase in half-life in patients with severe renal impairment. Close monitoring of cardiovascular parameters in patients with impaired renal function is advised if they are candidates for topical Apraclonidine therapy. Close monitoring of cardiovascular parameters in patients with impaired liver function is also advised as the systemic dosage form of clonidine is partly metabolized in the liver.

While the topical administration of IOPIDINE 0.5% Ophthalmic Solution had minimal effect on heart rate or blood pressure in clinical studies evaluating glaucoma patients, the preclinical pharmacology profile of this drug suggest that caution should be observed in treating patients with severe, uncontrolled cardiovascular disease, including hypertension.

IOPIDINE 0.5% Ophthalmic Solution should be used with caution in patients with coronary insufficiency, recent myocardial infarction, cerebrovascular disease, chronic renal failure, Raynaud's disease, or thromboangiitis obliterans. Caution and monitoring of depressed patients are advised since Apraclonidine has been infrequently associated with depression.

Apraclonidine can cause dizziness and somnolence. Patients who engage in hazardous activities requiring mental alertness should be warned of the potential for a decrease in mental alertness while using Apraclonidine.

Topical ocular administration of two drops of 0.5, 1.0 and 1.5% Apraclonidine Ophthalmic Solution to New Zealand albino rabbits three times daily for one month resulted in sporadic and transient instances of minimal corneal edema in the 1.5% group only; no histopathological changes were noted in thoses eyes.

Use of IOPIDINE 0.5% Ophthalmic Solution can lead to allergic-like reaction characterized wholly or in part by the symptoms of hyperemia, pruritus, discomfort, tearing, foreign body sensation, and edema of the lids and conjunctiva. If ocular allergic-like symptoms occur, IOPIDINE® 0.5% (Apraclonidine Ophthalmic Solution) therapy should be discontinued.

Patient Information: Do not touch dropper tip to any surface as this may contaminate the contents.

Drug Interactions: Apraclonidine should not be used in patients receiving MAO inhibitors. (See CONTRAINDICATIONS). Although no specific drug interactions with topical glaucoma drugs or systemic medications were identified in clinical studies of IOPIDINE 0.5% Ophthalmic Solution, the possibility of an additive or potentiating effect with CNS depressants (alcohol, barbiturates, opiates, sedatives, anesthetics) should be considered. Tricyclic antidepressants have been reported to blunt the hypotensive effect of systemic clonidine. It is not known whether the concurrent use of these agents with Apraclonidine can lead to a reduction in IOP lowering effect. No data on the level of circulating catecholamines after Apraclonidine withdrawal are available. Caution, however, is advised in patients taking tricyclic antidepressants which can affect the metabolism and uptake of circulating amines.

An additive hypotensive effect has been reported with the combination of systemic clonidine and neuroleptic therapy. Systemic clonidine may inhibit the production of catecholamines in response to insulin-induced hypoglycemia and mask the signs and symptoms of hypoglycemia.

Since Aproclonidine may reduce pulse and blood pressure, caution in using drugs such as beta-blockers (ophthalmic and systemic), antihypertensives, and cardiac glycosides is advised. Patients using cardiovascular drugs concurrently with IOPIDINE 0.5% Ophthalmic Solution should have pulse and blood pressures frequently monitored. Caution should be exercised with simultaneous use of clonidine and other similar pharmacologic agents.

Carcinogenesis, Mutagenesis, Impairment of Fertility: No significant change in tumor incidence or type was observed following two years of oral administration of apraclonidine HCl to rats and mice at dosages of 1.0 and 0.6 mg/kg, up to 20 and 12 times, respectively, the maximum dose recommended for human topical ocular use.

Apraclonidine HCl was not mutagenic in a series of *in vitro* mutagenicity tests, including the Ames test, a mouse lymphoma forward mutation assay, a chromosome aberration assay in cultured Chinese hamster ovary (CHO) cells, a sister chromatid exchange assay in (CHO) cells, and a cell transformation assay. An *in vivo* mouse micronucleus assay conducted with apraclonidine HCl also provided no evidence of mutagenicity.

Reproduction and fertility studies in rats showed no adverse effect on male or female fertility at a dose of 0.5 mg/kg (5 to 10 times the maximum recommended human dose).

Pregnancy: Pregnancy Category C: Apraclonidine HCl has been shown to have an embryocidal effect in rabbits when given in an oral dose of 3.0 mg/kg (60 times the maximum recommended human dose). Dose related maternal toxicity was observed in pregnant rats at 0.3 mg/kg (6 times the maximum recommended human dose). There are no adequate and well controlled studies in pregnant women. IOPIDINE 0.5% Ophthalmic Solution should be used during pregnancy only if the potential benefit justifies the potential risk to the fetus.

Nursing Mothers: It is not known whether this drug is excreted in human milk. Because many drugs are excreted in human milk, caution should be exercised when IOPIDINE 0.5% Ophthalmic Solution is administered to a nursing woman.

Pediatric Use: Safety and effectiveness in children have not been established.

Adverse Reactions: Use of IOPIDINE 0.5% Ophthalmic Solution can lead to an allergic-like reaction characterized wholly or in part by the symptoms of hyperemia, pruritus, discomfort, tearing, foreign body sensation and edema of the lids and conjunctiva. If ocular allergic-like symptoms occur, IOPIDINE 0.5% Ophthalmic Solution therapy should be discontinued.

In clinical studies the overall discontinuation rate related to IOPIDINE 0.5% Ophthalmic Solution was 15%. The most commonly reported events leading to discontinuation included (in decreasing order of frequency) hyperemia, pruritus, tearing, discomfort, lid edema, dry mouth, and foreign body sensation.

The following adverse reactions (incidences) were reported in clinical studies of IOPIDINE 0.5% (Apraclonidine Ophthalmic Solution) as being possibly, probably, or definitely related to therapy:

Ocular

Hyperemia (13%), pruritus (10%), discomfort (6%), tearing (4%). The following adverse reactions were reported in less than 3% of the patients: lid edema, blurred vision, foreign body sensation, dry eye, conjunctivitis, discharge, blanching. The following adverse reactions were reported in less than 1% of the patients: lid margin crusting, conjunctival follicles, conjunctival edema, edema, abnormal vision,

Continued on next page

Alcon—Cont.

pain, lid disorder, keratitis, blepharitis, photophobia, corneal staining, lid erythema, blepharoconjunctivitis, irritation, corneal erosion, corneal infiltrate, keratopathy, lid scales, lid retraction.

Nonocular

Body As A Whole: The following adverse reactions were reported in less than 3% of the patients: headache, asthenia. The following adverse reactions (incidences) were reported in less than 1% of the patients: chest pain, abnormal coordination, malaise, facial edema.

Cardiovascular: The following adverse reactions were reported in less than 1% of the patients: peripheral edema, arrhythmia. Although no reports of bradycardia related to IOPIDINE 0.5% Ophthalmic Solution were available from clinical studies, the possibility of its occurrence based on Apraclonidine's alpha-2-agonist effect should be considered (See Clinical Pharmacology Section).

Central Nervous System

The following adverse reactions were reported in less than 1% of the patients: somnolence, dizziness, nervousness, depression, insomnia, paresthesia.

Digestive System: Dry mouth (10%). The following adverse reactions were reported in less than 1% of the patients: constipation, nausea.

Musculoskeletal: Myalgia (0.2%).

Respiratory System: Dry nose (2%). The following adverse reactions were reported in less than 1% of the patients: rhinitis, dyspnea, pharyngitis, asthma.

Skin: The following adverse reactions were reported in less than 1% of the patients: contact dermatitis, dermatitis.

Special Senses: Taste perversion (3%), parosmia (0.2%).

Overdosage: While no instances of human ingestion of IOPIDINE 0.5% Ophthalmic Solution are known, overdose with the oral form of clonidine has been reported to cause hypotension, transient hypertension, asthenia, vomiting, irritabiity, diminished or absent reflexes, lethargy, somnolence, sedation or coma, pallor, hypothermia, bradycardia, conduction defects, arrhythmias, dryness of the mouth, miosis, apnea, respiratory depression, hypoventilation, and seizure. Treatment of an oral overdose includes supportive and symptomatic therapy; a patent airway should be maintained. Hemodialysis is of limited value, since a maximum of 5% of circulating drug is removed.

Dosage and Administration: One to two drops of IOPIDINE 0.5% Ophthalmic Solution should be instilled in the affected eye(s) three times daily. Since IOPIDINE 0.5% Ophthalmic Solution will be used with other ocular glaucoma therapies, an approximate 5 minute interval between instillation of each medication should be practiced to prevent washout of the previous dose. NOT FOR INJECTION INTO THE EYE. NOT FOR ORAL INGESTION.

How Supplied: IOPIDINE 0.5% Ophthalmic Solution as base in a sterile, isotonic, aqueous solution containing apraclonidine hydrochloride.

Supplied in plastic ophthalmic DROP-TAINER® dispenser as follows:

5 mL NDC 0065-0665-05

Storage: Store between 2–27°C (36–80°F). Protect from freezing and light.

U.S. Patent No. 4,517,199

CAUTION: Federal (USA) Law Prohibits Dispensing Without A Prescription.

ISOPTO® ATROPINE ℞
(atropine sulfate)
Ophthalmic Solution

Description: ISOPTO® ATROPINE (atropine sulfate) is an anticholinergic prepared as a sterile topical ophthalmic solution supplied in two strengths. The active ingredient is represented by the chemical structure:

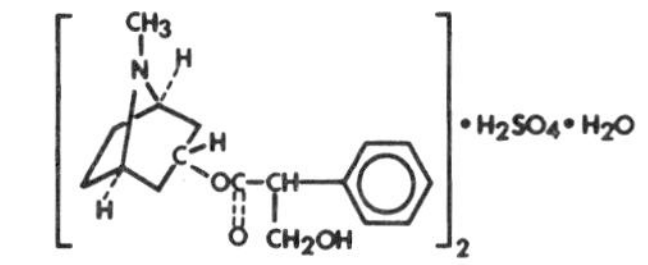

Established name:
Atropine Sulfate

Chemical name:
Benzeneacetic acid, α-(hydroxymethyl)-, 8-methyl-8-aza-bicyclo-[3.2.1]oct-3-yl ester, *endo* -(±)-, sulfate (2:1) (salt), monohydrate.

Each mL contains: **Active:** Atropine Sulfate 0.5%, 1.0%. **Preservative:** Benzalkonium Chloride 0.01%. **Vehicle:** 0.5% Hydroxypropyl Methylcellulose 2910. **Inactive:** Boric Acid, Sodium Hydroxide and/or Hydrochloric Acid (to adjust pH), Purified Water.

Clinical Pharmacology: This anticholinergic preparation blocks the responses of the sphincter muscle of the iris and the accommodative muscle of the ciliary body to cholinergic stimulation, producing pupillary dilation (mydriasis) and paralysis of accommodation (cycloplegia).

Indications and Usage: For mydriasis and/or cycloplegia. For cycloplegic refraction, for pupillary dilation desired in inflammatory conditions of the iris and uveal tract.

Contraindications: Contraindicated in persons with primary glaucoma or a tendency toward glaucoma, e.g., narrow anterior chamber angle, and in those persons showing hypersensitivity to any component of this preparation.

Warnings: For topical use only—not for injection. In infants and small children, use with extreme caution. Excessive use in children or in certain individuals with a previous history of susceptibility to belladonna alkaloids may produce systemic symptoms of atropine poisoning.

Precautions: General: To avoid excessive systemic absorption, the lacrimal sac should be compressed by digital pressure for two to three minutes after instillation. To avoid inducing angle closure glaucoma, an estimation of the depth of the angle of the anterior chamber should be made. Administration of atropine in infants requires great caution.

Information for Patients: Do not touch dropper tip to any surface, as this may contaminate the solution.

Carcinogenesis, mutagenesis, impairment of fertility: No studies have been conducted in animals or in humans to evaluate the potential of these effects.

Pregnancy Category C: Animal reproduction studies have not been performed with atropine. It is also not known whether atropine can cause fetal harm when administered to a pregnant woman or can affect reproduction capacity. Atropine should be given to pregnant women only if clearly needed.

Nursing Mothers: It is not known whether this drug is excreted in human milk. Because many drugs are excreted in human milk, caution should be exercised when atropine is administered to a nursing woman.

Patient Warning: Patient should be advised not to drive or engage in other hazardous activities while pupils are dilated. Patient may experience sensitivity to light and should protect eyes in bright illumination during dilation. Parents should be warned not to get this preparation in their child's mouth and to wash their own hands and the child's hands following administration.

Adverse Reactions: Prolonged use may produce local irritation characterized by follicular conjunctivitis, vascular congestion, edema, exudate, and an eczematoid dermatitis. Severe reactions are manifested by hypotension with progressive respiratory depression. Coma and death have been reported in the very young.

Overdosage: Excessive dosage may produce exaggerated symptoms as noted in ADVERSE REACTIONS. When drug administration is discontinued, patients usually recover spontaneously. In the case of severe manifestations of toxicity, parenteral administration of physostigmine as an antidote may be indicated.[1–4]

Dosage and Administration: Adults: For uveitis, administer one or two drops topically to the eye(s) up to four times daily.

Children: For refraction, administer one or two drops of 0.5% solution to each eye twice daily for one to three days prior to examination. For uveitis, administer one or two drops of 0.5% solution to each eye up to three times daily. The lacrimal sac should be compressed by digital pressure for two to three minutes after instillation. Heavily pigmented irides may require larger doses.

How Supplied: In 5mL (1% also available in 15mL) plastic DROP-TAINER® dispenser.

0.5%: 5mL: NDC 0998-0302-05
1%: 5mL: NDC 0998-0303-05
15mL: NDC 0998-0303-15

Storage: Store at 8°–27°C (46°–80°F).

Caution: Federal (USA) law prohibits dispensing without prescription.

References:

1. Litovitz, T. L. The anecdotal antidotes. Emergency Clinics of North America 1984; 2(1): 145–158.
2. Kulig K. Initial management of ingestions of toxic substances. New England Journal of Medicine 1992; 326(25): 1677–1681.
3. Smilkstein, M. J. As the pendulum swings. Journal of Emergency Medicine. 1991; 9(4): 275–277.
4. Klaasen, C. D., Amdur M. O., Doull J. (eds) *Casarett and Doull's Toxicology. The Basic Science of Poisons.* Third edition, New York, NY, Macmillan Publishing Company: 1986, p. 887.

ISOPTO® CARBACHOL ℞
(carbachol)
Sterile Ophthalmic Solution

Description: ISOPTO® CARBACHOL is a cholinergic prepared as a sterile topical ophthalmic solution. The active ingredient is represented by the chemical structure: $[NH_2COOCH_2CH_2N(CH_3)_3]^+Cl^-$

Established name: Carbachol

Chemical name: 2-[(Aminocarbonyl)oxy]-*N,N,N*-trimethylethanaminium chloride.

Each mL contains: Active: Carbachol 0.75%, 1.5%, 2.25%, or 3.0%. **Preservative:** Benzalkonium Chloride 0.005%. **Vehicle:** Hydroxypropyl Methylcellulose 1.0%. **Inactive:** Boric Acid, Sodium Chloride, Sodium Borate, Purified Water.

Clinical Pharmacology: A cholinergic (parasympathomimetic) agent. Carbachol has a double action, it not only stimulates the motor endplate of the muscle cell, as do all cholinesters, but it also partially inhibits cholinesterase.

Indications and Usage: For lowering intraocular pressure in the treatment of glaucoma.

Contraindications: Miotics are contraindicated where constriction is undesirable such as acute iritis. Contraindicated in those persons showing hypersensitivity to any component of this preparation.

Warnings: For topical use only. Not for injection. Carbachol should be used with caution in the presence of corneal abrasion to avoid excessive penetration which can produce systemic toxicity; and in patients with acute cardiac failure, bronchial asthma, active peptic ulcer, hyperthyroidism, gastrointestinal spasm, urinary tract obstruction. Parkinson's disease, recent myocardial infarct, systemic hypertension or hypotension. As with all miotics, retinal detachment has been reported when used in certain susceptible individuals.
Precautions: General: Avoid overdosage.
Information for Patients: The miosis usually causes difficulty in dark adaptation. Patient should be advised to exercise caution in night driving and other hazardous occupations in poor light. Do not touch dropper tip to any surface, as this may contaminate the solution.
Carcinogenesis, Mutagenesis, Impairment of Fertility. There have been no long-term studies done using carbachol in animals to evaluate carcinogenic potential.
Pregnancy. Pregnancy Category C. Animal reproduction studies have not been conducted with carbachol. It is also not known whether carbachol can cause fetal harm when administered to a pregnant woman or can affect reproduction capacity. Carbachol should be given to a pregnant woman only if clearly needed.
Nursing Mothers. It is not known whether this drug is excreted in human milk. Because many drugs are excreted in human milk, caution should be exercised when carbachol is administered to a nursing woman.
Adverse Reactions: Transient symptoms of stinging and burning may occur. This preparation is capable of producing systemic symptoms of a cholinesterase inhibitor even when the epithelium is intact. Transient ciliary and conjunctival injection, headache, and ciliary spasm with resultant temporary decrease of visual acuity may occur. Salivation, syncope, cardiac arrhythmia, gastrointestinal cramping, vomiting, asthma, hypotension, diarrhea, frequent urge to urinate, increased sweating, and irritation of eyes may occur.
Overdosage: Atropine should be administered parenterally (for dosage refer to Goodman & Gilman or other pharmacology reference).
Dosage and Administration: Instill two drops topically in the eye(s) up to three times daily or as indicated by physician.
How Supplied: 15mL and 30mL in plastic DROP-TAINER® Dispensers.

0.75%: 15 mL NDC 0998-0221-15
1.5%: 15 mL NDC 0998-0223-15
30 mL NDC 0998-0223-30
2.25%: 15 mL NDC 0998-0224-15
3%: 15 mL NDC 0998-0225-15
30 mL NDC 0998-0225-30

Storage: Store at 46°–80°F (8°–27°C).
Caution: Federal (USA) law prohibits dispensing without prescription.

ISOPTO® CARPINE ℞
(pilocarpine hydrochloride)
Sterile Ophthalmic Solution

Description: ISOPTO® CARPINE (Pilocarpine Hydrochloride) is a cholinergic prepared as a sterile topical ophthalmic solution. The active ingredient is represented by the chemical structure:

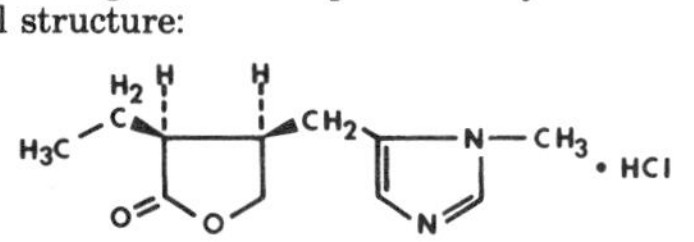

Established name:
Pilocarpine Hydrochloride
Chemical name:
2(3*H*)-Furanone, 3-ethyldihydro-4-[(1-methyl-1*H*-imidazol-5-yl)-methyl]-, monohydrochloride, (3*S*-*cis*)-.

Each mL contains: Active: Pilocarpine Hydrochloride 0.25%, 0.5%, 1%, 2%, 3%, 4%, 5%, 6%, 8% or 10%. **Preservative:** Benzalkonium Chloride 0.01%. **Vehicle:** 0.5% Hydroxypropyl Methycellulose 2910. **Inactive:** Boric Acid, Sodium Citrate, Sodium Chloride (present in 0.25%, 0.5%, and 1% only); Hydrochloric Acid and/or Sodium Hydroxide (to adjust pH in 1%, 2%, 3%, 4%, 5%, 6%, 8% and 10%); Citric Acid, Hydrochloric Acid and/or Sodium Hydroxide (to adjust pH in 0.25% and 0.5%); Purified Water.
Clinical Pharmacology: Pilocarpine is a direct acting cholinergic parasympathomimetic agent which acts through direct stimulation of muscarinic neuro receptors and smooth muscle such as the iris and secretory glands. Pilocarpine produces miosis through contraction of the iris sphincter, causing increased tension on the scleral spur and opening of the trabecular mesh work spaces to facilitate outflow of aqueous humor. Outflow resistance is thereby reduced, lowering intraocular pressure.
Indications and Usage: Pilocarpine Hydrochloride is a miotic (parasympathomimetic) used to control intraocular pressure. It may be used in combination with other miotics, beta blockers, carbonic anhydrase inhibitors, sympathomimetics, or hyperosmotic agents.
Contraindications: Miotics are contraindicated where constriction is undesirable such as in acute iritis, in those persons showing hypersensitivity to any of their components, and in pupillary block glaucoma.

Warnings: For topical use only. NOT FOR INJECTION.
Precautions: General. The miosis usually causes difficulty in dark adaptation. Patient should be advised to exercise caution in night driving and other hazardous occupations in poor illumination.
Carcinogenesis, Mutagenesis, Impairment of Fertility: There have been no long-term studies done using pilocarpine in animals to evaluate carcinogenic potential.
Pregnancy: Pregnancy Category C. Animal reproduction studies have not been conducted with pilocarpine. It is also not known whether pilocarpine can cause fetal harm when administered to a pregnant woman or can affect reproduction capacity. Pilocarpine should be given to a pregnant woman only if clearly needed.
Nursing Mothers: It is not known whether this drug is excreted in human milk. Because many drugs are excreted in human milk, caution should be exercised when pilocarpine is administered to a nursing woman.
Information for Patients: Do not touch dropper tip to any surface, as this may contaminate the solution.

Adverse Reactions: Transient symptoms of stinging and burning may occur. Ciliary spasm, conjunctival vascular congestion, temporal or supraorbital headache, and induced myopia may occur. This is especially true in younger individuals who have recently started administration. Reduced visual acuity in poor illumination is frequently experienced by older individuals and individuals with lens opacity. As with all miotics, rare cases of retinal detachment have been reported when used in certain susceptible individuals. Lens opacity may occur with prolonged use of pilocarpine.
Overdosage: Systemic toxicity following topical ocular administration of pilocarpine is rare, but occasional patients are peculiarly sensitive and develop sweating and gastrointestinal overactivity following suggested dosage and administration. Overdosage can produce sweating, salivation, nausea, tremors and slowing of the pulse and a decrease in blood pressure. In moderate overdosage, spontaneous recovery is to be expected and is aided by intravenous fluids to compensate for dehydration. For cases demonstrating severe poisoning, atropine is the pharmacologic antagonist to pilocarpine.[1]
A topical ocular overdose of an ophthalmic product containing pilocarpine may be flushed from the eye(s) with warm tap water.
Dosage and Administration: Two drops topically in the eye(s) up to three or four times daily as directed by a physician. Under selected conditions, more frequent instillations may be indicated. Individuals with heavily pigmented irides may require higher strengths.
How Supplied: In 15mL and 30mL plastic DROP-TAINER® dispensers.

0.25%—15mL: NDC 0998-0201-15
0.5%—15mL: NDC 0998-0202-15
1%—15mL: NDC 0998-0203-15
30mL: NDC 0998-0203-30
2%—15mL: NDC 0998-0204-15
30mL: NDC 0998-0204-30
3%—15mL: NDC 0998-0205-15
30mL: NDC 0998-0205-30
4%—15mL: NDC 0998-0206-15
30mL: NDC 0998-0206-30
5%—15mL: NDC 0998-0207-15
6%—15mL: NDC 0998-0208-15
30mL: NDC 0998-0208-30
8%—15mL: NDC 0998-0209-15
10%—15mL: NDC 0998-0211-15

Storage: Store at 46° to 80°F.
Caution: Federal (USA) law prohibits dispensing without prescription.

[1] Grant, W. M., Toxicology Of The Eye, 3rd Edition (1986). Charles Thomas Publishing, Springfield, Il.

CETAMIDE™ ℞
(sulfacetamide sodium ophthalmic ointment, USP)
10%
Sterile

ISOPTO CETAMIDE® ℞
(sulfacetamide sodium ophthalmic solution, USP) 15%
Sterile

Description: ISOPTO CETAMIDE® (sulfacetamide sodium ophthalmic solution, USP) 15% and CETAMIDE™ (sulfacetamide sodium ophthalmic ointment, USP) 10% are sterile topical antibacterial agents for ophthalmic use. The active ingredient is represented by the following structural formula:

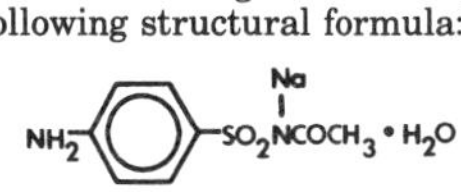

$C_8H_9N_2NaO_3S \cdot H_2O$ **MW=254.24**

Chemical name: *N*-Sulfanilylacetamide monosodium salt monohydrate
Each mL of solution contains: **Active:** Sulfacetamide Sodium 15% (150 mg/mL). **Preservatives:** Methylparaben 0.05%, Propylparaben 0.01%. **Vehicle:** 0.5% Hydroxypropyl Methylcellulose 2910 (viscosity type, 4000 cps). **Inactive:** Sodium Thiosulfate 0.3%, Dibasic Sodium Phosphate and/or Monobasic Sodium Phosphate (to adjust pH), Purified Water. pH range between 7.0 and 7.8.
Each gram of ointment contains: **Active:** Sulfacetamide Sodium 10% (100 mg). **Preservatives:** Methylparaben 0.05%, Propylparaben 0.01%. **Inactive:** White Petrolatum, Anhydrous Liquid Lanolin, Mineral Oil.
Clinical Pharmacology: Microbiology: The sulfonamides are bacteriostatic agents and the spectrum of activity is similar for all. Sulfona-

Continued on next page

Alcon—Cont.

mides inhibit bacterial synthesis of dihydrofolic acid by preventing the condensation of the pteridine with aminobenzoic acid through competitive inhibition of the enzyme dihydropteroate synthetase. Resistant strains have altered dihydropteroate synthetase with reduced affinity for sulfonamides or produce increased quantities of aminobenzoic acid. Topically applied sulfonamides are considered active against susceptible strains of the following common bacterial eye pathogens: *Escherichia coli, Staphylococcus aureus, Streptococcus pneumoniae, Streptococcus* (viridans group), *Haemophilus influenzae, Klebsiella* species, and *Enterobacter* species. Topically applied sulfonamides do not provide adequate coverage against *Neisseria* species, *Serratia marcescens* and *Pseudomonoas aeruginosa.* A significant percentage of Staphylococcai isolates are completely resistant to sulfa drugs.

Indications and Usage: Solution: For the treatment of conjunctivitis and other superficial ocular infections due to susceptible microorganisms and as an adjunctive in systemic sulfonamide therapy of trachoma: *Escherichia coli, Staphylococcus aureaus, Streptococcus pneumoniae, Streptococcus* (viridans group), *Haemophilus influenzae, Klebsiella* species, and *Enterobacter* species.

Ointment: For the treatment of conjunctivitis and other superficial ocular infections due to susceptible microorganisms. Topically applied sulfonamides do not provide adequate coverage against *Neisseria* species, *Serratia marcescens* and *Pseudomonas aeruginosa.* A significant percentage of staphylococcal isolates are completely resistant to sulfa drugs.

Contraindications: Hypersensitivity to sulfonamides or to any ingredient of the preparation.

Warnings: FOR TOPICAL EYE USE ONLY—NOT FOR INJECTION. FATALITIES HAVE OCCURRED, ALTHOUGH RARELY, DUE TO SEVERE REACTIONS TO SULFONAMIDES INCLUDES STEVENS-JOHNSON SYNDROME, TOXIC EPIDERMAL NECROLYSIS, FULMINANT HEPATIC NECROSIS, AGRANULOCYTOSIS, APLASTIC ANEMIA AND OTHER BLOOD DYSCRASIAS. Sensitizations may recur when a sulfonamide is readministered, irrespective of the route of administration. Sensitivity reactions have been reported in individuals with no prior history of sulfonamide hypersensitivity. At the first sign of hypersensitivity, skin rash or other serious reaction, discontinue use of this preparation.

Precautions: General: Prolonged use of topical anti-bacterial agents may give rise to overgrowth of nonsusceptible organisms including fungi. Bacterial resistance to sulfonamides may also develop. Ophthalmic ointments may retard corneal wound healing. The effectiveness of sulfonamides may be reduced by the para-aminobenzoic acid present in purulent exudates. Sensitization may recur when a sulfonamide is readministered irrespective of the route of administration, and cross-sensitivity between different sulfonamides may occur. At the first sign of hypersensitivity, increase in purulent discharge, or aggravation of inflammation or pain, the patient should discontinue use of the medication and consult a physician (see WARNINGS).

Information for patients: To avoid contamination, do not touch tip of container to eye, eyelid or any surface.

Drug Interactions: Sulfacetamide preparations are incompatible with silver preparations.

Carcinogenesis, Mutagenesis, Impairment of Fertility: No studies have been conducted in animals or in humans to evaluate the possibility of these effects with ocularly administered sulfacetamide. Rats appear to be especially susceptible to the goitrogenic effects of sulfonamides, and long-term oral administration of sulfonamides has resulted in thyroid malignancies in these animals.

Pregnancy: Pregnancy Category C. Animal reproduction studies have not been conducted with sulfonamide ophthalmic preparations. Kernicterus may occur in the newborn as a result of treatment of a pregnant woman at term with orally administered sulfonamides. There are no adequate and well controlled studies of sulfonamide ophthalmic preparations in pregnant women and it is not known whether topically applied sulfonamides can cause fetal harm when administered to a pregnant woman. This product should be used in pregnancy only if the potential benefit justifies the potential risk to the fetus.

Nursing Mothers: Systemically administered sulfonamides are capable of producing kernicterus in infants of lactating women. Because of the potential for the development of kernicterus in neonates, a decision should be made whether to discontinue nursing or discontinue the drug taking into account the importance of the drug to the mother.

Pediatric Use: Safety and effectiveness in children below the age of two months have not been established.

Adverse Reactions: Bacterial and fungal corneal ulcers have developed during treatment with sulfonamide ophthalmic preparations. The most frequently reported reactions are local irritation, stinging and burning. Less commonly reported reactions include non-specific conjunctivitis, conjunctival hyperemia, secondary infections and allergic reactions. Fatalities have occurred, although rarely, due to severe reactions to sulfonamides including Stevens-Johnson syndrome, toxic epidermal necrolysis, fulminant hepatic necrosis, agranulocytosis, aplastic anemia, and other blood dyscrasias (see WARNINGS).

Dosage and Administration: For conjunctivitis and other superficial ocular infections:
Solution: Instill one or two drops into the conjunctival sac(s) of the affected eye(s) every two to three hours initially. Dosages may be tapered by increasing the time interval between doses as the condition responds. The usual duration of treatment is seven to ten days.
Ointment: Apply a small amount (approximately one-half inch ribbon) into the conjunctival sac(s) of the affected eye(s) every three to four hours and at bedtime. Dosages may be tapered by increasing the time interval between doses as the condition responds. The ointment may be used as adjunct to the solution. The usual duration of treatment is seven to ten days.

How to apply CETAMIDE™ Ointment:
1. Tilt your head back.
2. Place a finger on your cheek just under your eye and gently pull down until a "V" pocket is formed between your eyeball and your lower lid.
3. Place a small amount (about ½ inch) of CETAMIDE™ Ointment in the "V" pocket. Do not let the tip of the tube touch your eye.
4. Look downward before closing your eye.

For Trachoma:
Solution: Instill two drops into the conjunctival sac(s) of the affected eye(s) every two hours. Topical administration must be accompanied by systemic administration.

How Supplied: Solution in 5mL and 15mL plastic DROP-TAINER® Dispensers.
Ointment in 3.5g ophthalmic tubes.
5 mL solution—NDC 0998-0522-05
15 mL solution—NDC 0998-0522-15
3.5 g ointment—NDC 0065-0526-35

Storage: Solution—Store at 8°–24°C (46°–75°F). Protect from light. Do not use if solution is discolored (dark brown). Sulfonamide solutions, on long standing, will darken in color and should be discarded.
Ointment—Store at 8°–27°C (46°–80°F).

Caution: Federal (USA) law prohibits dispensing without prescription.

ISOPTO® CETAPRED® ℞
(Sulfacetamide Sodium and Prednisolone Acetate Ophthalmic Suspension USP) 10%/0.25%

CETAPRED® ℞
(Sulfacetamide Sodium and Prednisolone Acetate Ophthalmic Ointment USP) 10%/0.25%

Description: Isopto® Cetapred® (sulfacetamide sodium and prednisolone acetate ophthalmic suspension) and **Cetapred®** (sulfacetamide sodium and prednisolone acetate ophthalmic ointment) are sterile topical ophthalmic suspension/ointment combining an antibacterial and a corticosteroid which have the following composition:

Sulfacetamide Sodium .... 100 mg/mL (g)
(bacteriostatic antibacterial)
Prednisolone Acetate ....2.5 mg/mL (g)
(corticosteroid/anti-inflammatory)

The chemical name for sulfacetamide sodium is *N*-sulfanilylacetamide monosodium salt monohydrate. The chemical name for prednisolone acetate is 11β,17,21-trihydroxypregna-1, 4-diene-3, 20-dione, 21-acetate. They have the following structural formulas:

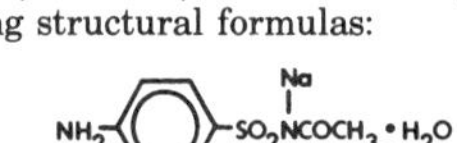

Sulfacetamide Sodium
MW=254.24 $C_8H_9N_2NaO_3S \cdot H_2O$

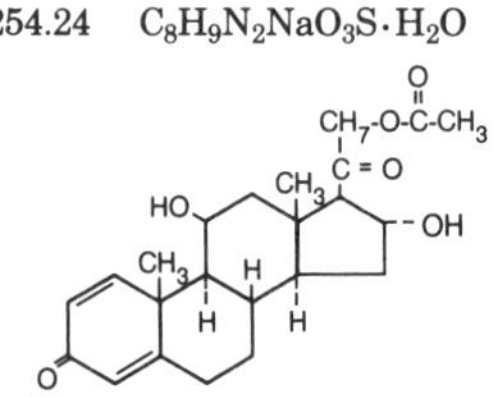

Prednisolone Acetate
MW=402.49 $C_{23}H_{30}O_6$

Each mL of suspension contains: Active: Sulfacetamide Sodium 100mg (10%), Prednisolone Acetate 2.5mg (0.25%). **Preservatives:** Benzalkonium Chloride 0.025%, Methylparaben 0.05%, Propylparaben 0.01%. **Vehicle:** 0.5% Hydroxypropyl Methylcellulose 2910. **Inactive:** Dibasic Sodium Phosphate, Monobasic Sodium Phosphate, Sodium Thiosulfate, Polysorbate 80, Edetate Disodium, HCl and/or NaOH to adjust pH, (6.6 to 7.4) Purified Water.

Each gram of ointment contains: Active: Sulfacetamide Sodium 100mg (10%), Prednisolone Acetate 2.5mg (0.25%). **Preservatives:** Methylparaben 0.05%, Propylparaben 0.01%. **Inactive:** White Petrolatum, Lanolin Oil, Mineral Oil.

Clinical Pharmacology: Corticosteroids suppress the inflammatory response to a variety of agents and they probably delay or slow healing. Since corticosteroids may inhibit the body's defense mechanism against infection, a concomitant antibacterial drug may be used when this inhibition is considered to be clinically significant in a particular case.
When a decision to administer both a corticosteroid and an antibacterial is made, the administration of such drugs in combination has the advantage of greater patient compliance and convenience, with the added assurance that the appropriate dosage of both drugs is administered, plus assured compatibility of

ingredients when both types of drugs are in the same formulation and, particularly, that the correct volume of drug is delivered and retained.

The relative potency of corticosteroids depends on the molecular structure, concentration and release from the vehicle.

Microbiology: Sulfacetamide exerts a bacteriostatic effect against susceptible bacteria by restricting the synthesis of folic acid required for growth through competition with p-aminobenzoic acid. Some strains of these bacteria may be resistant to sulfacetamide or resistant strains may emerge *in vivo.*

The anti-infective component in these products is included to provide action against specific organisms susceptible to it. Sulfacetamide sodium is active *in vitro* against susceptible strains of the following microorganisms: *Escherichia coli, Staphylococcus aureus, Streptococcus pneumoniae, Streptococcus* (viridans group), *Haemophilus influenzae, Klebsiella* species, and *Enterobacter* species. These products do not provide adequate coverage against: *Neisseria* species, *Pseudomonas* species, *Serratia marcescens.* (See **INDICATIONS AND USAGE**).

Indications and Usage: Sulfacetamide sodium and prednisolone acetate ophthalmic suspension/ointment is indicated for steroid-responsive inflammatory ocular conditions for which a corticosteroid is indicated and where superficial bacterial ocular infection or a risk of bacterial ocular infection exists.

Ocular corticosteroids are indicated in inflammatory conditions of the palpebral and bulbar conjunctiva, cornea, and anterior segment of the globe where the inherent risk of corticosteroid use in certain infective conjunctivitides is accepted to obtain a diminution in edema and inflammation. They are also indicated in chronic anterior uveitis and corneal injury from chemical, radiation or thermal burns or penetration of foreign bodies.

The use of a combination drug with an anti-infective component is indicated where the risk of superficial ocular infection is high or where there is an expectation that potentially dangerous numbers of bacteria will be present in the eye.

The particular antibacterial drug in this product is active against the following common bacterial eye pathogens: *Escherichia coli, Staphylococcus aureus, Streptococcus pneumoniae, Streptococcus (viridans* group), *Haemophilus influenzae, Klebsiella* species, and *Enterobacter* species.

The product does not provide adequate coverage against: *Neisseria* species, *Pseudomonas* species, and *Serratia marcescens.* A significant percentage of *staphylococcal* isolates are completely resistant to sulfa drugs.

Contraindications: Sulfacetamide sodium and prednisolone acetate ophthalmic suspension/ointment is contraindicated in most viral diseases of the cornea and conjunctiva including epithelial herpes simplex keratitis (dendritic keratitis), vaccinia, varicella, and also in mycobacterial infection of the eye and fungal diseases of ocular structures. This product is also contraindicated in individuals with known or suspected hypersensitivity to any of the ingredients of this preparation, to other sulfonamides and to other corticosteroids. **SEE WARNINGS.** (Hypersensitivity to the antimicrobial component occurs at a higher rate than for other components.)

Warnings: NOT FOR INJECTION INTO THE EYE. Prolonged use of corticosteroids may result in ocular hypertension/glaucoma with damage to the optic nerve, defects in visual acuity and fields of vision, and in posterior subcapsular cataract formation. Acute anterior uveitis may occur in susceptible individuals, primarily Blacks. Prolonged use of sulfacetamide soidum and prednisolone acetate ophthalmic suspension/ointment may suppress the host response and thus increase the hazard of secondary ocular infections. In those diseases causing thinning of the cornea or sclera, perforation has been known to occur with the use of topical corticosteroids. In acute purulent conditions of the eye, corticosteroids may mask infection or enhance existing infection. If the product is used for 10 days or longer, intraocular pressure should be routinely monitored even though it may be difficult in children and uncooperative patients. Corticosteroids should be used with caution in the presence of glaucoma. Intraocular pressure should be checked frequently. A significant percentage of staphylococcal isolates are completely resistant to sulfonamides. The use of steroids after cataract surgery may delay healing and increase the incidence of filtering blebs. The use of ocular corticosteroids may prolong the course and may exacerbate the severity of many viral infections of the eye (including herpes simplex).

Employment of corticosteroid medication in the treatment of herpes simplex requires great caution.

Topical steroids are not effective in mustard gas keratitis and Sjögren's kerato-conjunctivitis. Fatalities have occurred, although rarely, due to severe reactions to sulfonamides including Stevens-Johnson syndrome, toxic epidermal necrolysis, fulminant hepatic necrosis, agranulocytosis, aplastic anemia and other blood dyscrasias. Sensitizations may recur when a sulfonamide is readministered, irrespective of the route of administration. If signs of hypersensitivity or other serious reactions occur, discontinue use of this preparation. Cross-sensitivity among corticosteroids has been demonstrated (see **ADVERSE REACTIONS**).

Precautions: General: The initial prescription and renewal of the medication order beyond 8 g of ointment or 20 mL of suspension should be made by a physician only after examination of the patient with the aid of magnification, such as slit-lamp biomicroscopy and, where appropriate fluorescein staining. If signs and symptoms fail to improve after two days, the patient should be revaluated.

The possibility of fungal infections of the cornea should be considered after prolonged corticosteroid dosing. Use with caution in patients with severe dry eye. Fungal cultures should be taken when appropriate. The p-aminobenzoic acid present in purulent exudates competes with sulfonamides and can reduce their effectiveness. Ophthalmic ointments may retard corneal healing.

Information for Patients: If inflammation or pain persists longer than 48 hours or becomes aggravated, the patient should be advised to discontinue use of medication and consult a physician (See **WARNINGS**).

The product is sterile when packaged. To prevent contamination, care should be taken to avoid touching the dropper/tube tip to eyelids or to any other surface. The use of this dropper bottle/tube by more than one person may spread infection. Keep bottle/tube tightly closed when not in use. Protect from light. Sulfonamide solutions darken on prolonged standing and exposure to heat and light. Do not use if solution has darkened. Yellowing does not affect activity. Keep out of reach of children.

Laboratory Tests: Eyelid cultures and tests to determine the susceptibility of organisms to sulfacetamide may be indicated if signs and symptoms persist or recur in spite of the recommended course of treatment with sulfacetamide sodium and prednisolone acetate ophthalmic suspension/ointment.

Drug Interactions: Sulfacetamide sodium and prednisolone acetate ophthalmic suspension/ointment is incompatible with silver preparations. Local anesthetics related to p-aminobenzoic acid may antagonize the action of the sulfonamides.

Carcinogenesis, Mutagenesis, Impairment of Fertility: Prednisolone has been reported to be noncarcinogenic. Long-term animal studies for carcinogenic potential have not been performed with sulfacetamide. One author detected chromosomal nondisjunction in the yeast *Saccharomyces cerevisiae* following application of sulfacetamide sodium. The significance of this finding to topical ophthalmic use of sulfacetamide sodium in the human is unknown. Mutagenic studies with prednisolone have been negative. Studies on reproduction and fertility have not been performed with sulfacetamide. A long-term chronic toxicity study in dogs showed that high oral doses of prednisolone prevented estrus. A decrease in fertility was seen in male and female rats that were mated following oral dosing with another glucocorticosteroid.

Pregnancy: ***Teratogenic effects:*** Pregnancy Category C: Animal reproduction studies have not been conducted with sulfacetamide sodium. Prednisolone has been shown to be teratogenic in rabbits, hamsters, and mice. In mice, prednisolone has been shown to be teratogenic when given in doses 1 to 10 times the human ocular dose. Dexamethasone, hydrocortisone and prednisolone were ocularly applied to both eyes of pregnant mice five times per day on days 10 through 13 of gestation. A significant increase in the incidence of cleft palate was observed in the fetuses of the treated mice. There are no adequate well-controlled studies in pregnant women dosed with corticosteroids. Kernicterus may be precipitated in infants by sulfonamides being given systemically during the third trimester of pregnancy. It is not known whether sulfacetamide sodium can cause fetal harm when administered to a pregnant woman or whether it can affect reproductive capacity. Sulfacetamide sodium and prednisolone acetate ophthalmic suspension/ointment should be used during pregnancy only if the potential benefit justifies the potential risk to the fetus.

Nursing Mothers: It is not known whether topical administration of corticosteroids could result in sufficient systemic absorption to produce detectable quantities in human breast milk. Systemically administered corticosteroids appear in human breast milk and could suppress growth, interfere with endogenous corticosteroid production, or cause other untoward effects. Systemically administered sufonamides are capable of producing kernicterus in infants of lactating women. Because of the potential for serious adverse reactions in nursing infants from sulfacetamide sodium and prednisolone acetate ophthalmic suspension/ointment, a decision should be made whether to discontinue nursing or to discontinue the medication.

Pediatric Use: Safety and effectiveness in children below the age of six have not been established.

Adverse Reactions: Adverse reactions have occurred with corticosteroid/antibacterial combination drugs which can be attributed to the corticosteroid component, the antibacterial component, or the combination. Exact incidence figures are not available since no denominator of treated patients is available.

Reactions occurring most often from the presence of the antibacterial ingredient are allergic sensitizations. Fatalities have occurred, although rarely, due to severe reactions to sulfonamides including Stevens-Johnson syndrome, toxic epidermal necrolysis, fulminant hepatic necrosis, agranulocytosis, aplastic anemia, and other blood dyscrasias (See **WARNINGS**). Sulfacetamide sodium may cause local irritation. The reactions due to the corticoste-

Continued on next page

Alcon—Cont.

roid component in decreasing order of frequency are: elevation of intraocular pressure (IOP) with possible development of glaucoma and infrequent optic nerve damage; posterior subcapsular cataract formation; and delayed wound healing. Although systemic effects are extremely uncommon, there have been rare occurrences of systemic hypercorticoidism after use of topical steroids. Corticosteroid-containing preparations can also cause acute interior uveitis or perforation of the globe. Mydriasis, loss of accommodation and ptosis have occasionally been reported following local use of corticosteroids.

Secondary infection: The development of secondary infection has occurred after use of combinations containing corticosteroids and antibacterials. Fungal and viral infections of the cornea are particularly prone to develop coincidentally with long-term applications of corticosteroid. The possibility of fungal invasion must be considered in any persistent corneal ulceration where corticosteroid treatment has been used. Secondary bacterial ocular infection following suppression of host responses also occurs.

Dosage and Administration: Sulfacetamide sodium and prednisolone acetate ophthalmic suspension: SHAKE WELL BEFORE USING. Instill two drops topically in the eye(s) every four hours. Not more than 20 mL should be prescribed initially.

Sulfacetamide sodium and prednisolone acetate ophthalmic ointment: A small amount, approximately ½ inch ribbon of ointment, should be applied in the conjunctival sac three or four times daily and once or twice at night. Not more than 8 g should be prescribed initially. The dosing of sulfacetamide sodium and prednisolone acetate ophthalmic suspension/ointment may be reduced, but care should be taken not to discontinue therapy prematurely. In chronic conditions, withdrawal of treatment should be carried out by gradually decreasing the frequency of application. If signs and symptoms fail to improve after two days, the patient should be re-evaluated. (see **PRECAUTIONS**).

How Supplied: Isopto® Cetapred® sulfacetamide sodium and prednisolone acetate ophthalmic suspension USP, 10%/0.25%; 5 mL and 15 mL in plastic **DROP-TAINER®** dispensers.

Cetapred® sulfacetamide sodium and prednisolone acetate ophthalmic ointment USP, 10%/0.25%; 3.5 g in ophthalmic tubes.

5 mL	suspension—	NDC 0998-0613-05
15 mL	suspension—	NDC 0998-0613-15
3.5 g	ointment—	NDC 0065-0607-35

Storage: Store **ISOPTO CETAPRED** Suspension upright away from heat at 8°–24°C (46°–75°F) as clumping may occur on long standing at high temperatures. Store **CETAPRED** Ointment at controlled room temperature 15°–30°C (59°–86°F).

Caution: Federal (USA) law prohibits dispensing without prescription.

ISOPTO® HOMATROPINE ℞

(homatropine hydrobromide)
Sterile Ophthalmic Solution

Description: ISOPTO® HOMATROPINE (homatropine hydrobromide) is an anticholinergic prepared as a sterile topical ophthalmic solution supplied in two strengths. The active ingredient is represented by the chemical structure:

[See chemical structure at top of next column.]

Established name:
Homatropine Hydrobromide

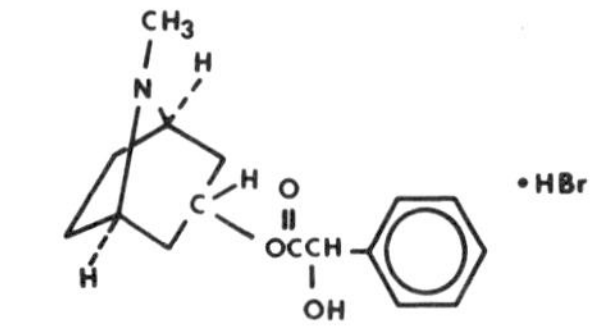

Chemical name:
Benzeneacetic acid, α-hydroxy-, 8-methyl-8-azabicyclo[3.2.1]-oct-3-yl ester, hydrobromide, *endo*-(±)-.

Each mL contains: Active: Homatropine Hydrobromide 2.0% or 5.0%. Preservatives: Benzalkonium Chloride 0.01% in 2% strength, Benzethonium Chloride 0.005% in 5% strength. Vehicle: Hydroxypropyl Methylcellulose 0.5%. Inactive: Sodium Chloride, Polysorbate 80 (in 2% strength), Sodium Hydroxide and/or Hydrochloric Acid (to adjust pH), Purified Water.

Clinical Pharmacology: This anticholinergic preparation blocks the responses of the sphincter muscle of the iris and the accommodative muscle of the ciliary body to cholinergic stimulation, producing pupillary dilation (mydriasis) and paralysis of accommodation (cycloplegia).

Indications and Usage: A moderately long-acting mydriatic and cycloplegic for cycloplegic refraction and in the treatment of inflammatory conditions of the uveal tract. For pre- and postoperative states when mydriasis is required. Use as an optical aid in some cases of axial lens opacities.

Contraindications: Contraindicated in persons with primary glaucoma or a tendency toward glaucoma, e.g., narrow anterior chamber angle, and in those persons showing hypersensitivity to any component of this preparation.

Warnings: For topical use only—not for injection. Risk-benefit should be considered when the following medical problems exist: keratoconus (homatropine may produce fixed dilated pupil); Down's syndrome, children with brain damage and the elderly (increased susceptibility). In infants and small children, use with extreme caution.

Precautions: General. To avoid excessive systemic absorption, the lacrimal sac should be compressed by digital pressure for two to three minutes after instillation. To avoid inducing angle closure glaucoma, an estimation of the depth of the angle of the anterior chamber should be made. Excessive topical use of this drug can potentially lead to a confusional state characterized by delirium, agitation, and rarely coma. This state is more apt to occur in the pediatric and geriatric age groups. The specific anti-dote for this systemic anticholinergic syndrome is injectable physostigmine salicylate.

Information for Patients. Patient should be advised not to drive or engage in other hazardous activities while pupils are dilated. Patient may experience sensitivity to light and should protect eyes in bright illumination during dilation. Parents should be warned not to get this preparation in their child's mouth and to wash their own hands and the child's hands following administration. Do not touch dropper tip to any surface, as this may contaminate the solution.

Carcinogenesis, Mutagenesis, Impairment of Fertility. There have been no long-term studies done using homatropine hydrobromide in animals to evaluate carcinogenic potential.

Pregnancy. Pregnancy Category C. Animal reproduction studies have not been conducted with homatropine hydrobromide. It is also not known whether homatropine hydrobromide can cause fetal harm when administered to a pregnant woman or can affect reproduction capacity. Homatropine hydrobromide should be given to a pregnant woman only if clearly needed.

Nursing Mothers. It is not known whether this drug is excreted in human milk. Because many drugs are excreted in human milk, caution should be exercised when homatropine hydrobromide is administered to a nursing woman.

Adverse Reactions: Transient symptoms of stinging and burning may occur. Prolonged use may produce local irritation characterized by follicular conjunctivitis, vascular congestion, edema, exudate, and an eczematoid dermatitis. Thirst or dryness of mouth, eye irritation not present before therapy, or increased sensitivity of eyes to light may occur.

Dosage and Administration: For refraction, instill one or two drops topically in the eye(s). May be repeated in five to ten minutes if necessary. For uveitis, instill one or two drops topically up to every three to four hours. Individuals with heavily pigmented irides may require larger doses. Only the 2% strength should be used in pediatric patients.

How Supplied: In 5mL and 15mL plastic DROP-TAINER® dispensers.
2% ISOPTO® HOMATROPINE
5mL NDC 0998-0311-05
15mL NDC 0998-0311-15
5% ISOPTO® HOMATROPINE
5mL NDC 0998-0315-05
15mL NDC 0998-0315-15

Storage: Store at 8°–24°C (46°–75°F).

Caution: Federal (USA) law prohibits dispensing without prescription.

ISOPTO® HYOSCINE ℞

(scopolamine hydrobromide)
Sterile Ophthalmic Solution

Description: ISOPTO® HYOSCINE (Scopolamine Hydrobromide) is an anticholinergic prepared as a sterile topical ophthalmic solution. The active ingredient is represented by the chemical structure:

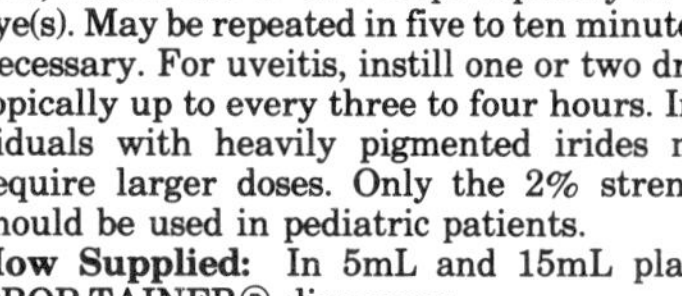

Established name:
Scopolamine Hydrobromide

Chemical name:
Benzeneacetic acid, α-(hydroxymethyl)-, 9-methyl-3-oxa-9-azatricyclo[3.3.1.0^{2,4}]non-7-yl ester, hydrobromide, trihydrate, [7(*S*)-(1α,2β,4β,5α,7β)]-.

Each mL contains: Active: Scopolamine Hydrobromide 0.25%. Preservative: Benzalkonium Chloride 0.01%. Vehicle: Hydroxypropyl Methylcellulose 0.5%. Inactive: Sodium Chloride, Glacial Acetic Acid, Sodium Acetate (to adjust pH), Purified Water.

Clinical Pharmacology: This anticholinergic preparation blocks the responses of the sphincter muscle of the iris and the accommodative muscle of the ciliary body to cholinergic stimulation, producing pupillary dilation (mydriasis) and paralysis of accommodation (cycloplegia).

Indications and Usage: For mydriasis and cycloplegia in diagnostic procedures. For some pre- and postoperative states when a mydriatic and cycloplegic is needed in the treatment of iridocyclitis.

Contraindications: Contraindicated in persons with primary glaucoma or a tendency toward glaucoma, e.g., narrow anterior chamber angle; and in those showing hypersensitivity to any component of this preparation.

Warnings: Do not touch dropper tip to any surface, as this may contaminate the solution. For topical use only—not for injection. In infants and small children, use with extreme caution.
Precautions: To avoid excessive absorption, the lacrimal sac should be compressed by digital pressure for two to three minutes after instillation. To avoid inducing angle closure glaucoma, an estimation of the depth of the angle of the anterior chamber should be made.
Patient Warning: Patient should be advised not to drive or engage in other hazardous activities when drowsy or while pupils are dilated. Patient may experience sensitivity to light and should protect eyes in bright illumination during dilation. Parents should be warned not to get this preparation in their child's mouth and to wash their own hands and the child's hands following administration.
Adverse Reactions: Prolonged use may produce local irritation, characterized by follicular conjunctivitis, vascular congestion, edema, exudate, and an eczematoid dermatitis. Somnolence, dryness of the mouth, or visual hallucinations may occur.
Dosage and Administration: For refraction, administer one or two drops topically in the eye(s) one hour before refracting. For uveitis, administer one or two drops topically in the eye(s) up to four times daily.
How Supplied: In 5 mL and 15mL plastic DROP-TAINER® dispensers.
5mL NDC 0998-0331-05
15mL NDC 0998-0331-15
Storage: Store at 46° to 80°F. Protect from light.

MAXIDEX® ℞
(dexamethasone sodium phosphate Ophthalmic Ointment, USP)
0.05% Dexamethasone Phosphate Equivalent
Sterile

Description: Dexamethasone Sodium Phosphate is 9-fluoro-11β, 17-dihydroxy-16α-methyl -21- (phosphonooxy)pregna -1,4 - diene-3,20-dione disodium salt. Its molecular formula is $C_{22}H_{28}FNa_2O_8P$ and its structural formula is:

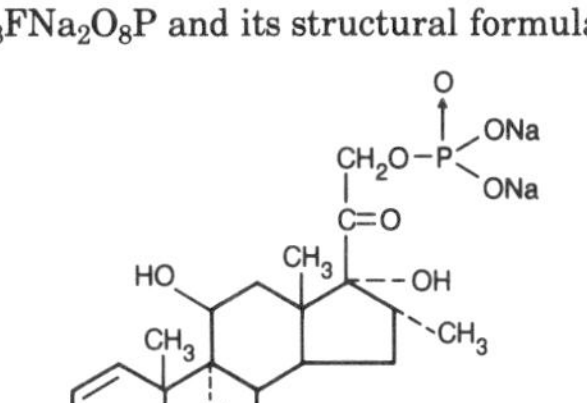

Glucocorticoids are adrenocortical steroids, both naturally occurring and synthetic. Dexamethasone is a synthetic analog of naturally occurring glucocorticoids (hydrocortisone and cortisone). Dexamethasone sodium phosphate is a water soluble, inorganic ester of dexamethasone. Its molecular weight is 516.41.
Sterile MAXIDEX (Dexamethasone Sodium Phosphate Ophthalmic Ointment, USP) is a topical steroid ointment containing dexamethasone sodium phosphate equivalent to 0.5 mg (0.05%) dexamethasone phosphate in each gram. Inactive ingredients: white petrolatum and mineral oil.
Clinical Pharmacology: Dexamethasone sodium phosphate suppresses the inflammatory response to a variety of agents and it probably delays or slows healing. No generally accepted explanation of these steroid properties has been advanced.
Indications and Usage: For the treatment of the following conditions: Steroid responsive inflammatory conditions of the palpebral and bulbar conjunctiva, cornea, and anterior segment of the globe, such as allergic conjunctivitis, acne rosacea, superficial punctate keratitis, herpes zoster keratitis, iritis, cyclitis, selected infective conjunctivitises when the inherent hazard of steroid use is accepted to obtain an advisable diminution in edema and inflammation; corneal injury from chemical or thermal burns, or penetration of foreign bodies.
Contraindications: Epithelial herpes simplex keratitis (dendritic keratitis). Acute infectious stages of vaccinia, varicella and many other viral diseases of the cornea and conjunctiva. Mycobacterial infection of the eye. Fungal disease of ocular structures. Hypersensitivity to a component of the preparation.
Warnings: Prolonged use may result in ocular hypertension and/or glaucoma, with damage to the optic nerve, defects in visual acuity and fields of vision, and posterior subcapsular cataract formation. Prolonged use may suppress the host response and thus increase the hazard of secondary ocular infections. In those diseases causing thinning of the cornea or sclera, perforations have been known to occur with the use of topical corticosteroids. In acute purulent conditions of the eye, corticosteroids may mask infection or enhance existing infection. If these products are used for 10 days or longer, intraocular pressure should be routinely monitored even though it may be difficult in children and uncooperative patients. Employment of corticosteroid medication in the treatment of herpes simplex other than epithelial herpes simplex keratitis, in which it is contraindicated, requires great caution; periodic slit-lamp microscopy is essential.
Precautions:
General:
The possibility of persistent fungal infections of the cornea should be considered after prolonged corticosteroid dosing.
There have been reports of bacterial keratitis associated with the use of multiple dose containers of topical ophthalmic products. These containers had been inadvertently contaminated by patients who, in most cases, had a concurrent corneal disease or a disruption of the ocular epithelial surface.
(See PRECAUTIONS, *Information for Patients.*)
Information for Patients: Patients should be instructed to avoid allowing the tip of the dispensing container to contact the eye or surrounding structures.
Patients should also be instructed that ocular preparations, if handled improperly, can become contaminated by common bacteria known to cause ocular infections. Serious damage to the eye and subsequent loss of vision may result from using contaminated preparations. (See PRECAUTIONS, *General.*)
Patients should also be advised that if they develop an intercurrent ocular condition (e.g., trauma, ocular surgery or infection), they should immediately seek their physician's advice concerning the continued use of the present multi-dose container.
Carcinogenesis, Mutagenesis, Impairment of Fertility: Long-term animal studies have not been performed to evaluate the carcinogenic potential or the effect on fertility of MAXIDEX® (Dexamethasone Sodium Phosphate Ophthalmic Ointment, USP).
Pregnancy: Pregnancy Category C. Dexamethasone has been shown to be teratogenic in mice and rabbits following topical ophthalmic application in multiples of the therapeutic dose. In the mouse, corticosteroids produce fetal resorptions and a specific abnormality, cleft palate. In the rabbit, corticosteroids have produced fetal resorptions and multiple abnormalities involving the head, ears, limbs, palate, etc. There are no adequate or well-controlled studies in pregnant women. MAXIDEX (Dexamethasone Sodium Phosphate Ophthalmic Ointment, USP) should be used during pregnancy only if the potential benefit to the mother justifies the potential risk to the embryo or fetus. Infants born of mothers who have received substantial doses of corticosteroids during pregnancy should be observed carefully for signs of hypoadrenalism.
Nursing Mothers: Topically applied steroids are absorbed systemically. Therefore, because of the potential for serious adverse reactions in nursing infants from dexamethasone sodium phosphate, a decision should be made whether to discontinue nursing or discontinue the drug, taking into account the importance of the drug to the mother.
Pediatric Use: Safety and effectiveness in children have not been established.
Adverse Reactions: Glaucoma with optic nerve damage, visual acuity and field defects, posterior subcapsular cataract formation, secondary ocular infections from pathogens including herpes simplex, and perforation of the globe. Rarely, filtering blebs have been reported when topical steroids have been used following cataract surgery. Rarely, stinging or burning may occur.
Dosage and Administration: The duration of treatment will vary with the type of lesion and may extend from a few days to several weeks, according to therapeutic response. Relapses, more common in chronic active lesions than in self-limited conditions, usually respond to retreatment.
Apply a thin coating of ointment three or four times a day. When a favorable response is observed, reduce the number of daily applications to two, and later to one a day as a maintenance dose if this is sufficient to control symptoms.
MAXIDEX® (Dexamethasone Sodium Phosphate Ophthalmic Ointment, USP) is particulaly convenient when an eye pad is used. It may also be the preparation of choice for patients in whom therapeutic benefit depends on prolonged contact of the active ingredients with ocular tissues.
How To Apply MAXIDEX® OINTMENT:
1. Tilt your head back.
2. Place a finger on your cheek just under your eye and gently pull down until a "V" pocket is formed between your eyeball and your lower lid.
3. Place a small amount (about ½ inch) of MAXIDEX® in the "V" pocket. Do not let the tip of the tube touch your eye.
4. Look downward before closing your eye.

How Supplied: MAXIDEX (Dexamethasone Sodium Phosphate Ophthalmic Ointment, USP) 0.05% Dexamethasone Phosphate Equivalent is a clear unctuous ointment and is supplied as follows:
NDC 0065-0616-35 in 3.5 g ophthalmic tubes (6505-00-961-5508, 0.05% 3.5g).
Storage: Store at 8°–27°C (46° to 80°F).
Caution: Federal (USA) law prohibits dispensing without prescription.

MAXIDEX® ℞
(dexamethasone 0.1%)
Sterile Ophthalmic Suspension

Description: MAXIDEX® (dexamethasone 0.1%) is an adrenocortical steroid prepared as a sterile topical ophthalmic suspension. The active ingredient is represented by the chemical structure:
[See chemical structure at top of next column.]
Established name:
Dexamethasone
Chemical name:
Pregna-1,4-diene-3,20-dione, 9-fluoro-11,17,21-trihydroxy-16-methyl-, (11β,16α)-.

Continued on next page

Alcon—Cont.

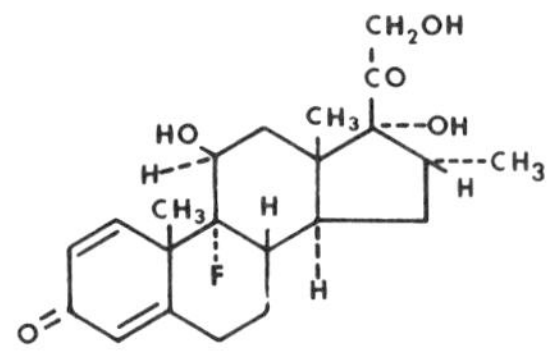

Each mL contains: **Active:** Dexamethasone 0.1%. **Preservative:** Benzalkonium Chloride 0.01%. **Vehicle:** Hydroxypropyl Methylcellulose 0.5%. **Inactive:** Sodium Chloride, Dibasic Sodium Phosphate, Polysorbate 80, Edetate Disodium, Citric Acid and/or Sodium Hydroxide (to adjust pH), Purified Water.

Clinical Pharmacology: Dexamethasone suppresses the inflammatory response to a variety of agents and it probably delays or slows healing. No generally accepted explanation of these steroid properties has been advanced.

Indications and Usage: Steroid responsive inflammatory conditions of the palpebral and bulbar conjunctiva, cornea, and anterior segment of the globe such as allergic conjunctivitis, acne rosacea, superficial punctate keratitis, herpes zoster keratitis, iritis, cyclitis, selected infective conjunctivitides when the inherent hazard of steroid use is accepted to obtain an advisable dimunition in edema and inflammation; corneal injury from chemical, radiation or thermal burns, or penetration of foreign bodies.

Contraindications: Contraindicated in epithelial herpes simplex (dendritic keratitis), vaccinia, varicella, and most other viral diseases of the cornea and conjunctiva; tuberculosis of the eye; fungal disease of ocular structures; and in those persons who have shown hypersensitivity to any component of this preparation. Steroids should not be used after uncomplicated removal of a corneal foreign body.

Warnings: Prolonged use may result in ocular hypertension and/or glaucoma, with damage to the optic nerve, defects in visual acuity and fields of vision, and posterior subcapsular cataract formation. Prolonged use may suppress the host response and thus increase the hazard of secondary ocular infections. In those diseases causing thinning of the cornea or sclera, perforations have been known to occur with the use of topical corticosteroids. In acute purulent conditions of the eye, corticosteroids may mask infection or enhance existing infection. If these products are used for 10 days or longer, intraocular pressure should be routinely monitored even though it may be difficult in children and uncooperative patients.
Employment of corticosteroid medication in the treatment of herpes simplex other than epithelial herpes simplex keratitis, in which it is contraindicated, requires great caution; periodic slit-lamp microscopy is essential.

Precautions: General. For topical use only. The possibility of persistent fungal infections of the cornea should be considered after prolonged corticosteroid dosing.

Information for Patients. Do not touch dropper tip to any surface, as this may contaminate the contents.

Carcinogenesis, Mutagenesis, Impairment of Fertility. Long-term animal studies have not been performed to evaluate the carcinogenic potential or the effect on fertility of MAXIDEX® Suspension.

Pregnancy. Pregnancy Category C. Dexamethasone has been shown to be teratogenic in mice and rabbits following topical ophthalmic application in multiples of the therapeutic dose.
In the mouse, corticosteroids produce fetal resorptions and a specific abnormality, cleft palate. In the rabbit, corticosteroids have produced fetal resorptions and multiple abnormalities involving the head, ears, limbs, palate, etc.
There are no adequate or well-controlled studies in pregnant women. MAXIDEX Suspension should be used during pregnancy only if the potential benefit to the mother justifies the potential risk to the embryo or fetus. Infants born to mothers who have received substantial doses of corticosteroids during pregnancy should be observed carefully for signs of hypoadrenalism.

Nursing Mothers. Topically applied steroids are absorbed systemically. Therefore, because of the potential for serious adverse reactions in nursing infants from dexamethasone, a decision should be made whether to discontinue nursing or discontinue the drug, taking into account the importance of the drug to the mother.

Pediatric Use. Safety and effectiveness in children have not been established.

Adverse Reactions: Glaucoma with optic nerve damage, visual acuity and field defects; cataract formation; secondary ocular infection following suppression of host response; and perforation of the globe may occur.

Dosage and Administration: SHAKE WELL BEFORE USING. One or two drops topically in the conjunctival sac(s). In severe disease, drops may be used hourly, being tapered to discontinuation as the inflammation subsides. In mild disease, drops may be used up to four to six times daily.

How Supplied: MAXIDEX ophthalmic suspension in plastic DROP-TAINER® dispensers: 5 mL NDC 0998-0615-05, 15 mL NDC 0998-0615-15.

Storage: Store upright at 8°–27°C (46°–80°F).

Caution: Federal (USA) law prohibits dispensing without prescription.

MAXITROL® ℞
(neomycin and polymyxin b sulfates and dexamethasone)
Sterile Ophthalmic
Suspension and Ointment

Description: MAXITROL® (Neomycin and Polymyxin B Sulfates and Dexamethasone) is a multiple dose anti-infective steroid combination in sterile suspension and sterile ointment forms for topical application. The chemical structure for the active ingredient, Dexamethasone, is:

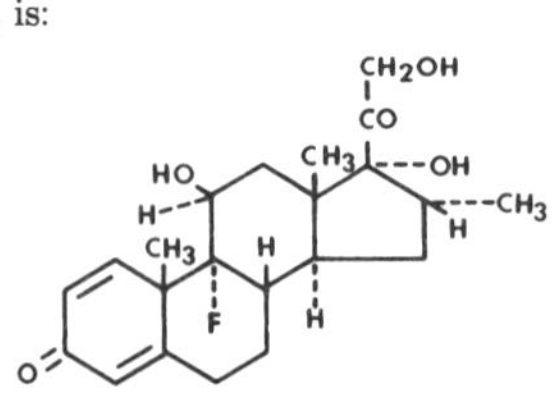

Established name:
Dexamethasone

Chemical name:
Pregna-1,4-diene-3,20-dione, 9-fluoro-11,17,21-trihydroxy-16-methyl-, (11β,16α)-.

The other active ingredients are Neomycin Sulfate and Polymyxin B Sulfate.
Each mL of suspension contains: Active: Neomycin Sulfate equivalent to Neomycin 3.5 mg, Polymyxin B Sulfate 10,000 units, Dexamethasone 0.1%. Preservative: Benzalkonium Chloride 0.004%. Vehicle: Hydroxypropyl Methylcellulose 2910 0.5%. Inactive: Sodium Chloride, Polysorbate 20, Hydrochloric Acid and/or Sodium Hydroxide (to adjust pH), Purified Water.
Each gram of ointment contains: Active: Neomycin Sulfate equivalent to Neomycin 3.5 mg, Polymyxin B Sulfate 10,000 units, Dexamethasone 0.1%. Preservatives: Methylparaben 0.05%, Propylparaben 0.01%. Inactive: White Petrolatum, Anhydrous Liquid Lanolin.

Clinical Pharmacology: Corticoids suppress the inflammatory response to a variety of agents and they probably delay or slow healing. Since corticoids may inhibit the body's defense mechanism against infection, a concomitant antimicrobial drug may be used when this inhibition is considered to be clinically significant in a particular case.
When a decision to administer both a corticoid and an antimicrobial is made, the administration of such drugs in combination has the advantage of greater patient compliance and convenience, with the added assurance that the appropriate dosage of both drugs is administered, plus assured compatibility of ingredients when both types of drugs are in the same formulation and, particularly, that the correct volume of drug is delivered and retained.
The relative potency of corticosteroids depends on the molecular structure, concentration and release from the vehicle.

Indications and Usage: For steroid-responsive inflammatory ocular conditions for which a corticosteroid is indicated and where bacterial infection or a risk of bacterial ocular infection exists.
Ocular steroids are indicated in inflammatory conditions of the palpebral and bulbar conjunctiva, cornea, and anterior segment of the globe where the inherent risk of steroid use in certain infective conjunctivitises is accepted to obtain a diminution in edema and inflammation. They are also indicated in chronic anterior uveitis and corneal injury from chemical, radiation or thermal burns; or penetration of foreign bodies.
The use of a combination drug with an anti-infective component is indicated where the risk of infection is high or where there is an expectation that potentially dangerous numbers of bacteria will be present in the eye.
The particular anti-infective drug in this product is active against the following common bacterial eye pathogens: *Staphylococcus aureus, Escherichia coli, Haemophilus influenzae, Klebsiella/Enterobacter* species, *Neisseria* species, and *Pseudomonas aeruginosa.*
This product does not provide adequate coverage against: *Serratia marcescens* and Streptococci, including *Streptococcus pneumoniae.*

Contraindications: Epithelial herpes simplex keratitis (dendritic keratitis), vaccinia, varicella, and many other viral diseases of the cornea and conjunctiva. Mycobacterial infection of the eye. Fungal diseases of ocular structures. Hypersensitivity to a component of the medication. (Hypersensitivity to the antibiotic component occurs at a higher rate than for other components.)
The use of these combinations is always contraindicated after uncomplicated removal of a corneal foreign body.

Warnings: NOT FOR INJECTION. Do not touch dropper or tube tip to any surface, as this may contaminate the contents. Prolonged use may result in glaucoma, with damage to the optic nerve, defects in visual acuity and fields of vision, and posterior subcapsular cataract formation. Prolonged use may suppress the host response and thus increase the hazard of secondary ocular infections. In those diseases causing thinning of the cornea or sclera, perforations have been known to occur with the use of topical steroids. In acute purulent conditions of the eye, steroids may mask infection or enhance existing infection. If these products are used for 10 days or longer, intraocular pressure should be routinely monitored even though it may be difficult in children and uncooperative patients.

Products containing neomycin sulfate may cause cutaneous sensitization.

Employment of steroid medication in the treatment of herpes simplex requires great caution.

Precautions: The initial prescription and renewal of the medication order beyond 20 mL or 8 g should be made by a physician only after examination of the patient with the aid of magnification, such as slit lamp biomicroscopy and, where appropriate, fluorescein staining.

The possibility of persistent fungal infections of the cornea should be considered after prolonged steroid dosing.

Usage in Pregnancy: The safety of intensive or protracted use of topical steroids in pregnancy has not been studied.

Adverse Reactions: Adverse reactions have occurred with steroid/anti-infective combination drugs which can be attributed to the steroid component, the anti-infective component, or the combination. Exact incidence figures are not available since no denominator of treated patients is available.

Reactions occurring most often from the presence of the anti-infective ingredient are allergic sensitizations. The reactions due to the steroid component are: elevation of intraocular pressure (IOP) with possible development of glaucoma, and infrequent optic nerve damage; posterior subcapsular cataract formation; and delayed wound healing.

Secondary Infection: The development of secondary infection has occurred after use of combinations containing steroids and antimicrobials. Fungal infections of the cornea are particularly prone to develop coincidentally with long-term applications of steroid. The possibility of fungal invasion must be considered in any persistent corneal ulceration where steroid treatment has been used.

Secondary bacterial ocular infection following suppression of host responses also occurs.

Dosage and Administration:

MAXITROL ® Suspension: One to two drops topically in the conjunctival sac(s). In severe disease, drops may be used hourly, being tapered to discontinuation as the inflammation subsides. In mild disease, drops may be used up to four to six times daily. *MAXITROL ® Ointment:* Apply a small amount into the conjunctival sac(s) up to three or four times daily, or may be used adjunctively with drops at bedtime.

How to apply MAXITROL Ointment:

1. Tilt your head back.
2. Place a finger on your cheek just under your eye and gently pull down until a "V" pocket is formed between your eyeball and your lower lid.
3. Place a small amount (about ½ inch) of MAXITROL Ointment in the "V" pocket. Do not let the tip of the tube touch your eye.
4. Look downward before closing your eye.

Not more than 20 mL or 8 g should be prescribed initially and the prescription should not be refilled without further evaluation as outlined in PRECAUTIONS above.

How Supplied:

Suspension (**NDC** 0998-0630-06) in 5 mL plastic DROP-TAINER® dispenser.

Ointment (**NDC** 0065-0631-36) in 3.5 g ophthalmic tube.

Storage: Store at 46°–80°F.

MYDFRIN® 2.5% ℞
(phenylephrine hydrochloride Ophthalmic Solution)
Vasoconstrictor and Mydriatic
For Use in Ophthalmology

WARNING: PHYSICIANS SHOULD COMPLETELY FAMILIARIZE THEMSELVES WITH THE COMPLETE CONTENTS OF THIS LEAFLET BEFORE PRESCRIBING PHENYLEPHRINE HYDROCHLORIDE.

Description: MYDFRIN® 2.5% is a sterile topical ophthalmic solution. The active ingredient is represented by the chemical structure:

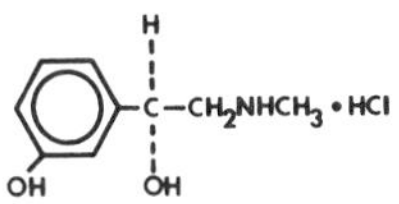

Established name:
Phenylephrine Hydrochloride

Chemical name:
Benzenemethanol, 3-hydroxy-α-[(methylamino)methyl]-, hydrochloride (*R*)-.

Each mL contains: Active: Penylephrine HCl 2.5%. **Preservative:** Benzalkonium Chloride 0.01%. **Inactive:** Boric Acid, Sodium Bisulfite, Edetate Disodium, Sodium Hydroxide and/or Hydrochloric Acid (to adjust pH), Purified Water.

Clinical Pharmacology: MYDFRIN 2.5% Ophthalmic Solution is an alpha receptor sympathetic agonist used in local ocular disorders because of its vasoconstrictor and mydriatic action. It exhibits rapid and moderately prolonged action, and it produces little rebound vasodilation. Systemic side effects are uncommon.

Indications and Usage: MYDFRIN 2.5% Ophthalmic Solution is recommended as a vasoconstrictor, decongestant, and mydriatic in a variety of ophthalmic conditions and procedures. Some of its uses are for pupillary dilation in uveitis (to prevent or aid in the disruption of posterior synechia formation), for many ophthalmic surgical procedures and for refraction without cycloplegia. MYDFRIN 2.5% Ophthalmic Solution may also be used for funduscopy and other diagnostic procedures.

Contraindications: Ophthalmic solutions of phenylephrine HCl are contraindicated in patients with anatomically narrow angles or narrow angle glaucoma. Phenylephrine HCl may be contraindicated in low birth weight infants and in some elderly adults with severe arteriosclerotic cardiovascular or cerebrovascular disease. Phenylephrine HCl may be contraindicated during intraocular operative procedures when the corneal epithelial barrier has been disturbed. This preparation is also contraindicated in persons with a known sensitivity to phenylephrine HCl or any of its components.

Warnings: Not for intraocular use. As with other adrenergic drugs, when MYDFRIN 2.5% Ophthalmic Solution is administered simultaneously with, or up to 21 days after, administration of monoamine oxidase (MAO) inhibitors, careful supervision and adjustment of dosages are required since exaggerated adrenergic effects may result. The pressor response of adrenergic agents may also be potentiated by tricyclic antidepressants. Systemic side effects are more common in patients taking beta adrenergic blocking agents such as propanolol. Concomitant use of phenylephrine and atropine may enhance the pressor effects and induce tachycardia in some patients, especially infants.[1] Contains sodium bisulfite, a sulfite that may cause allergic-type reactions including anaphylactic symptoms and life-threatening or less severe asthmatic episodes in certain susceptible people. The overall prevalence of sulfite sensitivity in the general population is unknown and probably low. Sulfite sensitivity is seen more frequently in asthmatic than in nonasthmatic people.

Precautions: Ordinarily, any mydriatic, including phenylephrine HCl, is contraindicated in patients with glaucoma, since it may occasionally raise intraocular pressure. However, when temporary dilation of the pupil may free adhesions, this advantage may temporarily outweigh the danger from coincident dilation of the pupil. Rebound miosis has been reported in older persons one day after receiving phenylephrine HCl ophthalmic solutions, and reinstillation of the drug may produce less mydriasis than previously. This may be of clinical importance in dilating the pupils of older subjects prior to retinal detachment or cataract surgery. The lacrimal sac should be compressed by digital pressure for two to three minutes after instillation to avoid excessive systemic absorption.

Due to a strong action of the drug on the dilator muscle, older individuals may also develop transient pigment floaters in the aqueous humor 40 to 45 minutes following the administration of phenylephrine HCl ophthalmic solution. The appearance may be similar to anterior uveitis or to a microscopic hyphema. To prevent pain, a drop of suitable topical anesthetic may be applied before using MYDFRIN 2.5% Ophthalmic Solution. Prolonged exposure to air or strong light may cause oxidation and discoloration. Do not use if solution is brown or contains a precipitate. Monitor blood pressure in geriatric patients with known cardiac disease. Use caution in infants with known cardiac anomalies.

Exceeding recommended dosages or applying MYDFRIN® 2.5% Ophthalmic Solution to the instrumented, traumatized, diseased or post-surgical eye or adnexa, or to patients with suppressed lacrimation, as during anesthesia, may result in the absorption of sufficient quantities of phenylephrine to produce a systemic vasopressor response.

Information for Patients: Do not touch dropper tip to any surface, as this may contaminate the solution.

Carcinogenesis, Mutagenesis, Impairment of Fertility: There have been no long-term studies done using phenylephrine HCl in animals to evaluate carcinogenic potential.

Pregnancy: Pregnancy Category C. Animal reproduction studies have not been conducted with phenylephrine HCl. It is also not known whether phenylephrine HCl can cause fetal harm when administered to a pregnant woman or can affect reproduction capacity. MYDFRIN Ophthalmic Solution should be given to a pregnant woman only if clearly needed.

Nursing Mothers: It is not known whether these drugs are excreted in human milk. Because many drugs are excreted in human milk, caution should be exercised when MYDFRIN Ophthalmic Solution is administered to a nursing woman.

Adverse Reactions: A marked increase in blood pressure has been reported in low-weight premature neonates, infants and adult patients with idiopathic orthostatic hypotension. Cardiovascular reactions which have occurred primarily in elderly patients include marked increase in blood pressure, syncope, myocardial infarction, tachycardia, arrythmia, and fatal subarachnoid hemorrhage.[2]

Dosage and Administration:

Vasoconstriction and Pupil Dilation:
MYDFRIN 2.5% Ophthalmic Solution is especially useful when rapid and powerful dilation of the pupil without cycloplegia and reduction of congestion in the capillary bed are desired. A drop of a suitable topical anesthetic may be applied, followed in a few minutes by 1 drop of MYDFRIN 2.5% Ophthalmic Solution on the upper limbus. The anesthetic prevents stinging and consequent dilution of the solution by lacrimation. It may occasionally be necessary to repeat the instillation after one hour, again preceded by the use of the topical anesthetic.

Uveitis: Posterior Synechiae: MYDFRIN 2.5% Ophthalmic Solution may be used in patients with uveitis when synechiae are present or

Continued on next page

Alcon—Cont.

may develop. The formation of synechiae may be prevented by the use of this solution and atropine or other cycloplegics to produce wide dilation of the pupil. For recently formed posterior synechiae one drop of MYDFRIN 2.5% Ophthalmic Solution may be applied to the upper surface of the cornea and be repeated as necessary, not to exceed three times. Treatment may be continued the following day, if necessary. Atropine sulfate and the application of hot compresses should also be used if indicated.

Glaucoma: MYDFRIN 2.5% Ophthalmic Solution may be used with miotics in patients with open angle glaucoma. It reduces the difficulties experienced by the patient because of the small field produced by miosis, and still it permits and often supports the effect of the miotic in lowering the intraocular pressure in open angle glaucoma. Hence, there may be marked improvement in visual acuity after using MYDFRIN 2.5% Ophthalmic Solution in conjunction with miotic drugs.

Surgery: When a short-acting mydriatic is needed for wide dilation of the pupil before intraocular surgery, MYDFRIN 2.5% Ophthalmic Solution may be applied topically from 30 to 60 minutes before the operation.

Refraction: MYDFRIN 2.5% Ophthalmic Solution may be used effectively to increase mydriasis with homatropine hydrobromide, cyclopentolate hydrochloride, tropicamide hydrochloride and atropine sulfate.

FOR ADULTS:

One drop of the preferred cycloplegic is placed in each eye, followed in 5 minutes by one drop of MYDFRIN 2.5% Ophthalmic Solution. Since adequate cycloplegia is achieved at different time intervals after the instillation of the necessary number of drops, different cycloplegics will require different waiting periods to achieve adequate cycloplegia.

FOR CHILDREN:

For a "one application method,"MYDFRIN 2.5% Ophthalmic Solution may be combined with one of the preferred rapid acting cycloplegics to produce adequate cycloplegia.

Ophthalmoscopic Examination: One drop of MYDFRIN 2.5% Ophthalmic Solution is placed in each eye. Sufficient mydriasis to permit examination is produced in 15 to 30 minutes. Dilation lasts from one to three hours.

Diagnostic Procedures: Provocative Test for Angle Closure Glaucoma: MYDFRIN 2.5% Ophthalmic Solution may be used cautiously as a provocative test when interval narrow angle closure glaucoma is suspected. Intraocular tension and gonioscopy are performed prior to and after dilation of the pupil with phenylephrine HCl. A "significant" intraocular pressure (IOP) rise combined with gonioscopic evidence of angle closure indicates an anterior segment anatomy capable of angle closure. A negative test does not rule this out. This pharmacologically induced angle closure glaucoma may not simulate real life conditions and other causes for transient elevations of IOP should be excluded.

Retinoscopy (Shadow Test): When dilation of the pupil without cycloplegic action is desired for retinoscopy, MYDFRIN 2.5% Ophthalmic Solution may be used.

NOTE: Heavily pigmented irides may require larger doses in all of the above procedures.

Blanching Test: One or two drops of MYDFRIN 2.5% Ophthalmic Solution should be applied to the injected eye. After five minutes, examine for perilimbal blanching. If blanching occurs, the congestion is superficial and probably does not indicate iridocyclitis.

How Supplied: MYDFRIN 2.5% Ophthalmic Solution in plastic DROP-TAINER® dispensers:
3 mL: NDC 0065-0342-03
5 mL: NDC 0998-0342-05

Storage: Store at 36° to 80°F. Protect from light and excessive heat.

References:

1. Fraunfelder, F. T., and Meyer, S. M.: Possible Cardiovascular Effects Secondary to Topical Ophthalmic 2.5% Phenylephrine, *Am. J. Oph.* 99:3:362, 1985.
2. Ibid.

Caution: Federal (USA) law prohibits dispensing without prescription.

MYDRIACYL® ℞
Tropicamide
Sterile Ophthalmic Solution, USP

Description: MYDRIACYL® (Tropicamide ophthalmic solution, USP) is an anticholinergic prepared as a sterile topical ophthalmic solution in two strengths. The active ingredient is represented by the chemical structure:

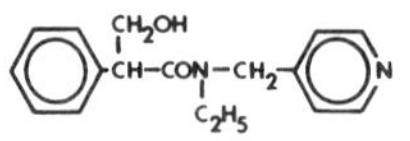

Established name:
Tropicamide

Chemical name:
Benzeneacetamide, *N*-ethyl-α-(hydroxymethyl)-*N*-(4-pyridinylmethyl)-.

Each mL contains: **Active:** Tropicamide 0.5% or 1%. **Preservative:** Benzalkonium Chloride 0.01%. **Inactive:** Sodium Chloride, Edetate Disodium, Hydrochloric Acid and/or Sodium Hydroxide (to adjust pH), Purified Water. pH range 4.0–5.8.

Clinical Pharmacology: This anticholinergic preparation blocks the responses of the sphincter muscle of the iris and the ciliary muscle to cholinergic stimulation, dilating the pupil (mydriasis). The stronger preparation (1%) also paralyzes accommodation. This preparation acts rapidly and the duration of activity is relatively short. The weaker strength may be useful in producing mydriasis with only slight cycloplegia.

Indications and Usage: For mydriasis and cycloplegia for diagnostic procedures.

Contraindications: Contraindicated in persons with primary glaucoma or a tendency toward glaucoma (e.g. narrow anterior chamber angle), and in persons showing hypersensitivity to any component of this preparation.

Warnings: For topical use only—not for injection. Reproductive studies have not been performed in animals. There is not adequate information on whether this drug may affect fertility in human males or females or have a teratogenic potential or other adverse effect on the fetus. This preparation may cause CNS disturbances which may be dangerous in infants and children. Possibility of occurrence of psychotic reaction and behavioral disturbance due to hypersensitivity to anticholinergic drugs should be borne in mind.

Precautions: In the elderly and others where increased intraocular pressure may be encountered, mydriatics and cycloplegics should be used cautiously. To avoid inducing angle closure glaucoma, an estimation of the depth of the angle of the anterior chamber should be made. The lacrimal sac should be compressed by digital pressure for two to three minutes after instillation to avoid excessive systemic absorption.

Patient Warning: Do not touch dropper tip to any surface, as this may contaminate the solution. Patient should be advised not to drive or engage in other hazardous activities while pupils are dilated. Patient may experience sensitivity to light and should protect eyes in bright illumination during dilation. Parents should be warned not to get this preparation in their child's mouth and to wash their own hands and the child's hands following administration.

Adverse Reactions: Increased intraocular pressure. Psychotic reactions, behavioral disturbances, and cardiorespiratory collapse in children and some adults with this class of drugs have been reported. Transient stinging, dryness of the mouth, blurred vision, photophobia with or without corneal staining, tachycardia, headache, parasympathetic stimulation, or allergic reaction may occur.

Dosage and Administration: For refraction, one or two drops of 1% solution in the eye(s), repeated in five minutes. If patient is not seen within 20 to 30 minutes, an additional drop may be instilled to prolong mydriatic effect. For examination of fundus, one or two drops of 0.5% solution 15 to 20 minutes prior to examination. Individuals with heavily pigmented irides may require larger doses.

How Supplied: 0.5% and 1% in 15 mL plastic DROP-TAINER® dispensers.
0.5% NDC 0998-0354-15
1% NDC 0998-0355-15
1% in 3 mL plastic DROP-TAINER® dispensers.
1% NDC 0065-0355-03

Storage: Store at 8°–27°C (46°–80° F). Do not refrigerate or store at high temperatures. Keep container tightly closed.

Caution: Federal (USA) law prohibits dispensing without prescription.

NAPHCON® OTC
(Naphazoline Hydrochloride Ophthalmic Solution)
Redness Reliever Eye Drops
Sterile

Ingredients: Each mL contains: **Active:** Naphazoline Hydrochloride 0.012%. **Preservative:** Benzalkonium Chloride 0.01%. **Inactives:** Boric Acid, Sodium Chloride, Potassium Chloride, Edetate Disodium, Sodium Carbonate and/or Hydrochloric Acid (to adjust pH), Purified Water.

Indications:

FDA APPROVED USE
Relieves redness of the eye due to minor eye irritations.

FOR TOPICAL EYE USE ONLY.

Warnings: Remove contact lenses before using. If you experience eye pain, changes in vision, continued redness or irritation of the eye, or if the condition worsens or persists for more than 72 hours, discontinue use and consult a doctor. If you have glaucoma, do not use this product except under the advice and supervision of a doctor. Overuse of this product may produce increased redness of the eye. If solution changes color or becomes cloudy, do not use.

To avoid contamination, do not touch tip of container to any surface. Replace cap after using. Keep this and all drugs out of the reach of children. In case of accidental ingestion, seek professional assistance or contact a Poison Control Center immediately.

Directions: Instill 1 to 2 drops in the affected eye(s) up to four times daily.

How Supplied: In 15 mL DROP-TAINER® dispenser. NDC 0998-0078-15

Storage: Store at room temperature.

NAPHCON® FORTE ℞

(Naphazoline Hydrochloride Ophthalmic Solution, USP), 0.1%

Description: NAPHCON® FORTE (Naphazoline Hydrochloride Ophthalmic Solution, USP) 0.1% is a sterile preparation. Naphazoline HCl, an ocular vasoconstrictor, is an imidazoline derivative sympathomimetic amine. It occurs as a white, odorless crystalline powder having a bitter taste and is freely soluble in water and in alcohol. The active ingredient is represented by the structural formula:

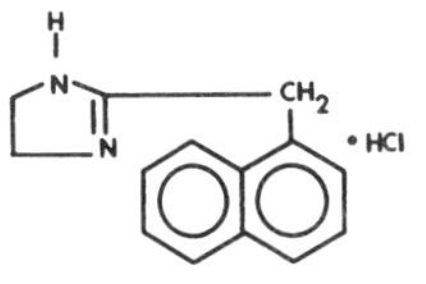

$C_{14}H_{14}N_2HCl$

Chemical name: MW = 246.74
2-(1-naphthylmethyl)-2-imidazoline monohydrochloride

Each mL contains: Active: Naphazoline Hydrochloride 0.1%. Preservative: Benzalkonium Chloride 0.01%. Inactive: Boric Acid, Sodium Chloride, Potassium Chloride, Edetate Disodium, Sodium Carbonate and/or Hydrochloric Acid (to adjust pH), Purified Water. The solution has a pH of 5.5 to 7.0.

Clinical Pharmacology: Naphazoline constricts the vascular system of the conjunctiva. It is presumed that this effect is due to direct stimulation action of the drug upon the alpha adrenergic receptors in the arterioles of the conjunctiva resulting in decreased conjunctival congestion. Naphazoline belongs to the imidazoline class of sympathomimetics.

Indications and Usage: NAPHCON® FORTE (Naphazoline Hydrochloride Ophthalmic Solution, USP), 0.1% is indicated for use as a topical ocular vasoconstrictor.

Contraindications: Contraindicated in the presence of an anatomically narrow angle or in narrow angle glaucoma or in persons who have shown hypersensitivity to any component of this preparation.

Warnings: NOT FOR INJECTION—FOR OPHTHALMIC USE ONLY. Patients under therapy with MAO inhibitors may experience a severe hypertensive crisis if given a sympathomimetic drug. Use in children, especially infants, may result in CNS depression leading to coma and marked reduction in body temperature.

Precautions:

General: For topical ophthalmic use only. Use with caution in the presence of hypertension, cardiovascular abnormalities, hyperglycemia (diabetes), hyperthyroidism, infection or injury.

Information For Patients: Patients should be advised to discontinue the drug and consult a physician if relief is not obtained within 48 hours of therapy, if irritation, blurring or redness persists, or increases, or if symptoms of systemic absorption occur, i.e., dizziness, headache, nausea, decrease in body temperature, or drowsiness.

To prevent contaminating the dropper tip and solution, do not touch the eyelids or the surrounding area with the dropper tip of the bottle. If solution changes color or becomes cloudy, do not use.

Drug Interactions: Concurrent use of maprotiline or tricyclic antidepressants and naphazoline may potentiate the pressor effect of naphazoline. Patients under therapy with MAO inhibitors may experience a severe hypertensive crisis if given a sympathomimetic drug. (See WARNINGS).

Pregnancy Category C: Animal reproduction studies have not been conducted with naphazoline. It is also not known whether naphazoline can cause fetal harm when administered to a pregnant woman or can affect reproduction capacity. Naphazoline should be given to a pregnant woman only if clearly needed.

Nursing Mothers: It is not known whether naphazoline is excreted in human milk. Because many drugs are excreted in human milk, caution should be exercised when naphazoline is administered to a nursing woman.

Pediatric Use: Safety and effectiveness in children have not been established. See "WARNINGS" and "CONTRAINDICATIONS."

Adverse Reactions:

Ocular: Mydriasis, increased redness, irritation, discomfort, blurring, punctate keratitis, lacrimation, increased intraocular pressure.

Systemic: Dizziness, headache, nausea, sweating, nervousness, drowsiness, weakness, hypertension, cardiac irregularities, and hyperglycemia.

Dosage and Administration: Instill one or two drops in the conjunctival sac(s) every three to four hours as needed.

How Supplied: NAPHCON® FORTE (Naphazoline Hydrochloride Ophthalmic Solution, USP), 0.1% is available in 15 mL DROP-TAINER® dispenser.
NDC 0998-0079-15.

Storage: Store at 8°–27°C (46°–80°F).

Caution: Federal (USA) law prohibits dispensing without prescription.

NAPHCON-A® ℞

(naphazoline hydrochloride and pheniramine maleate)
Sterile Ophthalmic Solution

Description: NAPHCON-A® (naphazoline hydrochloride, pheniramine maleate) is a combination of an antihistamine and a decongestant prepared as a sterile topical ophthalmic solution. The active ingredients are represented by the chemical structures:

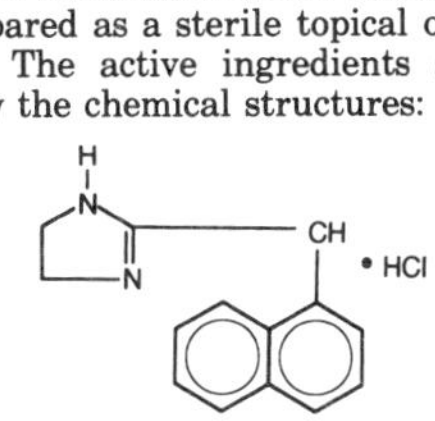

Established name:
Naphazoline Hydrochloride

Chemical Name:
1*H*-Imidazole, 4,5-dihydro-2-(1-naphthalenylmethyl)-, monohydrochloride.

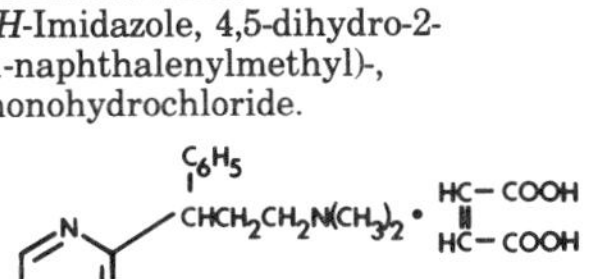

Established name:
Pheniramine Maleate

Chemical name:
N,N-Dimethyl-γ-phenyl-2-pyridine-propanamine, (*Z*)-Butenedioic acid.

Each mL contains: Active: Naphazoline Hydrochloride 0.025%, Pheniramine Maleate 0.3%. Preservative: Benzalkonium Chloride 0.01%. Inactive: Boric Acid, Sodium Borate, Edetate Disodium, Sodium Chloride, Sodium Hydroxide and/or Hydrochloric Acid (to adjust pH), and Purified Water.

Clinical Pharmacology: NAPHCON-A® combines the effects of the antihistamine, pheniramine maleate, and the decongestant, naphazoline.

Indications and Usage: Based on a review of a related combination of drugs by the National Academy of Sciences—National Research Council and/or other information, FDA has classified the indications as follows: "Possibly" effective: For relief of ocular irritation and/or congestion or for the treatment of allergic or inflammatory ocular conditions. Final classification of the less-than-effective indication requires further investigation.

Contraindications: Hypersensitivity to one or more of the components of this preparation. Do not use in the presence of narrow angle glaucoma or in patients predisposed to narrow angle glaucoma.

Warnings: Patients under MAO inhibitors may experience a severe hypertensive crisis if given a sympathomimctic drug such as Naphazoline HCl. Use in infants and children may result in CNS depression leading to coma and marked reduction in body temperature.

Precautions: General. For topical eye use only—not for injection. This preparation should be used with caution in patients with severe cardiovascular disease including cardiac arrhythmias, patients with poorly controlled hypertension, patients with diabetes, especially those with a tendency toward diabetic ketoacidosis.

Information for Patients: To prevent contaminating the dropper tip and solution, care should be taken not to touch the eyelids or surrounding area with the dropper tip of the bottle.

Carcinogenesis, Mutagenesis, Impairment of Fertility: There have been no long-term studies done using naphazoline hydrochloride and/or pheniramine maleate in animals to evaluate carcinogenic potential.

Pregnancy: Pregnancy Category C. Animal reproduction studies have not been conducted with naphazoline hydrochloride and/or pheniramine maleate. It is also not known whether naphazoline hydrochloride and/or pheniramine maleate can cause fetal harm when administered to a pregnant woman or can affect reproduction capacity. NAPHCON-A® Ophthalmic Solution should be given to a pregnant woman only if clearly needed.

Nursing Mothers: It is not known whether these drugs are excreted in human milk. Because many drugs are excreted in human milk, caution should be exercised when NAPHCON-A Ophthalmic Solution is administered to a nursing woman.

Adverse Reactions: The following adverse reactions may occur: Pupillary dilation, increase in intraocular pressure, systemic effects due to absorption (i.e., hypertension, cardiac irregularities, hyperglycemia). Drowsiness may be experienced by some patients.

Dosage and Administration: One or two drops instilled in each eye every 3 to 4 hours or less frequently, as required to relieve symptoms.

How Supplied: In 15 mL plastic DROP-TAINER® Dispenser.
NDC 0998-0080-15.

Storage: Store at 2°–27°C (36°–80°F). Keep bottle tightly closed when not in use. Protect from light and excessive heat.

Caution: Federal (USA) law prohibits dispensing without prescription.

Continued on next page

Alcon—Cont.

NATACYN® ℞

(natamycin ophthalmic suspension, USP) 5% Sterile

Description: NATACYN® (natamycin sterile ophthalmic suspension, USP) 5% is a sterile, antifungal drug for topical ophthalmic administration. The active ingredient is represented by the chemical structure:

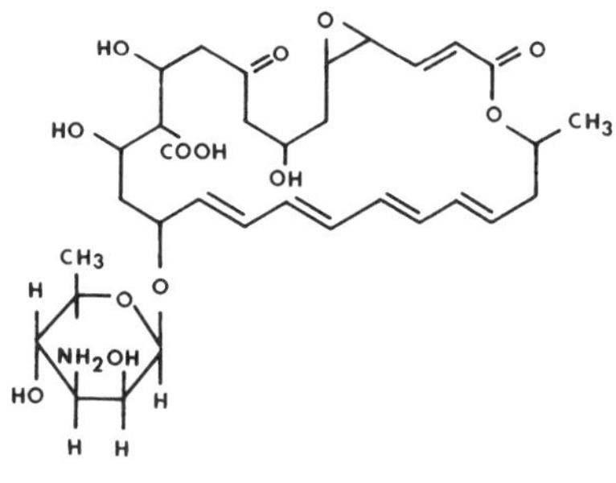

Established name:
Natamycin

Chemical name:
Stereoisomer of 22-[(3-amino-3,6-dideoxy-β-D-mannopyranosyl)oxy]-1,3,26-trihydroxy-12-methyl-10-oxo-6,11,28-trioxatricyclo[22.3.1.$0^{5,7}$]octacosa-8,14,16,18,20-pentaene-25-carboxylic acid.
Other: Pimaricin

Each mL of the suspension contains: **Active:** Natamycin 5% (50mg). **Preservative:** Benzalkonium Chloride 0.02%. **Inactive:** Sodium Hydroxide and/or Hydrochloric Acid (neutralized to adjust the pH), Purified Water.

Clinical Pharmacology: Natamycin is a tetraene polyene antibiotic derived from *Streptomyces natalensis.* It possesses *in vitro* activity against a variety of yeast and filamentous fungi, including *Candida, Aspergillus, Cephalosporium, Fusarium* and *Penicillium.* The mechanism of action appears to be through binding of the molecule to the sterol moiety of the fungal cell membrane. The polyenesterol complex alters the permeability of the membrane to produce depletion of essential cellular constituents. Although the activity against fungi is dose-related, natamycin is predominantly fungicidal.* Natamycin is not effective *in vitro* against gram-positive or gram-negative bacteria. Topical administration appears to produce effective concentrations of natamycin within the corneal stroma, but not in intraocular fluid. Systemic absorption should not be expected following topical administration of NATACYN (natamycin ophthalmic suspension USP) 5%. As with other polyene antibiotics, absorption from the gastrointestinal tract is very poor. Studies in rabbits receiving topical natamycin revealed no measurable compound in the aqueous humor or sera, but the sensitivity of the measurement was no greater than 2 mg/mL.

Indications and Usage: NATACYN (natamycin ophthalmic suspension USP) 5% is indicated for the treatment of fungal blepharitis, conjunctivitis, and keratitis caused by susceptible organisms including *Fusarium solani* keratitis. As in other forms of suppurative keratitis, initial and sustained therapy of fungal keratitis should be determined by the clinical diagnosis, laboratory diagnosis by smear and culture of corneal scrapings and drug response. Whenever possible, the *in vitro* activity of natamycin against the responsible fungus should be determined. The effectiveness of natamycin as a single agent in fungal endophthalmitis has not been established.

Contraindication: NATACYN (natamycin ophthalmic suspension USP) 5% is contraindicated in individuals with a history of hypersensitivity to any of its components.

Precautions: General. For topical eye use only—NOT FOR INJECTION. Failure of improvement of keratitis following 7–10 days of administration of the drug suggests that the infection may be caused by a microorganism not susceptible to natamycin.

Continuation of therapy should be based on clinical re-evaluation and additional laboratory studies.

Adherence of the suspension to areas of epithelial ulceration or retention of the suspension in the fornices occurs regularly. There has only been a limited number of cases in which natamycin has been used; therefore, it is possible that adverse reactions of which we have no knowledge at present may occur. For this reason, patients on this drug should be monitored at least twice weekly. Should suspicion of drug toxicity occur, the drug should be discontinued.

Information for Patients: Do not touch dropper tip to any surface, as this may contaminate the suspension.

Carcinogenesis, Mutagenesis, Impairment of Fertility: There have been no long term studies done using natamycin in animals to evaluate carcinogenesis, mutagenesis, or impairment of fertility.

Pregnancy: Pregnancy Category C. Animal reproduction studies have not been conducted with natamycin. It is also not known whether natamycin can cause fetal harm when administered to a pregnant woman or can affect reproduction capacity. NATACYN (natamycin ophthalmic suspension USP) 5% should be given to a pregnant woman only if clearly needed.

Nursing Mothers: It is not known whether these drugs are excreted in human milk. Because many drugs are excreted in human milk, caution should be exercised when natamycin is administered to a nursing woman.

Pediatric Use: Safety and effectiveness in children have not been establised.

Adverse Reactions: One case of conjunctival chemosis and hyperemia, thought to be allergic in nature, has been reported.

Dosage and Administration: SHAKE WELL BEFORE USING. The preferred initial dosage in fungal keratitis is one drop of NATACYN (natamycin ophthalmic suspension USP) 5% instilled in the conjunctival sac at hourly or two-hourly intervals. The frequency of application can usually be reduced to one drop 6 to 8 times daily after the first 3 to 4 days. Therapy should generally be continued for 14 to 21 days or until there is resolution of active fungal keratitis. In many cases, it may be helpful to reduce the dosage gradually at 4 to 7 day intervals to assure that the replicating organism has been eliminated. Less frequent initial dosage (4 to 6 daily applications) may be sufficient in fungal blepharitis and conjunctivitis.

How Supplied: 15 mL in glass bottles with sterile dropper assembly. **NDC** 0065-0645-15.

Storage: May be stored in refrigerator [(36°–46° F) (2°–8°C)] or at room temperature [(46°–75° F) (8°–24°C)]. *Do not freeze.* Avoid exposure to light and excessive heat.

CAUTION: Federal (USA) Law Prohibits Dispensing Without Prescription.

*Laupen, J.O.; McLellan, W.L.; El Nakeeb, M.A.: "Antibiotics and Fungal Physiology," Antimicrobial Agents and Chemotherapy, 1965:1006, 1965.

References:

1. Barckhausen, B.: Die Behandlung der Probleminfektionen das vorderen Augenabschnittes in der Praxis. Landarzt 46:842, 1970.
2. Cuendet, J.F.; Nouri, A.: Traitement local en ophthalmologie par un nouvel antibiotique fungicide, la "pimaricine". Ophthalmologica 145:297, 1963.
3. Forster, R.K.; Rebell, G.: "The Diagnosis and Management of Keratomycoses" Arch. Ophth. 93:1134, 1975.
4. Francois, J.; de Vos, El: Traitement des mycoses oculaires par la pimaricine. Bull. Soc. Belge Ophthal. 131:382, 1962.
5. Jones, D.B.; Sexton, R.; Rebell, G.: "Mycotic keratitis in South Florida: A Review of Thirty-nine Cases." Transactions ophthal. Soc. U.K. 89:781, 1969.
6. Jones, D.B.; Forster, R.K.; Rebell, G.: "*Fusarium solani* keratitis treated with Natamycin (pimaricin), 18 consecutive cases." Arch. Ophth. 88:147, 1972.
7. L'Editeur: Traitement des mycoses oculaires. Presse med. 77:147, 1969.
8. Vozza, R.; Bagolini, B.: Su di un caso di grave ulcerazione bilaterale delle palpebra de Candida albicans. Bol. Oculist. 43:433, 1964.

Manufactured Under License From Gist-Brocades, N.V., Delft, Holland

---

PILOPINE HS® GEL ℞

(pilocarpine hydrochloride) 4% Sterile Ophthalmic Gel

Description: PILOPINE HS® (Pilocarpine Hydrochloride) 4% Gel is a sterile topical ophthalmic aqueous gel which contains more than 90% water and employs CARBOPOL 940, a synthetic high molecular weight cross-linked polymer of acrylic acid, to impart a high viscosity. The active ingredient, Pilocarpine Hydrochloride, is a cholinergic and is represented by the chemical structure:

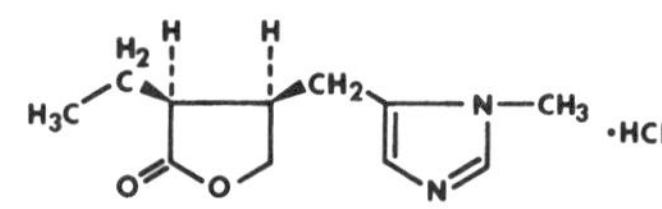

Established name:
Pilocarpine Hydrochloride
Chemical name:
2(3*H*)-Furanone, 3-ethyldihydro-4-[(1-methyl-1*H*-imidazol-5-yl)-methyl]-, monohydrochloride, (3*S-cis*)-.

PILOPINE HS Gel—Each Gram Contains: **Active:** Pilocarpine Hydrochloride 4% (40 mg). **Preservative:** Benzalkonium Chloride 0.008%. **Inactive:** Carbopol 940, Edetate Disodium, Hydrochloric Acid and/or Sodium Hydroxide (to adjust pH) and Purified Water.

Clinical Pharmacology: Pilocarpine is a direct acting cholinergic parasympathomimetic agent which acts through direct stimulation of muscarinic neuro receptors and smooth muscle such as the iris and secretory glands. Pilocarpine produces miosis through contraction of the iris sphincter, causing increased tension on the scleral spur and opening of the trabecular meshwork spaces to facilitate outflow of aqueous humor. Outflow resistance is thereby reduced, lowering intraocular pressure.

Indications and Usage: Pilocarpine Hydrochloride is a miotic (parasympathomimetic) used to control intraocular pressure. It may be used in combination with other miotics, beta blockers, carbonic anhydrase inhibitors, sympathomimetics or hyperosmotic agents.

Contraindications: Miotics are contraindicated where constriction is undesirable, such as in acute iritis, and in those persons showing hypersensitivity to any of their components.

Warnings: For topical use only.

Precautions: General: The miosis usually causes difficulty in dark adaptation. Patient should be advised to exercise caution in night driving and other hazardous occupations in poor illumination.

Information For Patients: Do not touch tube tip to any surface, as this may contaminate the gel.
Carcinogenesis, Mutagenesis, Impairment of Fertility: There have been no long-term studies done using Pilocarpine Hydrochloride in animals to evaluate carcinogenic potential.
Pregnancy: Pregnancy Category C. Animal reproduction studies have not been conducted with Pilocarpine Hydrochloride. It is also not known whether Pilocarpine Hydrochloride can cause fetal harm when administered to a pregnant woman or can affect reproduction capacity. PILOPINE HS Gel should be given to a pregnant woman only if clearly needed.
Nursing Mothers: It is not known whether this drug is excreted in human milk. Because many drugs are excreted in human milk, caution should be exercised when Pilocarpine Hydrochloride is administered to a nursing woman.
Pediatric Use: Safety and effectiveness in children have not been established.
Adverse Reactions: The following adverse experiences associated with pilocarpine therapy have been reported: lacrimation, burning or discomfort, temporal or periorbital headache, ciliary spasm, conjunctival vascular congestion, superficial keratitis and induced myopia. Systemic reactions following topical administration are extremely rare, but occasional patients are peculiarly sensitive to develop sweating and gastrointestinal overactivity following suggested dosage and administration. Ocular reactions usually occur during initiation of therapy and often will not persist with continued therapy. Reduced visual acuity in poor illumination is frequently experienced by older individuals and in those with lens opacity. A subtle corneal granularity was observed in about 10% of patients treated with PILOPINE HS Gel. Cases of retinal detachment have been reported during treatment with miotic agents; especially in young myopic patients. Lens opacity may occur with prolonged use of pilocarpine.
Overdosage: Overdosage can produce sweating, salivation, nausea, tremors, and slowing of the pulse and a decrease in blood pressure. Bronchial constriction may develop in asthmatic patients. In moderate overdosage, spontaneous recovery is to be expected and is aided by intravenous fluids to compensate for dehydration. For cases demonstrating severe poisoning, atropine is the pharmacologic antagonist to pilocarpine.
A topical ocular overdose of an ophthalmic product containing pilocarpine may be flushed from the eye(s) with warm tap water.
Dosage and Administration: Apply a one-half inch ribbon in the lower conjunctival sac of the affected eye(s) once a day at bedtime.
How Supplied: PILOPINE HS Gel is supplied as a 4% sterile aqueous gel in 4 gram tubes with ophthalmic tip.
4 gram: NDC 0065-0215-35
Storage: Store at room temperature (36°F–80°F). Avoid excessive heat. Do not freeze.
Caution: Federal (USA) law prohibits dispensing without prescription.
Reference:
1. Grant, W.M., Toxicology Of the Eye, 3rd Edition (1986), Charles Thomas Publishing, Springfield, IL.
Patented: U.S. Patent No. 4,271,143

TEARS NATURALE® II — OTC
Lubricant Eye Drops
TEARS NATURALE FREE®
Lubricant Eye Drops

Description: TEARS NATURALE II is the only lubricant eye drop preserved with safe, nonsensitizing POLYQUAD 0.001%. *In vitro* studies have shown that POLYQUAD substantially avoids the damaging effects of epithelial cell toxicity possible with other tear substitute preservatives and allows epithelial cell growth. POLYQUAD has been shown to be 99% reaction-free in normal subjects and 97% reaction-free in subjects known to be preservative sensitive. TEARS NATURALE FREE is a preservative-free version of TEARS NATURALE II.
With their unique mucin like polymeric formulation, and with their natural pH, low viscosity, and isotonicity, TEARS NATURALE II and TEARS NATURALE FREE provide dry eye patients with comfort and prompt relief of dry eye symptoms.
Sterile-For Topical Eye Use Only
Ingredients: TEARS NATURALE II: Each mL contains:
Active: DUASORB®, a water soluble polymeric system containing Dextran 70 0.1% and Hydroxypropyl Methylcellulose 2910 0.3%.
Preservative: POLYQUAD® (Polyquaternium-1) 0.001%. **Inactive:** Sodium Borate, Potassium Chloride, Sodium Chloride, Purified Water. May contain Hydrochloric Acid and/or Sodium Hydroxide to adjust pH.
TEARS NATURALE FREE: Each mL contains:
Active: DUASORB, a water soluble polymeric system containing Dextran 70 0.1% and Hydroxypropyl Methylcellulose 2910 0.3%.
Inactive: Sodium Borate, Potassium Chloride, Sodium Chloride, Purified Water. May contain Hydrochloric Acid and/or Sodium Hydroxide to adjust pH.
Indications: For the temporary relief of burning and irritation due to dryness of the eye and for use as a protectant against further irritation. For temporary relief of discomfort due to minor irritations of the eye or to exposure to wind or sun.
Warnings: Remove contact lenses before using. If you experience eye pain, changes in vision, continued redness or irritation of the eye, or if the condition worsens or persists for more than 72 hours, discontinue use and consult a doctor.
If solution changes color or becomes cloudy, do not use.
To avoid contamination, do not touch tip of container to any surface. TEARS NATURALE II: Replace cap after using. TEARS NATURALE FREE: Do not reuse. Once opened, discard. Keep this and all drugs out of the reach of children. In case of accidental ingestion, seek professional assistance or contact a Poison Control Center immediately.
Directions: TEARS NATURALE II: Instill 1 or 2 drops in the affected eye(s) as needed. TEARS NATURALE FREE: Completely twist off tab: do not pull. Instill 1 or 2 drops in the affected eye(s) as needed.
How Supplied: TEARS NATURALE II Lubricant Eye Drops are supplied in 15 mL and 30 mL plastic DROP-TAINER® bottles.
15 mL NDC 0065-0418-15
30 mL NDC 0065-0418-32
TEARS NATURALE FREE Lubricant Eye Drops are supplied in boxes of 32 0.02 fl. oz. single-use containers.
NDC 0065-0416-32
Storage: Store at room temperature.

TOBRADEX® — ℞
(Tobramycin and Dexamethasone)
Sterile Ophthalmic Suspension and Ointment

Description: TOBRADEX® (Tobramycin and Dexamethasone) Ophthalmic Suspension and Ointment are sterile, multiple dose antibiotic and steroid combinations for topical ophthalmic use.
The chemical structures for tobramycin and dexamethasone are presented below:
[See structure at top of next column.]

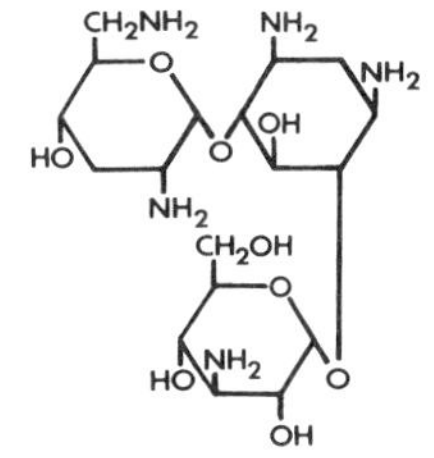

Tobramycin
Empirical Formula: $C_{18}H_{37}N_5O_9$
Chemical name:
O-3-Amino-3-deoxy-α-D-glucopyranosyl-(1→4)-*O*-[2,6-diamino-2,3,6-trideoxy-α-D-*ribo*-hexopyranosyl-(1→6)]-2-deoxy-L-streptamine

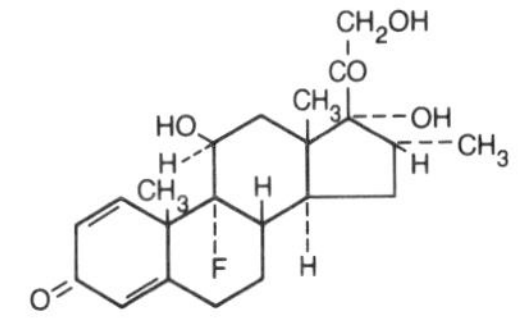

Dexamethasone
Empirical Formula: $C_{22}H_{29}F\ O_5$
Chemical Name:
9-Fluoro-11β,17,21-trihydroxy-16α-methylpregna-1,4-diene-3,20-dione
Each mL of TOBRADEX® Suspension contains: Active: Tobramycin 0.3% (3 mg) and Dexamethasone 0.1% (1 mg). Preservative: Benzalkonium Chloride 0.01%. Inactive: Tyloxapol, Edetate Disodium, Sodium Chloride, Hydroxyethyl Cellulose, Sodium Sulfate, Sulfuric Acid and/or Sodium Hydroxide (to adjust pH) and Purified Water.
Each gram of TOBRADEX® Ointment contains: Active: Tobramycin 0.3% (3 mg) and Dexamethasone 0.1% (1 mg). Preservative: Chlorobutanol 0.5%. Inactive: Mineral Oil and White Petrolatum.
Clinical Pharmacology: Corticoids suppress the inflammatory response to a variety of agents and they probably delay or slow healing. Since corticoids may inhibit the body's defense mechanism against infection, a concomitant antimicrobial drug may be used when this inhibition is considered to be clinically significant. Dexamethasone is a potent corticoid.
The antibiotic component in the combination (tobramycin) is included to provide action against susceptible organisms. *In vitro* studies have demonstrated that tobramycin is active against susceptible strains of the following microorganisms:
Staphylococci, including *S. aureus* and *S. epidermidis* (coagulase-positive and coagulase-negative), including penicillin-resistant strains.
Streptococci, including some of the Group A beta-hemolytic species, some nonhemolytic species, and some *Streptococcus pneumoniae*.
Pseudomonas aeruginosa, Escherichia coli, Klebsiella pneumoniae, Enterobacter aerogenes, Proteus mirabilis, Morganella morganii, most *Proteus vulgaris* strains, *Haemophilus influenzae* and *H. aegyptius, Moraxella lacunata,* and *Acinetobacter calcoaceticus* and some *Neisseria* species.
Bacterial susceptibility studies demonstrate that in some cases microorganisms resistant to gentamicin remain susceptible to tobramycin. A significant bacterial population resistant to tobramycin has not yet emerged; however, bacterial resistance may develop upon prolonged use.
No data are available on the extent of systemic absorption from TOBRADEX® Ophthalmic

Continued on next page

Alcon—Cont.

Suspension or Ointment; however, it is known that some systemic absorption can occur with ocularly applied drugs. If the maximum dose of TOBRADEX Ophthalmic Suspension is given for the first 48 hours (two drops in each eye every 2 hours) and complete systemic absorption occurs, which is highly unlikely, the daily dose of dexamethasone would be 2.4 mg. The usual physiologic replacement dose is 0.75 mg daily. If TOBRADEX Ophthalmic Suspension is given after the first 48 hours as two drops in each eye every 4 hours, the administered dose of dexamethasone would be 1.2 mg daily. The administered dose for TOBRADEX Ophthalmic Ointment in both eyes four times daily would be 0.4 mg of dexamethasone daily.

Indications and Usage: TOBRADEX® Ophthalmic Suspension and Ointment are indicated for steroid-responsive inflammatory ocular conditions for which a corticosteroid is indicated and where superficial bacterial ocular infection or a risk of bacterial ocular infection exists.

Ocular steroids are indicated in inflammatory conditions of the palpebral and bulbar conjunctiva, cornea and anterior segment of the globe where the inherent risk of steroid use in certain infective conjunctivitides is accepted to obtain a diminution in edema and inflammation. They are also indicated in chronic anterior uveitis and corneal injury from chemical, radiation or thermal burns, or penetration of foreign bodies.

The use of a combination drug with an anti-infective component is indicated where the risk of superficial ocular infection is high or where there is an expectation that potentially dangerous numbers of bacteria will be present in the eye.

The particular anti-infective drug in this product is active against the following common bacterial eye pathogens:

Staphylococci, including *S. aureus* and *S. epidermidis* (coagulase-positive and coagulase-negative), including penicillin-resistant strains.

Streptococci, including some of the Group A beta-hemolytic species, some nonhemolytic species, and some *Streptococcus pneumoniae.*

Pseudomonas aeruginosa, Escherichia coli, Klebsiella pneumoniae, Enterobacter aerogenes, Proteus mirabilis, Morganella morganii, most *Proteus vulgaris* strains, *Haemophilus influenzae* and *H. aegyptius, Moraxella lacunata,* and *Acinetobacter calcoaceticus* and some *Neisseria* species.

Contraindications: Epithelial herpes simplex keratitis (dendritic keratitis), vaccinia, varicella, and many other viral diseases of the cornea and conjunctiva. Mycobacterial infection of the eye. Fungal diseases of ocular structures. Hypersensitivity to a component of the medication.

The use of this combination is always contraindicated after uncomplicated removal of a corneal foreign body.

Warnings: NOT FOR INJECTION INTO THE EYE. Sensitivity to topically applied aminoglycosides may occur in some patients. If a sensitivity reaction does occur, discontinue use.

Prolonged use of steroids may result in glaucoma, with damage to the optic nerve, defects in visual acuity and fields of vision, and posterior subcapsular cataract formation. Intraocular pressure should be routinely monitored even though it may be difficult in children and uncooperative patients. Prolonged use may suppress the host response and thus increase the hazard of secondary ocular infections. In those diseases causing thinning of the cornea or sclera, perforations have been known to occur with the use of topical steroids. In acute purulent conditions of the eye, steroids may mask infection or enhance existing infection.

Precautions:

General. The possibility of fungal infections of the cornea should be considered after long-term steroid dosing. As with other antibiotic preparations, prolonged use may result in overgrowth of nonsusceptible organisms, including fungi. If superinfection occurs, appropriate therapy should be initiated. When multiple prescriptions are required, or whenever clinical judgement dictates, the patient should be examined with the aid of magnification, such as slit lamp biomicroscopy and, where appropriate, fluorescein staining.

Information for Patients: Do not touch dropper or tube tip to any surface, as this may contaminate the contents.

Carcinogenesis, Mutagenesis, Impairment of Fertility. No studies have been conducted to evaluate the carcinogenic or mutagenic potential. No impairment of fertility was noted in studies of subcutaneous tobramycin in rats at doses of 50 and 100 mg/kg/day.

Pregnancy Category C. Corticosteroids have been found to be teratogenic in animal studies. Ocular administration of 0.1% dexamethasone resulted in 15.6% and 32.3% incidence of fetal anomalies in two groups of pregnant rabbits. Fetal growth retardation and increased mortality rates have been observed in rats with chronic dexamethasone therapy. Reproduction studies have been performed in rats and rabbits with tobramycin at doses up to 100 mg/kg/day parenterally and have revealed no evidence of impaired fertility or harm to the fetus. There are no adequate and well-controlled studies in pregnant women. TOBRADEX® Ophthalmic Suspension and Ointment should be used during pregnancy only if the potential benefit justifies the potential risk to the fetus.

Nursing Mothers. It is not known whether this drug is excreted in human milk. Because many drugs are excreted in human milk, a decision should be considered to discontinue nursing temporarily while using TOBRADEX Ophthalmic Suspension or Ointment.

Pediatric Use. Safety and effectiveness in children have not been established.

Adverse Reactions: Adverse reactions have occurred with steroid/anti-infective combination drugs which can be attributed to the steroid component, the anti-infective component, or the combination. Exact incidence figures are not available. The most frequent adverse reactions to topical ocular tobramycin (TOBREX®) are hypersensitivity and localized ocular toxicity, including lid itching and swelling, and conjunctival erythema. These reactions occur in less than 4% of patients. Similar reactions may occur with the topical use of other aminoglycoside antibiotics. Other adverse reactions have not been reported; however, if topical ocular tobramycin is administered concomitantly with systemic aminoglycoside antibiotics, care should be taken to monitor the total serum concentration. The reactions due to the steroid component are: elevation of intraocular pressure (IOP) with possible development of glaucoma, and infrequent optic nerve damage; posterior subcapsular cataract formation; and delayed wound healing.

Secondary Infection. The development of secondary infection has occurred after use of combinations containing steroids and antimicrobials. Fungal infections of the cornea are particularly prone to develop coincidentally with long-term applications of steroids. The possibility of fungal invasion must be considered in any persistent corneal ulceration where steroid treatment has been used. Secondary bacterial ocular infection following suppression of host responses also occurs.

Dosage and Administration: Suspension: One or two drops instilled into the conjunctival sac(s) every four to six hours. During the initial 24 to 48 hours, the dosage may be increased to one or two drops every two (2) hours. Frequency should be decreased gradually as warranted by improvement in clinical signs. Care should be taken not to discontinue therapy prematurely. **Ointment:** Apply a small amount (approximately ½ inch ribbon) into the conjunctival sac(s) up to three or four times daily. TOBRADEX Ophthalmic Ointment may be used at bedtime in conjunction with TOBRADEX Ophthalmic Suspension used during the day. Not more than 20 mL or 8 g should be prescribed initially and the prescription should not be refilled without further evaluation as outlined in PRECAUTIONS above.

How Supplied: Sterile ophthalmic suspension in 2.5 mL (NDC 0065-0647-25) and 5 mL (NDC 0065-0647-05) DROP-TAINER® dispensers. Sterile ophthalmic ointment in 3.5 g ophthalmic tube (NDC 0065-0648-35).

Storage: Store 8° to 27°C (46° to 80°F).

Store suspension upright and shake well before using.

U.S. Patent No. 5,149,694

Caution: Federal (USA) law prohibits dispensing without prescription.

TOBREX® ℞
(tobramycin 0.3%)
Ophthalmic Solution and Ointment

Description: TOBREX® (tobramycin 0.3%) is a sterile topical ophthalmic antibiotic formulation prepared specifically for topical therapy of external ophthalmic infections. This product is supplied in solution and ointment forms.

Each mL of TOBREX Ophthalmic solution contains: Active: Tobramycin 0.3% (3 mg). Preservative: Benzalkonium Chloride 0.01% (0.1 mg). Inactive: Boric Acid, Sodium Sulfate, Sodium Chloride, Tyloxapol, Sodium Hydroxide and/or Sulfuric Acid (to adjust pH), Purified Water.

Each gram of TOBREX Ophthalmic ointment contains: Active: Tobramycin 0.3% (3 mg). Preservative: Chlorobutanol 0.5%. Inactive: Mineral Oil, White Petrolatum.

The chemical structure of tobramycin is presented below.

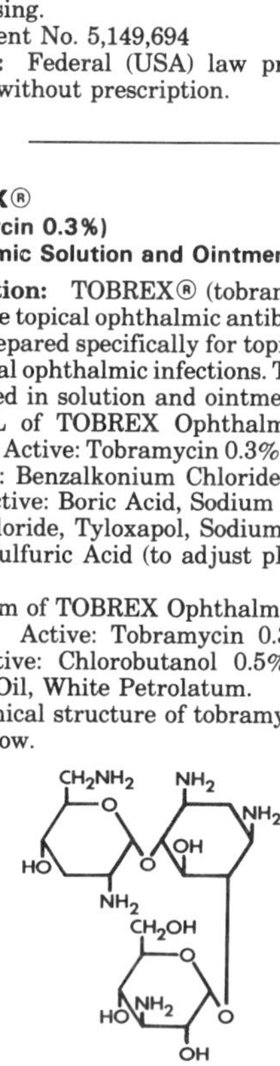

Chemical name: 0-{3-amino-3-deoxy-α-D-gluco-pyranosyl-(1→4)} -0- {2,6-diamino-2,3,6- trideoxy-α -D- ribohexo-pyranosyl-(1→6)} -2- deoxy-streptamine.

Tobramycin is a water-soluble aminoglycoside antibiotic active against a wide variety of gram-negative and gram-positive ophthalmic pathogens.

Clinical Pharmacology: *In Vitro Data: In vitro* studies have demonstrated tobramycin is active against susceptible strains of the following microorganisms:

Staphylococci, including *S. aureus* and *S. epidermidis* (coagulase-positive and coagulase-negative), including penicillin-resistant strains.

Streptococci, including some of the Group A beta-hemolytic species, some nonhemolytic species, and some *Streptococcus pneumoniae.*

Pseudomonas aeruginosa, Escherichia coli, Klebsiella pneumoniae, Enterobacter aerogenes, Proteus mirabilis, Morganella morganii, most

Proteus vulgaris strains, *Haemophilus influenzae* and *H. aegyptius, Moraxella lacunata, Acinetobacter calcoaceticus* and some *Neisseria* species. Bacterial susceptibility studies demonstrate that in some cases, microorganisms resistant to gentamicin retain susceptibility to tobramycin.
Indications and Usage: TOBREX® is a topical antibiotic indicated in the treatment of external infections of the eye and its adnexa caused by susceptible bacteria. Appropriate monitoring of bacterial response to topical antibiotic therapy should accompany the use of TOBREX. Clinical studies have shown tobramycin to be safe and effective for use in children.
Contraindications: TOBREX Ophthalmic Solution and Ointment are contraindicated in patients with known hypersensitivity to any of their components.
Warnings: NOT FOR INJECTION INTO THE EYE. Sensitivity to topically applied aminoglycosides may occur in some patients. If a sensitivity reaction to TOBREX occurs, discontinue use.
Precautions: As with other antibiotic preparations, prolonged use may result in overgrowth of nonsusceptible organisms, including fungi. If superinfection occurs, appropriate therapy should be initiated. Ophthalmic ointments may retard corneal wound healing.
Information For Patients: Do not touch dropper or tube tip to any surface, as this may contaminate the contents.
Pregnancy Category B. Reproduction studies in three types of animals at doses up to thirty-three times the normal human systemic dose have revealed no evidence of impaired fertility or harm to the fetus due to tobramycin. There are, however, no adequate and well-controlled studies in pregnant women. Because animal studies are not always predictive of human response, this drug should be used during pregnancy only if clearly needed.
Nursing Mothers: Because of the potential for adverse reactions in nursing infants from TOBREX, a decision should be made whether to discontinue nursing the infant or discontinue the drug, taking into account the importance of the drug to the mother.
Adverse Reactions: The most frequent adverse reactions to TOBREX Ophthalmic Solution and Ointment are hypersensitivity and localized ocular toxicity, including lid itching and swelling, and conjunctival erythema. These reactions occur in less than three of 100 patients treated with TOBREX. Similar reactions may occur with the topical use of other aminoglycoside antibiotics. Other adverse reactions have not been reported from TOBREX therapy; however, if topical ocular tobramycin is administered concomitantly with systemic aminoglycoside antibiotics, care should be taken to monitor the total serum concentration.
In clinical trials, TOBREX Ophthalmic Ointment produced significantly fewer adverse reactions (3.7%) than did GARAMYCIN® Ophthalmic Ointment (10.6%).
Overdosage: Clinically apparent signs and symptoms of an overdose of TOBREX Ophthalmic Solution or Ointment (punctate keratitis, erythema, increased lacrimation, edema and lid itching) may be similar to adverse reaction effects seen in some patients.
Dosage and Administration: Solution: In mild to moderate disease, instill one or two drops into the affected eye(s) every four hours. In severe infections, instill two drops into the eye(s) hourly until improvement, following which treatment should be reduced prior to discontinuation.
Ointment: In mild to moderate disease, apply a half-inch ribbon into the affected eye(s) two or three times per day. In severe infections, instill a half-inch ribbon into the affected eye(s) every three to four hours until improvement, following which treatment should be reduced prior to discontinuation.

How to Apply TOBREX® Ointment

1. Tilt your head back.
2. Place a finger on your cheek just under your eye and gently pull down until a "V" pocket is formed between your eyeball and your lower lid.
3. Place a small amount (about ½ inch) of TOBREX in the "V" pocket. Do not let the tip of the tube touch your eye.
4. Look downward before closing your eye.

Tobrex Ointment may be used in conjunction with Tobrex Solution.
How Supplied: 5 mL STERILE solution in DROP-TAINER® dispenser (NDC 0065-0643-05), containing tobramycin 0.3% (3 mg/mL) and 3.5 g STERILE ointment in ophthalmic tube (NDC 0065-0644-35), containing tobramycin 0.3% (3 mg/g).
Storage: Store at 8°–27°C (46°–80°F).
Caution: Federal (USA) law prohibits dispensing without prescription.

ZINCFRIN® OTC
Redness Reliever/Astringent Eye Drops

Ingredients: Each mL contains: Active: Zinc Sulfate 0.25%, Phenylephrine Hydrochloride 0.12%. **Preservative:** Benzalkonium Chloride 0.01%. **Inactives:** Sodium Citrate, Polysorbate 80, Citric Acid and/or Sodium Hydroxide (to adjust pH), Purified Water.
Indications: For the temporary relief of redness and discomfort due to minor eye irritations.
Sterile—FOR TOPICAL EYE USE ONLY.
Warnings: Remove contact lenses before using. If you experience eye pain, changes in vision, continued redness or irritation of the eye, or if the condition worsens or persists for more than 72 hours, discontinue use and consult a doctor. If you have glaucoma, do not use this product except under the advice and supervision of a doctor. Overuse of this product may produce increased redness of the eye. If solution changes color or becomes cloudy, do not use. To avoid contamination, do not touch tip of container to any surface. Replace cap after using. Keep this and all drugs out of the reach of children. In case of accidental ingestion, seek professional assistance or contact a Poison Control Center immediately.
Directions: Instill 1 to 2 drops in the affected eye(s) up to four times daily.
How Supplied: In ½ fl. oz. (15 mL) DROP-TAINER® dispenser.
NDC 0998-0512-15
Storage: Store at 8°–27°C (46° to 80° F).

Alcon Surgical
6201 SOUTH FREEWAY
FT. WORTH, TX 76134

BSS® ℞
Sterile Irrigating Solution
(balanced salt solution)

Description: BSS® Sterile Irrigating Solution is a sterile physiological balanced salt solution, each mL containing Sodium Chloride (NaCl) 0.64%, Potassium Chloride (KCl) 0.075%, Calcium Chloride Dihydrate ($CaCl_2 \cdot 2H_2O$) 0.048%, Magnesium Chloride Hexahydrate ($MgCl_2 \cdot 6H_2O$) 0.03%, Sodium Acetate Trihydrate ($C_2H_3NaO_2 \cdot 3H_2O$) 0.39%, Sodium Citrate Dihydrate ($C_6H_5Na_3O_7 \cdot 2H_2O$) 0.17%, Sodium Hydroxide and/or Hydrochloric Acid (to adjust pH), and Water for Injection. BSS Sterile Irrigating Solution is isotonic to the tissues of the eyes. It is a lint-free solution containing essential ions for normal cell metabolism.
Clinical Pharmacology: A physiologic irrigating solution.
Indications and Usage: For irrigation during various surgical procedures of the eyes, ears, nose, and/or throat.
Warnings: If blister or paper backing is damaged or broken, sterility of the enclosed bottle cannot be assured. Open under aseptic conditions only.
NOT FOR INJECTION OR INTRAVENOUS INFUSION.
Precautions: This solution contains no preservative and should not be used for more than one patient. Prior to use, check the following: tip should be firmly in place, irrigating needle should be properly seated; squeeze out several drops before inserting into anterior chamber. The needle should be removed from the anterior chamber prior to releasing pressure to prevent suction.
The addition of any medication to BSS solution may result in damage to intraocular tissue. Studies suggest that intraocular irrigating solutions which are iso-osmotic with normal aqueous fluids should be used with caution in diabetic patients undergoing vitrectomy since intraoperative lens changes have been observed.[1,2]
There have been reports of corneal clouding or edema following ocular surgery in which BSS solution was used as an irrigating solution. As in all surgical procedures appropriate measures should be taken to minimize trauma to the cornea and other ocular tissues.
Adverse Reactions: When the corneal endothelium is abnormal, irrigation or any other trauma may result in bullous keratopathy. Postoperative inflammatory reactions as well as incidents of corneal edema and corneal decompensation have been reported. Their relationship to the use of BSS solution has not been established.
Dosage and Administration: The adapter plug is designed to accept an irrigating needle. Tissues may be irrigated by attaching the needle to the DROP-TAINER® bottle as explained below. External irrigation may be done without the irrigating needle.
Method of using Adapter Plug for LUER-LOK* Hub Ophthalmic Irrigating Needle:

1. Aseptically remove DROP-TAINER bottle from blister by peeling paper backing.
2. Snap on surgeon's sterile irrigation needle. Push until firmly in place and twist slightly.
3. Test assembly for proper function before use.

*NOTE: LUER-LOK is a registered trademark of Becton, Dickinson and Company.
How Supplied: In 15 mL and 30 mL sterile DROP-TAINER bottles.
15 mL NDC 0065-0795-15
30 mL NDC 0065-0795-30
Storage: Store at 46° to 80° F (8° to 27° C).
References:

1. Faulborn, J., Conway, B.P., Machemer, R., Surgical Complications of Pars Plana Vitreous Surgery. Ophthalmology 85: 116–125, 1978.
2. Haimann, M.H. and Abrams, G. W., Prevention of Lens Opacification During Diabetic Vitrectomy. Ophthalmology 91: 116–121, 1984.

Caution: Federal Law prohibits dispensing without prescription.

BSS® ℞
Sterile Irrigating Solution
(balanced salt solution)
(250 mL and 500 mL)

Description: BSS® Sterile Irrigating Solution is a sterile physiological balanced salt solution, each mL containing Sodium Chloride

Continued on next page

Alcon Surgical—Cont.

(NaCl) 0.64%, Potassium Chloride (KCl) 0.075%, Calcium Chloride Dihydrate ($CaCl_2 \cdot 2H_2O$) 0.048%, Magnesium Chloride Hexahydrate ($MgCl_2 \cdot 6H_2O$) 0.03%, Sodium Acetate Trihydrate ($C_2H_3NaO_2 \cdot 3H_2O$) 0.39%, Sodium Citrate Dihydrate ($C_6H_5Na_3O_7 \cdot 2H_2O$) 0.17%, Sodium Hydroxide and/or Hydrochloric Acid (to adjust pH), and Water for Injection.

BSS Sterile Irrigating Solution is isotonic to the tissues of the eyes. It is a lint-free solution containing essential ions for normal cell metabolism.

Clinical Pharmacology: A physiologic irrigation solution.

Indications and Usage: For irrigation during various surgical procedures of the eyes, ears, nose and/or throat.

Warnings: NOT FOR INJECTION OR INTRAVENOUS INFUSION. Do not use unless product is clear, seal is intact, vacuum is present and container is undamaged. Do not use if product is discolored or contains a precipitate.

Precautions: Discard unused contents. **Do not use this container for more than one patient. Do not use additives with this product. Tissue damage could result if other drugs are added to product.** This solution contains no preservative.

Studies suggest that intraocular irrigating solutions which are iso-osmotic with normal aqueous fluids should be used with caution in diabetic patients undergoing vitrectomy since intraoperative lens changes have been observed.[1,2] There have been reports of corneal clouding or edema following ocular surgery in which BSS sterile irrigating solution was used as an irrigating solution. As in all surgical procedures appropriate measures should be taken to minimize trauma to the cornea and other ocular tissues.

Adverse Reactions: When the corneal endothelium is abnormal, irrigation or any other trauma may result in bullous keratopathy. Postoperative inflammatory reactions as well as incidents of corneal edema and corneal decompensation have been reported. Their relationship to the use of BSS sterile irrigating solution has not been established.

Dosage and Administration: This irrigating solution should be used according to standard format for each surgical procedure.

Note:

Use an administration set with an air inlet in the plastic spike since the bottle does not contain a separate airway tube. Follow directions of the particular administration set to be used. Pull the tab to remove the outer aluminum ring and dust cover. Insert the spike aseptically into the bottle through the target area of the rubber stopper. Allow the fluid to flow and remove air from the tubing before irrigation begins.

How Supplied: In 250 mL and 500 mL bottles. 250 mL: **NDC** 0065-0795-25. 500 mL: **NDC** 0065-0795-50.

Storage: Store at 46° to 80° F (8° to 27° C).

References:

1. Faulborn, J., Conway, B.P., Machemer, R., Surgical Complications of Pars Plana Vitreous Surgery. Ophthalmology 85: 116–125, 1978.
2. Haimann, M.H. and Abrams, G. W., Prevention of Lens Opacification During Diabetic Vitrectomy. Ophthalmology 91: 116–121, 1984.

BSS PLUS® ℞
STERILE INTRAOCULAR IRRIGATING SOLUTION
(Balanced Salt Solution Enriched with Bicarbonate, Dextrose and Glutathione)
U.S. Patents Nos. 4,443,432 and 4,550,022

Description: BSS PLUS® is a sterile intraocular irrigating solution for use during all intraocular surgical procedures, even those requiring a relatively long intraocular perfusion time (e.g., pars plana vitrectomy, phacoemulsification, extracapsular cataract extraction/lens aspiration, anterior segment reconstruction, etc.). The solution does not contain a preservative and should be prepared just prior to use in surgery.

Part I: Part I is a sterile 480 mL solution in a 500 mL single-dose bottle to which the Part II concentrate is added. Each mL of Part I contains: Sodium Chloride 7.44 mg, Potassium Chloride 0.395 mg, Dibasic Sodium Phosphate 0.433 mg, Sodium Bicarbonate 2.19 mg, Hydrochloric Acid and/or Sodium Hydroxide (to adjust pH), in Water for Injection.

Part II: Part II is a sterile concentrate in a 20 mL single-dose vial for addition to Part I. Each mL of Part II contains: Calcium Chloride Dihydrate 3.85 mg, Magnesium Chloride Hexahydrate 5 mg, Dextrose 23 mg, Glutathione Disulfide (Oxidized Glutathione) 4.6 mg, in Water for Injection.

After addition of BSS PLUS® Part II to the Part I bottle, each mL of the reconstituted product contains: Sodium Chloride 7.14 mg, Potassium Chloride 0.38 mg, Calcium Chloride Dihydrate 0.154 mg, Magnesium Chloride Hexahydrate 0.2 mg, Dibasic Sodium Phosphate 0.42 mg, Sodium Bicarbonate 2.1 mg, Dextrose 0.92 mg, Glutathione Disulfide (Oxidized Glutathione) 0.184 mg, Hydrochloric Acid and/or Sodium Hydroxide (to adjust pH), in Water for Injection.

The reconstituted product has a pH of approximately 7.4. Osmolality is approximately 305 mOsm.

Clinical Pharmacology: None of the components of BSS PLUS are foreign to the eye, and BSS PLUS has no pharmacological action. Human perfused cornea studies[1-3] have shown BSS PLUS to be an effective irrigation solution for providing corneal detumescence and maintaining corneal endothelial integrity during intraocular perfusion. An *in vivo* study[4] in rabbits has shown that BSS PLUS is more suitable than normal saline or Balanced Salt Solution for intravitreal irrigation because BSS PLUS contains the appropriate bicarbonate, pH, and ionic composition necessary for the maintenance of normal retinal electrical activity. Human *in vivo* studies have demonstrated BSS PLUS to be safe and effective when used during surgical procedures such as pars plana vitrectomy, phacoemulsification, cataract extraction/lens aspiration and anterior segment reconstruction.

Indications and Usage: BSS PLUS is indicated for use as an intraocular irrigating solution during intraocular surgical procedures involving perfusion of the eye.

Contraindications: There are no specific contraindications to the use of BSS PLUS, however, contraindications for the surgical procedure during which BSS PLUS is to be used should be strictly adhered to.

Warnings: For IRRIGATION during ophthalmic surgery only. Not for injection or intravenous infusion. Do not use unless product is clear, seal is intact, vacuum is present and container is undamaged. Do not use if product is discolored or contains a precipitate.

Precautions: DO NOT USE BSS PLUS UNTIL RECONSTITUTED. **Discard unused contents. BSS PLUS does not contain a preservative, therefore, do not use this container for more than one patient.** Do not use additives other than BSS PLUS Concentrate Part II (20 mL) with this product. Tissue damage could result if other drugs are added to product. DISCARD ANY UNUSED PORTION SIX HOURS AFTER PREPARATION. Studies suggest that intraocular irrigating solutions which are iso-osmotic with normal aqueous fluids should be used with caution in diabetic patients undergoing vitrectomy since intraoperative lens changes have been observed.[5,6]

There have been reports of corneal clouding or edema following ocular surgery in which BSS PLUS was used as an irrigating solution. As in all surgical procedures appropriate measures should be taken to minimize trauma to the cornea and other ocular tissues.

Preparation: Reconstitute BSS PLUS® just prior to use in surgery. Follow the same strict aseptic procedures in the reconstitution of BSS PLUS as is used for intravenous additives. Pull the tab to remove the outer aluminum ring and dust cover from the BSS PLUS Part I (480 mL) bottle. Remove the blue flip-off seal from the BSS PLUS Part II (20 mL) vial. Clean and disinfect the rubber stoppers on both containers by using sterile alcohol wipes. Transfer the contents of the Part II vial to the Part I bottle using a BSS PLUS Vacuum Transfer Device (provided). An alternative method of solution transfer may be accomplished by using a 20 mL syringe to remove the Part II solution from the vial and transferring exactly 20 mL to the Part I container through the target area of the rubber stopper. An excess volume of Part II is provided in each vial. Gently agitate the contents to mix the solution. Place a sterile cap on the bottle. Remove the tear-off portion of the label. Record the time and date of reconstitution and the patient's name on the bottle label.

Adverse Reactions: Postoperative inflammatory reactions as well as incidents of corneal edema and corneal decompensation have been reported. Their relationship to the use of BSS PLUS has not been established.

Overdosage: The solution has no pharmacological action and thus has no potential for overdosage. However, as with any intraocular surgical procedure, the duration of intraocular manipulation should be kept to a minimum.

Dosage and Administration: The solution should be used according to the technique standardly employed by the operating surgeon. Use an administration set with an air inlet in the plastic spike since the bottle does not contain a separate airway tube. Follow the directions for the particular administration set to be used. Insert the spike aseptically into the bottle through the target area of the rubber stopper. Allow the fluid to flow to remove air from the tubing before intraocular irrigation begins. If a second bottle is necessary to complete the surgical procedure, insure that the vacuum is vented from the second bottle BEFORE attachment to the administration set.

How Supplied: BSS PLUS is supplied in two packages for reconstitution prior to use: a 500 mL bottle containing 480 mL (Part I) and a 20 mL vial (Part II). See the **Precautions** and **Preparation** sections for information concerning reconstitution of the solution.

NDC 0065-0800-50.

Storage: Store Part I and Part II at 46°–80°F (8°–27°C). Discard prepared solution after six hours.

Caution: Federal (USA) law prohibits dispensing without prescription.

References:

1. Edelhauser, H. F., Van Horn, D. L., Hyndiuk, R. A., Schultz, R. O., Intraocular Irrigation Solutions: Their Effect on the Corneal Endothelium. **Arch. Ophthalmol., 93,** 648, 1975.
2. Edelhauser, H. F., Van Horn, D. L., Schultz, R. O., Hyndiuk, R. A., Comparative Toxicity of Intraocular Irrigating Solutions on the

Corneal Endothelium, **Am. J. Ophthalmol., 81,** 473, 1976.
3 Edelhauser, H. F., Gonnering, R., Van Horn, D. L., Intraocular Irrigating Solutions: A Comparative Study of BSS PLUS and Lactated Ringer's Solution, **Arch. Ophthalmol., 96,** 516, 1978.
4 Moorhead, L. C., Redburn, D. A., Merritt, J., Garcia, C. A., The Effects of Intravitreal Irrigation During Vitrectomy on the Electroretinogram, **Am. J. Ophthalmol., 88,** 239, 1979.
5 Faulborn, J., Conway, B. P., Machemer, R., Surgical Complications of Pars Plana Vitreous Surgery. **Ophthalmology 85:** 116–125, 1978.
6 Haimann, M. H., and Abrams, G. W., Prevention of Lens Opacification During Diabetic Vitrectomy. **Ophthalmology, 91:**116–121, 1984.

RECONSTITUTION INSTRUCTIONS

Directions: Use Aseptic Technique

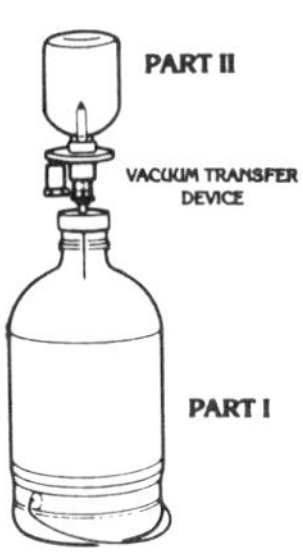

1. Pull the tab to remove the outer aluminum ring and dust cover from the BSS PLUS® Part I (480mL) bottle. Remove the blue flip-off seal from the BSS PLUS Part II (20mL) vial. Prepare the stoppers on both parts by using sterile alcohol wipes.
2. Peel open a BSS PLUS Vacuum Transfer Device package (supplied) and remove the sterile transfer spike.
NOTE: This device is vented permitting air to enter vial during solution transfer, thereby preventing the creation of a vacuum inside the vial. An air-inlet filter is provided to protect the system. Do not remove the air-inlet filter.
3. Remove protector from the white plastic piercing pin.
4. Firmly grasp device from behind the flange and insert the white plastic piercing pin into the upright rubber stopper of the BSS PLUS Part II (20mL) vial.
5. Remove guard from filter needle. Firmly grasp vial in the palm of one hand and with thumb and index finger, hold plastic flange against top of vial.
6. Invert vial and immediately insert filter needle into the rubber injection site of the BSS PLUS Part I (480mL) bottle.
(See illustration.)
7. Fluid will automatically transfer from the vial into the large vacuum bottle unless filter becomes occluded or loss of vacuum occurs. NOTE: An excess amount of BSS PLUS Part II is provided in each vial. A non-transferred solution residual of approximately 0.3mL can be expected to remain in the vial.
8. Immediately remove needle from the BSS PLUS® Part I container and discard it after solution transfer has been completed.
9. Place a sterile safety cap over the rubber stopper of Part I if the solution is not going to be used immediately. Mix the solution gently until uniform. Peel off the right-hand side of Part I bottle label (fully reconstituted BSS PLUS Solution). Record the patient's name and the date and time of reconstitution.
BSS PLUS Solution is now ready for use.
Caution: Reconstituted BSS PLUS Solution must be used within six hours of mixing. Discard any solution which has aged beyond that time. Never use the same bottle of BSS PLUS Solution on more than one patient.

Alternative Transfer Method

If preferred, the contents of the BSS PLUS Part II component may be aspirated with an 18-gauge cannula attached to a 20mL syringe and then transferred into the Part I bottle.

ENUCLENE® OTC

Cleaning/Lubricating Solution for Artificial Eyes

Ingredients: Each mL contains: Active: Tyloxapol 0.25%, Benzalkonium Chloride 0.02%.

Description: ENUCLENE® is a sterile, buffered, isotonic solution formulated especially for artificial eye wearers. ENUCLENE Solution lubricates, cleans, and wets the artificial eye, thereby increasing the wearing comfort to the patient. In addition, ENUCLENE Solution contains sufficient concentration of the antibacterial agent, Benzalkonium Chloride, to kill most germs which are commonly found in the eye socket of artificial eye wearers.

ENUCLENE Solution contains a special ingredient, Tyloxapol, which is a detergent. It liquefies the solid matter so that it is less irritating. Laboratory tests show that ENUCLENE Solution causes no harmful effects to artificial eyes. Benzalkonium Chloride, in addition to its germ killing action, aids Tyloxapol in wetting the artificial eye so that it is completely covered. This combination of wetting, cleansing, and lubricating, and also the softening of thickened matter, makes ENUCLENE Solution an ideal product for artificial eye wearers.

ENUCLENE Solution is recommended for wearers of artificial eyes. In clinical studies, the use of this preparation was found to improve the wearing effects of the artificial eye by its soothing action, thus reducing the undesirable effects of secretions of the glands in the mucous membrane of the eye socket.

Contraindications: Contraindicated in those persons who have shown hypersensitivity to any component of this preparation.

Caution: If irritation persists or increases, discontinue use and consult physician. Keep container tightly closed. Keep out of reach of children.

Warning: Do not touch dropper tip to any surface since this may contaminate solution.

Directions: The drops should be used just as ordinary eye drops are used. With the artificial eye in place, drop 1 or 2 drops onto it, 3 or 4 times daily. The artificial eye may be removed periodically if advised by the physician and 2 or 3 drops applied to remove oily or mucous materials. The artificial eye is then rubbed between the fingers and rinsed with tap water. Then 1 or 2 drops may then be applied to the artificial eye, either prior to or after reinsertion.

How Supplied: ½ fl. oz. (15 mL) in sterile DROP-TAINER® Dispenser.

Storage: Store at 46°–80°F (8°–27°C).

ISMOTIC® ℞

(Isosorbide Solution)
45% w/v Solution

Description: ISMOTIC® is a 45% w/v solution of isosorbide in a vanilla-mint flavored vehicle. ISMOTIC is a caramel colored aqueous solution that is chemically stable at room temperature.

Each mL contains: Isosorbide 45% w/v (Isosorbide Concentrate 60.6%), Alcohol 0.3% w/v, Caramel, Creme de Menthe, Malic Acid, Potassium Citrate, Potassium Sorbate, Saccharin Calcium, Sodium Citrate, Sorbitol Solution, Vanilla Concentrate Imitation #20, Potassium Hydroxide (to adjust pH) and Purified Water.

Typical analysis of electrolyte content:
4.6 meq. of Sodium/220 mL ISMOTIC Solution
0.9 meq. of Potassium/220 mL ISMOTIC Solution

Isosorbide, the osmotic agent in ISMOTIC, is a dihydric alcohol with the formula $C_6H_{10}O_4$ represented by the structure:

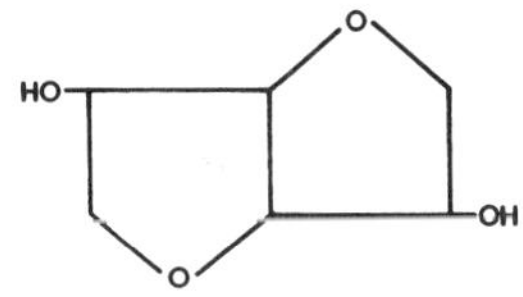

Established name:
Isosorbide

Chemical name:
1,4:3,6-dianhydro-D-glucitol

Clinical Pharmacology: Isosorbide is rapidly absorbed after oral administration. It is essentially non-metabolized, and in the circulation, it contributes to the tonicity of the blood until it is eliminated by the kidney unchanged. While in the blood, isosorbide acts as an osmotic agent to promote redistribution of water toward the circulation with ultimate elimination in the urine. The physical action of ISMOTIC is similar to that of other osmotic drugs.

Indications and Usage: For the short-term reduction of intraocular pressure. May be used prior to and after intraocular surgery. May be used to interrupt an acute attack of glaucoma. Use where less risk of nausea and vomiting than that posed by other oral hyperosmotic agents is needed.

Contraindications:
1. Well-established anuria.
2. Severe dehydration.
3. Frank or impending acute pulmonary edema.
4. Severe cardiac decompensation.
5. Hypersensitivity to any component of this preparation.

Warnings:
1. With repeated doses, consideration should be given to maintenance of adequate fluid and electrolyte balance.
2. If urinary output continues to decrease, the patient's clinical status should be closely reviewed. Accumulation of ISMOTIC may result in over-expansion of the extracellular fluid.

As with all medications, keep out of the reach of children.

Precautions: For oral use only—not for injection. Repetitive doses should be used with caution particularly in patients with diseases associated with salt retention. Ensure that patient's bladder has been emptied prior to surgery.

Usage in Pregnancy: Pregnancy Category B: Reproduction studies have been performed in rats and rabbits and there was no evidence of impaired fertility or harm to the animal fetus due to isosorbide. There are no adequate or well controlled studies on whether this drug may affect fertility in human males or females or have a teratogenic potential or other adverse effect on the fetus. Because animal reproduction studies are not always predictive of human responses, this drug should be used during pregnancy only if clearly needed.

Adverse Reactions: Nausea, vomiting, headache, confusion and disorientation may occur. Occurrences of syncope, gastric discomfort, lethargy, vertigo, thirst, dizziness, hiccups, hypernatremia, hyperosmolarity, irritability, rash, and light-headedness have been reported.

Dosage and Administration: The recommended initial dose 1.5 gm/kg body weight of

Continued on next page

Alcon Surgical—Cont.

isosorbide (equivalent to 1.5 mL/lb. of body weight). The onset of action is usually within 30 minutes while the maximum effect is expected at 1 to 1½ hours. The useful dose range is 1 to 3 gm/kg body weight and the drug effect will persist up to 5 to 6 hours. Use two to four times a day as indicated. Palatability may be improved if the medication is poured over cracked ice and sipped.

RECOMMENDED DOSAGES ARE:

POUNDS	MILLI-LITERS	POUNDS	MILLI-LITERS
100	150	155	235
105	155	160	240
110	165	165	250
115	170	170	255
120	180	175	265
125	190	180	270
130	195	185	280
135	205	190	285
140	210	195	295
145	220	200	300
150	225		

Storage: Store at room temperature.
How Supplied: Disposable plastic bottles of 220 mL (100 gm of isosorbide/220 mL) for oral use only. NDC 0065-0034-08
Caution: Federal (USA) law prohibits dispensing without prescription.

MIOSTAT® ℞
(CARBACHOL 0.01%)
INTRAOCULAR SOLUTION

Description: MIOSTAT® (Carbachol 0.01%) is a sterile balanced salt solution of Carbachol for intraocular injection. The active ingredient is represented by the chemical structure:

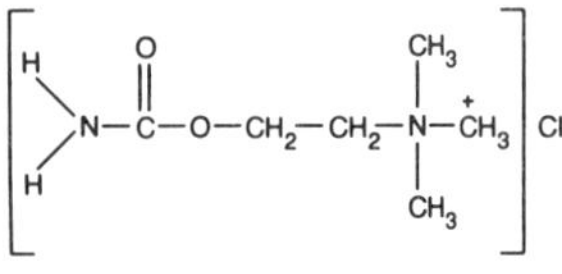

Established name: Carbachol
Chemical name: Ethanaminium, 2-[(aminocarbonyl)oxy]-*N,N,N*-trimethyl-, chloride.
Each mL contains: Active: Carbachol 0.01%. Inactives: Sodium Chloride 0.64%, Potassium Chloride 0.075%, Calcium Chloride Dihydrate 0.048%, Magnesium Chloride Hexahydrate 0.03%, Sodium Acetate Trihydrate 0.39%, Sodium Citrate Dihydrate 0.17%, Sodium Hydroxide and/or Hydrochloric Acid (to adjust pH) and Water for Injection.
Clinical Pharmacology: Carbachol is a potent cholinergic (parasympathomimetic) agent.
Indications and Usage: Intraocular use for miosis during surgery.
Contraindications: Should not be used in those persons showing hypersensitivity to any of the components of this preparation.
Warnings: For single-dose intraocular use only. Discard unused portion. Intraocular carbachol 0.01% should be used with caution in patients with acute cardiac failure, bronchial asthma, peptic ulcer, hyperthyroidism, G. I. spasm, urinary tract obstruction and Parkinson's disease.
Adverse Reactions: Side effects such as flushing, sweating, epigastric distress, abdominal cramps, tightness in urinary bladder, and headache have been reported after systemic or topical use of carbachol. These symptoms were not reported following intraocular use of carbachol 0.01% in pre-marketing studies. Corneal clouding, persistent bullous keratopathy and post-operative iritis following cataract extraction with utilization of intraocular carbachol have been reported in an occasional patient. As with all miotics, retinal detachment has been reported when miotics are used in certain susceptible individuals.
Overdosage: Atropine should be administered parenterally (for dosage refer to Goodman & Gilman or other pharmacology reference).
Dosage and Administration: Aseptically remove the sterile vial from the blister package by peeling the backing paper and dropping the vial onto a sterile tray. Withdraw the contents into a dry sterile syringe, and replace the needle with an atraumatic cannula prior to intraocular irrigation. **No more than one-half milliliter** should be gently instilled into the anterior chamber for the production of satisfactory miosis. It may be instilled before or after securing sutures. Miosis is usually maximal within two to five minutes after application.
How Supplied: In 1.5 mL sterile glass vials packaged twelve to a carton.
NDC 0065-0023-15
Storage: Store at controlled room temperature 15°–30°C (59°–86°F).
Caution: Federal (USA) law prohibits dispensing without prescription.

OSMOGLYN® ℞
[50% Glycerin (volume/volume)]
Oral Osmotic Agent

OSMOGLYN® Oral Osmotic Agent is a 50% v/v (0.628 g/mL) solution of Glycerin in a pleasantly lime flavored aqueous vehicle. It is administered orally, thereby avoiding the hazards of hypertonic agents that must be given intravenously.
Description: Active: glycerin 50% v/v (0.628 g/mL). Preservative: potassium sorbate 0.05%. Inactive: lime flavor, purified water.
Linear structure of Glycerin is: $CH_2OH \cdot CHOH \cdot CH_2OH$.
Chemical name: 1,2,3-Propanetriol.
CAUTION: FEDERAL (USA) LAW PROHIBITS DISPENSING WITHOUT PRESCRIPTION.
Clinical Pharmacology: An oral osmotic agent for reducing intraocular pressure. It adds to the tonicity of the blood until metabolized and eliminated by the kidneys.
Indications and Usage: For the short term reduction of intraocular pressure. May be used prior to and after intraocular surgery. May be used to interrupt an acute attack of glaucoma.
Contraindications: Contraindicated in patients with well-established anuria; severe dehydration; frank or impending acute pulmonary edema; severe cardiac decompensation; and in those with hypersensitivity to any component of this preparation.
Warnings: For oral use only. Not for injection. Caution should be exercised in hypervolemia, confused mental states, and congestive heart disease; and in the dehydrated patient, e.g., certain diabetics.
Precautions: When administered prior to surgery, ensure that the patient's bladder is emptied. Prolonged use may cause excess weight gain. Glycerin should be administered with caution to patients with cardiac, renal or hepatic diseases. Altered hydration may lead to pulmonary edema and/or congestive heart failure.
PREGNACY CATEGORY C. Animal reproduction studies have not been conducted with OSMOGLYN®. It is also not known whether OSMOGLYN can cause fetal harm when administered to a pregnant woman or can affect reproduction capacity. This drug should be given to a pregnant woman only if clearly needed.
Adverse Reactions: Nausea, vomiting, headache, confusion, and disorientation may occur. Severe dehydration, cardiac arrhythmia, or hyperosmolar nonketotic coma which can result in death have been reported.
Dosage and Administration: Usual dosage is 2 to 3 mL of OSMOGLYN per kg of body weight (approximately 4 to 6 oz. per individual), given 1 to 1½ hours prior to surgery. Serving over cracked ice with a soda straw improves palatability.
Storage: Store at room temperature.
How Supplied: 220 mL NDC 0065-0035-08.

PROFENAL® 1% ℞
(Suprofen)
Sterile Ophthalmic Solution

Description: PROFENAL® (suprofen) 1% ophthalmic solution is a topical nonsteroidal anti-inflammatory product for ophthalmic use. Suprofen chemically is α-methyl-4-(2-thienylcarbonyl) benzeneacetic acid, with an empirical formula of $C_{14}H_{12}O_3S$, and a molecular weight of 260.3. The chemical structure of suprofen is:

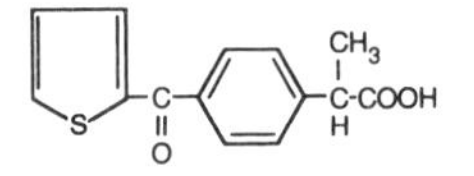

PROFENAL Sterile Ophthalmic Solution contains suprofen 1.0% (10 mg/mL), thimerosal 0.005% (0.05 mg/mL), caffeine 2% (20 mg/mL), edetate disodium, dibasic sodium phosphate, monobasic sodium phosphate, sodium chloride, sodium hydroxide and/or hydrochloric acid (to adjust pH to 7.4) and purified water.
Clincal Pharmacology: Suprofen is one of a series of phenylalkanoic acids that have shown analgesic, antipyretic, and anti-inflammatory activity in animal inflammatory diseases. Its mechanism of action is believed to be through inhibition of the cyclo-oxygenase enzyme that is essential in the biosynthesis of prostaglandins.
Prostaglandins have been shown in many animal models to be mediators of certain kinds of intraocular inflammation. In studies performed on animal eyes, prostaglandins have been shown to produce disruption of the blood-aqueous humor barrier, vasodilatation, increased vascular permeability, leukocytosis, and increased intraocular pressure. Prostaglandins appear to play a role in the miotic response produced during ocular surgery by constricting the iris sphincter independently of cholinergic mechanisms. In clinical studies, PROFENAL has been shown to inhibit the miosis induced during the course of cataract surgery. PROFENAL could possibly interfere with the miotic effect of intraoperatively administered acetylcholine chloride.
Results from clinical studies indicate that PROFENAL Ophthalmic Solution has no significant effect on intraocular pressure.
There are no data available on the systemic absorption of ocularly applied suprofen. The oral dose of suprofen is 200 mg every four to six hours. If PROFENAL 1% Ophthalmic Solution is applied as two drops (1 mg suprofen) to one eye five times on the day prior to surgery and three times on the day of surgery, the total applied dose over the two days would be about 25 times less than a single 200 mg oral dose.
Indications and Usage: PROFENAL Ophthalmic Solution is indicated for inhibition of intraoperative miosis.
Contraindications: PROFENAL is contraindicated in epithelial herpes simplex keratitis (dendritic keratitis) and in individuals hypersensitive to any component of the medication.
Warnings: The potential exists for cross sensitivity to acetylsalicylic acid and other nonsteroidal anti-inflammatory drugs. Therefore, caution should be used when treating individu-

als who have previously exhibited sensitivities to these drugs.

With nonsteroidal anti-inflammatory drugs, the potential exists for increased bleeding time due to interference with thrombocyte aggregation. There have been reports that ocularly applied nonsteroidal anti-inflammatory drugs may cause increased bleeding tendency of ocular tissues in conjunction with ocular surgery.

Precautions:

General. Use of oral suprofen has been associated with a syndrome of acute flank pain and generally reversible renal insufficiency, which may present as acute uric acid nephropathy. This syndrome occurs in approximately 1 in 3500 patients and has been reported with as few as one to two doses of a 200 mg capsule. If PROFENAL 1% Ophthalmic Solution is applied as two drops (1 mg suprofen) to one eye five times on the day prior to surgery and three times on the day of surgery, the total applied dose over the two days would be about 25 times less than a single 200 mg oral dose. Do not touch dropper tip to any surface, as this may contaminate the solution.

Ocular. Patients with histories of herpes simplex keratitis should be monitored closely. PROFENAL is contraindicated in patients with active herpes simplex keratitis.

The possibility of increased ocular bleeding during surgery associated with nonsteroidal anti-inflammatory drugs should be considered.

Carcinogenesis, Mutagenesis, Impairment of Fertility. In an 18-month study in mice, an increased incidence of benign hepatomas occurred in females at a dose of 40 mg/kg/day. Male mice, treated at doses of 2, 5, 10 and 40 mg/kg/day, also had an increased incidence of hepatomas when compared to control animals. No evidence of carcinogenicity was found in long term studies in doses as high as 40 mg/kg/day in the rat and mouse. Based on a battery of mutagenicity tests (Ames, micronucleus, and dominant lethal) suprofen does not appear to have mutagenic potential. Reproductive studies in rats at a dose of up to 40 mg/kg/day revealed no impairment of fertility and only slight reductions of fertility at doses of 80 mg/kg/day. However, testicular atrophy/hypoplasia was observed in a six-month dog study (at 80 mg/kg/day) and a 12-month rat study (at 40 mg/kg/day).

Pregnancy Category C. Reproductive studies have been performed in rabbits at doses up to 200 mg/kg/day and in rats at doses up to 80 mg/kg/day. In rats, doses of 40 mg/kg/day and above, and in rabbits, doses of 80 mg/kg/day and above, resulted in an increased incidence of fetal resorption associated with maternal toxicity. There was an increase in stillbirths and a decrease in postnatal survival in pregnant rats treated with suprofen at 2.5 mg/kg/day and above. An increased incidence of delayed parturition occurred in rats. As there are no adequate and well-controlled studies in pregnant women, this drug should be used during pregnancy only if the potential benefit justifies the potential risk to the fetus. Because of the known effect of nonsteroidal anti-inflammatory drugs on the fetal cardiovascular system (closure of ductus arteriosus), use during late pregnancy should be avoided.

Nursing Mothers. Suprofen is excreted in human milk after a single oral dose. Based on measurements of plasma and milk levels in women taking oral suprofen, the milk concentration is about 1% of the plasma level. Because systemic absorption may occur from topical ocular administration, a decision should be considered to discontinue nursing while receiving PROFENAL, since the safety of suprofen in human neonates has not been established.

Pediatric Use. Safety and effectiveness in children have not been established.

Drug Interations. Clinical studies with acetylcholine chloride revealed no interference, and there is no known pharmacological basis for such an interaction. However, with other topical nonsteroidal anti-inflammatory products, there have been reports that acetylcholine chloride and carbachol have been ineffective when used in patients treated with these agents.

Interaction of PROFENAL with other topical ophthalmic medications has not been fully investigated.

Adverse Reactions: **Ocular**—The most frequent adverse reactions reported are burning and stinging of short duration. Instances of discomfort, itching and redness have been reported. Other reactions occurring in less than 0.5% of patients include allergy, iritis, pain, chemosis, photophobia, irritation, and punctate epithelial staining.

Systemic—Systemic reactions related to therapy were not reported in the clinical studies. It is known that some systemic absorption does occur with ocularly applied drugs, and that nonsteroidal anti-inflammatory drugs have been shown to increase bleeding time by interference with thrombocyte aggregation. It is recommended that PROFENAL be used with caution in patients with bleeding tendencies and those taking anticoagulants.

Overdosage: Overdosage will not ordinarily cause acute problems. If accidently ingested, drink fluids to dilute.

Dosage and Administration: On the day of surgery, instill two drops into the conjunctival sac at three, two and one hour prior to surgery. Two drops may be instilled into the conjunctival sac every four hours, while awake, the day preceding surgery.

How Supplied: Sterile ophthalmic solution, 2.5 mL in plastic DROP-TAINER® dispensers.

2.5mL NDC 0065-0348-25

Storage: Store at room temperature.

Caution: Federal (USA) law prohibits dispensing without prescription.

U.S. Patent Nos. 4,035,376; 4,559,343.

PROSHIELD® ℞

Collagen Corneal Shield

Description: The ProShield® Collagen Corneal Shield is a transparent, thin, pliable collegen film. The source of the collagen is bovine tissue. The 12 hour shield has a base curve of 8.8 mm and a diameter of 14.6 mm. The 24 hour shield has a base curve of 8.8 mm and a diameter of 16.0 mm.

Actions: The shield is designed to provide comfort for post-surgical traumatic and non-traumatic ocular surface conditions by providing a barrier film that temporarily separates the compromised ocular surface from eyelid movements.

When hydrated and applied to the eye, the shield conforms to the ocular surface. The slow dissolution of the shield (over approximately 12 or 24 hours) provides a lubricating layer while normal healing occurs.

Indications for Use: The ProShield® Collagen Corneal Shield is indicated for relief of discomfort from post-surgical, traumatic and non-traumatic corneal conditions.

Contraindications: The ProShield® Collagen Corneal Shield must not be used on infected wounds.

Physicians should exercise professional judgment in using the ProShield® Collagen Corneal Shield on patients who demonstrate the following conditions:

- Corneal Anesthesia
- Evidence of Acute External Ocular Infections
- Intraocular Infection
- Monocular Patients
- Dysthyroid Ophthalmopathy
- Nasal Lacrimal Obstruction
- Blepharitis
- Chalazion
- Lax Lids
- Dry Eye Syndrome
- Allergic Reaction to Collagen
- Allergic Reaction to Bovine-Derived Products

Precautions: The sterile, sealed package containing the ProShield® Collagen Corneal Shield should be stored at room temperature. Avoid heat above 40°C (104°F), or temperature at or below freezing.

Do not resterilize. Discard all open and unused shields.

Physicians should use care in screening their patients for any known allergies to collagen or bovine-derived products. In addition, patients should be monitored for reactions to the ProShield® Collagen Corneal Shield, (i.e., conjunctival hyperemia and edema, erythema, lacrimation, and pruritus).

Recommended Instructions for Use: Fill the well that surrounds the shield with BSS® (Balanced Salt Solution) sterile irrigating solution so that the shield is completely immersed. Hydrate the shield for a minimum of ten minutes. Remove the shield from the well and place over the ocular surface as you would a soft contact lens. If desired, one or two drops of hydrating fluid may be placed in the bowl of the shield just prior to placement. The eye should be patched.

Lubricating solutions may be used while the shield is in place. Unpreserved solutions are recommended.

The physician should exercise professional judgment in using the ProShield® Collagen Corneal Shield for repeated application.

How Supplied: Each shield is sterile and supplied in a sterile tray. The tray is marked with the lot number and expiration date.

ProShield® 12 Hour Collagen Corneal Shield
CAT. NO. 8065-1014-01
ProShield® 24 Hour Collagen Corneal Shield
CAT. NO. 8065-1017-01

STERI-UNITS® Solutions ℞

Description:

STERILE OPHTHALMIC SOLUTIONS FOR SINGLE USE ONLY.

Packaged in pre-sterilized ready to use units.
Sterile unless opened or damaged
Except for 2% Fluorescein Sodium, no preservatives are added to the solutions.

Ophthalmic solutions available in STERI-UNITS containers are:

1% or 2% Atropine Sulfate
1%, 2%, 4%, or 8% Pilocarpine Hydrochloride
0.5% Tetracaine Hydrochloride
15% Sulfacetamide Sodium
5% Homatropine Hydrobromide
2% Fluorescein Sodium

How Supplied: In 2 mL sterile blister packs, packaged 12 to a carton.

The Indices are divided into five parts –
Part I Manufacturers' Index,
Part II Product Name Index,
Part III Product Category Index,
Part IV Active Ingredients Index,
Part V Instrumentation Index.

Allergan, Inc.
Medical Optics Division
9701 JERONIMO ROAD
IRVINE, CA 92718-2020

AMO®ENDOSOL® ℞
(Balanced Salt Solution)

Description: **AMO®ENDOSOL®** is a sterile, physiologically balanced salt solution containing essential ions (Na^+, K^+, Ca^{++}, Mg^{++}, Cl^-, acetate and citrate) to irrigate and help maintain the integrity of the ocular tissues during ophthalmic surgical procedures.

AMO®ENDOSOL® contains:

Sodium Chloride (NaCl)	0.64%
Potassium Chloride (KCl)	0.075%
Calcium Chloride, Dihydrate ($CaCl_2 \cdot 2H_2O$)	0.048%
Magnesium Chloride, Hexahydrate ($MgCl_2 \cdot 6H_2O$)	0.03%
Sodium Acetate, Trihydrate ($C_2H_3NaO_2 \cdot 3H_2O$)	0.39%
Sodium Citrate, Dihydrate ($C_6H_5Na_3O_7 \cdot 2H_2O$)	0.17%

and Water for Injection, with Sodium Hydroxide and/or Hydrochloric Acid to adjust the solution to physiologic pH. The solution is isotonic and has the following electrolyte content (mEq/liter): Na^+ 156, K^+ 10, Ca^{++} 6.5, Mg^{++} 3, Cl^- 129, acetate 29, and citrate 17.

AMO®ENDOSOL® contains no bacteriostat or antimicrobial agent and is intended for use only as a single-dose or short procedure irrigant.

Clinical Pharmacology:
AMO®ENDOSOL® is a physiological irrigation solution. It does not contain organic agents with pharmacological activity.

Indications and Usage: For irrigation during ophthalmic surgery, and surgical procedures of ears, nose or throat requiring a physiological irrigant.

Warnings: Not for parenteral injection or infusion.

Precautions: **AMO®ENDOSOL®** does not contain a preservative and should not be reused after opening. Do not use if seal assembly or bottle is damaged. Do not use 18 mL bottle if blister package is opened or damaged. Open only under aseptic conditions. Do not use the product unless product is clear.

Adverse Reactions: When used for intraocular surgery in cases where the corneal endothelium is abnormal, excessive intraocular irrigation (as well as other intraocular manipulations) may contribute to endothelial damage and result in bullous keratopathy.

Dosage and Administration:
AMO®ENDOSOL® should be used according to standard format for each surgical procedure. Irrigating solutions should be visually inspected for particulate matter and discoloration prior to administration, whenever solution container permits.
Tissue damage could result if other drugs are added to product.

• **For 500 mL plastic bottles**
An administration set equipped with an air inlet device in the plastic spike end should be used since the container does not have an airway tube.
1. Flip off plastic cap from the aluminum seal assembly.
2. Using aseptic technique, it is recommended to insert the spike through the larger circular, indented area of the rubber plug.
3. Prior to irrigating, invert the bottle and allow solution to flow entire length of tubing so air is purged from the tubing.

• **For 18 mL plastic bottles**
The Luer-Lok® adapter is designed to accept a needle or other device with reciprocal fitting. For external irrigation, attachment of any device may not be necessary. To use the container in an aseptic field:
1. Remove the backing material to expose the container of **AMO®ENDOSOL®**.
2. Aseptically transfer the container out of the plastic tray and remove the protective cap with a brisk twist to reveal the adapter.
3. Attach needle or appropriate attachment by pushing it firmly onto the adapter and twisting into place.
4. Prior to use, test the assembly to ensure proper function.

How Supplied: **AMO®ENDOSOL®** is supplied in sterile plastic bottles:
18 mL NDC 0023-0850-02
500 mL NDC 0023-0850-50

Caution: Federal (U.S.A.) law prohibits dispensing without prescription.

Recommended storage: Room temperature ranges from 46°F to 80°F (8°C–27°C). Avoid excessive heat. Protect from freezing.

Luer-Lok® is a registered trademark of Becton-Dickinson.

AMO®ENDOSOL *EXTRA*® ℞
(Balanced Salt Solution Enriched with Bicarbonate, Dextrose and Glutathione)

Description: **AMO®ENDOSOL *EXTRA*®** is a sterile intraocular irrigating solution for use during surgical procedures, including those requiring a relatively long intraocular perfusion time (e.g., pars plana vitrectomy, phacoemulsification, extracapsular cataract extraction/lens aspiration, anterior segment reconstruction, etc.). **The solution does not contain a preservative and should be prepared just prior to use in surgery.**

Part I:
Part I is a sterile 515 mL solution in a 515 mL single use bottle to which the Part II sterile powdered concentrate is added. Each mL of Part I contains: Sodium Chloride 7.14 mg, Potassium Chloride 0.38 mg, Calcium Chloride Dihydrate 0.154 mg, Magnesium Chloride Hexahydrate 0.20 mg, Dextrose 0.92 mg, Hydrochloric Acid and/or Sodium Hydroxide (to adjust pH), in Water for Injection.

Part II:
Part II is a sterile lyophilized powder in a 60 mL vial for addition to Part I. Part II contains: Sodium Bicarbonate 1,081 mg, Dibasic, Sodium Phosphate (Anhy) 216 mg, Glutathione Disulfide (Oxidized Glutathione) 95 mg.

After addition of **AMO®ENDOSOL *EXTRA*®** Part II to the Part I bottle, each mL of the reconstituted product contains: Sodium Chloride 7.14 mg, Potassium Chloride 0.38 mg, Calcium Chloride Dihydrate 0.154 mg, Magnesium Chloride Hexahydrate 0.20 mg, Dibasic, Sodium Phosphate (Anhy) 0.42 mg, Sodium Bicarbonate 2.1 mg, Dextrose 0.92 mg, Glutathione Disulfide (Oxidized Glutathione) 0.184 mg, Hydrochloric Acid and/or Sodium Hydroxide (to adjust pH), in Water for Injection.

The reconstituted product has pH of approximately 7.4. Osmolarity is approximately 305 mOsmol/L.

Clinical Pharmacology: In human perfused cornea studies, the components of **AMO®ENDOSOL *EXTRA*®** have been shown to be effective in providing corneal detumescence and maintaining corneal endothelial integrity. Human in vivo studies have demonstrated the components of **AMO®ENDOSOL *EXTRA*®** to be safe and effective when used during surgical procedures such as pars plana vitrectomy, phacoemulsification, cataract extraction, and anterior segment reconstruction.

Indication and Usage: **AMO®ENDOSOL *EXTRA*®** is indicated for use as an intraocular irrigating solution during intraocular surgical procedures involving perfusion of the eye.

Contraindications: None known.

Warnings: For irrigation during ophthalmic surgery only; **AMO®ENDOSOL *EXTRA*®** is NOT for injection or intravenous infusion.
Reconstituted **AMO®ENDOSOL *EXTRA*®** must be used within 6 hours of mixing. Discard any solution which has aged beyond that time. Never use the same bottle of **AMO®ENDOSOL *EXTRA*®** on more than one patient.
NEVER use Part 1 (515 mL) Solution at any time without reconstitution with Part II Small Volume vial. This could result in damage to the eye.

Precautions:
General: DO NOT USE **AMO®ENDOSOL *EXTRA*®** UNTIL RECONSTITUTED. DO NOT USE ADDITIVES OTHER THAN PART II. NOT FOR INJECTION. Do not use if the reconstituted solution is discolored or contains a precipitate. SINCE **AMO®ENDOSOL *EXTRA*®** IS INTENDED FOR INTRAOCULAR IRRIGATION, IT DOES NOT CONTAIN A PRESERVATIVE AND THEREFORE, SHOULD NOT BE USED FOR MORE THAN ONE PATIENT. DISCARD ANY UNUSED PORTION SIX HOURS AFTER PREPARATION. Studies suggest that intraocular irrigating solutions which are isosmotic with normal aqueous fluids should be used with caution in diabetic patients undergoing vitrectomy since intraoperative lens changes have been observed.

Carcinogenesis, mutagenesis, impairment of fertility: No long term studies in animals have been performed to evaluate the carcinogenic potential.

Pregnancy: Teratogenic effects. Pregnancy Category C. Animal reproduction studies have not been conducted with **AMO®ENDOSOL *EXTRA*®**. It is also not known whether **AMO®ENDOSOL *EXTRA*®** can cause fetal harm when administered to a pregnant woman or can affect reproductive capacity. **AMO®ENDOSOL *EXTRA*®** should be given to pregnant women only if clearly needed.

Nursing mothers: Caution should be exercised when **AMO®ENDOSOL *EXTRA*®** is administered to a nursing mother.

Pediatric use: Safety and effectiveness in children have not been established.

Adverse Reactions: There have been reports of corneal clouding and edema following ocular surgery in which irrigating solutions have been used.

Dosage and Administration: The solution should be used, according to the technique standardly employed by the operating surgeon. Use an administration set with an air inlet in the plastic spike since the bottle does not contain a separate airway tube.
Follow the directions for the particular administration set to be used. Insert the spike aseptically into the bottle through the target area of the rubber stopper. Allow the fluid to flow to remove air from the tubing before intraocular irrigation begins.
Reconstitute **AMO®ENDOSOL *EXTRA*®** just prior to use in surgery. Follow the same strict aseptic procedures in the reconstitution of **AMO®ENDOSOL *EXTRA*®** as is used for intravenous additives.
Peel open an **AMO®ENDOSOL *EXTRA*®** Part II/Transfer Spike Package (supplied) and remove the sterile transfer spike. To mix the two parts, remove the blue cap from the Part I Large Volume (515 mL) solution bottle and the blue flip-off cap from the Part II Small Volume powder vial. Prepare the stoppers on both parts by using sterile alcohol wipes. Remove one protector from either white plastic spike. Note: Leave the other white spike protector in place until ready for use. Firmly grasp the transfer spike from behind the flange and insert the white, exposed, plastic spike into the upright rubber stopper of the

AMO®ENDOSOL *EXTRA*® Part II Small Volume vial. Remove the spike protector from the remaining white plastic spike. Invert Part II Small Volume vial and immediately insert exposed plastic spike into the rubber stopper of the Part I (515 mL) bottle. Squeeze the large Part I bottle to force fluid into the vial and then release. The fluid and powder (already partly dissolved) will then return to the large bottle. Repeat this "squeeze and release" several times to flush all contents of the Part II Small Volume vial into the Large Volume bottle. In order to prevent solution from dripping out of the transfer spike, first invert the large bottle (Part I) and then remove the small vial (Part II) with transfer spike. Manually agitate the large bottle (Part I) for five (5) seconds or until all of the powder from the small vial (Part II) has gone into solution. Peel off the right section of the Part I label (fully reconstituted **AMO®ENDOSOL *EXTRA*®**) at the perforation. Record the patient's name and the date and time of reconstitution on the space provided on the label. The solution is now ready for use.

How Supplied: AMO®ENDOSOL *EXTRA*® (NDC 0023-0005-51) is supplied in two parts for reconstitution prior to use: a 515 mL bottle containing solution (Part I) and a vial containing lyophilized powder (Part II) along with a sterile transfer spike for mixing Part I and Part II. See the PRECAUTIONS and DOSAGE AND ADMINISTRATION sections for information concerning reconstitution of the solution.

Store Part I and Part II at 8–27°C (46–80°F).

Discard prepared solution after six (6) hours.

Caution: Federal (U.S.A.) law prohibits dispensing without prescription.

Part I Manufactured By:
ALLERGAN, INC.
Irvine, CA 92718, U.S.A.
(714) 951-0455 (800) 366-6554
Part II Manufactured By:
Ben Venue Laboratories, Inc.
Bedford, OH 44146, U.S.A.

AMO®VITRAX® VISCOELASTIC SOLUTION (SODIUM HYALURONATE) FOR USE IN ANTERIOR SEGMENT SURGERY ONLY ℞

Description: AMO®VITRAX® Viscoelastic Solution is a sterile, nonpyrogenic, viscoelastic preparation of a highly purified, noninflammatory, fraction of sodium hyaluronate. AMO®VITRAX® contains 30 mg/mL of sodium hyaluronate, dissolved in a physiological balanced salt solution (pH 7.0 to 7.5). This polymer is made up of repeating disaccharide units of N-acetylglucosamine and sodium glucuronate linked by glycosidic bonds.

Sodium hyaluronate is a physiological substance that is widely distributed in the extracellular matrix of connective tissues in both animals and man. For example, it is present in the vitreous and aqueous humor of the eye, the synovial fluid, the skin and the umbilical cord. Sodium hyaluronates prepared from various human and animal tissues are not chemically different from each other.

AMO®VITRAX® SODIUM HYALURONATE HAS BEEN DEVELOPED AS AN OPHTHALMIC SURGICAL AID FOR USE IN ANTERIOR SEGMENT SURGERY.

Indications: AMO®VITRAX® sodium hyaluronate is indicated for use as a surgical aid in the following ophthalmic surgical procedures:

- Cataract surgery with an intraocular lens
- Cataract surgery without an intraocular lens
- Secondary intraocular lens implantation
- Corneal transplant surgery
- Glaucoma filtration surgery

AMO®VITRAX® aids in filling space left by the loss of ocular fluid or tissues during or after these surgical procedures and reduces endothelial cell damage during these procedures by acting as a protective layer, reducing endothelial trauma from instruments or intraocular lens touch.

Contraindications: There are no known contraindications for the use of AMO®VITRAX® sodium hyaluronate, other than contraindications for the specific surgical procedure.

Applications:

1. **Cataract Surgery and IOL Implantation**
   The required amount of AMO®VITRAX® is slowly infused through a needle or cannula into the anterior chamber. The protective effect of AMO®VITRAX® as an aid is optimized when the injection is performed prior to cataract extraction and insertion of the IOL and may be performed prior to both intra- and extra-capsular cataract procedures. AMO®VITRAX® may also be used to coat surgical instruments and the IOL prior to insertion. Additional AMO®VITRAX® may be injected during surgery to replace any that is lost during manipulation (see **Precautions**).
2. **Corneal Transplant Surgery**
   The corneal button is removed and the anterior chamber filled with AMO®VITRAX® until it is level with the surface of the cornea. The donor graft is then placed on top of the AMO®VITRAX® and sutured into place. Additional AMO®VITRAX® can be used as required to aid in the surgical procedure (see **Precautions**).
3. **Glaucoma Filtration Surgery**
   AMO®VITRAX® is injected through a corneal paracentesis to restore and maintain the anterior chamber volume during the performance of the trabeculectomy. Additional AMO®VITRAX® can be used as required to aid in the surgical procedure (see **Precautions**).

Precautions: Those precautions normally considered during ophthalmic surgical procedure are recommended. There have been reports of significantly increased intraocular pressure following the use of sodium hyaluronate as an ophthalmic surgical aid. For this reason, the following precautions should be considered:

- The intraocular pressure of postoperative patients should be carefully monitored.
- An excess quantity of AMO®VITRAX® should not be used.
- AMO®VITRAX® should be removed from the anterior chamber at the end of surgery by irrigation or aspiration.
- If the postoperative intraocular pressure increases above expected values, correcting therapy should be administered.

Denaturation and particulate formation in viscoelastics with the repeated use of a reusable cannula has been reported in some studies. A single use cannula such as the one provided in this package should be used when instilling AMO®VITRAX® into the eye.

Because AMO®VITRAX® is a highly purified fraction extracted from avian tissues and may contain minute amounts of protein, the physician should be aware of potential risks of the type that can occur with the injection of biological material.

Adverse Reactions: The following adverse reactions have been reported following the use of sodium hyaluronate: increased intraocular pressure, secondary glaucoma, postoperative inflammatory reactions.

How Supplied: AMO®VITRAX® is a sterile, non-pyrogenic viscoelastic preparation of sodium hyaluronate. It is supplied in a disposable glass syringe delivering 0.65 mL sodium hyaluronate dissolved in a balanced salt solution. Each 1 mL of AMO®VITRAX® contains 30 mg sodium hyaluronate, 3.2 mg sodium chloride, 0.75 mg potassium chloride, 0.48 mg calcium chloride, 0.30 mg magnesium chloride, 3.9 mg sodium acetate, 1.7 mg sodium citrate and sterile water for injection USP. The viscosity of AMO®VITRAX® is approximately 40,000 cp and the osmolality is nominally 310 mOsm/kg. AMO®VITRAX® syringes are aseptically filled and terminally sterilized using ethylene oxide. A single use, 23 gauge blunt tip cannula is also included in the package.

NOTE: Cannula should be fastened securely to syringe; however, overtightening may cause hub to weaken and cannula, rarely, to detach. Extrusion of a test droplet is recommended prior to entering eye, and excessive force on plunger should be avoided.

FOR INTRAOCULAR USE

Store at room temperature: 15 – 30°C (59 – 86°F).

Protect from freezing.

Protect from light.

References:

1. Bourne, W., Liesegang, T., Walter, R., Illstrup, D: "The effect of sodium hyaluronate on endothelial cell damage during extracapsular cataract extraction and posterior chamber lens implantation," **Am. J. Ophthalmol,** 98:759–762, 1984.
2. Genstler, D., Keates, R.: "Am-Visc in extracapsular cataract extraction," **J. Am. Intraocul. Implant Soc.,** 9:317–320, 1983.
3. Miller, D., Stegmann, R.: "Use of Na-hyaluronate in anterior segment eye surgery," **Am. Intra-Ocular Implant Soc. J.,** 6:13–15, 1980.
4. Richter, W.: "Non-immunogenicity of purified hyaluronic acid preparations tested by passive cutaneous anaphylaxis," **Int. Arch. All,** 47:211–217, 1974.
5. Richter, W., Ryde, M., Zetterstron, O.: "Non-immunogenicity of a purified sodium hyaluronate preparation in man," **Int. Arch Appl Immun,** 59:45-48, 1979.
6. Swann, D.A.: "Studies on Hyaluronic Acid. 1. The preparation and properties of rooster comb hyaluronic acid." **Biochim, Biophys. Acta,** 156:17–30, 1968.

Caution: Federal (USA) law restricts this device to sale, distribution, or use by or on the order of a physician.

Distributed By:
ALLERGAN, INC.
Irvine, CA 92718, U.S.A.
Telephone: 1 (800) 366-6554
In Canada Distributed By:
ALLERGAN MEDICAL OPTICS
Div. of ALLERGAN Inc.
625 Cochrane Drive, Suite 1000,
Markham, Ontario, Canada, L3R 9R9
Telephone: 1-800-668-6472

OCUFEN® ℞
(flurbiprofen sodium) 0.03%
Liquifilm®
sterile ophthalmic solution

Description: OCUFEN® (flurbiprofen sodium) 0.03% Liquifilm® sterile ophthalmic solution is a topical nonsteroidal anti-inflammatory product for ophthalmic use.

Chemical Name: Sodium (±)-2-fluoro-α-methyl-4-biphenyl-acetate dihydrate.

Contains: flurbiprofen sodium ....0.03% with: Liquifilm® (polyvinyl alcohol) 1.4%; thimerosal 0.005%; edetate disodium; potassium chloride; sodium chloride; sodium citrate; citric acid; hydrochloric acid and/or sodium hydroxide to adjust the pH; and purified water.

Continued on next page

Allergan, Inc.—Cont.

Clinical Pharmacology: Flurbiprofen sodium is one of a series of phenylalkanoic acids that have shown analgesic, antipyretic, and anti-inflammatory activity in animal inflammatory diseases. Its mechanism of action is believed to be through inhibition of the cyclo-oxygenase enzyme that is essential in the biosynthesis of prostaglandins.

Prostaglandins have been shown in many animal models to be mediators of certain kinds of intraocular inflammation. In studies performed on animal eyes, prostaglandins have been shown to produce disruption of the blood-aqueous humor barrier, vasodilatation, increased vascular permeability, leukocytosis, and increased intraocular pressure.

Prostaglandins also appear to play a role in the miotic response produced during ocular surgery by constricting the iris sphincter independently of cholinergic mechanisms. In clinical studies, OCUFEN® has been shown to inhibit the miosis induced during the course of cataract surgery.

Results from clinical studies indicate that flurbiprofen sodium has no significant effect upon intraocular pressure.

Indications and Usage: OCUFEN® is indicated for the inhibition of intraoperative miosis.

Contraindications: OCUFEN® is contraindicated in individuals who are hypersensitive to any components of the medication.

Warnings: With nonsteroidal anti-inflammatory drugs, there exists the potential for increased bleeding due to interference with thrombocyte aggregation. There have been reports that OCUFEN® may cause increased bleeding of ocular tissues (including hyphemas) in conjunction with ocular surgery. There exists the potential for cross-sensitivity to acetylsalicylic acid and other nonsteroidal anti-inflammatory drugs. Therefore, caution should be used when treating individuals who have previously exhibited sensitivities to these drugs.

Precautions: General: Wound healing may be delayed with the use of OCUFEN®. It is recommended that OCUFEN® (flurbiprofen sodium) 0.03% Liquifilm® sterile ophthalmic solution be used with caution in surgical patients with known bleeding tendencies or who are receiving other medications which may prolong bleeding time.

Drug Interactions: Interaction of OCUFEN® with other topical ophthalmic medications has not been fully investigated.

Although clinical studies with acetylcholine chloride and animal studies with acetylcholine chloride or carbachol revealed no interference, and there is no known pharmacological basis for an interaction, there have been reports that acetylcholine chloride and carbachol have been ineffective when used in patients treated with OCUFEN®.

Carcinogenesis, mutagenesis, impairment of fertility: Long-term studies in mice and/or rats have shown no evidence of carcinogenicity or impairment of fertility with flurbiprofen.

Long-term mutagenicity studies in animals have not been performed.

Pregnancy:

Pregnancy category C. Flurbiprofen has been shown to be embryocidal, delay parturition, prolong gestation, reduce weight, and/or slightly retard growth of fetuses when given to rats in daily oral doses of 0.4 mg/kg (approximately 185 times the human daily topical dose) and above. There are no adequate and well-controlled studies in pregnant women. OCUFEN® should be used during pregnancy only if the potential benefit justifies the potential risk to the fetus.

Nursing Mothers: It is not known whether this drug is excreted in human milk. Because many drugs are excreted in human milk and because of the potential for serious adverse reactions in nursing infants from flurbiprofen sodium, a decision should be made whether to discontinue nursing or to discontinue the drug, taking into account the importance of the drug to the mother.

Pediatric use: Safety and effectiveness in children have not been established.

Adverse Reactions: The most frequent adverse reactions reported with the use of OCUFEN® are transient burning and stinging upon instillation and other minor symptoms of ocular irritation.

Increased bleeding tendency of ocular tissues in conjunction with ocular surgery has also been reported.

Overdosage: Overdosage will not ordinarily cause acute problems. If accidentally ingested, drink fluids to dilute.

Dosage and Administration: A total of four (4) drops of OCUFEN® should be administered by instilling 1 drop approximately every ½ hour beginning 2 hours before surgery.

How Supplied: OCUFEN® (flurbiprofen sodium) 0.03% solution is supplied in plastic dropper bottles in the following size:

2.5 mL—NDC 11980-801-03

Note: Store at room temperature.

Caution: Federal (U.S.A.) law prohibits dispensing without prescription.

Allergan, Inc.

Pharmaceutical Division
2525 DUPONT DRIVE
P.O. BOX 19534
IRVINE, CA 92713-9534

ACULAR® ℞

(ketorolac tromethamine) 0.5%
Sterile Ophthalmic Solution

Description: ACULAR® (ketorolac tromethamine) is a member of the pyrrolo-pyrolle group of nonsteroidal anti-inflammatory drugs (NSAIDs) for ophthalmic use. Its chemical name is (±)-5-benzoyl-2, 3-dihydro-1*H*-pyrrolizine-1-carboxylic acid compound with 2-amino-2-(hydroxymethyl)-1,3-propanediol (1:1).

ACULAR® is supplied as a sterile isotonic aqueous 0.5% solution, with a pH of 7.4. ACULAR® is a racemic mixture of R-(+)- and S-(−)- ketorolac tromethamine. Ketorolac tromethamine may exist in three crystal forms. All forms are equally soluble in water. The pKa of ketorolac is 3.5. This white to off-white crystalline substance discolors on prolonged exposure to light. The molecular weight of ketorolac tromethamine is 376.41. Each mL of ACULAR® ophthalmic solution contains ketorolac tromethamine 0.5%, benzalkonium chloride 0.01%, edetate disodium 0.1%, octoxynol 40, sodium chloride, hydrochloric acid and/or sodium hydroxide to adjust the pH, and purified water. The osmolality of ACULAR® is 290 mOsmol/kg.

Animal Pharmacology: Ketorolac tromethamine prevented the development of increased intraocular pressure induced in rabbits with topically applied arachidonic acid. Ketorolac did not inhibit rabbit lens aldose reductase *in vitro*.

Ketorolac tromethamine ophthalmic solution did not enhance the spread of ocular infections induced in rabbits with *Candida albicans, Herpes simplex* virus type one, or *Pseudomonas aeruginosa*.

Clinical Pharmacology: Ketorolac tromethamine is a nonsteroidal anti-inflammatory drug which, when administered systemically, has demonstrated analgesic, anti-inflammatory and anti-pyretic activity. The mechanism of its action is thought to be due, in part, to its ability to inhibit prostaglandin biosynthesis. Ocular administration of ketorolac tromethamine reduces prostaglandin E_2 levels in aqueous humor. The mean concentration of PGE_2 was 80 pg/mL in the aqueous humor of eyes receiving vehicle and 28 pg/mL in the eyes receiving 0.5% ACULAR® ophthalmic solution. Ketorolac tromethamine given systemically does not cause pupil constriction.

Results from clinical studies indicate that ACULAR® ophthalmic solution has no significant effect upon intraocular pressure.

Two controlled clinical studies showed that ACULAR® ophthalmic solution was significantly more effective than its vehicle in relieving ocular itching caused by seasonal allergic conjunctivitis. Two drops (0.1 mL) of 0.5% ACULAR® ophthalmic solution instilled into the eyes of patients 12 hours and 1 hour prior to cataract extraction achieved measurable levels in 8 of 9 patients' eyes (mean ketorolac concentration 95 ng/mL aqueous humor, range 40 to 170 ng/mL).

One drop (0.05 mL) of 0.5% ACULAR® ophthalmic solution was instilled into one eye and one drop of vehicle into the other eye tid in 26 normal subjects. Only 5 of 26 subjects had a detectable amount of ketorolac in their plasma (range 10.7 to 22.5 ng/mL) at Day 10 during topical ocular treatment. When ketorolac tromethamine 10 mg is administered systemically every 6 hours, peak plasma levels at steady state are around 960 ng/mL. ACULAR® ophthalmic solution has been safely administered in conjunction with other ophthalmic medications, such as antibiotics, beta blockers, carbonic anhydrase inhibitors, cycloplegics, and mydriatics.

Indications and Usage: ACULAR® ophthalmic solution is indicated for the relief of ocular itching due to seasonal allergic conjunctivitis.

Contraindications: ACULAR® ophthalmic solution is contraindicated in patients while wearing soft contact lenses and in patients with previously demonstrated hypersensitivity to any of the ingredients in the formulation.

Warnings: There is the potential for cross-sensitivity to acetylsalicylic acid, phenylacetic acid derivatives, and other nonsteroidal anti-inflammatory agents. Therefore, caution should be used when treating individuals who have previously exhibited sensitivities to these drugs.

With some nonsteroidal anti-inflammatory drugs, there exists the potential for increased bleeding time due to interference with thrombocyte aggregation. There have been reports that ocularly applied nonsteroidal anti-inflammatory drugs may cause increased bleeding of ocular tissues (including hyphemas) in conjunction with ocular surgery.

Precautions: General: It is recommended that ACULAR® ophthalmic solution be used with caution in patients with known bleeding tendencies or who are receiving other medications which may prolong bleeding time.

Carcinogenesis, Mutagenesis, and Impairment of Fertility: An 18-month study in mice at oral doses of ketorolac tromethamine equal to the parenteral MRHD (Maximum Recommended Human Dose) and a 24-month study in rats at oral doses 2.5 times the parenteral MRHD, showed no evidence of tumorigenicity. Ketorolac tromethamine was not mutagenic in Ames test, unscheduled DNA synthesis and repair, and in forward mutation assays. Ketorolac did not cause chromosome breakage in the *in vivo* mouse micronucleus assay. At 1590 ug/mL (approximately 1000 times the average human plasma levels) and at higher concentrations, ketorolac tromethamine increased the incidence of chromosomal aberrations in Chinese hamster ovarian cells.

Impairment of fertility did not occur in male or female rats at oral doses of 9 mg/kg (53.1 mg/m^2) and 16 mg/kg (94.4 mg/m^2) respectively.
Pregnancy: Pregnancy Category C. Reproduction studies have been performed in rabbits, using daily oral doses at 3.6 mg/kg (42.35 mg/m^2) and in rats at 10 mg/kg (59 mg/m^2) during organogenesis. Results of these studies did not reveal evidence of teratogenicity to the fetus. Oral doses of ketorolac tromethamine at 1.5 mg/kg (8.8 mg/m^2), which was half of the human oral exposure, administered after gestation day 17 caused dystocia and higher pup mortality in rats. There are no adequate and well-controlled studies in pregnant women. Ketorolac tromethamine should be used during pregnancy only if the potential benefit justifies the potential risk to the fetus.
Nursing Mothers: Caution should be exercised when ACULAR® is administered to a nursing woman.
Pediatric Use: Safety and efficacy in children have not been established.
Adverse Reactions: In patients with allergic conjunctivitis, the most frequent adverse events reported with the use of ACULAR® ophthalmic solution have been transient stinging and burning on instillation. These events were reported by approximately 40% of patients treated with ACULAR® ophthalmic solution. In all development studies conducted, other adverse events reported during treatment with ACULAR® include ocular irritation (3%), allergic reactions (3%), superficial ocular infections (0.5%) and superficial keratitis (1%).
Dosage and Administration: The recommended dose of ACULAR® ophthalmic solution is one drop (0.25 mg) four times a day for relief of ocular itching due to seasonal allergic conjunctivitis. The efficacy of ACULAR® ophthalmic solution has not been established beyond one week of therapy.
How Supplied: ACULAR® (ketorolac tromethamine) ophthalmic solution is available for topical ophthalmic administration as a 0.5% sterile solution, and is supplied in a white opaque plastic bottle (5 mL fill) with a controlled dropper tip (NDC 0023-2181-05). Store at controlled room temperature 15–30°C (59–86°F) with protection from light.
CAUTION: Federal (U.S.A.) law prohibits dispensing without prescription.
U.S. Patent Nos. 4,089,969; 4,454,151; 5,110,493

ACULAR®, a registered trademark of Syntex (U.S.A.) Inc., is manufactured and distributed by Allergan, Inc. under license from its developer, Syntex (U.S.A.) Inc., Palo Alto, California, U.S.A.
ALLERGAN
Irvine, CA 92715
***FISONS* Pharmaceuticals**
Fisons Corporation
Rochester, NY 14623 U.S.A.

ALBALON® ℞
(naphazoline hydrochloride ophthalmic solution) 0.1% with Liquifilm® (polyvinyl alcohol) 1.4% sterile

Description: Naphazoline hydrochloride, an ocular vasoconstrictor, is an imidazoline derivative sympathomimetic amine. It occurs as a white, odorless crystalline powder having a bitter taste and is freely soluble in water and in alcohol.
Chemical Name:
2-(1-Naphthylmethyl)-2-imidazoline monohydrochloride
Contains:
naphazoline HCl..0.1%
with: Liquifilm (polyvinyl alcohol) 1.4%; benzalkonium chloride 0.004%; edetate disodium; citric acid, monohydrate; sodium citrate, dihydrate; sodium chloride; sodium hydroxide to adjust the pH; and purified water. It has a pH of 5.5 to 7.0.
Clinical Pharmacology: Naphazoline constricts the vascular system of the conjunctiva. It is presumed that this effect is due to direct stimulation action of the drug upon the alpha-adrenergic receptors in the arterioles of the conjunctiva, resulting in decreased conjunctival congestion. Naphazoline belongs to the imidazoline class of sympathomimetics.
Indications and Usage: Albalon (naphazoline hydrochloride ophthalmic solution) 0.1% is indicated for use as a topical ocular vasoconstrictor.
Contraindications: Albalon ophthalmic solution is contraindicated in the presence of an anatomically narrow angle or in narrow-angle glaucoma or in persons who have shown hypersensitivity to any component of this preparation.
Warnings: Patients under therapy with MAO inhibitors may experience a severe hypertensive crisis if given a sympathomimetic drug. Use in children, especially infants, may result in CNS depression leading to coma and marked reduction in body temperature.
Precautions:
General: Use with caution in the presence of hypertension, cardiovascular abnormalities, hyperglycemia (diabetes), hyperthyroidism, infection or injury.
Patient Information: Patients should be advised to discontinue the drug and consult a physician if relief is not obtained within 48 hours of therapy, if irritation, blurring or redness persists or increases, or if symptoms of systemic absorption occur, i.e., dizziness, headache, nausea, decrease in body temperature, or drowsiness.
To prevent contaminating the dropper tip and solution, do not touch the eyelids or the surrounding area with the dropper tip of the bottle. If solution changes color or becomes cloudy, do not use.
Drug Interactions: Concurrent use of maprotiline or tricyclic antidepressants and naphazoline may potentiate the pressor effect of naphazoline. Patients under therapy with MAO inhibitors may experience a severe hypertensive crisis if given a sympathomimetic drug. (See WARNINGS).
Pregnancy: Pregnancy Category C: Animal reproduction studies have not been conducted with naphazoline. It is also not known whether naphazoline can cause fetal harm when administered to a pregnant woman or can affect reproduction capacity. Naphazoline should be given to a pregnant woman only if clearly needed.
Nursing Mothers: It is not known whether naphazoline is excreted in human milk. Because many drugs are excreted in human milk, caution should be exercised when naphazoline is administered to a nursing woman.
Pediatric Use: Safety and effectiveness in children have not been established. See "WARNINGS" AND "CONTRAINDICATIONS."
Adverse Reactions:
Ocular: Mydriasis, increased redness, irritation, discomfort, blurring, punctate keratitis, lacrimation, increased intraocular pressure.
Systemic: Dizziness, headache, nausea, sweating, nervousness, drowsiness, weakness, hypertension, cardiac irregularities, and hyperglycemia.
Dosage and Administration: Instill one or two drops in the conjunctival sac(s) every three to four hours as needed.
How Supplied: Albalon® (naphazoline hydrochloride ophthalmic solution) 0.1% with Liquifilm® (polyvinyl alcohol) 1.4% is supplied sterile in plastic dropper bottles in the following size:

15 mL—NDC 11980-154-15

Note: Store at room temperature.
Caution: Federal (U.S.A.) law prohibits dispensing without prescription.

ATROPINE SULFATE ℞
sterile ophthalmic solution
and
ATROPINE SULFATE S.O.P.®
sterile ophthalmic ointment

Description: ATROPINE SULFATE sterile ophthalmic solution and sterile ophthalmic ointment are topical anticholinergics for ophthalmic use.
Chemical Name: Benzeneacetic acid, α-(hydroxymethyl)-,8-methyl-8-azabicyclo-[3.2.1]oct-3-yl ester, endo-(±)-, sulfate (2:1) (salt), monohydrate.
ATROPINE SULFATE sterile ophthalmic solution contains:
atropine sulfate 1%
with: chlorobutanol (chloral deriv.) 0.5%, boric acid, sodium citrate, hydrochloric acid and/or sodium hydroxide to adjust the pH, and purified water.
ATROPINE SULFATE S.O.P. sterile ophthalmic ointment contains:
atropine sulfate 0.5%, 1%
with: chlorobutanol (chloral deriv.) 0.5%, white petrolatum, mineral oil, petrolatum (and) lanolin alcohol, and purified water.
Clinical Pharmacology: Anticholinergics act directly on the smooth muscles and secretory glands innervated by postganglionic cholinergic nerves. They act by blocking the parasympathomimetic (muscarinic) effects of acetylcholine and parasympathomimetic drugs at these sites.
Indications and Usage: ATROPINE SULFATE is used to produce mydriasis and cycloplegia for refraction, or for iris dilation and relaxation of the ciliary muscle desirable in acute inflammatory conditions of the anterior uveal tract.
Contraindications: Should not be used in patients with glaucoma or a predisposition to narrow-angle glaucoma. Should not be used in children who have previously had a severe systemic reaction to atropine.
Warnings: Excessive use in children and certain susceptible individuals may produce general toxic symptoms. If this occurs, discontinue medication and use appropriate therapy as outlined in "Overdosage" section.
Precautions: Information for patients: Keep out of the reach of children.
Carcinogenesis, mutagenesis, impairment of fertility: No studies have been conducted in animals or in humans to evaluate the potential of these effects.
Pregnancy Category C: Animal reproduction studies have not been performed with atropine. It is also not known whether atropine can cause fetal harm when administered to a pregnant woman or can affect reproduction capacity. Atropine should be given to pregnant women only if clearly needed.
Pediatric use: See "Contraindications" and "Warnings" sections.
Adverse Reactions: Prolonged use may cause general systemic reactions, allergic lid reactions, local irritation, hyperemia, edema, follicular conjunctivitis or dermatitis.
Overdosage: General signs and symptoms of atropine toxicity include dryness of mouth and skin, fever, irritability or delirium, tachycardia, and flushing of the face. Should overdos-

Continued on next page

Allergan Pharm—Cont.

age in the eye(s) occur, flush the eye(s) with water or normal saline. Use of a topical miotic may be required.
If accidentally ingested induce emesis or gastric lavage with 4% tannic acid. Five mg of pilocarpine should be administered orally at repeated intervals until the mouth is moist. General supportive measures should be used if needed as listed below:
respiratory depression—oxygen and artificial respiration
urinary retention—catheterization
fever—alcohol sponge baths.
Use extreme caution when employing short-acting barbiturates to control excitement.
Dosage and Administration: **Solution:** 1 or 2 drops in the eyes three times a day or as directed by physician.
Ointment: A small amount in the conjunctival sac once or twice a day or as directed by physician.
How Supplied: ATROPINE SULFATE sterile ophthalmic solution is supplied in plastic dropper bottles in the following concentration and size:
1%–15 mL—NDC 11980-002-15
ATROPINE SULFATE S.O.P.® sterile ophthalmic ointment is supplied in ophthalmic ointment tubes in the following concentrations and sizes:
½%–3.5 g—NDC 0023-0306-04
1%–3.5 g—NDC 0023-0305-04
Note: Store ointment away from heat.
Caution: Federal (U.S.A.) law prohibits dispensing without prescription.

BETAGAN® ℞
(levobunolol HCl)
Liquifilm®
sterile ophthalmic solution
with C CAP® Compliance Cap Q.D. and B.I.D.

Description: BETAGAN® (levobunolol HCl) Liquifilm® sterile ophthalmic solution is a noncardioselective beta-adrenoceptor blocking agent for ophthalmic use.
Chemical Name: (-)-5-[3-(*tert*-Butylamino)-2-hydroxypropoxy]-3,4-dihydro-1(2*H*)-naphthalenone hydrochloride.
Contains:
levobunolol HCl 0.25%, 0.5%
with: Liquifilm® (polyvinyl alcohol) 1.4%; benzalkonium chloride 0.004%; edetate disodium; sodium metabisulfite; sodium phosphate, dibasic; potassium phosphate, monobasic; sodium chloride; hydrochloric acid or sodium hydroxide to adjust the pH; and purified water.
Clinical Pharmacology: Levobunolol HCl is a noncardioselective beta-adrenoceptor blocking agent, equipotent at both $beta_1$ and $beta_2$ receptors. Levobunolol HCl is greater than 60 times more potent than its dextro isomer in its beta-blocking activity, yet equipotent in its potential for direct myocardial depression. Accordingly, the levo isomer, levobunolol HCl, is used. Levobunolol HCl does not have significant local anesthetic (membrane-stabilizing) or intrinsic sympathomimetic activity.
Beta-adrenergic receptor blockade reduces cardiac output in both healthy subjects and patients with heart disease. In patients with severe impairment of myocardial function, beta-adrenergic receptor blockade may inhibit the stimulatory effect of the sympathetic nervous system necessary to maintain adequate cardiac function.
Beta-adrenergic receptor blockade in the bronchi and bronchioles results in increased airway resistance from unopposed para-sympathetic activity. Such an effect in patients with asthma or other bronchospastic conditions is potentially dangerous.
BETAGAN® (levobunolol HCl) has been shown to be an active agent in lowering elevated as well as normal intraocular pressure (IOP) whether or not accompanied by glaucoma. Elevated IOP presents a major risk factor in glaucomatous field loss. The higher the level of IOP, the greater the likelihood of optic nerve damage and visual field loss.
The onset of action with one drop of BETAGAN® can be detected within one hour after treatment, with maximum effect seen between 2 and 6 hours.
A significant decrease in IOP can be maintained for up to 24 hours following a single dose.
In two, separate, controlled studies (one three month and one up to 12 months duration) BETAGAN® 0.25% b.i.d. controlled the IOP of approximately 64% and 70% of the subjects. The overall mean decrease from baseline was 5.4 mm Hg and 5.1 mm Hg respectively. In an open-label study, BETAGAN® 0.25% q.d. controlled the IOP of 72% of the subjects while achieving an overall mean decrease of 5.9 mm Hg.
In controlled clinical studies of approximately two years duration, intraocular pressure was well-controlled in approximately 80% of subjects treated with BETAGAN® 0.5% b.i.d. The mean IOP decrease from baseline was between 6.87 mm Hg and 7.81 mm Hg. No significant effects on pupil size, tear production or corneal sensitivity were observed. BETAGAN® at the concentrations tested, when applied topically, decreased heart rate and blood pressure in some patients. The IOP-lowering effect of BETAGAN® was well maintained over the course of these studies.
In a three month clinical study, a single daily application of BETAGAN® 0.5% controlled the IOP of 72% of subjects achieving an overall mean decrease in IOP of 7.0 mm Hg.
The primary mechanism of the ocular hypotensive action of levobunolol HCl in reducing IOP is most likely a decrease in aqueous humor production. BETAGAN® reduces IOP with little or no effect on pupil size or accommodation in contrast to the miosis which cholinergic agents are known to produce. The blurred vision and night blindness often associated with miotics would not be expected and have not been reported with the use of BETAGAN®. This is particularly important in cataract patients with central lens opacities who would experience decreased visual acuity with pupillary constriction.
Indications and Usage: BETAGAN® has been shown to be effective in lowering intraocular pressure and may be used in patients with chronic open-angle glaucoma or ocular hypertension.
Contraindications: BETAGAN® is contraindicated in those individuals with bronchial asthma or with a history of bronchial asthma, or severe chronic obstructive pulmonary disease (see WARNINGS); sinus bradycardia; second and third degree atrioventricular block; overt cardiac failure (see WARNINGS); cardiogenic shock; or hypersensitivity to any component of these products.
Warnings: As with other topically applied ophthalmic drugs, BETAGAN® may be absorbed systemically. The same adverse reactions found with systemic administration of beta-adrenergic blocking agents may occur with topical administration. For example, severe respiratory reactions and cardiac reactions, including death due to bronchospasm in patients with asthma, and rarely death in association with cardiac failure, have been reported with topical application of beta-adrenergic blocking agents (see CONTRAINDICATIONS).
Cardiac Failure: Sympathetic stimulation may be essential for support of the circulation in individuals with diminished myocardial contractility, and its inhibition by beta-adrenergic receptor blockade may precipitate more severe failure.
In Patients Without a History of Cardiac Failure: Continued depression of the myocardium with beta-blocking agents over a period of time can, in some cases, lead to cardiac failure. At the first sign or symptom of cardiac failure, BETAGAN® should be discontinued.
Obstructive Pulmonary Disease:
PATIENTS WITH CHRONIC OBSTRUCTIVE PULMONARY DISEASE (e.g., CHRONIC BRONCHITIS, EMPHYSEMA) OF MILD OR MODERATE SEVERITY, BRONCHOSPASTIC DISEASE OR A HISTORY OF BRONCHOSPASTIC DISEASE (OTHER THAN BRONCHIAL ASTHMA OR A HISTORY OF BRONCHIAL ASTHMA, IN WHICH BETAGAN® IS CONTRAINDICATED, See CONTRAINDICATIONS), SHOULD IN GENERAL NOT RECEIVE BETA BLOCKERS, INCLUDING BETAGAN®. However, if BETAGAN® is deemed necessary in such patients, then it should be administered cautiously since it may block bronchodilation produced by endogenous and exogenous catecholamine stimulation of $beta_2$ receptors.
Major Surgery: The necessity or desirability of withdrawal of beta-adrenergic blocking agents prior to major surgery is controversial. Beta-adrenergic receptor blockade impairs the ability of the heart to respond to beta-adrenergically mediated reflex stimuli. This may augment the risk of general anesthesia in surgical procedures. Some patients receiving beta-adrenergic receptor blocking agents have been subject to protracted severe hypotension during anesthesia. Difficulty in restarting and maintaining the heartbeat has also been reported. For these reasons, in patients undergoing elective surgery, gradual withdrawal of beta-adrenergic receptor blocking agents may be appropriate.
If necessary during surgery, the effects of beta-adrenergic blocking agents may be reversed by sufficient doses of such agonists as isoproterenol, dopamine, dobutamine or levarterenol (See OVERDOSAGE).
Diabetes Mellitus: Beta-adrenergic blocking agents should be administered with caution in patients subject to spontaneous hypoglycemia or to diabetic patients (especially those with labile diabetes) who are receiving insulin or oral hypoglycemic agents. Beta-adrenergic receptor blocking agents may mask the signs and symptoms of acute hypoglycemia.
Thyrotoxicosis: Beta-adrenergic blocking agents may mask certain clinical signs (e.g., tachycardia) of hyperthyroidism. Patients suspected of developing thyrotoxicosis should be managed carefully to avoid abrupt withdrawal of beta-adrenergic blocking agents, which might precipitate a thyroid storm.
These products contain sodium metabisulfite, a sulfite that may cause allergic-type reactions including anaphylactic symptoms and life-threatening or less severe asthmatic episodes in certain susceptible people. The overall prevalence of sulfite sensitivity in the general population is unknown and probably low. Sulfite sensitivity is seen more frequently in asthmatic than in nonasthmatic people.
Precautions:
General: BETAGAN® should be used with caution in patients with known hypersensitivity to other beta-adrenoceptor blocking agents. Use with caution in patients with known diminished pulmonary function.
BETAGAN® should be used with caution in patients who are receiving a beta-adrenergic blocking agent orally, because of the potential for additive effects on systemic beta-blockade or on intraocular pressure. Patients should not

typically use two or more topical ophthalmic beta-adrenergic blocking agents simultaneously.

Because of the potential effects of beta-adrenergic blocking agents on blood pressure and pulse rates, these medications must be used cautiously in patients with cerebrovascular insufficiency. Should signs or symptoms develop that suggest reduced cerebral blood flow while using BETAGAN®, alternative therapy should be considered.

In patients with angle-closure glaucoma, the immediate objective of treatment is to reopen the angle. This requires, in most cases, constricting the pupil with a miotic. BETAGAN® has little or no effect on the pupil. When BETAGAN® is used to reduce elevated intraocular pressure in angle-closure glaucoma, it should be followed with a miotic and not alone.

Muscle Weakness: Beta-adrenergic blockade has been reported to potentiate muscle weakness consistent with certain myasthenic symptoms (e.g., diplopia, ptosis and generalized weakness).

Drug Interactions: Although BETAGAN® used alone has little or no effect on pupil size, mydriasis resulting from concomitant therapy with BETAGAN® and epinephrine may occur.

Close observation of the patient is recommended when a beta-blocker is administered to patients receiving catecholamine-depleting drugs such as reserpine, because of possible additive effects and the production of hypotension and/or marked bradycardia, which may produce vertigo, syncope, or postural hypotension.

Patients receiving beta-adrenergic blocking agents along with either oral or intravenous calcium antagonists should be monitored for possible atrioventricular conduction disturbances, left ventricular failure and hypotension. In patients with impaired cardiac function, simultaneous use should be avoided altogether.

The concomitant use of beta-adrenergic blocking agents with digitalis and calcium antagonists may have additive effects on prolonging atrioventricular conduction time.

Phenothiazine-related compounds and beta-adrenergic blocking agents may have additive hypotensive effects due to the inhibition of each other's metabolism.

Risk of anaphylactic reaction: While taking beta-blockers, patients with a history of severe anaphylactic reaction to a variety of allergens may be more reactive to repeated challenge, either accidental, diagnostic, or therapeutic. Such patients may be unresponsive to the usual doses of epinephrine used to treat allergic reaction.

Animal Studies: No adverse ocular effects were observed in rabbits administered BETAGAN® topically in studies lasting one year in concentrations up to 10 times the human dose concentration.

Carcinogenesis, mutagenesis, impairment of fertility: In a lifetime oral study in mice, there were statistically significant ($p \leq 0.05$) increases in the incidence of benign leiomyomas in female mice at 200 mg/kg/day (14,000 times the recommended human dose for glaucoma), but not at 12 or 50 mg/kg/day (850 and 3,500 times the human dose). In a two-year oral study of levobunolol HCl in rats, there was a statistically significant ($p \leq 0.05$) increase in the incidence of benign hepatomas in male rats administered 12,800 times the recommended human dose for glaucoma. Similar differences were not observed in rats administered oral doses equivalent to 350 times to 2,000 times the recommended human dose for glaucoma.

Levobunolol did not show evidence of mutagenic activity in a battery of microbiological and mammalian *in vitro* and *in vivo* assays. Reproduction and fertility studies in rats showed no adverse effect on male or female fertility at doses up to 1,800 times the recommended human dose for glaucoma.

Pregnancy Category C: Fetotoxicity (as evidenced by a greater number of resorption sites) has been observed in rabbits when doses of levobunolol HCl equivalent to 200 and 700 times the recommended dose for the treatment of glaucoma were given. No fetotoxic effects have been observed in similar studies with rats at up to 1,800 times the human dose for glaucoma. Teratogenic studies with levobunolol in rats at doses up to 25 mg/kg/day (1,800 times the recommended human dose for glaucoma) showed no evidence of fetal malformations. There were no adverse effects on postnatal development of offspring. It appears when results from studies using rats and studies with other beta-adrenergic blockers are examined, that the rabbit may be a particularly sensitive species. There are no adequate and well-controlled studies in pregnant women. BETAGAN® should be used during pregnancy only if the potential benefit justifies the potential risk to the fetus.

Nursing Mothers: It is not known whether this drug is excreted in human milk. Systemic beta-blockers and topical timolol maleate are known to be excreted in human milk. Caution should be exercised when BETAGAN® is administered to a nursing woman.

Pediatric Use: Safety and effectiveness in children have not been established.

Adverse Reactions: In clinical trials, the use of BETAGAN® has been associated with transient ocular burning and stinging in up to 1 in 3 patients, and with blepharoconjunctivitis in up to 1 in 20 patients. Decreases in heart rate and blood pressure have been reported (see CONTRAINDICATIONS and WARNINGS).

The following adverse effects have been reported rarely with the use of BETAGAN®: iridocyclitis, headache, transient ataxia, dizziness, lethargy, urticaria and pruritus.

Decreased corneal sensitivity has been noted in a small number of patients. Although levobunolol has minimal membrane-stabilizing activity, there remains a possibility of decreased corneal sensitivity after prolonged use.

The following additional adverse reactions have been reported either with BETAGAN® or ophthalmic use of other beta-adrenergic receptor blocking agents:

BODY AS A WHOLE: Headache, asthenia, chest pain. CARDIOVASCULAR: Bradycardia, arrhythmia, hypotension, syncope, heart block, cerebral vascular accident, cerebral ischemia, congestive heart failure, palpitation, cardiac arrest. DIGESTIVE: Nausea, diarrhea. PSYCHIATRIC: Depression, increase in signs and symptoms of myasthenia gravis, paresthesia. SKIN: Hypersensitivity, including localized and generalized rash. RESPIRATORY: Bronchospasm (predominantly in patients with pre-existing bronchospastic disease), respiratory failure, dyspnea, nasal congestion. ENDOCRINE: Masked symptoms of hypoglycemia in insulin-dependent diabetics (see WARNINGS). SPECIAL SENSES: Signs and symptoms of keratitis, blepharoptosis, visual disturbances including refractive changes (due to withdrawal of miotic therapy in some cases), diplopia, ptosis.

Other reactions associated with the oral use of non-selective adrenergic receptor blocking agents should be considered potential effects with ophthalmic use of these agents.

Overdosage: No data are available regarding overdosage in humans. Should accidental ocular overdosage occur, flush eye(s) with water or normal saline. If accidentally ingested, efforts to decrease further absorption may be appropriate (gastric lavage).

The most common signs and symptoms to be expected with overdosage with administration of a systemic beta-adrenergic blocking agent are symptomatic bradycardia, hypotension, bronchospasm, and acute cardiac failure. Should these symptoms occur, discontinue BETAGAN® therapy and initiate appropriate supportive therapy. The following supportive measures should be considered:

1. Symptomatic bradycardia: Use atropine sulfate intravenously in a dosage of 0.25 mg to 2 mg to induce vagal blockade. If bradycardia persists, intravenous isoproterenol hydrochloride should be administered cautiously. In refractory cases, the use of a transvenous cardiac pacemaker should be considered.
2. Hypotension: Use sympathomimetic pressor drug therapy, such as dopamine, dobutamine or levarterenol. In refractory cases, the use of glucagon hydrochloride may be useful.
3. Bronchospasm: Use isoproterenol hydrochloride. Additional therapy with aminophylline may be considered.
4. Acute cardiac failure: Conventional therapy with digitalis, diuretics and oxygen should be instituted immediately. In refractory cases, the use of intravenous aminophylline is suggested. This may be followed, if necessary, by glucagon hydrochloride, which may be useful.
5. Heart block (second or third degree): Use isoproterenol hydrochloride or a transvenous cardiac pacemaker.

Dosage and Administration: The recommended starting dose is one to two drops of BETAGAN® 0.5% in the affected eye(s) once a day. Typical dosing with BETAGAN® 0.25% is one to two drops twice daily. In patients with more severe or uncontrolled glaucoma, BETAGAN® 0.5% can be administered b.i.d. As with any new medication, careful monitoring of patients is advised.

Dosages above one drop of BETAGAN® 0.5% b.i.d. are not generally more effective. If the patient's IOP is not at a satisfactory level on this regimen, concomitant therapy with dipivefrin and/or epinephrine, and/or pilocarpine and other miotics, and/or systemically administered carbonic anhydrase inhibitors, such as acetazolamide, can be instituted. Patients should not typically use two or more topical ophthalmic beta-adrenergic blocking agents simultaneously.

How Supplied: BETAGAN® (levobunolol HCl) Liquifilm® sterile ophthalmic solution is supplied in white opaque plastic dropper bottles as follows:

BETAGAN 0.25%:
C CAP® Compliance Cap
B.I.D. (twice daily)
5 mL—11980-469-25
10 mL—11980-469-20

BETAGAN 0.5%:
Standard Cap
2 mL—NDC 11980-252-02
C CAP® Compliance Cap
Q.D. (once daily)
5 mL—NDC 11980-252-65
10 mL—NDC 11980-252-60
15 mL—NDC 11980-252-61
C CAP® Compliance Cap
B.I.D. (twice daily)
5 mL—NDC 11980-252-25
10 mL—NDC 11980-252-20
15 mL—NDC 11980-252-21

NOTE: Protect from light. Store at controlled room temperature 15°–30°C (59°–86°F).

Caution: Federal (U.S.A.) law prohibits dispensing without prescription.

C CAP® Compliance Cap Patient Instructions

Instructions for use:

1. On the first usage, make sure the number "1" or the correct day of the week appears in

Continued on next page

Allergan Pharm—Cont.

the window. If not, click the cap to the right station.
2. Remove the cap and apply medication.
3. Replace the cap. Hold the C CAP® between your thumb and forefinger. Now rotate the bottle until the cap clicks to the next station.
4. When it's time to take your next dose, repeat steps 2 and 3.

Important Notes: Don't try to catch up on missed doses by applying more than one dose at a time. Each time you replace the cap, turn it until you hear the click. The number in the window specifies your next dosage.

Shown in Product Identification Guide, page 103

BLEPH®-10 ℞
(sulfacetamide sodium ophthalmic solution, USP) 10%

BLEPH®-10
(sulfacetamide sodium ophthalmic ointment, USP) 10%

Description: BLEPH®-10 (sulfacetamide sodium ophthalmic solution and ointment USP) 10% are sterile topical antibacterial agents for ophthalmic use.

Chemical Name:
N-Sulfanilylacetamide monosodium salt monohydrate.

Contains:
BLEPH®-10 solution:
Active: Sulfacetamide sodium .... 10% (100 mg/mL)
Preservative: benzalkonium chloride (0.005%)
Inactives: polyvinyl alcohol 1.4%; sodium thiosulfate; sodium phosphate dibasic; sodium phosphate monobasic; edetate disodium; polysorbate 80; hydrochloric acid and/or sodium hydroxide to adjust the pH; and purified water.
BLEPH®-10 ointment:
Active: Sulfacetamide sodium .... 10% (100 mg/g)
Preservative: phenylmercuric acetate (0.0008%)
Inactives: white petrolatum, mineral oil, and petrolatum (and) lanolin alcohol.

Clinical Pharmacology:
Microbiology: The sulfonamides are bacteriostatic agents and the spectrum of activity is similar for all. Sulfonamides inhibit bacterial synthesis of dihydrofolic acid by preventing the condensation of the pteridine with aminobenzoic acid through competitive inhibition of the enzyme dihydropteroate synthetase. Resistant strains have altered dihydropteroate synthetase with reduced affinity for sulfonamides or produce increased quantities of aminobenzoic acid.

Topically applied sulfonamides are considered active against susceptible strains of the following common bacterial eye pathogens: *Escherichia coli, Staphylococcus aureus, Streptococcus pneumoniae, Streptococcus* (viridans group), *Haemophilus influenzae, Klebsiella* species, and *Enterobacter* species.

Topically applied sulfonamides do not provide adequate coverage against *Neisseria* species, *Serratia marcescens* and *Pseudomonas aeruginosa.* A significant percentage of staphylococcal isolates are completely resistant to sulfa drugs.

Indications and Usage: BLEPH®-10 solution and ointment are indicated for the treatment of conjunctivitis and other superficial ocular infections due to the following susceptible microorganisms. BLEPH®-10 solution is also indicated as an adjunctive in systemic sulfonamide therapy of trachoma:
Escherichia coli, Staphylococcus aureus, Streptococcus pneumoniae, Streptococcus (viridans group), *Haemophilus influenza, Klebsiella* species, and *Enterobacter* species.

Topically applied sulfonamides do not provide adequate coverage against *Neisseria* species, *Serratia marcescens* and *Pseudomonas aeruginosa.* A significant percentage of staphylococcal isolates are completely resistant to sulfa drugs.

Contraindications: BLEPH®-10 solution and ointment are contraindicated in individuals who have a hypersensitivity to sulfonamides or to any ingredient of the preparations.

Warnings: FOR TOPICAL EYE USE ONLY—NOT FOR INJECTION.
FATALITIES HAVE OCCURRED, ALTHOUGH RARELY, DUE TO SEVERE REACTIONS TO SULFONAMIDES INCLUDING STEVENS-JOHNSON SYNDROME, TOXIC EPIDERMAL NECROLYSIS, FULMINANT HEPATIC NECROSIS, AGRANULOCYTOSIS, APLASTIC ANEMIA AND OTHER BLOOD DYSCRASIAS. Sensitizations may recur when a sulfonamide is readministered, irrespective of the route of administration. Sensitivity reactions have been reported in individuals with no prior history of sulfonamide hypersensitivity. At the first sign of hypersensitivity, skin rash or other serious reaction, discontinue use of these preparations.

Precautions: General: Prolonged use of topical antibacterial agents may give rise to overgrowth of nonsusceptible organisms including fungi. Bacterial resistance to sulfonamides may also develop.

The effectiveness of sulfonamides may be reduced by the para-aminobenzoic acid present in purulent exudates.

Ophthalmic ointments may retard corneal wound healing.

Sensitization may recur when a sulfonamide is readministered irrespective of the route of administration, and cross-sensitivity between different sulfonamides may occur.

At the first sign of hypersensitivity, increase in purulent discharge, or aggravation of inflammation or pain, the patient should discontinue use of the medication and consult a physician (see WARNINGS).

Information for patients: To avoid contamination, do not touch tip of container to the eye, eyelid or any surface.

Drug interactions: Sulfacetamide preparations are incompatible with silver preparations.

Carcinogenesis, Mutagenesis, Impairment of Fertility: No studies have been conducted in animals or in humans to evaluate the possibility of these effects with ocularly administered sulfacetamide. Rats appear to be especially susceptible to the goitrogenic effects of sulfonamides, and long-term oral administration of sulfonamides has resulted in thyroid malignancies in these animals.

Pregnancy: Pregnancy Category C. Animal reproduction studies have not been conducted with sulfonamide ophthalmic preparations. Kernicterus may occur in the newborn as a result of treatment of a pregnant woman at term with orally administered sulfonamides. There are no adequate and well controlled studies of sulfonamide ophthalmic preparations in pregnant women and it is not known whether topically applied sulfonamides can cause fetal harm when administered to a pregnant woman. This product should be used in pregnancy only if the potential benefit justifies the potential risk to the fetus.

Nursing mothers: Systematically administered sulfonamides are capable of producing kernicterus in infants of lactating women. Because of the potential for the development of kernicterus in neonates, a decision should be made whether to discontinue nursing or discontinue the drug taking into account the importance of the drug to the mother.

Pediatric Use: Safety and effectiveness in children below the age of two months have not been established.

Adverse Reactions: Bacterial and fungal corneal ulcers have developed during treatment with sulfonamide ophthalmic preparations.

The most frequently reported reactions are local irritation, stinging and burning. Less commonly reported reactions include non-specific conjunctivitis, conjunctival hyperemia, secondary infections and allergic reactions.

Fatalities have occurred, although rarely, due to severe reactions to sulfonamides including Stevens-Johnson syndrome, toxic epidermal necrolysis, fulminant hepatic necrosis, agranulocytosis, aplastic anemia, and other blood dyscrasias (see WARNINGS).

Dosage and Administration: For conjunctivitis and other superficial ocular infections:
BLEPH®-10 solution:
Instill one or two drops into the conjunctival sac(s) of the affected eye(s) every two to three hours initially. Dosages may be tapered by increasing the time interval between doses as the condition responds. The usual duration of treatment is seven to ten days.
BLEPH®-10 ointment:
Apply a small amount (approximately one-half inch ribbon) into the conjunctival sac(s) of the affected eye(s) every three to four hours and at bedtime. Dosages may be tapered by increasing the time interval between doses as the condition responds. The ointment may be used as adjunct to the solution. The usual duration of treatment is seven to ten days.
For trachoma:
BLEPH®-10 solution:
Instill two drops into the conjunctival sac(s) of the affected eye(s) every two hours. Topical administration must be accompanied by systemic administration.

BLEPH®-10 (sulfacetamide sodium ophthalmic solution, USP) 10% is supplied sterile in plastic bottles in the following sizes:

2.5 mL—NDC 11980-011-03
5 mL—NDC 11980-011-05
15 mL—NDC 11980-011-15

Note: Store between 8°-25°C (46°-77°F). Protect from light. Sulfonamide solutions, on long standing, will darken in color and should be discarded.

BLEPH®-10 (sulfacetamide sodium ophthalmic ointment, USP) 10% is supplied sterile in ophthalmic ointment tubes in the following size:

3.5 g—NDC 0023-0311-04

Note: Store away from heat.
Caution: Federal (U.S.A.) law prohibits dispensing without prescription.

BLEPHAMIDE® ℞
(sulfacetamide sodium—prednisolone acetate)
LIQUIFILM®
sterile ophthalmic suspension

Description: BLEPHAMIDE® LIQUIFILM® sterile ophthalmic suspension is a topical anti-inflammatory/anti-infective combination product for ophthalmic use.

Chemical Names:
Sulfacetamide sodium: N-Sulfanilylacetamide monosodium salt monohydrate.
Prednisolone acetate: 11β, 17, 21-Trihydroxypregna-1, 4-diene-3, 20-dione 21-acetate.

Contains:
sulfacetamide sodium 10.0%
prednisolone acetate
(microfine suspension) 0.2%
with: LIQUIFILM® (polyvinyl alcohol) 1.4%; benzalkonium chloride; polysorbate 80; edetate disodium; sodium phosphate, dibasic; potassium phosphate, monobasic; sodium thiosulfate; hydrochloric acid and/or sodium hydroxide to adjust the pH; and purified water.

Clinical Pharmacology: Corticosteroids suppress the inflammatory response to a variety of agents and they probably delay or slow healing. Since corticosteroids may inhibit the body's defense mechanism against infection, a concomitant antimicrobial drug may be used when this inhibition is considered to be clinically significant in a particular case.

The anti-infective component in BLEPHAMIDE® is included to provide action against specific organisms susceptible to it. Sulfacetamide sodium is considered active against the following microorganisms: **Escherichia coli, Staphylococcus aureus, Streptococcus pneumoniae, Streptococcus (viridans group), Pseudomonas** species, **Haemophilus influenzae, Klebsiella** species, and **Enterobacter** species.

When a decision to administer both a corticosteroid and an antimicrobial is made, the administration of such drugs in combination has the advantage of greater patient compliance and convenience, with the added assurance that the appropriate dosage of both drugs is administered. When both types of drugs are in the same formulation, compatibility of ingredients is assured and the correct volume of drug is delivered and retained. The relative potency of corticosteroids depends on the molecular structure, concentration, and release from the vehicle.

Indications and Usage: A steroid/anti-infective combination is indicated for steroid-responsive inflammatory ocular conditions for which a corticosteroid is indicated and where bacterial infection or a risk of bacterial ocular infection exists.

Ocular steroids are indicated in inflammatory conditions of the palpebral and bulbar conjunctiva, cornea, and anterior segment of the globe where the inherent risk of steroid use in certain infective conjunctivitides is accepted to obtain a diminution in edema and inflammation. They are also indicated in chronic anterior uveitis and corneal injury from chemical, radiation, or thermal burns or penetration of foreign bodies.

The use of a combination drug with an anti-infective component is indicated where the risk of infection is high or where there is an expectation that potentially dangerous numbers of bacteria will be present in the eye.

The particular anti-infective drug in this product is active against the following common bacterial eye pathogens: **Escherichia coli, Staphylococcus aureus, Streptococcus pneumoniae, Streptococcus (viridans group), Pseudomonas** species, **Haemophilus influenzae, Klebsiella** species, and **Enterobacter** species. This product does not provide adequate coverage against **Neisseria** species and **Serratia marcescens.**

Contraindications: Epithelial herpes simplex keratitis (dendritic keratitis), vaccinia, varicella, and many other viral diseases of the cornea and conjunctiva. Mycobacterial infection of the eye. Fungal diseases of the ocular structures. Hypersensitivity to a component of the medication. (Hypersensitivity to the antimicrobial component occurs at a higher rate than for other components.)

The use of these combinations is always contraindicated after uncomplicated removal of a corneal foreign body.

Warnings: Prolonged use may result in glaucoma, with damage to the optic nerve, defects in visual acuity and fields of vision, and in posterior subcapsular cataract formation. Prolonged use may suppress the host response and thus increase the hazard of secondary ocular infections. In those diseases causing thinning of the cornea or sclera, perforations have been known to occur with the use of topical steroids. In acute purulent conditions of the eye, steroids may mask infection or enhance existing infection. If these products are used for 10 days or longer, intraocular pressure should be routinely monitored even though it may be difficult in children and uncooperative patients. Employment of a steroid medication in the treatment of herpes simplex requires great caution.

A significant percentage of staphylococcal isolates are completely resistant to sulfa drugs.

Precautions: The initial prescription and renewal of the medication order beyond 20 milliliters should be made by a physician only after examination of the patient with the aid of magnification, such as slit lamp biomicroscopy and, where appropriate, fluorescein staining. The possibility of fungal infections of the cornea should be considered after prolonged steroid dosing.

Adverse Reactions: Adverse reactions have occurred with steroid/anti-infective combination drugs which can be attributed to the steroid component, the anti-infective component, or the combination. Exact incidence figures are not available since no denominator of treated patients is available.

Reactions occurring most often from the presence of the anti-infective ingredient are allergic sensitizations. The reactions due to the steroid component in decreasing order of frequency are: elevation of intraocular pressure (IOP) with possible development of glaucoma, and infrequent optic nerve damage; posterior subcapsular cataract formation; and delayed wound healing.

Secondary infection: The development of secondary infection has occurred after use of combinations containing steroids and antimicrobials. Fungal infections of the cornea are particularly prone to develop coincidentally with long-term applications of steroid. The possibility of fungal invasion must be considered in any persistent corneal ulceration where steroid treatment has been used.

Secondary bacterial ocular infection following suppression of host responses also occurs.

Dosage and Administration: Optimal dosage is 1 drop two to four times daily, depending upon the severity of the condition.

In general, during early or acute stages of blepharitis, BLEPHAMIDE® LIQUIFILM® sterile ophthalmic suspension produces results most rapidly—and most efficiently—with instillation directly into the eye, with the excess spread on the lid (Method I). When the condition is confined to the lid, however, BLEPHAMIDE® may be applied directly to the site of the lesions (Method II).

METHOD I: In the Eye and On the Lid

1. Wash hands carefully. Tilt head back and drop **1 drop** into the eye.
2. Close the eye and spread the excess medication present after closing the eye on the full length of the upper and lower lids.
3. Do not wipe any of the medication off the lids. It will dry completely in 4 or 5 minutes to a clear film that remains on the lids for several hours—it cannot be seen by others, nor will it interfere with vision.
4. The medication should be washed off the lids once or twice a day. **However, it should be reapplied after each washing.**

METHOD II: On the Lid

1. Wash hands carefully. With head tilted back and **eye closed,** drop 1 drop onto the lid—preferably at the corner of the eye close to the nose.
2. Spread the medication over the full length of the upper and lower lids.
3. Do not wipe away any medication—it will dry in 4 to 5 minutes to a clear, invisible film which will remain on the lids for several hours.
4. The medication should be washed off the lids once or twice a day. **However, it should be reapplied after each washing.**

Not more than 20 milliliters should be prescribed initially and the prescription should not be refilled without further evaluation as outlined in PRECAUTIONS above.

How Supplied: BLEPHAMIDE® LIQUIFILM® is supplied in plastic dropper bottles in the following sizes:

2.5 mL—NDC 11980-022-03
5 mL—NDC 11980-022-05
10 mL—NDC 11980-022-10

Note: Protect from freezing. **Shake well before using.**

Caution: Federal (U.S.A.) law prohibits dispensing without prescription.

ALLERGAN AMERICA,
Hormiguerous, Puerto Rico 00660

BLEPHAMIDE® ℞
(sulfacetamide sodium and prednisolone acetate ophthalmic ointment USP)
10%/0.2% sterile

Description: BLEPHAMIDE® (sulfacetamide sodium and prednisolone acetate ophthalmic ointment USP) is a sterile topical ophthalmic ointment combining an antibacterial and a corticosteroid which has the following composition:

Sulfacetamide Sodium .... 10% (100 mg/g)
(bacteriostatic antibacterial)
Prednisolone Acetate .... 0.2% (2 mg/g)
(corticosteroid/anti-inflammatory)

with: phenylmercuric acetate (0.0008%); mineral oil; white petrolatum; and petrolatum (and) lanolin alcohol.

Chemical Names:

Sulfacetamide sodium: N-sulfanilylacetamide monosodium salt monohydrate.

Prednisolone acetate: 11β, 17, 21-trihydroxypregna-1,4-diene-3, 20-dione, 21-acetate.

Clinical Pharmacology: Corticosteroids suppress the inflammatory response to a variety of agents and they probably delay or slow healing. Since corticosteroids may inhibit the body's defense mechanism against infection, a concomitant antibacterial drug may be used when this inhibition is considered to be clinically significant in a particular case.

When a decision to administer both a corticosteroid and an antibacterial is made, the administration of such drugs in combination has the advantage of greater patient compliance and convenience, with the added assurance that the appropriate dosage of both drugs is administered, plus assured compatibility of ingredients when both types of drugs are in the same formulation and, particularly, that the correct volume of drug is delivered and retained.

The relative potency of corticosteroids depends on the molecular structure, concentration and release from the vehicle.

Microbiology: Sulfacetamide exerts a bacteriostatic effect against susceptible bacteria by restricting the synthesis of folic acid required for growth through competition with p-amino benzoic acid.

Some strains of these bacteria may be resistant to sulfacetamide or resistant strains may emerge *in vivo.*

The anti-infective component in BLEPHAMIDE® ointment is included to provide action against specific organisms susceptible to it. Sulfacetamide sodium is active *in vitro* against susceptible strains of the following microorganisms: *Escherichia coli, Staphylococcus aureus, Streptococcus pneumoniae, Streptococcus* (viridans group), *Haemophilus influenzae, Klebsiella* species, and *Enterobacter* species. This product does not provide adequate coverage against: *Neisseria* species, *Pseudomonas* species, and *Serratia marcescens* (see **INDICATIONS AND USAGE**).

Continued on next page

Allergan Pharm—Cont.

Indications and Usage: BLEPHAMIDE® ophthalmic ointment is indicated for steroid-responsive inflammatory ocular conditions for which a corticosteroid is indicated and where superficial bacterial ocular infection or a risk of bacterial ocular infection exists.

Ocular corticosteroids are indicated in inflammatory conditions of the palpebral and bulbar conjunctiva, cornea, and anterior segment of the globe where the inherent risk of corticosteroid use in certain infective conjunctivitides is accepted to obtain diminution in edema and inflammation. They are also indicated in chronic anterior uveitis and corneal injury from chemical, radiation or thermal burns or penetration of foreign bodies.

The use of a combination drug with an anti-infective component is indicated where the risk of superficial ocular infection is high or where there is an expectation that potentially dangerous numbers of bacteria will be present in the eye.

The particular antibacterial drug in this product is active against the following common bacterial eye pathogens: *Escherichia coli, Staphylococcus aureus, Streptococcus pneumoniae, Streptococcus* (viridans group), *Haemophilus influenzae, Klebsiella* species, and *Enterobacter* species.

The product does not provide adequate coverage against: *Neisseria* species, *Pseudomonas* species, and *Serratia marcescens.*

A significant percentage of staphylococcal isolates are completely resistant to sulfa drugs.

Contraindications: BLEPHAMIDE® ophthalmic ointment is contraindicated in most viral diseases of the cornea and conjunctiva including epithelial herpes simplex keratitis (dendritic keratitis), vaccinia, and varicella, and also in mycobacterial infection of the eye and fungal diseases of ocular structures.

This product is also contraindicated in individuals with known or suspected hypersensitivity to any of the ingredients of this preparation, to other sulfonamides and to other corticosteroids. See **WARNINGS.** (Hypersensitivity to the antimicrobial component occurs at a higher rate than for other components).

Warnings: NOT FOR INJECTION INTO THE EYE. Prolonged use of corticosteroids may result in ocular hypertension/glaucoma with damage to the optic nerve, defects in visual acuity and fields of vision, and in posterior subcapsular cataract formation.

Acute anterior uveitis may occur in susceptible individuals, primarily Blacks.

Prolonged use of BLEPHAMIDE® ophthalmic ointment may suppress the host response and thus increase the hazard of secondary ocular infections. In those diseases causing thinning of the cornea or sclera, perforation has been known to occur with the use of topical corticosteroids. In acute purulent conditions of the eye, corticosteroids may mask infection or enhance existing infection.

If the product is used for 10 days or longer, intraocular pressure should be routinely monitored even though it may be difficult in children and uncooperative patients. Corticosteroids should be used with caution in the presence of glaucoma. Intraocular pressure should be checked frequently.

A significant percentage of staphylococcal isolates are completely resistant to sulfonamides.

The use of steroids after cataract surgery may delay healing and increase the incidence of filtering blebs.

The use of ocular corticosteroids may prolong the course and may exacerbate the severity of many viral infections of the eye (including herpes simplex). Employment of corticosteroid medication in the treatment of herpes simplex requires great caution.

Topical steroids are not effective in mustard gas keratitis and Sjogren's keratoconjunctivitis.

Fatalities have occurred, although rarely, due to severe reactions to sulfonamides including Stevens-Johnson syndrome, toxic epidermal necrolysis, fulminant hepatic necrosis, agranulocytosis, aplastic anemia and other blood dyscrasias. Sensitization may recur when a sulfonamide is readministered, irrespective of the route of administration.

If signs of hypersensitivity or other serious reactions occur, discontinue use of this preparation. Cross-sensitivity among corticosteroids has been demonstrated (see **ADVERSE REACTIONS**).

Precautions: General: The initial prescription and renewal of the medication order beyond 8 g of ointment should be made by a physician only after examination of the patient with the aid of magnification, such as slit lamp biomicroscopy and, where appropriate, fluorescein staining. If signs and symptoms fail to improve after two days, the patient should be re-evaluated. The possibility of fungal infections of the cornea should be considered after prolonged corticosteroid dosing. Use with caution in patients with severe dry eye. Fungal cultures should be taken when appropriate.

The p-amino benzoic acid present in purulent exudates competes with sulfonamides and can reduce their effectiveness. Ophthalmic ointments may retard corneal healing.

Information for Patients: If inflammation or pain persists longer than 48 hours or becomes aggravated, the patient should be advised to discontinue use of the medication and consult a physician (see **WARNINGS**).

This product is sterile when packaged. To prevent contamination, care should be taken to avoid touching the tube tip to eyelids or to any other surface. The use of this tube by more than one person may spread infection. Keep tube tightly closed when not in use. Keep out of the reach of children.

Laboratory Tests: Eyelid cultures and tests to determine the susceptibility of organisms to sulfacetamide may be indicated if signs and symptoms persist or recur in spite of the recommended course of treatment with BLEPHAMIDE® ophthalmic ointment.

Drug Interactions: BLEPHAMIDE® ophthalmic ointment is incompatible with silver preparations. Local anesthetics related to p-amino benzoic acid may antagonize the action of the sulfonamides.

Carcinogenesis, Mutagenesis, Impairment of Fertility: Prednisolone has been reported to be noncarcinogenic. Long-term animal studies for carcinogenic potential have not been performed with sulfacetamide.

One author detected chromosomal nondisjunction in the yeast *Saccharomyces cerevisiae* following application of sulfacetamide sodium. The significance of this finding to topical ophthalmic use of sulfacetamide sodium in the human is unknown.

Mutagenic studies with prednisolone have been negative. Studies on reproduction and fertility have not been performed with sulfacetamide. A long-term chronic toxicity study in dogs showed that high oral doses of prednisolone prevented estrus. A decrease in fertility was seen in male and female rats that were mated following oral dosing with another glucocorticosteroid.

Pregnancy: Teratogenic Effects: Pregnancy Category C. Animal reproduction studies have not been conducted with sulfacetamide sodium. Prednisolone has been shown to be teratogenic in rabbits, hamsters, and mice. In mice, prednisolone has been shown to be teratogenic when given in doses 1 to 10 times the human ocular dose. Dexamethasone, hydrocortisone and prednisolone were ocularly applied to both eyes of pregnant mice five times per day on days 10 through 13 of gestation. A significant increase in the incidence of cleft palate was observed in the fetuses of the treated mice. There are no adequate well-controlled studies in pregnant women dosed with corticosteroids.

Kernicterus may be precipitated in infants by sulfonamides being given systemically during the third trimester of pregnancy. It is not known whether sulfacetamide sodium can cause fetal harm when administered to a pregnant woman or whether it can affect reproductive capacity.

BLEPHAMIDE® ophthalmic ointment should be used during pregnancy only if the potential benefit justifies the potential risk to the fetus.

Nursing Mothers: It is not known whether topical administration of corticosteroids could result in sufficient systemic absorption to produce detectable quantities in human milk. Systemically administered corticosteroids appear in human milk and could suppress growth, interfere with endogenous corticosteroid production, or cause other untoward effects. Systemically administered sulfonamides are capable of producing kernicterus in infants of lactating women. Because of the potential for serious adverse reactions in nursing infants from sulfacetamide sodium and prednisolone acetate ophthalmic ointments, a decision should be made whether to discontinue nursing or to discontinue the medication.

Pediatric Use: Safety and effectiveness in children below the age of six have not been established.

Adverse Reactions: Adverse reactions have occurred with corticosteroid/antibacterial combination drugs which can be attributed to the corticosteroid component, the antibacterial component, or the combination. Exact incidence figures are not available since no denominator of treated patients is available.

Reactions occurring most often from the presence of the antibacterial ingredient are allergic sensitizations. Fatalities have occurred, although rarely, due to severe reactions to sulfonamides including Stevens-Johnson syndrome, toxic epidermal necrolysis, fulminant hepatic necroses, agranulocytosis, aplastic anemia, and other blood dyscrasias (See **WARNINGS**).

Sulfacetamide sodium may cause local irritation.

The reactions due to the corticosteroid component in decreasing order of frequency are: elevation of intraocular pressure (IOP) with possible development of glaucoma and infrequent optic nerve damage, posterior subcapsular cataract formation, and delayed wound healing.

Although systemic effects are extremely uncommon, there have been rare occurrences of systemic hypercorticoidism after use of topical steroids.

Corticosteroid-containing preparations can also cause acute anterior uveitis or perforation of the globe. Mydriasis, loss of accommodation and ptosis have occasionally been reported following local use of corticosteroids.

Secondary Infection: The development of secondary infection has occurred after use of combinations containing corticosteroids and antibacterials. Fungal and viral infections of the cornea are particularly prone to develop coincidentally with long-term applications of corticosteroid. The possibility of fungal invasion must be considered in any persistent corneal ulceration where corticosteroid treatment has been used.

Secondary bacterial ocular infection following suppression of host responses also occurs.

Dosage and Administration: A small amount, approximately ½ inch ribbon of ointment, should be applied in the conjunctival sac three or four times daily and once or twice at night.

Not more than 8 g should be prescribed initially.
The dosing of BLEPHAMIDE® ophthalmic ointment may be reduced, but care should be taken not to discontinue therapy prematurely. In chronic conditions, withdrawal of treatment should be carried out by gradually decreasing the frequency of application.
If signs and symptoms fail to improve after two days, the patient should be re-evaluated (see **PRECAUTIONS**).
How Supplied: BLEPHAMIDE® (sulfacetamide sodium and prednisolone acetate ophthalmic ointment USP) 10%/0.2% is supplied sterile in 3.5 gram ointment tubes: NDC 0023-0313-04.
Note: Store away from heat.
Caution: Federal (U.S.A.) law prohibits dispensing without prescription.

CHLOROPTIC®* ℞
(chloramphenicol 0.5%)
sterile ophthalmic solution

Contains:
chloramphenicol .... 0.5% (5 mg/mL)
with: chlorobutanol (chloral deriv. as a preservative) 0.5%; polyethylene glycol 300; polyoxyl 40 stearate; sodium hydroxide or hydrochloric acid to adjust the pH and purified water.
Actions: CHLOROPTIC® (chloramphenicol) has a wide spectrum of antimicrobial activity and is effective against many gram-negative and gram-positive organisms such as **Escherichia coli, Haemophilus influenzae, Staphylococcus aureus, Streptococcus hemolyticus,** and **Moraxella lacunata** (Morax-Axenfeld bacillus).
Indications: For the treatment of superficial ocular infections involving the conjunctiva and/or cornea caused by chloramphenicol-susceptible organisms.
Contraindications: Contraindicated in patients who are hypersensitive to chloramphenicol.
Warnings: As with other antibiotics, prolonged use may result in overgrowth of non-susceptible organisms. If superinfection occurs, or if clinical improvement is not noted within a reasonable period, discontinue use and institute appropriate therapy. Sensitivity reactions such as stinging, itching, angioneurotic edema, urticaria, vesicular and maculopapular dermatitis may also occur in some patients. Occasionally one sees hematopoietic toxicity with the use of systemic chloramphenicol, and rarely with topical administration. This type of blood dyscrasia is generally a dose-related toxic effect on bone marrow and is usually reversible on cessation of the drug. Rare cases of aplastic anemia have been reported with prolonged (months to years) or frequent intermittent (over months and years) use of topical chloramphenicol.
Adverse Reactions: The most serious reaction reported following prolonged or frequent intermittent use of topical chloramphenicol is bone marrow aplasia.
Dosage and Administration: One or two drops 4 to 6 times a day for the first 72 hours, depending upon the severity of the condition. Intervals between applications may be increased after the first two days. Since the action of the drug is primarily bacteriostatic, therapy should be continued for 48 hours after an apparent cure has been attained.
How Supplied: CHLOROPTIC® (chloramphenicol) sterile ophthalmic solution is supplied in plastic dropper bottles in the following sizes:
2.5 mL—NDC 11980-109-03
7.5 mL—NDC 11980-109-08
Refrigerate until dispensed.
Caution: Federal (U.S.A.) law prohibits dispensing without prescription.

*U.S. Patent 3,702,364

CHLOROPTIC® ℞
(chloramphenicol) 1.0%
S.O.P.®
sterile ophthalmic ointment

Description: CHLOROPTIC® (chloramphenicol) 1.0% S.O.P.® sterile ophthalmic ointment is a topical anti-infective product for ophthalmic use.
Chemical Name: D-*threo* -(-)-2,2-Dichloro-N-[β-hydroxy-α-(hydroxymethyl)-p-nitrophenethyl] acetamide
Contains:
chloramphenicol .... 1.0% (10 mg/g)
with: chlorobutanol (chloral deriv.) 0.5%; white petrolatum; mineral oil; polyoxyl 40 stearate; polyethylene glycol 300; and petrolatum (and) lanolin alcohol.
Clinical Pharmacology: Chloramphenicol inhibits protein synthesis by interfering with the transfer of activated amino acids from soluble RNA to ribosomes. Chloramphenicol is a broad-spectrum antibiotic originally isolated from **Streptomyces venezuelae.** It is primarily bacteriostatic and useful in the treatment of bacterial infections caused by organisms such as **Haemophilus influenzae, Staphylococcus aureus, Streptococcus hemolyticus** and **Moraxella lacunata** (Morax-Axenfeld bacillus). Chloramphenicol also has an effect on the rickettsiae and the mycoplasma (PPLO) groups of organisms.
Indications and Usage: Chloramphenicol should be used only in those serious infections for which less potent drugs are ineffective or contraindicated.
CHLOROPTIC® is indicated for the treatment of ocular infections involving the conjunctiva and/or cornea caused by chloramphenicol-susceptible organisms.
The particular anti-infective drug in the product is active against the following common eye pathogens: **Staphylococcus aureus;** Streptococci, including **Streptococcus pneumoniae; Escherichia coli; Haemophilus influenzae; Klebsiella/Enterobacter** species; **Neisseria** species; **Moraxella lacunata** (Morax-Axenfeld bacillus).
The product does not provide adequate coverage against: **Pseudomonas aeruginosa** and **Serratia marcescens.**
Contraindications: This product is contraindicated in persons sensitive to any of the components.
Warnings: Occasionally one sees hematopoietic toxicity with the use of systemic chloramphenicol and rarely with topical administration. This type of blood dyscrasia is generally a dose-related toxic effect on bone marrow and is usually reversible on cessation of the drug. Rare cases of aplastic anemia have been reported with prolonged (months to years) or frequent intermittent (over months and years) use of topical chloramphenicol.
As with other antibiotics, prolonged use may result in overgrowth of non-susceptible organisms. If superinfection occurs, or if clinical improvement is not noted within a reasonable period, discontinue use and institute appropriate therapy.
Precautions: Ophthalmic ointments may retard corneal healing.
Adverse Reactions: Exact incidence figures are not available since no denominator of treated patients is available.
The most serious reaction occurring from the presence of chloramphenicol is bone marrow aplasia. Three cases, including one fatality, have been reported following prolonged or frequent intermittent use of topical chloramphenicol.
Reactions occurring most often from the use of topical anti-infectives are allergic sensitizations. These reactions include stinging, itching, angioneurotic edema, urticaria, vesicular and maculopapular dermatitis.
Dosage and Administration: Place a small amount of ointment in the conjunctival sac every 3 hours, or more often if required, day and night for the first 48 hours. Intervals between applications may be increased after the first two days. Since the action of chloramphenicol is primarily bacteriostatic, therapy should be continued for 48 hours after an apparent cure has been obtained.
How Supplied: CHLOROPTIC® (chloramphenicol) 1.0% S.O.P.® sterile ophthalmic ointment is supplied in ophthalmic ointment tubes in the following size:
3.5 g—**NDC** 0023-0301-04
Note: Store away from heat.
Caution: Federal (U.S.A.) law prohibits dispensing without prescription.

EPIFRIN® ℞
(epinephrine, USP)
sterile ophthalmic solution

Description: EPIFRIN® (epinephrine, USP) sterile ophthalmic solution is a topical sympathomimetic agent for ophthalmic use.
Chemical Name: 1,2-Benzenediol,4-[1-hydroxy-2-(methylamino)ethyl]-, (R)-.
Contains: epinephrine, USP 0.5%, 1%, 2% with: benzalkonium chloride; sodium metabisulfite; edetate disodium; hydrochloric acid; and purified water.
Clinical Pharmacology: Epinephrine is an adrenergic agonist that stimulates α- and β-adrenergic receptors. The capacity of EPIFRIN® (epinephrine, USP) to decrease the aqueous inflow in open-angle glaucoma has been well documented. Studies have also shown that prolonged topical epinephrine therapy offers significant improvement in the coefficient of aqueous outflow.
EPIFRIN® is effective alone in reducing intraocular pressure and is particularly useful in combination with miotics or beta-adrenergic blocking agents for the difficult-to-control patients. The addition of EPIFRIN® to the patient's regimen often provides better control of intraocular pressure than the original agent alone.
Indications and Usage: EPIFRIN® is indicated for the treatment of chronic simple glaucoma.
Contraindications: EPIFRIN® should not be used in patients who have had an attack of narrow-angle glaucoma, since dilation of the pupil may trigger an acute attack. Do not use if hypersensitive to any ingredient.
Warnings:
1. EPIFRIN® should be used with caution in patients with a narrow angle, since dilation of the pupil may trigger an acute attack of narrow-angle glaucoma.
2. Use with caution in patients with hypertensive cardiovascular disease or coronary artery disease.
3. Epinephrine has been reported to produce reversible macular edema in some aphakic patients and should be used with caution in these patients.

Contains sodium metabisulfite, a sulfite that may cause allergic-type reactions, including anaphylactic symptoms and life-threatening or less severe asthmatic episodes in certain susceptible people. The overall prevalence of sulfite sensitivity in the general population is

Continued on next page

Allergan Pharm—Cont.

unknown and probably low. Sulfite sensitivity is seen more frequently in asthmatic than in nonasthmatic people.

Precautions:

General: Epinephrine in any form is relatively uncomfortable upon instillation. However, discomfort lessens as the concentration of epinephrine decreases. EPIFRIN® is not for injection.

Carcinogenesis, mutagenesis and impairment of fertility: No studies have been conducted in animals or in humans to evaluate the potential of these effects.

Pregnancy Category C: Animal reproduction studies have not been conducted with epinephrine. It is also not known whether epinephrine can cause fetal harm when administered to a pregnant woman or if it can affect reproduction capacity. Epinephrine should be given to a pregnant woman only if clearly needed.

Pediatric Use: Safety and effectiveness in children have not been established.

Adverse Reactions: Undesirable reactions to topical epinephrine include eye pain or ache, browache, headache, conjunctival hyperemia and allergic lid reactions.

Adrenochrome deposits in the conjunctiva and cornea after prolonged epinephrine therapy have been reported. Topical epinephrine has been reported to produce reversible macular edema in some aphakic patients.

Overdosage: Accidental ingestion will not cause problems because pharmacologically active concentrations of epinephrine cannot be achieved orally in man. Should accidental overdosage in the eye(s) occur, flush eye(s) with water or normal saline.

Dosage and Administration: The usual dosage is 1 drop in the affected eye(s) once or twice daily. However, the dosage should be adjusted to meet the needs of the individual patients. This is made easier with EPIFRIN® (epinephrine, USP) sterile ophthalmic solution available in three strengths.

How Supplied: EPIFRIN® is available on prescription only in plastic dropper bottles in the following concentrations and sizes:

0.5%	15 mL—NDC 11980-119-15
1%	15 mL—NDC 11980-122-15
2%	15 mL—NDC 11980-058-15

Note: Protect from light and excessive heat. If the solution discolors or a precipitate forms, it should be discarded.

FML® ℞
(fluorometholone) 0.1%
LIQUIFILM®
sterile ophthalmic suspension

Description: FML® (fluorometholone) 0.1% LIQUIFILM sterile ophthalmic suspension is a topical anti-inflammatory agent for ophthalmic use.

Chemical Name: Fluorometholone: 9-Fluoro-11β,17-dihydroxy-6α-methylpregna-1,4-diene-3,20-dione.

Contains:

fluorometholone 0.1%

with: LIQUIFILM® (polyvinyl alcohol) 1.4%; benzalkonium chloride 0.004%; edetate disodium; sodium chloride; sodium phosphate, monobasic; sodium phosphate, dibasic; polysorbate 80; sodium hydroxide to adjust the pH, and purified water.

Clinical Pharmacology: Corticosteroids inhibit the inflammatory response to a variety of inciting agents and probably delay or slow healing. They inhibit the edema, fibrin deposition, capillary dilation, leukocyte migration, capillary proliferation, fibroblast proliferation, deposition of collagen, and scar formation associated with inflammation.

There is no generally accepted explanation for the mechanism of action of ocular corticosteroids. However, corticosteroids are thought to act by the induction of phospholipase A_2 inhibitory proteins, collectively called lipocortins. It is postulated that these proteins control the biosynthesis of potent mediators of inflammation such as prostaglandins and leukotrienes by inhibiting the release of their common precursor arachidonic acid. Arachidonic acid is released from membrane phospholipids by phospholipase A_2.

Corticosteroids are capable of producing a rise in intraocular pressure. In clinical studies on patients' eyes treated with both dexamethasone and fluorometholone 0.1% suspensions, fluorometholone demonstrated a lower propensity to increase intraocular pressure than did dexamethasone.

Indications and Usage: FML® suspension is indicated for the treatment of corticosteroid-responsive inflammation of the palpebral and bulbar conjunctiva, cornea and anterior segment of the globe.

Contraindications: FML® suspension is contraindicated in most viral diseases of the cornea and conjunctiva, including epithelial herpes simplex keratitis (dendritic keratitis), vaccinia, and varicella and also in mycobacterial infection of the eye and fungal diseases of ocular structures. FML® suspension is also contraindicated in individuals with known or suspected hypersensitivity to any of the ingredients of this preparation and to other corticosteroids.

Warnings: Prolonged use of corticosteroids may result in glaucoma with damage to the optic nerve, defects in visual acuity and fields of vision, and/or in posterior subcapsular cataract formation. Prolonged use may also suppress the host immune response and thus increase the hazard of secondary ocular infections.

Various ocular diseases and long-term use of topical corticosteroids have been known to cause corneal and scleral thinning. Use of topical corticosteroids in the presence of thin corneal or scleral tissue may lead to perforation.

Acute purulent untreated infections of the eye may be masked or activity enhanced by presence of corticosteroid medication.

If this product is used for 10 days or longer, intraocular pressure should be routinely monitored even though it may be difficult in children and uncooperative patients. Steroids should be used with caution in the presence of glaucoma. Intraocular pressure should be checked frequently.

The use of steroids after cataract surgery may delay healing and increase the incidence of bleb formation.

Use of ocular steroids may prolong the course and may exacerbate the severity of many viral infections of the eye (including herpes simplex). Employment of a corticosteroid medication in the treatment of patients with a history of herpes simplex requires great caution; frequent slit lamp microscopy is recommended.

Corticosteroids are not effective in mustard gas keratitis and Sjogren's keratoconjunctivitis.

Precautions: General: The initial prescription and renewal of the medication order beyond 20 milliliters of FML® suspension should be made by a physician only after examination of the patient with the aid of magnification, such as slit lamp biomicroscopy and, where appropriate, fluorescein staining. If signs and symptoms fail to improve after two days, the patient should be re-evaluated.

As fungal infections of the cornea are particularly prone to develop coincidentally with long-term local corticosteroid applications, fungal invasion should be suspected in any persistent corneal ulceration where a corticosteroid has been used or is in use. Fungal cultures should be taken when appropriate.

If this product is used for 10 days or longer, intraocular pressure should be monitored (see WARNINGS).

Information for Patients: If inflammation or pain persists longer than 48 hours or becomes aggravated, the patient should be advised to discontinue use of the medication and consult a physician.

This product is sterile when packaged. To prevent contamination, care should be taken to avoid touching the bottle tip to eyelids or to any other surface. The use of this bottle by more than one person may spread infection. Keep bottle tightly closed when not in use. Keep out of the reach of children.

Carcinogenesis, mutagenesis, impairment of fertility: No studies have been conducted in animals or in humans to evaluate the possibility of these effects with fluorometholone.

Pregnancy: Teratogenic effects. Pregnancy Category C: Fluorometholone has been shown to be embryocidal and teratogenic in rabbits when administered at low multiples of the human ocular dose. Fluorometholone was applied ocularly to rabbits daily on days 6–18 of gestation, and dose-related fetal loss and fetal abnormalities including cleft palate, deformed rib cage, anomalous limbs and neural abnormalities such as encephalocele, craniorachischisis, and spina bifida were observed. There are no adequate and well-controlled studies of fluorometholone in pregnant women, and it is not known whether fluorometholone can cause fetal harm when administered to a pregnant woman. Fluorometholone should be used during pregnancy only if the potential benefit justifies the potential risk to the fetus.

Nursing Mothers: It is not known whether topical ophthalmic administration of corticosteroids could result in sufficient systemic absorption to produce detectable quantities in breast milk. Systemically administered corticosteroids appear in human milk and could suppress growth, interfere with endogenous corticosteroid production, or cause other untoward effects. Because of the potential for serious adverse reactions in nursing infants from fluoromethalone, a decision should be made whether to discontinue nursing or to discontinue the drug, taking into account the importance of the drug to the mother.

Pediatric Use: Safety and effectiveness in children below the age of two years have not been established.

Adverse Reactions: Adverse reactions include, in decreasing order of frequency, elevation of intraocular pressure (IOP) with possible development of glaucoma and infrequent optic nerve damage, posterior subcapsular cataract formation, and delayed wound healing.

Although systemic effects are extremely uncommon, there have been rare occurrences of systemic hypercorticoidism after use of topical steroids.

Corticosteroid-containing preparations have also been reported to cause acute anterior uveitis and perforation of the globe. Keratitis, conjunctivitis, corneal ulcers, mydriasis, conjunctival hyperemia, loss of accommodation and ptosis have occasionally been reported following local use of corticosteroids.

The development of secondary ocular infection (bacterial, fungal and viral) has occurred. Fungal and viral infections of the cornea are particularly prone to develop coincidentally with long-term applications of steroids. The possibility of fungal invasion should be considered in any persistent corneal ulceration where steroid treatment has been used (see WARNINGS).

Dosage and Administration: Instill one drop into the conjunctival sac two to four times daily. During the initial 24 to 48 hours, the dosage may be increased to one application every four hours. Care should be taken not to discontinue therapy prematurely.

If signs and symptoms fail to improve after two days, the patient should be re-evaluated (see PRECAUTIONS).

The dosing of FML® suspension may be reduced, but care should be taken not to discontinue therapy prematurely. In chronic conditions, withdrawal of treatment should be carried out by gradually decreasing the frequency of applications.

How Supplied: FML® (fluorometholone) 0.1% LIQUIFILM® sterile ophthalmic suspension is supplied in plastic dropper bottles in the following sizes:

1 mL—NDC 11980-211-01
5 mL—NDC 11980-211-05
10 mL—NDC 11980-211-10
15 mL—NDC 11980-211-15

Note: Store at or below 25°C (77°F); protect from freezing. **Shake well before using.**

Caution: Federal (U.S.A.) law prohibits dispensing without prescription.

FML® ℞
(fluorometholone) 0.1%
S.O.P.®
sterile ophthalmic ointment

Description: FML® (fluorometholone) 0.1% S.O.P.® sterile ophthalmic ointment is a topical anti-inflammatory agent for ophthalmic use.

Chemical Name: Fluorometholone:
9-Fluoro-11β,17-dihydroxy-6α-methylpregna-1,4-diene-3,20-dione.

Contains:
fluorometholone 0.1%
with: phenylmercuric acetate (0.0008%), white petrolatum, mineral oil, and petrolatum (and) lanolin alcohol.

Clinical Pharmacology: Corticosteroids inhibit the inflammatory response to a variety of inciting agents and probably delay or slow healing. They inhibit the edema, fibrin deposition, capillary dilation, leukocyte migration, capillary proliferation, fibroblast proliferation, deposition of collagen and scar formation associated with inflammation.

There is no generally accepted explanation for the mechanism of action of ocular corticosteroids. However, corticosteroids are thought to act by the induction of phospholipase A_2 inhibitory proteins, collectively called lipocortins. It is postulated that these proteins control the biosynthesis of potent mediators of inflammation such as prostaglandins and leukotrienes by inhibiting the release of their common precursor arachidonic acid. Arachidonic acid is released from membrane phospholipids by phospholipase A_2.

Corticosteroids are capable of producing a rise in intraocular pressure. In clinical studies on patients' eyes treated with both dexamethasone and fluorometholone 0.1% suspensions, fluorometholone demonstrated a lower propensity to increase intraocular pressure than did dexamethasone.

Indications and Usage: FML® ointment is indicated for the treatment of corticosteroid-responsive inflammation of the palpebral and bulbar conjunctiva, cornea and anterior segment of the globe.

Contraindications: FML® ointment is contraindicated in most viral diseases of the cornea and conjunctiva, including epithelial herpes simplex keratitis (dendritic keratitis), vaccinia, and varicella and also in mycobacterial infection of the eye and fungal diseases of ocular structures. FML® ointment is also contraindicated in individuals with known or suspected hypersensitivity to any of the ingredients of this preparation and to other corticosteroids.

Warnings: Prolonged use of corticosteroids may result in glaucoma with damage to the optic nerve, defects in visual acuity and field of vision, and in posterior subcapsular cataract formation. Prolonged use may also suppress the host immune response and thus increase the hazard of secondary ocular infections.

Various ocular diseases and long-term use of topical corticosteroids have been known to cause corneal and scleral thinning. Use of topical corticosteroids in the presence of thin corneal or scleral tissue may lead to perforation.

Acute purulent untreated infection of the eye may be masked or activity enhanced by presence of corticosteroid medication.

If this product is used for 10 days or longer, intraocular pressure should be routinely monitored even though it may be difficult in children and uncooperative patients. Steroids should be used with caution in the presence of glaucoma. Intraocular pressure should be checked frequently.

The use of steroids after cataract surgery may delay healing and increase the incidence of bleb formation.

Use of ocular steroids may prolong the course and may exacerbate the severity of many viral infections of the eye (including herpes simplex). Employment of a corticosteroid medication in the treatment of patients with a history of herpes simplex requires great caution; frequent slit lamp microscopy is recommended.

Corticosteroids are not effective in mustard gas keratitis and Sjogren's keratoconjunctivitis.

Precautions: General: The initial prescription and renewal of the medication order beyond 8 grams of FML® ointment should be made by a physician only after examination of the patient with the aid of magnification, such as slit lamp biomicroscopy and, where approriate, fluorescein staining. If signs and symptoms fail to improve after two days, the patient should be re-evaluated.

As fungal infections of the cornea are particularly prone to develop coincidentally with long-term local corticosteroid applications, fungal invasion should be suspected in any persistent corneal ulceration where a corticosteroid has been used or is in use. Fungal cultures should be taken when appropriate.

If this product is used for 10 days or longer, intraocular pressure should be monitored (see WARNINGS).

Ophthalmic ointments may retard corneal healing.

Information for Patients: If inflammation or pain persists longer than 48 hours or becomes aggravated, the patient should be advised to discontinue use of the medication and consult a physician.

This product is sterile when packaged. To prevent contamination, care should be taken to avoid touching the tube tip to eyelids or to any other surface. The use of this tube by more than one person may spread infection. Keep tube tightly closed when not in use. Keep out of the reach of children.

Carcinogenesis, mutagenesis, impairment of fertility: No studies have been conducted in animals or in humans to evaluate the possibility of these effects with fluorometholone.

Pregnancy: Teratogenic effects. Pregnancy Category C: Fluorometholone has been shown to be embryocidal and teratogenic in rabbits when administered at low multiples of the human ocular dose. Fluorometholone was applied ocularly to rabbits daily on days 6–18 of gestation, and dose-related fetal loss and fetal abnormalities including cleft palate, deformed rib cage, anamalous limbs and neural abnormalities such as encephalocele, craniorachischisis, and spina bifida were observed. There are no adequate and well-controlled studies of fluorometholone in pregnant women, and it is not known whether fluorometholone can cause fetal harm when administered to a pregnant woman. Fluorometholone should be used during pregnancy only if the potential benefit justifies the potential risk to the fetus.

Nursing Mothers: It is not known whether topical ophthalmic administration of corticosteroids could result in sufficient systemic absorption to produce detectable quantities in human milk. Systemically administered corticosteroids appear in human milk and could suppress growth, interfere with endogenous corticosteroid production, or cause other untoward effects. Because of the potential for serious adverse reactions in nursing infants from fluorometholone, a decision should be made whether to discontinue nursing or to discontinue the drug, taking into account the importance of the drug to the mother.

Pediatric Use: Safety and effectiveness in children below the age of two years have not been established.

Adverse Reactions: Adverse reactions include, in decreasing order of frequency, elevation of intraocular pressure (IOP) with possible development of glaucoma and infrequent optic nerve damage, posterior subcapsular cataract formation, and delayed wound healing.

Although systemic effects are extremely uncommon, there have been rare occurrences of systemic hypercorticoidism after use of topical steroids.

Corticosteroid-containing preparations have also been reported to cause acute anterior uveitis and perforation of the globe. Keratitis, conjunctivitis, corneal ulcers, mydriasis, conjunctival hyperemia, loss of accommodation and ptosis have occasionally been reported following local use of corticosteroids.

The development of secondary ocular infection (bacterial, fungal and viral) has occurred. Fungal and viral infections of the cornea are particularly prone to develop coincidentally with long-term applications of steroids. The possibility of fungal invasion should be considered in any persistent corneal ulceration where steroid treatment has been used (see WARNINGS).

Dosage and Administration: A small amount (approximately ½ inch ribbon) of ointment should be applied in the conjunctival sac one to three times daily. During the initial 24 to 48 hours, the frequency of dosing may be increased to one application every four hours. Care should be taken not to discontinue therapy prematurely.

If signs and symptoms fail to improve after two days, the patient should be re-evaluated (see PRECAUTIONS).

The dosing of FML® ointment may be reduced, but care should be taken not to discontinue therapy prematurely. In chronic conditions, withdrawal of treatment should be carried out by gradually decreasing the frequency of applications.

How Supplied: FML® (fluorometholone) 0.1% S.O.P.® sterile ophthalmic ointment is supplied in ophthalmic ointment tubes in the following size:

3.5 g—NDC 0023-0316-04

Note: Store at or below 25°C (77°F). Avoid exposure to temperatures above 40°C (104°F).

Caution: Federal (U.S.A.) law prohibits dispensing without prescription.

FML Forte® ℞
(fluorometholone) 0.25%
Liquifilm®
sterile ophthalmic suspension

Description: FML Forte® Liquifilm® sterile ophthalmic suspension is a topical anti-inflammatory product for ophthalmic use.

Continued on next page

Allergan Pharm—Cont.

Chemical Name:
Fluorometholone: 9-Fluoro-11β, 17-dihydroxy-6α-methylpregna-1,4-diene-3,20-dione.

Contains:
fluorometholone 0.25%
with: Liquifilm® (polyvinyl alcohol) 1.4%; benzalkonium chloride 0.005%; edetate disodium; sodium chloride; sodium phosphate, monobasic; sodium phosphate, dibasic; polysorbate 80; sodium hydroxide to adjust the pH; and purified water.

Clinical Pharmacology: Corticosteroids inhibit the inflammatory response to a variety of inciting agents and probably delay or slow healing. They inhibit the edema, fibrin deposition, capillary dilation, leukocyte migration, capillary proliferation, fibroblast proliferation, deposition of collagen, and scar formation associated with inflammation.
There is no generally accepted explanation for the mechanism of action of ocular corticosteroids. However, corticosteroids are thought to act by the induction of phospholipase A_2 inhibitory proteins, collectively called lipocortins. It is postulated that these proteins control the biosynthesis of potent mediators of inflammation such as prostaglandins and leukotrienes by inhibiting the release of their common precursor, arachidonic acid. Arachidonic acid is released from membrane phospholipids by phospholipase A_2.
Corticosteroids are capable of producing a rise in intraocular pressure. In clinical studies of documented steroid-responders, fluorometholone demonstrated a significantly longer average time to produce a rise in intraocular pressure than dexamethasone phosphate; however, in a small percentage of individuals a significant rise in intraocular pressure occurred within one week. The ultimate magnitude of the rise was equivalent for both drugs.

Indications and Usage: FML Forte® suspension is indicated for the treatment of corticosteroid-responsive inflammation of the palpebral and bulbar conjunctiva, cornea and anterior segment of the globe.

Contraindications: FML Forte® suspension is contraindicated in most viral diseases of the cornea and conjunctiva, including epithelial herpes simplex keratitis (dendritic keratitis), vaccinia, and varicella, and also in mycobacterial infection of the eye and fungal diseases of ocular structures. FML Forte® suspension is also contraindicated in individuals with known or suspected hypersensitivity to any of the ingredients of this preparation and to other corticosteroids.

Warnings: Prolonged use of corticosteroids may result in glaucoma, with damage to the optic nerve, defects in visual acuity and fields of vision, and in posterior subcapsular cataract formation. Prolonged use may also suppress the host immune response and thus increase the hazard of secondary ocular infections.
Various ocular diseases and long-term use of topical corticosteroids have been known to cause corneal and scleral thinning. Use of topical corticosteroids in the presence of thin corneal or scleral tissue may lead to perforation.
Acute purulent untreated infection of the eye may be masked or activity enhanced by the presence of corticosteroid medication.
If this product is used for 10 days or longer, intraocular pressure should be routinely monitored even though it may be difficult in children and uncooperative patients. Steroids should be used with caution in the presence of glaucoma. Intraocular pressure should be checked frequently.
The use of steroids after cataract surgery may delay healing and increase the incidence of bleb formation.
Use of ocular steroids may prolong the course and may exacerbate the severity of many viral infections of the eye (including herpes simplex). Employment of a corticosteroid medication in the treatment of patients with a history of herpes simplex requires great caution; frequent slit lamp microscopy is recommended.
Corticosteroids are not effective in mustard gas keratitis and Sjogren's keratoconjunctivitis.

Precautions: General: The initial prescription and renewal of the medication order beyond 20 milliliters of FML Forte® suspension should be made by a physician only after examination of the patient with the aid of magnification, such as slit lamp biomicroscopy and, where appropriate, fluorescein staining. If signs and symptoms fail to improve after two days, the patient should be re-evaluated.
As fungal infections of the cornea are particularly prone to develop coincidentally with long-term local corticosteroid applications, fungal invasion should be suspected in any persistent corneal ulceration where a corticosteroid has been used or is in use. Fungal cultures should be taken when appropriate.
If this product is used for 10 days or longer, intraocular pressure should be monitored (see WARNINGS).

Information for Patients: If inflammation or pain persists longer than 48 hours or becomes aggravated, the patient should be advised to discontinue use of the medication and consult a physician.
This product is sterile when packaged. To prevent contamination, care should be taken to avoid touching the bottle tip to eyelids or to any other surface. The use of this bottle by more than one person may spread infection. Keep bottle tightly closed when not in use. Keep out of reach of children.

Carcinogenesis, mutagenesis, impairment of fertility: No studies have been conducted in animals or in humans to evaluate the possibility of these effects with fluorometholone.

Pregnancy: Teratogenic effects. Pregnancy Category C: Fluorometholone has been shown to be embryocidal and teratogenic in rabbits when administered at low multiples of the human ocular dose. Fluorometholone was applied ocularly to rabbits daily on days 6–18 of gestation, and dose-related fetal loss and fetal abnormalities including cleft palate, deformed rib cage, anomalous limbs and neural abnormalities such as encephalocele, craniorachischisis, and spina bifida were observed. There are no adequate and well-controlled studies of fluorometholone in pregnant women, and it is not known whether fluorometholone can cause fetal harm when administered to a pregnant woman. Fluorometholone should be used during pregnancy only if the potential benefit justifies the potential risk to the fetus.

Nursing Mothers: It is not known whether topical ophthalmic adminstration of corticosteroids could result in sufficient systemic absorption to produce detectable quantities in human milk. Systemically administered corticosteroids appear in human milk and could suppress growth, interfere with endogenous corticosteroids production, or cause other untoward effects. Because of the potential for serious adverse reactions in nursing infants from fluorometholone, a decision should be made whether to discontinue nursing or to discontinue the drug, taking into account the importance of the drug to the mother.

Pediatric Use: Safety and effectiveness in children below the age of two years have not been established.

Adverse Reactions: Adverse reactions include, in decreasing order of frequency, elevation of intraocular pressure (IOP) with possible development of glaucoma and infrequent optic nerve damage, posterior subcapsular cataract formation, and delayed wound healing.
Although systemic effects are extremely uncommon, there have been rare occurrences of systemic hypercorticoidism after use of topical steroids.
Corticosteroid-containing preparations have also been reported to cause acute anterior uveitis and perforation of the globe. Keratitis, conjunctivitis, corneal ulcers, mydriasis, conjunctival hyperemia, loss of accommodation and ptosis have occasionally been reported following local use of corticosteroids.
The development of secondary ocular infection (bacterial, fungal and viral) has occurred. Fungal and viral infections of the cornea are particularly prone to develop coincidentally with long-term applications of steroids. The possibility of fungal invasion should be considered in any persistent corneal ulceration where steroid treatment has been used (see WARNINGS).

Dosage and Administration: Instill one drop into the conjunctival sac two to four times daily. Care should be taken not to discontinue therapy prematurely. If signs and symptoms fail to improve after two days, the patient should be re-evaluated (see PRECAUTIONS).
The dosing of FML Forte® suspension may be reduced, but care should be taken not to discontinue therapy prematurely. In chronic conditions, withdrawal of treatment should be carried out by gradually decreasing the frequency of applications.

How Supplied: FML Forte® (fluorometholone) 0.25% Liquifilm® sterile ophthalmic suspension is supplied in plastic dropper bottles in the following sizes:
2 mL—NDC 11980-228-02
5 mL—NDC 11980-228-05
10 mL—NDC 11980-228-10
15 mL—NDC 11980-228-15

Note: Store at or below 25°C (77°F); protect from freezing. **Shake well before using.**

Caution: Federal (U.S.A.) law prohibits dispensing without prescription.

FML-S® ℞
(fluorometholone, sulfacetamide sodium)
LIQUIFILM®
sterile ophthalmic suspension

Description: FML-S® LIQUIFILM sterile ophthalmic suspension is a topical anti-inflammatory/anti-infective combination product for ophthalmic use.

Chemical Names: Fluorometholone: 9-Fluoro-11β, 17-dihydroxy-6α-methylpregna-1,4-diene-3, 20-dione.
Sulfacetamide sodium: N-Sulfanilylacetamide monosodium salt monohydrate.

Contains:
fluorometholone 0.1%
sulfacetamide sodium 10%
with: LIQUIFILM® (polyvinyl alcohol) 1.4%; benzalkonium chloride 0.006%; edetate disodium; polysorbate 80; povidone; sodium chloride; sodium phosphate, dibasic; sodium phosphate, monobasic; sodium thiosulfate; hydrochloric acid and/or sodium hydroxide to adjust the pH; and purified water.

Clinical Pharmacology: Corticosteroids suppress the inflammatory response to a variety of agents and they probably delay or slow healing. Corticosteroids and their derivatives are capable of producing a rise in intraocular pressure. Since corticosteroids may inhibit the body's defense mechanism against infection, a concomitant antimicrobial drug may be used when this inhibition is considered to be clinically significant in a particular case.
In clinical studies of documented steroid-responders, fluorometholone demonstrated a significantly longer average time to produce a rise in intraocular pressure than dexametha-

sone phosphate; however, in a small percentage of individuals, a significant rise in intraocular pressure occurred within one week. The ultimate magnitude of the rise was equivalent for both drugs.

The anti-infective component in FML-S® is included to provide action against specific organisms susceptible to it. Sulfacetamide sodium is active *in-vitro* against susceptible strains of the following microorganisms: *Escherichia coli, Staphylococcus aureus, Streptococcus pneumoniae, Streptococcus* (viridans group), *Haemophilus influenzae, Klebsiella* species, and *Enterobacter* species. Some strains of these bacteria may be resistant to sulfacetamide or resistant strains may emerge *in vivo*.

When a decision to administer both a corticosteroid and an antimicrobial is made, the administration of such drugs in combination has the advantage of greater patient compliance and convenience, with the added assurance that the appropriate dosage of both drugs is administered. When both types of drugs are in the same formulation, compatibility of ingredients is assured and the correct volume of drug is delivered and retained.

The relative potency of corticosteroid formulations depends on the molecular structure, concentration, and release from the vehicle.

Indications and Usage: FML-S® is indicated for steroid-responsive inflammatory ocular conditions for which a corticosteroid is indicated and where superficial bacterial ocular infection or a risk of bacterial ocular infection exists.

Ocular steroids are indicated in inflammatory conditions of the palpebral and bulbar conjunctiva, cornea, and anterior segment of the globe where the inherent risk of steroid use in certain infective conjunctivitides is accepted to obtain a diminution in edema and inflammation. They are also indicated in chronic anterior uveitis and corneal injury from chemical, radiation or thermal burns or penetration of foreign bodies.

The use of a combination drug with an anti-infective component is indicated where the risk of superficial ocular infection is high or where there is an expectation that potentially dangerous numbers of bacteria will be present in the eye.

The anti-infective drug in this product, sulfacetamide, is active against the following common bacterial eye pathogens: *Escherichia coli, Staphylococcus aureus, Streptococcus pneumoniae, Streptococcus* (viridans group), *Haemophilus influenzae, Klebsiella* species, and *Enterobacter* species.

The product does not provide adequate coverage against: *Neisseria* species and *Serratia marcescens.* A significant percentage of Staphylococcal isolates are completely resistant to sulfa drugs.

Contraindications: Epithelial herpes simplex keratitis (dendritic keratitis), and vaccinia. Fungal diseases of the ocular structures. Hypersensitivity to any component of the medication.

Warnings: **NOT FOR INJECTION INTO THE EYE.**

Prolonged use of steroids may result in glaucoma, with damage to the optic nerve, defects in visual acuity and fields of vision, and in posterior subcapsular cataract formation. If used for longer than 10 days, intraocular pressure should be routinely monitored even though it may be difficult in children and uncooperative patients.

Prolonged use of steroids may suppress the host immune response in ocular tissues and thus increase the hazard of secondary ocular infections. Various ocular diseases and long-term use of topical corticosteroids have been known to cause corneal and scleral thinning. Use of topical corticosteroids in the presence of thin corneal or scleral tissue may lead to perforation. In acute purulent conditions of the eye, corticosteroids may mask infection or enhance existing infection.

Use of ocular steroids may prolong the course and may exacerbate the severity of many viral infections of the eye.

Employment of a corticosteroid medication in the treatment of patients with a history of herpes simplex requires great caution.

Fatalities have occurred, although rarely, due to severe reactions to sulfonamides including Stevens-Johnson syndrome, toxic epidermal necrolysis, fulminant hepatic necrosis, agranulocytosis, aplastic anemia, and other blood dyscrasias. Sensitizations may recur when a sulfonamide is readministered, irrespective of the route of administration. If signs of hypersensitivity or other serious reactions occur, discontinue use of this preparation (see **Adverse Reactions**). Cross-sensitivity among corticosteroids has been demonstrated.

A significant percentage of staphylococcal isolates are completely resistant to sulfa drugs.

Precautions: General: The initial prescription and renewal of the medication order beyond 20 milliliters should be made only by a physician after evaluation of the patient's intraocular pressure, examination of the patient with the aid of magnification, such as slit lamp biomicroscopy and, where appropriate, fluorescein staining.

Keep this and all drugs out of the reach of children.

Drug Interactions: Sulfacetamide preparations are incompatible with silver preparations.

Carcinogenesis, mutagenesis, impairment of fertility: No studies have been conducted in animals or in humans to evaluate the possibility of these effects with fluorometholone or sulfacetamide.

Pregnancy: **Pregnancy Category C:** Animal studies have not been conducted with FML-S® Liquifilm Ophthalmic Suspension. Fluorometholone has been shown to be embryocidal and teratogenic in rabbits when administered at low multiples of the human dose. Fluorometholone was applied ocularly to rabbits daily on days 6-18 of gestation, and dose-related fetal loss and fetal abnormalities including cleft palate, deformed rib cage, anomalous limbs and neural abnormalities such as encephalocele, craniorachischisis, and spina bifida were observed. Kernicterus may be precipitated in infants by sulfonamides being given systemically during the third trimester of pregnancy. There are no adequate and well-controlled studies of FML-S® Liquifilm Ophthalmic Suspension in pregnant women, and it is not known whether FML-S® can cause fetal harm when administered to a pregnant woman. FML-S® Liquifilm Ophthalmic Suspension should be used during pregnancy only if the potential benefit justifies the potential risk to the fetus.

Nursing Mothers: It is not known whether topical administration of corticosteroids could result in sufficient systemic absorption to produce detectable quantities in breast milk. Systemically administered corticosteroids appear in breast milk and could suppress growth, interfere with endogenous corticosteroid production, or cause other untoward effects. Systemically administered sulfonamides are capable of producing kernicterus in infants of lactating women. Because of the potential for serious adverse reactions in nursing infants from FML-S, a decision should be made whether to discontinue nursing or to discontinue the medication.

Pediatric Use: Safety and effectiveness in children have not been established.

Adverse Reactions: Adverse reactions have occurred with corticosteroid/anti-infective combination drugs which can be attributed to the corticosteroid component, the anti-infective component, or the combination. Exact incidence figures are not available since no denominator of treated patients is available.

Reactions occurring most often from the presence of the anti-infective ingredient are allergic sensitizations. Fatalities have occurred, although rarely, due to severe reactions to sulfonamides including Stevens-Johnson syndrome, toxic epidermal necrolysis, fulminant hepatic necrosis, agranulocytosis, aplastic anemia, and other blood dyscrasias (see **Warnings**). Sulfacetamide sodium may cause local irritation.

The reactions due to the corticosteroid component in decreasing order of frequency are: elevation of intraocular pressure (IOP) with possible development of glaucoma, and infrequent optic nerve damage; posterior subcapsular cataract formation; and delayed wound healing.

Secondary Infection: The development of secondary infection has occurred after use of combinations containing corticosteroids and antimicrobials. Fungal infections of the cornea are particularly prone to develop coincidentally with long-term application of corticosteroids. When signs of chronic ocular inflammation persist following prolonged corticosteroid dosing, the possibility of fungal infections of the cornea should be considered.

Secondary bacterial ocular infection following suppression of host responses also occurs.

Dosage and Administration: One drop of FML-S® should be instilled into the conjunctival sac four times daily. Care should be taken not to discontinue therapy prematurely.

Not more than 20 milliliters should be prescribed initially and the prescription should not be refilled without further evaluation as outlined in **Precautions** above.

How Supplied: FML-S® (fluorometholone, sulfacetamide sodium) Liquifilm® Sterile Ophthalmic Suspension is supplied in plastic dropper bottles in the following sizes:

5 mL—NDC 11980-422-05
10 mL—NDC 11980-422-10

Note: Store at controlled room temperature 15°–30°C (59°–86°F). Protect from freezing and light. **SHAKE WELL BEFORE USING.** Do not use suspension if it is dark brown.

Caution: Federal (U.S.A.) law prohibits dispensing without prescription.

GENOPTIC® ℞
(gentamicin sulfate ophthalmic solution, USP) 0.3%
Sterile
and

GENOPTIC® ℞
(gentamicin sulfate ophthalmic ointment, USP)
Sterile
Each gram contains gentamicin sulfate, USP equivalent to 3.0 mg gentamicin

Description: GENOPTIC® is a sterile, topical anti-infective agent for ophthalmic use. Gentamicin sulfate is a water-soluble antibiotic of the aminoglycoside group.

Gentamicin is obtained from cultures of *Micromonospora purpurea.* It is a mixture of the sulfate salts of gentamicin C_1, C_2, and C_{1A}. All three components appear to have similar antimicrobial activities. Gentamicin sulfate occurs as a white to buff powder and is soluble in water and insoluble in alcohol.

GENOPTIC® Solution:

Contains: Each mL contains gentamicin sulfate equivalent to 3 mg (0.3%) gentamicin base with: LIQUIFILM® (polyvinyl alcohol) 14 mg (1.4%); benzalkonium chloride; edetate disodium; sodium phosphate, dibasic; sodium chloride; hydrochloric acid and/or sodium hydroxide to adjust the pH; and purified water.

Continued on next page

Allergan Pharm—Cont.

The solution is an aqueous, buffered solution with a pH of 7.2–7.5.

GENOPTIC® Ointment:

Contains: Each gram contains gentamicin sulfate, USP (equivalent to 3.0 mg gentamicin) in a base of white petrolatum, with methylparaben (0.5 mg) and propylparaben (0.1 mg) as preservatives.

Clinical Pharmacology: Microbiology: Gentamicin sulfate is active *in vitro* against many strains of the following microorganisms: *Staphylococcus aureus, Staphylococcus epidermidis, Streptococcus pyogenes, Streptococcus pneumoniae, Enterobacter aerogenes, Escherichia coli, Haemophilus influenzae, Klebsiella pneumoniae, Neisseria gonorrhoeae, Pseudomonas aeruginosa*, and *Serratia marcescens.*

Indications and Usage: GENOPTIC® Ointment and Solution are indicated in the topical treatment of ocular bacterial infections including conjunctivitis, keratitis, keratoconjunctivitis, corneal ulcers, blepharitis, blepharoconjunctivitis, acute meibomianitis, and dacryocystitis, caused by susceptible strains of the following microorganisms: *Staphylococcus aureus, Staphylococcus epidermidis, Streptococcus pyogenes, Streptococcus pneumoniae, Enterobacter aerogenes, Escherichia coli, Haemophilus influenzae, Klebsiella pneumoniae, Neisseria gonorrhoeae, Pseudomonas aeruginosa, and Serratia marcescens.*

Contraindications: GENOPTIC® is contraindicated in patients with known hypersensitivity to any of the components.

Warnings: NOT FOR INJECTION INTO THE EYE.

Gentamicin sulfate ophthalmic ointment and solution are not for injection. They should never be injected subconjunctivally, nor should they be directly introduced into the anterior chamber of the eye.

Precautions:

General: Prolonged use of topical antibiotics may give rise to overgrowth of nonsusceptible organisms, including fungi. Bacterial resistance to gentamicin may also develop. If purulent discharge, inflammation or pain becomes aggravated, the patient should discontinue use of the medication and consult a physician.

If irritation or hypersensitivity to any component of the drug develops, the patient should discontinue use of this preparation, and appropriate therapy should be instituted.

Ophthalmic ointments may retard corneal healing.

Information for Patients: To avoid contamination, do not touch tip of container to the eye, eyelid or any surface.

Carcinogenesis, Mutagenesis, Impairment of Fertility: There are no published carcinogenicity or impairment of fertility studies on gentamicin. Aminoglycoside antibiotics have been found to be non-mutagenic.

Pregnancy: Pregnancy Category C. Gentamicin has been shown to depress body weights, kidney weights and median glomerular counts in newborn rats when administered systemically to pregnant rats in daily doses approximately 500 times the maximum recommended ophthalmic human dose. There are no adequate and well-controlled studies in pregnant women. Gentamicin should be used during pregnancy only if the potential benefit justifies the potential risk to the fetus.

Adverse Reactions: Bacterial and fungal corneal ulcers have developed during treatment with gentamicin ophthalmic preparations.

The most frequently reported adverse reactions are ocular burning and irritation upon drug instillation, non-specific conjunctivitis, conjunctival epithelial defects and conjunctival hyperemia.

Other adverse reactions which have occurred rarely are allergic reactions, thrombocytopenic purpura and hallucinations.

GENOPTIC® Solution:

Dosage and Administration: Instill one or two drops into the affected eye(s) every four hours. In severe infections, dosage may be increased to as much as two drops every hour.

How Supplied: GENOPTIC® (gentamicin sulfate ophthalmic solution, USP) 0.3% is supplied sterile in plastic dropper bottles in the following sizes:

1 mL—NDC 11980-117-01
5 mL—NDC 11980-117-05

Note: Store at or below 25°C (77°F). Avoid exposure to excessive heat (104°F/40°C or above).

GENOPTIC® Ointment:

Dosage and Administration: Apply a small amount (about ½ inch) to the affected eye two to three times a day.

How Supplied: GENOPTIC® (gentamicin sulfate ophthalmic ointment, USP) 0.3% is supplied sterile in a 3.5 gram tube (NDC 0023-0320-04).

Note: Store between 2° and 30°C (36° and 86°F).

Caution: Federal (U.S.A.) law prohibits dispensing without prescription.

HMS® ℞
(medrysone) 1.0%
LIQUIFILM®
sterile ophthalmic suspension

Description: HMS® (medrysone) 1.0% LIQUIFILM® sterile ophthalmic suspension is a topical anti-inflammatory agent for ophthalmic use.

Chemical Name: 11β-Hydroxy-6α-methylpregn-4-ene-3, 20-dione.

Contains:

medrysone....................1.0%

with: LIQUIFILM® (polyvinyl alcohol) 1.4%; benzalkonium chloride 0.004%; edetate disodium; sodium chloride; potassium chloride; sodium phosphate, monobasic; sodium phosphate, dibasic; hydroxypropyl methylcellulose; sodium hydroxide to adjust the pH; and purified water.

Clinical Pharmacology: HMS® (medrysone) is a synthetic corticosteroid with topical anti-inflammatory and anti-allergic activity. Corticosteroids inhibit the inflammatory response to inciting agents of mechanical, chemical, or immunological nature of edema, fibrin deposition, capillary dilation and leukocyte migration, capillary proliferation, deposition of collagen and scar formation. HMS® (medrysone) has less anti-inflammatory potency than 0.1% dexamethasone. Data from 2 uncontrolled studies[1-2] indicate that in patients with increased intraocular pressure and in those susceptible to a rise in intraocular pressure, there is less effect on pressure with HMS® than with dexamethasone or betamethasone.

Indications and Usage: HMS® (medrysone) is indicated for the treatment of allergic conjunctivitis, vernal conjunctivitis, episcleritis, and epinephrine sensitivity.

Contraindications: HMS® (medrysone) is contraindicated in the following conditions:

Acute superficial herpes simplex
Viral diseases of the conjunctiva and cornea
Ocular tuberculosis
Fungal diseases of the eye
Hypersensitivity to any of the components of the drug

Warnings:

Acute purulent untreated infections of the eye may be masked, enhanced or activated by the presence of corticosteroid medication.

Corneal or scleral perforation occasionally has been reported with prolonged use of topical corticosteroids. In high dosages, they have been associated with corneal thinning.

Prolonged use of topical corticosteroids may increase intraocular pressure, with resultant glaucoma, damage to the optic nerve, and defects in visual acuity and fields of vision. However, data from 2 uncontrolled studies[1-2] indicate that in patients with increased intraocular pressure and in those susceptible to a rise in intraocular pressure upon application of topical corticosteroids, there is less effect on pressure with HMS® than with dexamethasone or betamethasone.

Prolonged use of topical corticosteroids may rarely be associated with development of posterior subcapsular cataracts.

Systemic absorption and systemic side effects may result with the use of topical corticosteroids.

HMS® is not recommended for use in iritis and uveitis as its therapeutic effectiveness has not been demonstrated in these conditions.

Corticosteroid medication in the presence of stromal herpes simplex requires great caution; frequent slit-lamp microscopy is suggested.

Prolonged use may aid in the establishment of secondary ocular infections from fungi and viruses liberated from ocular tissue.

Precautions:

General: With prolonged use of HMS®, the intraocular pressure and the lens should be examined periodically.

In persistent corneal ulceration where a corticosteroid has been used, or is in use, fungal infection should be suspected.

Carcinogenesis, mutagenesis, impairment of fertility: No studies have been conducted in animals or in humans to evaluate the potential of these effects.

Pregnancy Category C: Medrysone has been shown to be embryocidal in rabbits when given in doses 10 and 30 times the human dose. Medrysone was ocularly applied to both eyes of pregnant rabbits 2 drops 4 times per day on day 6 through 18 of gestation. A significant increase in early resorptions was observed in the treated rabbits. There are no adequate or well-controlled studies in pregnant women. Medrysone should be used during pregnancy only if the potential benefit justifies the potential risk to the fetus.

Pediatric Use: Safety and effectiveness in children have not been established.

Adverse Reactions: Adverse reactions include occasional transient stinging and burning on instillation. Increased intraocular pressure, which may be associated with optic nerve damage and defects in the visual fields, and posterior subcapsular cataract formation have been reported rarely with the use of HMS®.

Overdosage: Overdosage will not ordinarily cause acute problems. If accidentally ingested, drink fluids to dilute.

Dosage and Administration: Shake well before using. Instill one drop in the conjunctival sac up to every four hours.

How Supplied: HMS® (medrysone) is supplied in plastic dropper bottles in the following sizes:

5 mL—NDC 11980-074-05
10 mL—NDC 11980-074-10

Note: Protect from freezing.

Caution: Federal (U.S.A.) law prohibits dispensing without a prescription.

References:

1. Becker B, Kolker AE. Intraocular pressure response to topical corticosteroids. In: Leopold IH, ed. Ocular therapy, complications and management. St. Louis: CV Mosby, 1967.
2. Spaeth G. Hydroxymethylprogesterone. *Arch Ophthalmol.* 1966;75:783–787.

HERPLEX® ℞
(idoxuridine) 0.1%
LIQUIFILM®
sterile ophthalmic solution

For Ophthalmic Use Only

Description: A topical ophthalmic antiviral chemotherapeutic preparation.
Chemical Name: 2′-Deoxy-5-iodouridine.
Contains:
idoxuridine 0.1%
with: LIQUIFILM® (polyvinyl alcohol) 1.4%, benzalkonium chloride, sodium chloride, edetate disodium, and purified water.
Clinical Pharmacology: In chemical structure, idoxuridine closely approximates the configuration of thymidine, one of the four building blocks of DNA—the genetic material of the herpes virus. As a result, idoxuridine is able to replace thymidine in the enzymatic step of viral replication or "growth". The consequent production of faulty DNA results in a pseudostructure which cannot infect or destroy tissue. In short, by preempting a vital building block in the genetic material of the herpes simplex virus, idoxuridine destroys the infective and destructive capacity of the viral material.
Indications and Usage: HERPLEX® LIQUIFILM® is indicated for the treatment of keratitis caused by the herpes simplex virus.
Contraindications: HERPLEX® LIQUIFILM® is contraindicated for those who have a hypersensitivity to the active ingredient or other components of this medication.
Warnings: Recurrence may occur if medication is not continued 5 to 7 days after lesion is apparently healed (does not stain).
Precautions: General: Some strains of herpes simplex virus appear resistant to the action of idoxuridine. If there is no lessening of fluorescein staining in 14 days, another form of therapy should be undertaken.
Drug Interactions: Boric acid should not be administered during the course of therapy. The potential exists for interaction between boric acid and ingredients in HERPLEX® LIQUIFILM® which may result in precipitate formation.
Carcinogenesis, mutagenesis, impairment of fertility: The studies performed to date on idoxuridine are inadequate for assessment of carcinogenicity. This cytotoxic drug should be regarded as being potentially carcinogenic. It can inhibit DNA synthesis or function and is incorporated into the DNA of mammalian cells as well as into the genome of DNA viruses. Idoxuridine has been reported to induce RNA tumor virus (type C particles) production from virus-negative mouse cells. The degree of oncogenic activity of idoxuridine-induced oncornaviruses has not been documented. However, several idoxuridine-activated oncornaviruses have caused *in vitro* cell transformation and induction of specific neoplasms (lymphatic leukemias and carcinomas) upon inoculation into syngeneic mice.
Idoxuridine has been reported to cause chromosome aberrations in mice and to be mutagenic in mammalian cells in culture (e.g., diploid human lymphoblasts and mouse lymphoma cells), Drosophila melanogaster and in host-mediated assay system utilizing mammalian cells.
Pregnancy Category C: Idoxuridine has been reported to cross the placental barrier and to produce fetal malformations in rabbits when administered topically to the eyes of pregnant females in doses similar to those used clinically. Idoxuridine has also been reported to produce fetal malformations in the rat after intraperitoneal and oral administration and in the mouse after subcutaneous administration. There are no adequate and well-controlled studies in pregnant women. Idoxuridine should be used during pregnancy only if the potential benefit justifies the potential risk to the fetus.
Nursing Mothers: It is not known whether this drug is excreted in human milk. Because of the potential for tumorigenicity shown for idoxuridine in animal studies, a decision should be made whether to discontinue nursing or to discontinue the drug, taking into account the importance of the drug to the mother.
Pediatric Use: Safety and effectiveness in children have not been established.
Adverse Reactions: Exact incidence figures are not available since no denominator of treated patients is available.
Adverse reactions associated with topical idoxuridine administration include occasional irritation, pain, pruritus, inflammation, edema of the eyes or lids, allergic reactions, photophobia, occasional corneal clouding, stippling, and punctate defects of the epithelium.
Overdosage: Overdosage will not ordinarily cause acute problems. Should accidental overdosage in the eye(s) occur, flush the eye(s) with water or normal saline. If accidentally ingested, drink fluids to dilute.
Dosage and Administration: For optimal results, the infected tissues should be kept "saturated" with HERPLEX® LIQUIFILM®. Under practical, clinical conditions, one of the following "high frequency" dosage schedules is recommended.

1. Instill one drop in the infected eye(s) every hour during the day. At night, the dosage may be reduced to one drop every other hour.
2. Instill one drop every minute for 5 minutes. This schedule should be repeated every four hours—night and day.

How Supplied: HERPLEX® (idoxuridine) 0.1% LIQUIFILM® sterile ophthalmic solution is supplied in plastic dropper bottles in the following size: 15 mL—NDC 0023-0033-15.
Note: Store at controlled room temperature (59°- 86°F). Protect from light.
Caution: Federal (U.S.A.) law prohibits dispensing without prescription.

OCUFLOX™ ℞
(ofloxacin ophthalmic solution) 0.3%
sterile

Description: Ocuflox™ (ofloxacin ophthalmic solution) 0.3% is a sterile ophthalmic solution. It is a fluorinated carboxyquinolone anti-infective for topical ophthalmic use.
Chemical name: (±)-9-Fluoro-2,3-dihydro-3-methyl-10-(4-methyl-1-piperazinyl)-7-oxo-7H-pyrido [1,2,3-e]-1,4 benzoxazine-6-carboxylic acid.
Contains: Ofloxacin .... 0.3% (3 mg/mL) with: Benzalkonium chloride (0.005%), sodium chloride and purified water. May also contain hydrochloric acid and/or sodium hydroxide to adjust pH.
Ocuflox™ solution is unbuffered and formulated with a pH of 6.4 (range–6.0 to 6.8). It has an osmolality of 300 mOsm/kg. Ofloxacin is a fluorinated 4-quinolone which differs from other fluorinated 4-quinolones in that there is a six member (pyridobenzoxazine) ring from positions 1 to 8 of the basic ring structure.
Clinical Pharmacology:
Pharmacokinetics: Serum, urine and tear film concentrations of ofloxacin were measured in 30 healthy women at various time points during a ten-day course of treatment with Ocuflox™ solution. The mean serum ofloxacin concentration ranged from 0.4 ng/mL to 1.9 ng/mL. Maximum ofloxacin concentration increased from 1.1 ng/mL on day one to 1.9 ng/mL on day 11 after QID dosing for 10 ½ days. Maximum serum ofloxacin concentrations after ten days of topical ophthalmic dosing were more than 1000 times lower than those reported after standard oral doses of ofloxacin.
Tear film ofloxacin concentrations ranged from 5.7 to 31 μg/g during the 40 minute period following the last dose on day 11. Mean tear film levels measured four hours after topical opththolmic dosing were 9.2 μg/g. Ofloxacin was excreted in the urine primarily unmodified.
Microbiology: Ofloxacin has *in vitro* activity against a broad range of gram-positive and gram-negative aerobic and anaerobic bacteria. Ofloxacin is bactericidal at concentrations equal to or slightly greater than inhibitory concentrations. Ofloxacin is thought to exert a bactericidal effect on susceptible bacterial cells by inhibiting DNA gyrase, an essential bacterial enzyme which is a critical catalyst in the duplication, transcription, and repair of bacterial DNA.
Cross resistance has been observed between ofloxacin and other fluoroquinolones. There is generally no cross-resistance between ofloxacin and other classes of antibacterial agents such as beta-lactams or aminoglycosides; therefore organisms resistant to these drugs may be susceptible to ofloxacin.
Organisms resistant to ofloxacin may also be susceptible to beta-lactams or aminoglycosides.
Ofloxacin has been shown to be active against most strains of the following organisms both *in vitro* and, clinically, in conjunctival infections as described in the **INDICATIONS AND USAGE section.**
AEROBES, GRAM-POSITIVE:
Staphylococcus aureus
Staphylococcus epidermidis
Streptococcus pneumoniae
AEROBES, GRAM-NEGATIVE:
Enterobacter cloacae
Haemophilus influenzae
Proteus mirabilis
Pseudomonas aeruginosa
The following *in vitro* data are also available: *but their clinical significance in ophthalmic infections is unknown.*
Ofloxacin exhibits *in vitro* minimal inhibitory concentrations (MIC's) of 2μg/mL or less against most (90%) strains of the following microorganisms; however, the safety and effectiveness of ofloxacin in treating ocular infections due to these microorganisms have not been established.
AEROBES, GRAM-POSITIVE:
Enterococcus faecalis
Listeria monocytogenes
Streptococcus pyogenes
AEROBES, GRAM-NEGATIVE
Acinetobacter calcoaceticus var. anitratus
Acinetobacter calcoaceticus var. Iwoffi
Citrobacter diversus
Citrobacter freundii
Enterobacter aerogenes
Escherichia coli
Klebsiella oxytoca
Klebsiella pneumoniae
Moraxella (Branhamella) catarrhalis
Morganella morganii
Neisseria gonorrhoeae
Pseudomonas acidovorans
Pseudomonas fluorescens
Serratia marcescens
Shigella sonnei
ANAEROBIC SPECIES:
Propionibacterium acnes
OTHER:
Chlamydia trachomatis
Clinical Studies: In a randomized, double-masked, multicenter clinical trial, Ocuflox™ solution was superior to its vehicle after 2 days of treatment in patients with conjunctivitis and positive conjunctival cultures. Clinical outcomes for the trial demonstrated a clinical improvement rate of 86% (54/63) for the oflox-

Continued on next page

Allergan Pharm—Cont.

acin treated group versus 72% (48/67) for the placebo treated group after 2 days of therapy. Microbiological outcomes for the same clinical trial demonstrated an eradication rate for causative pathogens of 65% (41/63) for the ofloxacin treated group versus 25% (17/67) for the vehicle treated group after 2 days of therapy. Please note that microbiologic eradication does not always correlate with clinical outcome in anti-infective trials.

Indications and Usage: Ocuflox™ solution is indicated for the treatment of conjunctivitis caused by susceptible strains of the following bacteria:

Gram-positive bacteria:
Staphylococcus aureus
Staphylococcus epidermidis
Streptococcus pneumoniae

Gram-negative bacteria:
Enterobacter cloacae
Haemophilus influenzae
Proteus mirabilis
Pseudomonas aeruginosa

Contraindications: Ocuflox™ solution is contraindicated in patients with a history of hypersensitivity to ofloxacin, to other quinolones, or to any of the components in this medication.

Warnings: NOT FOR INJECTION.
Ocuflox™ solution should not be injected subconjunctivally, nor should it be introduced directly into the anterior chamber of the eye. Serious and occasionally fatal hypersensitivity (anaphylactic) reactions, some following the first dose, have been reported in patients receiving systemic quinolones, including ofloxacin. Some reactions were accompanied by cardiovascular collapse, loss of consciousness, angioedema (including laryngeal, pharyngeal or facial edema), airway obstruction, dyspnea, urticaria, and itching. If an allergic reaction to ofloxacin occurs, discontinue the drug. Serious acute hypersensitivity reactions may require immediate emergency treatment. Oxygen and airway management, including intubation, should be administered as clinically indicated.

Precautions: General: As with other anti-infectives, prolonged use may result in overgrowth of nonsusceptible organisims, including fungi. If superinfection occurs or if clinical improvement is not noted within 7 days, discontinue use and institute appropriate therapy. Whenever clinical judgment dictates, the patient should be examined with the aid of magnification, such as slit lamp biomicroscopy and, where appropriate, fluorescein staining.
The systemic administration of quinolones, including ofloxacin, has led to lesions or erosions of the cartilage in weight-bearing joints and other signs of arthropathy in immature animals of various species. Ofloxacin, administered systemically at 10 mg/kg/day in young dogs (equivalent to 150 times the maximum recommended daily adult ophthalmic dose) has been associated with these types of effects.

Information for Patients: Avoid contaminating the applicator tip with material from the eye, fingers or other source.
Systemic quinolones, including ofloxacin, have been associated with hypersensitivity reactions, even following a single dose. Discontinue use immediately and contact your physician at the first sign of a rash or allergic reaction.

Drug Interactions: Specific drug interaction studies have not been conducted with Ocuflox™ solution.

Carcinogenesis, mutagenesis, impairment of fertility: Long term studies to determine the carcinogenic potential of ofloxacin have not been conducted.
Ofloxacin was not mutagenic in the Ames test, *in vitro* and *in vivo* cytogenic assay, sister chromatid exchange assay (Chinese hampster and human cell lines), unscheduled DNA synthesis (UDS) assay using human fibroblasts, the dominant lethal assay, or mouse micronucleus assay. Ofloxacin was positive in the UDS test using rat hepatocyte, and in the mouse lymphoma assay.
In fertility studies in rats, ofloxacin did not affect male or female fertility or morphological or reproductive performance at oral dosing up to 360 mg/kg/day (equivalent to 6000 times the maximum recommended daily ophthalmic dose).

Pregnancy: Teratogenic Effects. Pregnancy Category C: Ofloxacin has been shown to have an embryocidal effect in rats and in rabbits when given in doses of 810 mg/kg/day (equivalent to 13,500 times the maximum recommended daily ophthalmic dose) and 160 mg/kg/day (equivalent to 2600 times the maximum recommended daily ophthalmic dose). These dosages resulted in decreased fetal body weight and increased fetal mortality in rats and rabbits, respectively. Minor fetal skeletal variations were reported in rats receiving doses of 810 mg/kg/day. Ofloxacin has not been shown to be teratogenic at doses as high as 810 mg/kg/day and 160 mg/kg/day when administered to pregnant rats and rabbits, respectively.

Nonteratogenic Effects. Additional studies in rats with doses up to 360 mg/kg/day during late gestation showed no adverse effect on late fetal development, labor, delivery, lactation, neonatal viability, or growth of the newborn. There are, however, no adequate and well-controlled studies in pregnant women. Ocuflox™ solution should be used during pregnancy only if the potential benefit justifies the potential risk to the fetus.

Nursing Mothers: In nursing women a single 200 mg oral dose resulted in concentrations of ofloxacin in milk which were similar to those found in plasma. It is not known whether ofloxacin is excreted in human milk following topical ophthalmic administration. Because of the potential for serious adverse reactions from ofloxacin in nursing infants, a decision should be made whether to discontinue nursing or to discontinue the drug, taking into account the importance of the drug to the mother.

Pediatric Use: Safety and effectiveness in infants below the age of one year have not been established.
Quinolones, including ofloxacin, have been shown to cause arthropathy in immature animals after oral administration; however, topical ocular administration of ofloxacin to immature animals has not shown any arthropathy. There is no evidence that the ophthalmic dosage form of ofloxacin has any effect on weight bearing joints.

Adverse Reactions: Ophthalmic use: The most frequently reported drug-related adverse reaction was transient ocular burning or discomfort. Other reported reactions were stinging, redness, itching, photophobia, tearing, and dryness. One report of dizziness was also received.

Dosage and Administration: Instill one to two drops every two to four hours for the first two days, and then four times daily in the affected eye(s) for up to five additional days.

How Supplied: Ocuflox™ (ofloxacin ophthalmic solution) 0.3% is supplied sterile in plastic dropper bottles of the following size:
5 mL–NDC 11980-779-05

Note: Store at 15–25°C (59–77°F).

Caution: Federal (U.S.A.) law prohibits dispensing without prescription.
Licensed from Daiichi Pharmaceutical Co., Ltd., Tokyo, Japan and Santen Pharmaceutical Co., Ltd., Osaka, Japan
©Allergan Inc.

Shown in Product Identification Guide, page 103

OPHTHETIC® ℞
(proparacaine HCl) 0.5%
sterile ophthalmic solution

Description: OPHTHETIC® (proparacaine HCl) 0.5% sterile ophthalmic solution is a topical local anesthetic for ophthalmic use.

Chemical Name:
Benzoic acid, 3-amino-4-propoxy-,2-(diethylamino)ethyl ester, monohydrochloride.

Contains:
proparacaine HCl 0.5%
with: benzalkonium chloride (0.01%), glycerin, sodium chloride and purified water. pH may be adjusted with hydrochloric acid and/or sodium hydroxide.

Clinical Pharmacology: OPHTHETIC® sterile ophthalmic solution is a rapidly-acting topical anesthetic, with induced anesthesia lasting 15 minutes or longer.

Indications and Usage: OPHTHETIC® sterile ophthalmic solution is indicated for procedures in which a topical ophthalmic anesthetic is indicated: corneal anesthesia of short duration, e.g., tonometry, gonioscopy, removal of corneal foreign bodies, and for short corneal and conjunctival procedures.

Contraindications: OPHTHETIC® sterile ophthalmic solution should be considered contraindicated in patients with known hypersensitivity to any of the ingredients of this preparation.

Warnings: Prolonged use of a topical ocular anesthetic is not recommended. It may produce permanent corneal opacification with accompanying visual loss.

Precautions:

Carcinogenesis, Mutagenesis, Impairment of Fertility: Long-term studies in animals have not been performed to evaluate carcinogenic potential, mutagenicity, or possible impairment of fertility in males or females.

Pregnancy: Pregnancy Category C: Animal reproduction studies have not been conducted with OPHTHETIC® (proparacaine hydrochloride) ophthalmic solution. It is also not known whether proparacaine hydrochloride can cause fetal harm when administered to a pregnant woman or can affect reproduction capacity. Proparacaine hydrochloride should be administered to a pregnant woman only if clearly needed.

Nursing Mothers: It is not known whether this drug is excreted in human milk. Because many drugs are excreted in human milk, caution should be exercised when proparacaine hydrochloride is administered to a nursing mother.

Pediatric Use: Safety and effectiveness in children have not been established.

Adverse Reactions: Occasional temporary stinging, burning, and conjunctival redness may occur with the use of proparacaine. A rare, severe, immediate-type, apparently hyperallergic corneal reaction, characterized by acute, intense and diffuse epithelial keratitis, a gray, ground glass appearance, sloughing of large areas of necrotic epithelium, corneal filaments and sometimes, iritis with descemetitis has been reported.
Allergic contact dermatitis from proparacaine with drying and fissuring of the fingertips has also been reported.

Dosage and Administration:
Usual Dosage: Removal of foreign bodies and sutures, and for tonometry: 1 to 2 drops (in single instillations) in each eye before operating.
Deep Ophthalmic Anesthesia: 1 drop in each eye every 5 to 10 minutes for 5–7 doses.

Note: OPHTHETIC® should be clear to straw-color. If the solution becomes darker, discard the solution.

How Supplied:
OPHTHETIC® sterile ophthalmic solution is supplied in plastic dropper bottles in the following size:

15 mL—NDC 11980-048-15
Bottle must be stored in unit carton to protect contents from light. Store bottles under refrigeration at 2°C to 8°C (36°F to 46°F).
Caution: Federal (U.S.A.) law prohibits dispensing without prescription.

PAREMYD™ ℞
(hydroxyamphetamine hydrobromide/ tropicamide ophthalmic solution) 1%/0.25% sterile

PRODUCT OVERVIEW

PAREMYD™ sterile ophthalmic solution is a topical mydriatic combination product for ophthalmic use. It is a convenient combination of two separate, well-established agents.
PAREMYD™ Solution is indicated for mydriasis in routine diagnostic procedures and in conditions where short-term pupil dilation is desired. PAREMYD™ provides clinically significant mydriasis with only partial cycloplegia. Its minimal effect on cycloplegia is attributed to the low concentration of tropicamide in the combination drop.
The onset of action with PAREMYD™ occurs within 15 minutes, followed by maximum effect within 60 minutes after instillation of one drop.
Clinically significant dilation, inhibition of pupillary light response, and partial cycloplegia last 3 hours, with recovery beginning at approximately 90 minutes and with complete recovery occurring in most patients in 6–8 hours.
A clinical trial showed that PAREMYD™ Solution produced a significantly better combined response of pupillary dilation and diminished pupillary light response than either of its active ingredients alone and was as safe as either of its active components.[1]
Paremyd™ Solution is now available through distributors.
There is evidence that mydriatics may produce a transient elevation of intraocular pressure in patients with open-angle glaucoma.
Please see full prescribing information.
1. Data on file, Allergan, Inc.

PRESCRIBING INFORMATION

PAREMYD™ ℞
(hydroxyamphetamine hydrobromide 1% and tropicamide 0.25%) sterile ophthalmic solution

Description: PAREMYD™ sterile ophthalmic solution is a topical mydriatic combination product for ophthalmic use.
Chemical Name: Hydroxyamphetamine hydrobromide: Phenol, 4-(2-amino-propyl)-, hydrobromide. Tropicamide: Benzeneacetamide, N-ethyl-α-(hydroxymethyl)-N-(4-pyridinylmethyl).
Contains: Hydroxyamphetamine hydrobromide, USP 1.0%. Tropicamide, USP 0.25% with: benzalkonium chloride 0.005%; edetate disodium 0.015%; sodium chloride; and purified water. Hydrochloric acid and/or sodium hydroxide are added to adjust the pH. The pH of PAREMYD™ can range from 4.2 to 5.8 during its shelf life. The osmolality of PAREMYD™ is approximately 307 mOsm/l.
Clinical Pharmacology: PAREMYD™ Solution combines the effects of the adrenergic agent, hydroxyamphetamine hydrobromide, and the anticholinergic agent, tropicamide. Hydroxyamphetamine hydrobromide is an indirectly-acting sympathomimetic agent which, when applied topically to the eye, causes the release of endogenous norepinephrine from intact adrenergic nerve terminals, resulting in mydriasis. Since hydroxyamphetamine hydrobromide has little or no direct activity on the receptor site, dilation does not usually occur if there is damage to the presynaptic nerve terminal, e.g., Horner's Syndrome. However, it is not known whether damage to the presynaptic nerve terminal will influence the extent of mydriasis produced by PAREMYD™. Hydroxyamphetamine hydrobromide has minimal cycloplegic action. Tropicamide is a parasympatholytic agent which, when applied topically to the eye, blocks the responses of the sphincter muscle of the iris and ciliary muscle to cholinergic stimulation, producing dilation of the pupil and paralysis of the ciliary muscle. Tropicamide produces short-duration mydriasis. Although cycloplegia occurs with higher doses of tropicamide, there is evidence with 0.25% tropicamide that full cycloplegia does not occur. Since both these agents act on different effector sites, their simultaneous use produces an additive mydriatic effect. PARAMYD™ provides diminished pupil responsiveness to light, facilitating ophthalmoscopy. The onset of action with PAREMYD™ occurs within 15 minutes, followed by maximum effect within 60 minutes after instillation of one drop. Clinically significant dilation, inhibition of pupillary light response, and partial cycloplegia last 3 hours, with recovery beginning at approximately 90 minutes and with complete recovery occurring in most patients in 6 to 8 hours. However, in some cases, complete recovery may take up to 24 hours. Effectiveness may differ slightly in patients with light and dark irides, with those patients with light irides experiencing a slightly greater mydriasis.
Indications: PAREMYD™ Solution is indicated for mydriasis in routine diagnostic procedures and in conditions where short-term pupil dilation is desired. PAREMYD™ provides clinically significant mydriasis with partial cycloplegia.
Contraindications: PAREMYD™ Solution should not be used in patients with angle-closure glaucoma or in those with narrow angles in whom dilation of the pupil may precipitate an attack of angle-closure glaucoma. This product is also contraindicated in patients who are hypersensitive to any of its components.
Warnings: For topical ophthalmic use only, not for injection. There is evidence that mydriatics may produce a transient elevation of intraocular pressure in patients with open-angle glaucoma. This preparation rarely may cause CNS disturbances which may be particularly dangerous in infants, children or the aged. Psychotic reactions, behavioral disturbances and vasomotor or cardio-respiratory collapse in children have been reported with the use of anticholinergic drugs.
Precautions: **General:** Patients with hypertension, hyperthyroidism, diabetes or cardiac disease (i,e., arrhythmias or chronic ischemic heart disease) should be monitored after instillation. The elderly and others in whom glaucoma or increased intraocular pressure may be encountered following administration of PAREMYD™ Solution should also be monitored closely. To avoid inducing angle-closure glaucoma, an estimation of the depth of the angle of the anterior chamber should be made.
Information for Patients: Patients should be advised not to touch the dropper tip to any surface since this may contaminate the solution. Patients should be advised to use caution when driving or engaging in other hazardous activities while pupils are dilated. Patients may experience photophobia and/or blurred vision and should protect their eyes in bright illumination when pupils are dilated. Parents should be warned not to get this preparation in their child's mouth and to wash their own hands and the child's hands following administration.
Carcinogenesis, mutagenesis, impairment of fertility: No studies have been performed to evaluate the carcinogenic, mutagenic or impairment of fertility potential of PAREMYD™.
Pregnancy: Pregnancy Category C. Animal reproduction studies have not been conducted with PAREMYD™. It is also not known whether PAREMYD™ can cause fetal harm when administered to a pregnant woman or can affect reproduction capability. PAREMYD™ should be given to a pregnant woman only if clearly needed.
Nursing Mothers: It is not known whether this drug is excreted in human milk. Because many drugs are excreted in human milk, caution should be exercised when PAREMYD™ is administered to a nursing woman.
Pediatric Use: Safety and effectiveness in children have not been established, PAREMYD™ may rarely cause CNS disturbances which may be dangerous in infants and children. Psychotic reactions, behavioral disturbances and vasomotor or cardio-respiratory collapse in children have been reported with the use of anticholinergic drugs. (See **Warnings**). Keep this and all medications out of the reach of children.
Adverse Reactions: Increased intraocular pressure has been reported following use of mydriatics. Transient stinging, dryness of the mouth, blurred vision, photophobia with or without corneal staining, tachycardia, headache, allergic reactions, nausea, vomiting, pallor, and muscle rigidity have been reported with the use of tropicamide and/or hydroxyamphetamine hydrobromide, and thus may occur with PAREMYD™ Solution. Central nervous system disturbances have also been reported. Psychotic reactions, behavioral disturbances, and vasomotor or cardio-respiratory collapse in children have been reported with the use of anticholinergic drugs.
Overdosage: Ocular overdosage will cause dilation of the pupils. Systemic overdosage or ingestion of large doses may result in hypertension, cardiac arrhythmias, sub-sternal discomfort, headache, sweating, nausea, vomiting and gastrointestinal irritation. Patients with systemic overdosage should be carefully monitored and treated symptomatically.
Dosage and Administration: One to two drops in the conjunctival sac. The onset of action with PAREMYD™ Solution occurs within 15 minutes, followed by maximum effect within 60 minutes. Clinically significant dilation, inhibition of pupillary light response, and partial cycloplegia last 3 hours. Mydriasis will reverse spontaneously with time, typically in 6 to 8 hours. However, in some cases, complete recovery may take up to 24 hours.
How Supplied: PAREMYD™ (hydroxyamphetamine hydrobromide/tropicamide ophthalmic solution) 1%/0.25% is supplied in plastic dropper bottles in the following sizes: 5 mL—NDC 11980-289-05; 15 mL—NDC 11980-289-15.
Note: Protect from light. Store between 15°C to 25°C (59°F to 77°F).
Caution: Federal (U.S.A.) law prohibits dispensing without prescription.

PILAGAN® ℞
(pilocarpine nitrate)
Liquifilm®
sterile ophthalmic solution
with C CAP® Compliance Cap Q.I.D.

Description: **PILAGAN®** (pilocarpine nitrate) Liquifilm® sterile ophthalmic solution is a topical parasympathomimetic agent for ophthalmic use.
Chemical Name: 2(3*H*)-Furanone, 3-ethyldihydro-4-[(1-methyl-1*H*-imidazol-5-yl)methyl]-,(3*S*-*cis*)-,mononitrate.
Contains: pilocarpine nitrate ...1%, 2%, 4% with Liquifilm® (polyvinyl alcohol) 1.4%; chlorobutanol (chloral derivative) 0.5% as a

Continued on next page

Allergan Pharm—Cont.

preservative; sodium acetate; sodium chloride; citric acid; menthol; camphor; phenol; eucalyptol; and purified water.

Clinical Pharmacology: Pilocarpine is a direct-acting parasympathomimetic drug which duplicates the muscarinic effects of acetylcholine, but has no nicotinic effects. Pilocarpine stimulates secretory glands and smooth muscles and has no effect on striated muscle. Pilocarpine is effective in the treatment of glaucoma by improving the facility of outflow and by decreasing aqueous secretion.

Indications and Usage: PILAGAN® Liquifilm® is indicated for:

1. The control of intraocular pressure in glaucoma.
2. Emergency relief of mydriasis in an acutely glaucomatous situation.
3. To reverse mydriasis caused by cycloplegic agents.

Contraindications: PILAGAN® Liquifilm® is contraindicated in persons showing hypersensitivity to any of its ingredients.

Warnings: Pilocarpine is readily absorbed systemically through the conjunctiva. Excessive application (instillation) may elicit systemic toxicity symptoms in some individuals.

Precautions: **General:** Pilocarpine has been reported to elicit retinal detachment in individuals with pre-existing retinal disease or predisposed to retinal tears. Fundus examination is advised for all patients prior to initiation of pilocarpine therapy.

Carcinogenesis, mutagenesis and impairment of fertility: No studies have been conducted in animals or in humans to evaluate the potential of these effects.

Pregnancy Category C: Animal reproduction studies have not been conducted with pilocarpine. It is also not known whether pilocarpine can cause fetal harm when administered to a pregnant woman or can affect reproduction capacity. Pilocarpine should be given to a pregnant woman only if clearly needed.

Pediatric Use: Safety and effectiveness in children have not been established.

Adverse Reactions: Adverse reactions associated with topical pilocarpine therapy include: visual blurring due to miosis and accommodative spasm, poor dark adaptation caused by the failure of the pupil to dilate in reduced illumination, and conjunctival hyperemia.

Miotics have been reported to cause lens opacities in susceptible individuals after prolonged use.

Systemic reactions following topical use of pilocarpine are rare.

Overdosage: Should accidental overdosage in the eye(s) occur, flush eye(s) with water or normal saline. If accidentally ingested, induce emesis or perform gastric lavage. Observe patients for signs of pilocarpine toxicity, i.e., salivation, lacrimation, sweating, nausea, vomiting and diarrhea. If these occur, therapy with anticholinergics (atropine) may be necessary. Bronchial constriction may be a problem in asthmatic patients.

Dosage and Administration:

1. For glaucoma, the recommended dosage is 1 to 2 drops two or four times a day of the selected concentration; patient response may be variable.
2. To aid in emergency miosis, 1 to 2 drops of one of the higher concentrations should be used.
3. The dosage and strength required to reverse mydriasis depends on the cycloplegic used.

How Supplied: PILAGAN® (pilocarpine nitrate) Liquifilm® sterile ophthalmic solution is available in 15 mL plastic dropper bottles with the C CAP® Compliance Cap.

1%—NDC 11980-879-45
2%—NDC 11980-878-45
4%—NDC 11980-877-45

Note: Shake well before use. Protect from freezing. Keep out of the reach of children.

Caution: Federal (U.S.A.) law prohibits dispensing without prescription.

POLY-PRED® ℞

(prednisolone acetate, neomycin sulfate, polymyxin B sulfate)
Liquifilm®
sterile ophthalmic suspension

Description: POLY-PRED® Liquifilm® sterile ophthalmic suspension is a topical anti-inflammatory/anti-infective combination product for ophthalmic use.

Chemical Name: Prednisolone acetate: 11β, 17, 21-Trihydroxypregna-1, 4-diene-3, 20-dione 21-acetate.

Neomycin sulfate is the sulfate salt of neomycin B and neomycin C which are produced by the growth of **Streptomyces fradiae** (Fam. **Streptomycetaceae**). It has a potency equivalent to not less than 600 micrograms per milligram of neomycin base, calculated on an anhydrous basis.

Polymyxin B sulfate is the sulfate salt of polymyxin B_1 and polymyxin B_2 which are produced by the growth of **Bacillus polymyxa** (Prazmowski) Migula (Fam. **Bacillaceae**). It has a potency of not less than 6,000 polymyxin B units per milligram, calculated on an anhydrous basis.

Contains: prednisolone acetate (microfine suspension) 0.5%
neomycin sulfate equivalent to 0.35% neomycin base
polymyxin B sulfate ....10,000 units/mL
with: Liquifilm® (polyvinyl alcohol) 1.4%; thimerosal 0.001%; polysorbate 80; propylene glycol; sodium acetate; and purified water.

Clinical Pharmacology: Corticosteroids suppress the inflammatory response to a variety of agents and they probably delay or slow healing. Since corticosteroids may inhibit the body's defense mechanism against infection, a concomitant antimicrobial drug may be used when this inhibition is considered to be clinically significant in a particular case.

The anti-infective components in POLY-PRED® are included to provide action against specific organisms susceptible to them. Neomycin sulfate and polymyxin B sulfate are considered active against the following microorganisms: **Staphylococcus aureus; Escherichia coli; Haemophilus influenzae; Klebsiella/Enterobacter** species; **Neisseria** species; and **Pseudomonas aeruginosa.**

When a decision to administer both a corticosteroid and an antimicrobial is made, the administration of such drugs in combination has the advantage of greater patient compliance and convenience, with the added assurance that the appropriate dosage of both drugs is administered. When both types of drugs are in the same formulation, compatibility of ingredients is assured and the correct volume of drug is delivered and retained.

The relative potency of corticosteroids depends on the molecular structure, concentration and release from the vehicle.

Indications and Usage: A steroid/anti-infective combination is indicated for steroid-responsive inflammatory ocular conditions for which a corticosteroid is indicated and where bacterial infection or a risk of bacterial ocular infection exists.

Ocular steroids are indicated in inflammatory conditions of the palpebral and bulbar conjunctiva, cornea, and anterior segment of the globe where the inherent risk of steroid use in certain infective conjunctivitides is accepted to obtain a diminution in edema and inflammation. They are also indicated in chronic anterior uveitis and corneal injury from chemical, radiation or thermal burns or penetration of foreign bodies.

The use of a combination drug with an anti-infective component is indicated where the risk of infection is high or where there is an expectation that potentially dangerous numbers of bacteria will be present in the eye.

The particular anti-infective drugs in this product are active against the following common bacterial eye pathogens: **Staphylococcus aureus; Escherichia coli; Haemophilus influenzae; Klebsiella/Enterobacter** species; **Neisseria** species; and **Pseudomonas aeruginosa.**

The product does not provide adequate coverage against: **Serratia marcescens;** Streptococci, including **Streptococcus pneumoniae.**

Contraindications: Epithelial herpes simplex keratitis (dendritic keratitis), vaccinia, varicella, and many other viral diseases of the cornea and conjunctiva. Mycobacterial infection of the eye. Fungal diseases of the ocular structures. Hypersensitivity to a component of the medication. (Hypersensitivity to the antibiotic component occurs at a higher rate than for other components.)

The use of these combinations is always contraindicated after uncomplicated removal of a corneal foreign body.

Warnings: Prolonged use may result in glaucoma, with damage to the optic nerve, defects in visual acuity and fields of vision, and in posterior subcapsular cataract formation. Prolonged use may suppress the host response and thus increase the hazard of secondary ocular infections. In those diseases causing thinning of the cornea or sclera, perforations have been known to occur with the use of topical steroids. In acute purulent conditions of the eye, steroids may mask infection or enhance existing infection. If these products are used for 10 days or longer, intraocular pressure should be routinely monitored even though it may be difficult in children and uncooperative patients.

Employment of a steroid medication in the treatment of herpes simplex requires great caution.

There exists a potential for neomycin sulfate to cause cutaneous sensitization. The exact incidence of this reaction is unknown.

Precautions: The initial prescription and renewal of the medication order beyond 20 milliliters should be made by a physician only after examination of the patient with the aid of magnification, such as slit lamp biomicroscopy and, where appropriate, fluorescein staining.

The possibility of persistent fungal infections of the cornea should be considered after prolonged steroid dosing.

Adverse Reactions: Adverse reactions have occurred with steroid/anti-infective combination drugs which can be attributed to the steroid component, the anti-infective component, or the combination. Exact incidence figures are not available since no denominator of treated patients is available.

Reactions occurring most often from the presence of the anti-infective ingredients are allergic sensitizations. The reactions due to the steroid component in decreasing order of frequency are: elevation of intraocular pressure (IOP) with possible development of glaucoma, and infrequent optic nerve damage; posterior subcapsular cataract formation; and delayed wound healing.

Secondary Infection: The development of secondary infection has occurred after use of combinations containing steroids and antimicrobials. Fungal infections of the cornea are particularly prone to develop coincidentally with long-term applications of steroid. The possibility of fungal invasion must be considered in any persistent corneal ulceration where steroid treatment has been used.

Secondary bacterial ocular infection following suppression of host responses also occurs.

Dosage and Administration: TO TREAT THE EYE: 1 or 2 drops every 3 or 4 hours, or more frequently as required. Acute infections may require administration every 30 minutes, with frequency of administration reduced as the infection is brought under control. TO TREAT THE LIDS: Instill 1 or 2 drops in the eye every 3 to 4 hours, close the eye and rub the excess on the lids and lid margins.

Not more than 20 milliliters should be prescribed initially and the prescription should not be refilled without further evaluation as outlined in the **Precautions** section above.

How Supplied: POLY-PRED® Liquifilm® sterile ophthalmic suspension is supplied in plastic dropper bottles in the following sizes:

5 mL—NDC 0023-0028-05
10 mL—NDC 0023-0028-15

Note: Protect from freezing. **Shake well before using.**

Caution: Federal (U.S.A.) law prohibits dispensing without prescription.

POLYTRIM® OPHTHALMIC SOLUTION ℞
Sterile
(TRIMETHOPRIM SULFATE AND POLYMYXIN B SULFATE)

Description: POLYTRIM® Ophthalmic Solution (trimethoprim sulfate and polymyxin B sulfate) is a sterile antimicrobial solution for topical ophthalmic use. Each mL contains trimethoprim sulfate equivalent to 1 mg trimethoprim and polymyxin B sulfate 10,000 units. The vehicle contains benzalkonium chloride 0.004% (added as preservative) and the inactive ingredients sodium chloride, sodium hydroxide or sulfuric acid (added to adjust pH), and Water for Injection.

Trimethoprim sulfate, 2,4-diamino-5-(3,4,5-trimethoxybenzyl)pyrimidine sulfate (2:1), is a white, odorless, crystalline powder with a molecular weight of 678.72.

Polymyxin B sulfate is the sulfate salt of polymyxin B_1 and B_2 which are produced by the growth of *Bacillus polymyxa* (Prazmowski) Migula (Fam. Bacillaceae). It has a potency of not less than 6,000 polymyxin B units per mg, calculated on an anhydrous basis.

Clinical Pharmacology: Trimethoprim is a synthetic antibacterial drug active against a wide variety of aerobic gram-positive and gram-negative ophthalmic pathogens. Trimethoprim blocks the production of tetrahydrofolic acid from dihydrofolic acid by binding to and reversibly inhibiting the enzyme dihydrofolate reductase. This binding is very much stronger for the bacterial enzyme than for the corresponding mammalian enzyme. For that reason, trimethoprim selectively interferes with bacterial biosynthesis of nucleic acids and proteins.

Polymyxin B, a cyclic lipopeptide antibiotic, is rapidly bactericidal for a variety of gram-negative organisms, especially *Pseudomonas aeruginosa*. It increases the permeability of the bacterial cell membrane by interacting with the phospholipid components of the membrane.

When used topically, trimethoprim and polymyxin B absorption through intact skin and mucous membranes is insignificant.

Blood samples were obtained from 11 human volunteers at 20 minutes, 1 hour and 3 hours following instillation in the eye of 2 drops of ophthalmic solution containing 1 mg trimethoprim and 10,000 units polymyxin B per mL. Peak serum concentrations were approximately 0.03 µg/mL trimethoprim and 1 unit/mL polymyxin B.

Microbiology: *In vitro* studies have demonstrated that the anti-infective components of POLYTRIM® are active against the following bacterial pathogens that are capable of causing external infections of the eye:

Trimethoprim: *Staphylococcus aureus* and *Staphylococcus epidermidis, Streptococcus pyogenes, Streptococcus faecalis, Streptococcus pneumoniae, Haemophilus influenzae, Haemophilus aegyptius, Escherichia coli, Klebsiella pneumoniae, Proteus mirabilis* (indole-negative), *Proteus vulgaris* (indole-positive), *Enterobacter aerogenes,* and *Serratia marcescens.*

Polymyxin B: *Pseudomonas aeruginosa, Escherichia coli, Klebsiella pneumoniae, Enterobacter aerogenes* and *Haemophilus influenzae.*

Indications and Usage: POLYTRIM® Ophthalmic Solution is indicated in the treatment of surface ocular bacterial infections, including acute bacterial conjunctivitis, and blepharoconjunctivitis, caused by susceptible strains of the following microorganisms: *Staphylococcus aureus, Staphylococcus epidermidis, Streptococcus pneumoniae, Streptococcus viridans, Haemophilus influenzae* and *Pseudomonas aeruginosa.**

*Efficacy for this organism in this organ system was studied in fewer than 10 infections.

Contraindications: POLYTRIM® Ophthalmic Solution is contraindicated in patients with known hypersensitivity to any of its components.

Warnings: NOT FOR INJECTION INTO THE EYE. If a sensitivity reaction to POLYTRIM® occurs, discontinue use. POLYTRIM® Ophthalmic Solution is not indicated for the prophylaxis or treatment of ophthalmia neonatorum.

Precautions:

General: As with other antimicrobial preparations, prolonged use may result in overgrowth of nonsusceptible organisms, including fungi. If superinfection occurs, appropriate therapy should be initiated.

Information for Patients: Avoid contaminating the applicator tip with material from the eye, fingers, or other source. This precaution is necessary if the sterility of the drops is to be maintained.

If redness, irritation, swelling or pain persists or increases, discontinue use immediately and contact your physician.

Carcinogenesis, Mutagenesis, Impairment of Fertility:

Carcinogenesis: Long-term studies in animals to evaluate carcinogenic potential have not been conducted with polymyxin B sulfate or trimethoprim.

Mutagenesis: Trimethoprim was demonstrated to be non-mutagenic in the Ames assay. In studies at two laboratories no chromosomal damage was detected in cultured Chinese hamster ovary cells at concentrations approximately 500 times human plasma levels after oral administration; at concentrations approximately 1000 times human plasma levels after oral administration in these same cells a low level of chromosomal damage was induced at one of the laboratories. Studies to evaluate mutagenic potential have not been conducted with polymyxin B sulfate.

Impairment of Fertility: Polymyxin B sulfate has been reported to impair the motility of equine sperm, but its effects on male or female fertility are unknown.

No adverse effects on fertility or general reproductive performance were observed in rats given trimethoprim in oral dosages as high as 70 mg/kg/day for males and 14 mg/kg/day for females.

Pregnancy: ***Teratogenic Effects:*** Pregnancy Category C. Animal reproduction studies have not been conducted with polymyxin B sulfate. It is not known whether polymyxin B sulfate can cause fetal harm when administered to a pregnant woman or can affect reproduction capacity.

Trimethoprim has been shown to be teratogenic in the rat when given in oral doses 40 times the human dose. In some rabbit studies, the overall increase in fetal loss (dead and resorbed and malformed conceptuses) was associated with oral doses 6 times the human therapeutic dose.

While there are no large well-controlled studies on the use of trimethoprim in pregnant women, Brumfitt and Pursell, in a retrospective study, reported the outcome of 186 pregnancies during which the mother received either placebo or oral trimethoprim in combination with sulfamethoxazole. The incidence of congenital abnormalities was 4.5% (3 of 66) in those who received placebo and 3.3% (4 of 120) in those receiving trimethoprim and sulfamethoxazole. There were no abnormalities in the 10 children whose mothers received the drug during the first trimester. In a separate survey, Brumfitt and Pursell also found no congenital abnormalities in 35 children whose mothers had received oral trimethoprim and sulfamethoxazole at the time of conception or shortly thereafter.

Because trimethoprim may interfere with folic acid metabolism, trimethoprim should be used during pregnancy only if the potential benefit justifies the potential risk to the fetus.

Nonteratogenic Effects: The oral administration of trimethoprim to rats at a dose of 70 mg/kg/day commencing with the last third of gestation and continuing through parturition and lactation caused no deleterious effects on gestation or pup growth and survival.

Nursing Mothers: It is not known whether this drug is excreted in human milk. Because many drugs are excreted in human milk, caution should be exercised when POLYTRIM® Ophthalmic Solution is administered to a nursing woman.

Pediatric Use: Safety and effectiveness in children below the age of 2 months have not been established (see WARNINGS).

Adverse Reactions: The most frequent adverse reaction to POLYTRIM® Ophthalmic Solution is local irritation consisting of increased redness, burning, stinging, and/or itching. This may occur on instillation, within 48 hours, or at any time with extended use. There are also multiple reports of hypersensitivity reactions consisting of lid edema, itching, increased redness, tearing, and/or circumocular rash.

Photosensitivity has been reported in patients taking oral trimethoprim.

Dosage and Administration:

Adults: In mild to moderate infections, instill one drop in the affected eye(s) every three hours (maximum of 6 doses per day) for a period of 7 to 10 days.

Pediatric Use: Clinical studies have shown POLYTRIM® to be safe and effective for use in children over two months of age. The dosage regimen is the same as for adults.

How Supplied: A sterile ophthalmic solution, each mL contains trimethoprim sulfate** equivalent to 1 mg trimethoprim and polymyxin B sulfate 10,000 units in a plastic dropper bottle of 10 mL (NDC 0023-7824-10). Store at 15°–25°C (59°–77°F) and protect from light.

**Mfd. under U.S. Patent No. 3,956,327.

PRED FORTE® ℞
(prednisolone acetate) 1%
sterile ophthalmic suspension

Description: PRED FORTE® (prednisolone acetate) 1% sterile ophthalmic suspension is a topical anti-inflammatory agent for ophthalmic use.

Chemical Name: 11β, 17, 21-Trihydroxypregna-1,4-diene-3,20-dione 21-acetate.

Continued on next page

Allergan Pharm—Cont.

Contains: prednisolone acetate (microfine suspension) 1.0%
with: benzalkonium chloride, polysorbate 80, boric acid, sodium citrate, sodium bisulfite, sodium chloride, edetate disodium, hydroxypropyl methylcellulose and purified water.

Clinical Pharmacology: Prednisolone acetate is a glucocorticoid that, on the basis of weight, has 3 to 5 times the anti-inflammatory potency of hydrocortisone. Glucocorticoids inhibit the edema, fibrin deposition, capillary dilation and phagocytic migration of the acute inflammatory response as well as capillary proliferation, deposition of collagen and scar formation.

Indications and Usage: PRED FORTE® is indicated for the treatment of steroid responsive inflammation of the palpebral and bulbar conjunctiva, cornea and anterior segment of the globe.

Contraindications: PRED FORTE® is contraindicated in acute untreated purulent ocular infections, acute superficial herpes simplex (dendritic keratitis), vaccinia, varicella and most other viral diseases of the cornea and conjunctiva, ocular tuberculosis, and fungal diseases of the eye. It is also contraindicated for individuals sensitive to any components of the formulation.

Warnings: In those diseases causing thinning of the cornea, perforation has been reported with the use of topical steroids.

Since PRED FORTE® contains no antimicrobial, if infection is present, appropriate measures must be taken to counteract the organisms involved.

Acute purulent infections of the eye may be masked or enhanced by the use of topical steroids.

Use of steroid medication in the presence of stromal herpes simplex requires caution and should be followed by frequent mandatory slit-lamp microscopy.

As fungal infections of the cornea have been reported coincidentally with long-term local steroid applications, fungal invasion may be suspected in any persistent corneal ulceration where a steroid has been used, or is in use.

Use of topical corticosteroids may cause increased intraocular pressure in certain individuals. This may result in damage to the optic nerve, with defects in the visual fields. It is advisable that the intraocular pressure be checked frequently.

Posterior subcapsular cataract formation has been reported after heavy or protracted use of topical ophthalmic corticosteroids.

Contains sodium bisulfite, a sulfite that may cause allergic-type reactions, including anaphylactic symptoms and life-threatening or less severe asthmatic episodes in certain susceptible people. The overall prevalence of sulfite sensitivity in the general population is unknown and probably low. Sulfite sensitivity is seen more frequently in asthmatic than in nonasthmatic people.

Precautions: General: Patients with histories of herpes simplex keratitis should be treated with caution.

Carcinogenesis, mutagenesis, Impairment of fertility: No studies have been conducted in animals or in humans to evaluate the potential of these effects.

Pregnancy Category C: Prednisolone has been shown to be teratogenic in mice when given in doses 1–10 times the human dose. There are no adequate well-controlled studies in pregnant women. Prednisolone should be used during pregnancy only if the potential benefit justifies the potential risk to the fetus.

Dexamethasone, hydrocortisone and prednisolone were ocularly applied to both eyes of pregnant mice five times per day on days 10 through 13 of gestation. A significant increase in the incidence of cleft palate was observed in the fetuses of the treated mice.

Nursing Mothers: It is not known whether topical administration of corticosteroids could result in sufficient systemic absorption to produce detectable quantities in breast milk. Systemically administered corticosteroids are secreted into breast milk in quantities not likely to have a deleterious effect on the infant. Nevertheless, caution should be exercised when topical corticosteroids are administered to a nursing woman.

Pediatric Use: Safety and effectiveness in children have not been established.

Adverse Reactions: Adverse reactions include increased intraocular pressure, which may be associated with optic nerve damage and defects in the visual fields, posterior subcapsular cataract formation, secondary ocular infections from fungi or viruses liberated from ocular tissues; and perforation of the globe when used in conditions where there is thinning of the cornea or sclera. Systemic side effects may occur rarely with extensive use of topical steroids.

Overdosage: Overdosage will not ordinarily cause acute problems. If accidentally ingested, drink fluids to dilute.

Dosage and Administration: Shake well before using. Instill one to two drops into the conjunctival sac two to four times daily. During the initial 24 to 48 hours, the dosing frequency may be increased if necessary. Care should be taken not to discontinue therapy prematurely.

NOTE: Keep this and all medications out of the reach of children.

How Supplied: PRED FORTE® (prednisolone acetate) 1% sterile ophthalmic suspension is supplied in plastic dropper bottles in the following sizes:

1 mL—**NDC** 11980-180-01
5 mL—**NDC** 11980-180-05
10 mL—**NDC** 11980-180-10
15 mL—**NDC** 11980-180-15

Note: Protect from freezing.

Caution: Federal (U.S.A.) law prohibits dispensing without prescription.

PRED-G® ℞
(prednisolone acetate, gentamicin sulfate) Liquifilm®
sterile ophthalmic suspension

Description: PRED-G® Liquifilm® sterile ophthalmic suspension is a topical anti-inflammatory/anti-infective combination product for ophthalmic use.

Chemical Names: Prednisolone acetate: 11β, 17,21-Trihydroxypregna-1,4-diene-3,20-dione 21-acetate.

Gentamicin sulfate is the sulfate salt of gentamicin C_1, gentamicin C_2, and gentamicin C_{1A} which are produced by the growth of **Micromonospora purpurea.**

Contains: prednisolone acetate 1.0%
(microfine suspension)
gentamicin sulfate............................ equivalent to 0.3% gentamicin base
with: Liquifilm® (polyvinyl alcohol) 1.4%; benzalkonium chloride 0.005%; edetate disodium; hydroxypropyl methylcellulose; polysorbate 80; sodium citrate, dihydrate; sodium chloride; sodium hydroxide and/or hydrochloric acid to adjust the pH; and purified water.

Clinical Pharmacology: Corticosteroids suppress the inflammatory response to a variety of agents and they probably delay or slow healing. Since corticosteroids may inhibit the body's defense mechanism against infection, a concomitant antimicrobial drug may be used when this inhibition is considered to be clinically significant in a particular case.

The anti-infective component in PRED-G® is included to provide action against specific organisms susceptible to it. Gentamicin sulfate is active *in vitro* against susceptible strains of the following microorganisms: *Staphylococcus aureus, Streptococcus pyogenes, Streptococcus pneumoniae, Enterobacter aerogenes, Escherichia coli, Haemophilus influenzae, Klebsiella pneumoniae, Neisseria gonorrhoeae, Pseudomonas aeruginosa, and Serratia marcescens.*

When a decision to administer both a corticosteroid and an antimicrobial is made, the administration of such drugs in combination has the advantage of greater patient compliance and convenience, with the added assurance that the appropriate dosage of both drugs is administered. When both types of drugs are in the same formulation, compatibility of ingredients is assured and the correct volume of drug is delivered and retained.

The relative potency of corticosteroids depends on the molecular structure, concentration, and release from the vehicle.

Indications and Usage: PRED-G® suspension is indicated for steroid-responsive inflammatory ocular conditions for which a corticosteroid is indicated and where superficial bacterial ocular infection or a risk of bacterial ocular infection exists.

Ocular steroids are indicated in inflammatory conditions of the palpebral and bulbar conjunctiva, cornea, and anterior segment of the globe where the inherent risk of steroid use in certain infective conjunctivitides is accepted to obtain a diminution in edema and inflammation. They are also indicated in chronic anterior uveitis and corneal injury from chemical, radiation, or thermal burns or penetration of foreign bodies.

The use of a combination drug with an anti-infective component is indicated where the risk of superficial ocular infection is high or where there is an expectation that potentially dangerous numbers of bacteria will be present in the eye.

The particular anti-infective drug in this product is active against the following common bacterial eye pathogens: *Staphylococcus aureus, Streptococcus pyogenes, Streptococcus pneumoniae, Enterobacter aerogenes, Escherichia coli, Haemophilus influenzae, Klebsiella pneumoniae, Neisseria gonorrhoeae, Pseudomonas aeruginosa, and Serratia marcescens.*

Contraindications: PRED-G® suspension is contraindicated in most viral diseases of the cornea and conjunctiva including epithelial herpes simplex keratitis (dendritic keratitis), vaccinia, and varicella, and also in mycobacterial infection of the eye and fungal diseases of the ocular structures. PRED-G® suspension is also contraindicated in individuals with known or suspected hypersensitivity to any of the ingredients of this preparation or to other corticosteroids.

Warnings: Prolonged use of corticosteroids may result in glaucoma with damage to the optic nerve, defects in visual acuity and fields of vision, and in posterior subcapsular cataract formation. Prolonged use of corticosteroids may suppress the host response and thus increase the hazard of secondary ocular infections.

Various ocular diseases and long term use of topical corticosteroids have been known to cause corneal and scleral thinning. Use of topical corticosteroids in the presence of thin corneal or scleral tissue may lead to perforation.

Acute purulent infections of the eye may be masked or enhanced by the presence of corticosteroid medication.

If this product is used for 10 days or longer, intraocular pressure should be routinely monitored even though it may be difficult in children and uncooperative patients. Steroids should be used with caution in the presence of glaucoma. Intraocular pressure should be checked frequently.

The use of steroids after cataract surgery may delay healing and increase the incidence of bleb formation.

Use of ocular steroids may prolong the course and may exacerbate the severity of many viral infections of the eye (including herpes simplex). Employment of a corticosteroid medication in the treatment of patients with a history of herpes simplex requires great caution; frequent slit lamp microscopy is recommended.

PRED G® Liquifilm® sterile ophthalmic suspension is not for injection. It should never be injected subconjunctivally, nor should it be directly introduced into the anterior chamber of the eye.

Precautions: General: Ocular irritation and punctate keratitis have been associated with the use of PRED-G® suspension. The initial prescription and renewal of the medication order beyond 20 milliliters should be made by a physician only after examination of the patient's intraocular pressure, examination of the patient with the aid of magnification such as slit lamp biomicroscopy and, where appropriate, fluorescein staining.

As fungal infections of the cornea are particularly prone to develop coincidentally with long-term local corticosteroid applications, fungal invasion should be suspected in any persistent corneal ulceration where a corticosteroid has been used or is in use. Fungal cultures should be taken when appropriate.

Information for Patients: If inflammation or pain persists longer than 48 hours or becomes aggravated, the patient should be advised to discontinue use of the medication and consult a physician.

This product is sterile when packaged. To prevent contamination, care should be taken to avoid touching the bottle tip to eyelids or to any other surface. The use of this bottle by more than one person may spread infection. Protect from freezing and from heat of 40°C (104°F) and above. Keep out of the reach of children. Shake well before using.

Carcinogenesis, mutagenesis, impairment of fertility: There are no published carcinogenicity or impairment of fertility studies on gentamicin. Aminoglycoside antibiotics have been found to be non-mutagenic.

There are no published mutagenicity or impairment of fertility studies on prednisolone. Prednisolone has been reported to be non-carcinogenic.

Pregnancy: Pregnancy Category C. Gentamicin has been shown to depress body weight, kidney weight, and median glomerular counts in newborn rats when administered systemically to pregnant rats in daily doses approximately 500 times the maximum recommended ophthalmic human dose. There are no adequate and well-controlled studies in pregnant women. Gentamicin should be used during pregnancy only if the potential benefit justifies the potential risk to the fetus.

Prednisolone has been shown to be teratogenic in mice when given in doses 1–10 times the human ocular dose. Dexamethasone, hydrocortisone and prednisolone were applied to both eyes of pregnant mice five times per day on days 10 through 13 of gestation. A significant increase in the incidence of cleft palate was observed in the fetuses of the treated mice. There are no adequate well-controlled studies in pregnant women. PRED-G® suspension should be used during pregnancy only if the potential benefit justifies the potential risk to the fetus.

Nursing Mothers: It is not known whether topical administration of corticosteroids could result in sufficient systemic absorption to produce detectable quantities in human milk. Systemically administered corticosteroids appear in human milk and could suppress growth, interfere with endogenous corticosteroid production, or cause other untoward effects. Because of the potential for serious adverse reactions in nursing infants from PRED-G® suspension, a decision should be made whether to discontinue nursing while the drug is being administered or to discontinue the medication.

Pediatric Use: Safety and effectiveness in children have not been established.

Adverse Reactions: Adverse reactions have occurred with steroid/anti-infective combination drugs which can be attributed to the steroid component, the anti-infective component, or the combination. Exact incidence figures are not available since no denominator of treated patients is available.

Reactions occurring most often from the presence of the anti-infective ingredient are allergic sensitizations. The reactions due to the steroid component in decreasing order of frequency are: elevation of intraocular pressure (IOP) with possible development of glaucoma, and infrequent optic nerve damage; posterior subcapsular cataract formation; and delayed wound healing.

Burning, stinging and other symptoms of irritation have been reported with PRED-G.® Superficial punctate keratitis has been reported occasionally with onset occurring typically after several days of use.

Secondary Infection: The development of secondary infection has occurred after use of combinations containing steroids and antimicrobials. Fungal and viral infections of the cornea are particularly prone to develop coincidentally with long-term applications of steroid. The possibility of fungal invasion should be considered in any persistent corneal ulceration where steroid treatment has been used. (See WARNINGS)

Secondary bacterial ocular infection following suppression of host responses also occurs.

Dosage and Administration: Instill one drop into the conjunctival sac two to four times daily. During the initial 24 to 48 hours, the dosing frequency may be increased, if necessary, up to 1 drop every hour. Care should be taken not to discontinue therapy prematurely. If signs and symptoms fail to improve after two days, the patient should be re-evaluated. (See PRECAUTIONS)

Not more than 20 milliliters should be prescribed initially and the prescription should not be refilled without further evaluation as outlined in **Precautions** above.

How Supplied: PRED-G® (prednisolone acetate 1.0%, gentamicin sulfate—0.3% base) Liquifilm® sterile ophthalmic suspension is supplied in plastic dropper bottles in the following sizes:

2 mL—NDC 0023-0106-02
5 mL—NDC 0023-0106-05
10 mL—NDC 0023-0106-10

Note: Store at room temperature. Avoid excessive heat, 40° C (104° F) and above. Protect from freezing. **Shake well before using.**

Caution: Federal (U.S.A.) law prohibits dispensing without prescription.

PRED–G® ℞
(prednisolone acetate, gentamicin sulfate)
S.O.P.®
sterile ophthalmic ointment

Description: PRED-G® S.O.P.® sterile ophthalmic ointment is a topical anti-inflammatory/anti-infective combination product for ophthalmic use.

Chemical Names: Prednisolone acetate: 11β,17,21-Trihydroxypregna-1,4-diene-3, 20-dione 21-acetate.

Gentamicin sulfate is the sulfate salt of gentamicin C_1, gentamicin C_2, and gentamicin C_{1A} which are produced by the growth of *Micromonospora purpurea.*

Contains: prednisolone acetate 0.6%
gentamicin sulfate ....equivalent to 0.3% gentamicin base
with: chlorobutanol (chloral derivative) 0.5%; white petrolatum; mineral oil; petrolatum (and) lanolin alcohol; and purified water.

Clinical Pharmacology: Corticosteroids suppress the inflammatory response to a variety of agents and they probably delay or slow healing. Since corticosteroids may inhibit the body's defense mechanism against infection, a concomitant antimicrobial drug may be used when this inhibition is considered to be clinically significant in a particular case.

The anti-infective component in PRED-G® S.O.P.® is included to provide action against specific organisms susceptible to it. Gentamicin sulfate is active *in vitro* against susceptible strains of the following microorganisms: *Staphylococcus aureus, Streptococcus pyogenes, Streptococcus pneumoniae, Enterobacter aerogenes, Escherichia coli, Hemophilus influenzae, Klebsiella pneumoniae, Neisseria gonorrhoeae, Pseudomonas aeruginosa,* and *Serratia marcescens.*

When a decision to administer both a corticosteroid and an antimicrobial is made, the administration of such drugs in combination has the advantage of greater patient compliance and convenience, with the added assurance that the appropriate dosage of both drugs is administered. When both types of drugs are in the same formulation, compatibility of ingredients is assured and the correct volume of drug is delivered and retained.

The relative potency of corticosteroids depends on the molecular structure, concentration, and release from the vehicle.

Indications and Usage: PRED-G® S.O.P.® is indicated for steroid-responsive inflammatory ocular conditions for which a corticosteroid is indicated and where superficial bacterial ocular infection or a risk of bacterial ocular infection exists.

Ocular steroids are indicated in inflammatory conditions of the palpebral and bulbar conjunctiva, cornea, and anterior segment of the globe where the inherent risk of steroid use in certain infective conjunctivitides is accepted to obtain a diminution in edema and inflammation. They are also indicated in chronic anterior uveitis and corneal injury from chemical, radiation, or thermal burns or penetration of foreign bodies.

The use of a combination drug with an anti-infective component is indicated where the risk of superficial ocular infection is high or where there is an expectation that potentially dangerous numbers of bacteria will be present in the eye.

The particular anti-infective drug in this product is active against the following common bacterial eye pathogens: *Staphylococcus aureus, Streptococcus pyogenes, Streptococcus pneumoniae, Enterobacter aerogenes, Escherichia coli, Hemophilus influenzae, Klebsiella pneumoniae, Neisseria gonorrhoeae, Pseudomonas aeruginosa,* and *Serratia marcescens.*

Contraindications: Epithelial herpes simplex keratitis (dendritic keratitis), vaccinia, varicella, and many other viral diseases of the cornea and conjunctiva. Mycobacterial infection of the eye. Fungal diseases of the ocular structures. Hypersensitivity to a component of the medication. (Hypersensitivity to the antibiotic component occurs at a higher rate than for other components.)

PRED-G® S.O.P.® is always contraindicated after uncomplicated removal of a corneal foreign body.

Warnings: Prolonged use may result in glaucoma with damage to the optic nerve, defects in visual acuity and fields of vision, and in posterior subcapsular cataract formation. Pro-

Continued on next page

Allergan Pharm—Cont.

longed use may suppress the host immune response and thus increase the hazard of secondary ocular infections. In those diseases causing thinning of the cornea or sclera, perforations have been known to occur with the use of topical steroids. In acute purulent conditions of the eye, steroids may mask infection or enhance existing infection. If these products are used for 10 days or longer, intraocular pressure should be routinely monitored even though it may be difficult in children and uncooperative patients.

Employment of a steroid medication in the treatment of patients with a history of herpes simplex requires great caution. PRED-G® S.O.P. is contraindicated in patients with active herpes simplex keratitis.

Precautions: General: Ocular irritation and punctate keratitis have been associated with the use of PRED-G.® S.O.P. The initial prescription and renewal of the medication order beyond 8 grams should be made by a physician only after examination of the patient's intraocular pressure, examination of the patient with the aid of magnification, such as slit lamp biomicroscopy and, where appropriate, fluorescein staining. The possibility of fungal infections of the cornea should be considered after prolonged steroid dosing.

Carcinogenesis, mutagenesis, impairment of fertility: There are no published carcinogenicity or impairment of fertility studies on gentamicin. Aminoglycoside antibiotics have been found to be non-mutagenic.

There are no published mutagenicity or impairment of fertility studies on prednisolone. Prednisolone has been reported to be non-carcinogenic.

Pregnancy: Pregnancy Category C: Gentamicin has been shown to depress newborn body weights, kidney weights, nephron counts and shows evidence of glomeruli and proximal tubule nephrotoxicity in rats when administered systemically in daily doses of approximately 500 times the maximum recommended ophthalmic dose in humans.

Prednisolone has been shown to be teratogenic in mice when given in doses 1–10 times the human dose. Dexamethasone, hydrocortisone and prednisolone were ocularly applied to both eyes of pregnant mice five times per day on days 10 through 13 of gestation. A significant increase in the incidence of cleft palate was observed in the fetuses of the treated mice. There are no adequate well-controlled studies in pregnant women. PRED-G® S.O.P. should be used during pregnancy only if the potential benefit justifies the potential risk to the fetus.

Nursing Mothers: It is not known whether topical administration of corticosteroids could result in sufficient systemic absorption to produce detectable quantities in breast milk. Systemically administered corticosteroids appear in breast milk and could suppress growth, interfere with endogenous corticosteroid production, or cause other untoward effects. Because of the potential for serious adverse reactions in nursing infants from PRED-G® S.O.P. a decision should be made whether to discontinue nursing or to discontinue the medication.

Pediatric Use: Safety and effectiveness in children have not been established.

Adverse Reactions: Adverse reactions have occurred with steroid/anti-infective combination drugs which can be attributed to the steroid component, the anti-infective component, or the combination. Exact incidence figures are not available since no denominator of treated patients is available.

The most frequent reactions observed include ocular discomfort, irritation upon instillation of the medication and punctate keratitis. These reactions have resolved upon discontinuation of the medication.

Reactions occurring most often from the presence of the anti-infective ingredient are allergic sensitizations. The reactions due to the steroid component in decreasing order of frequency are: elevation of intraocular pressure (IOP) with possible development of glaucoma, and infrequent optic nerve damage; posterior subcapsular cataract formation; and delayed wound healing.

Secondary Infection: The development of secondary infection has occurred after use of combinations containing steroids and antimicrobials. Fungal infections of the cornea are particularly prone to develop coincidentally with long-term applications of steroid. The possibility of fungal invasion must be considered in any persistent corneal ulceration where steroid treatment has been used.

Secondary bacterial ocular infection following suppression of host responses also occurs.

Dosage and Administration: A small amount (½ inch ribbon) of ointment should be applied in the conjunctival sac one to three times daily. Care should be taken not to discontinue therapy prematurely.

Not more than 8 grams should be prescribed initially and the prescription should not be refilled without further evaluation as outlined in **Precautions** above.

How Supplied: PRED-G® (prednisolone acetate 0.6%, gentamicin sulfate-0.3% base) S.O.P.® sterile ophthalmic ointment is supplied in ophthalmic ointment tubes of the following size:

3.5 g—NDC 0023-0066-04

Note: Store at controlled room temperature between 15°–30°C (59°–86°F).

Caution: Federal (U.S.A.) law prohibits dispensing without prescription.

PRED MILD® ℞

(prednisolone acetate) 0.12%
sterile ophthalmic suspension

Description: PRED MILD® (prednisolone acetate) 0.12% sterile ophthalmic suspension is a topical anti-inflammatory agent for ophthalmic use.

Chemical Name: 11β,17,21-Trihydroxypregna-1,4-diene-3,20-dione 21-acetate.

Contains: prednisolone acetate (microfine suspension) 0.12%
with: benzalkonium chloride; polysorbate 80; boric acid; sodium citrate; sodium metabisulfite; sodium chloride; edetate disodium; hydroxypropyl methylcellulose; and purified water.

Clinical Pharmacology: Prednisolone acetate is a glucocorticoid that, on the basis of weight, has 3 to 5 times the anti-inflammatory potency of hydrocortisone. Glucocorticoids inhibit the edema, fibrin deposition, capillary dilation and phagocytic migration of the acute inflammatory response as well as capillary proliferation, deposition of collagen and scar formation.

Indications and Usage: PRED MILD® is indicated for the treatment of mild to moderate noninfectious allergic and inflammatory disorders of the lid, conjunctiva, cornea and sclera (including chemical and thermal burns).

Contraindications: PRED MILD® is contraindicated in acute untreated purulent ocular infections, acute superficial herpes simplex (dendritic keratitis), vaccinia, varicella and most other viral diseases of the cornea and conjunctiva, ocular tuberculosis, and fungal diseases of the eye. It is also contraindicated for individuals sensitive to any component of the formulation.

Warnings: In those diseases causing thinning of the cornea, perforation has been reported with the use of topical steroids. Since PRED MILD® contains no antimicrobial, if infection is present, appropriate measures must be taken to counteract the organisms involved. Acute purulent infections of the eye may be masked or enhanced by the use of topical steroids. Use of steroid medication in the presence of stromal herpes simplex requires caution and should be followed by frequent mandatory slit-lamp microscopy. As fungal infections of the cornea have been reported coincidentally with long-term local steroid applications, fungal invasion may be suspected in any persistent corneal ulceration where a steroid has been used, or is in use.

Use of topical corticosteroids may cause increased intraocular pressure in certain individuals. This may result in damage to the optic nerve with defects in the visual fields. It is advisable that the intraocular pressure be checked frequently. Posterior subcapsular cataract formation has been reported after heavy or protracted use of topical ophthalmic corticosteroids.

Contains sodium metabisulfite, a sulfite that may cause allergic-type reactions including anaphylactic symptoms and life-threatening or less severe asthmatic episodes in certain susceptible people. The overall prevalence of sulfite sensitivity in the general population is unknown and probably low. Sulfite sensitivity is seen more frequently in asthmatic than in nonasthmatic people.

Precautions: General: Patients with histories of herpes simplex keratitis should be treated with caution.

Carcinogenesis, mutagenesis, impairment of fertility: No studies have been conducted in animals or in humans to evaluate the potential of these effects.

Pregnancy Category C: Prednisolone has been shown to be teratogenic in mice when given in doses 1–10 times the human dose. There are no adequate well-controlled studies in pregnant women. Prednisolone should be used during the pregnancy only if the potential benefit justifies the potential risk to the fetus. Dexamethasone, hydrocortisone and prednisolone were ocularly applied to both eyes of pregnant mice five times per day on days 10 through 13 of gestation. A significant increase in the incidence of cleft palate was observed in the fetuses of the treated mice.

Nursing Mothers: It is not known whether topical administration of corticosteroids could result in sufficient systemic absorption to produce detectable quantities in breast milk. Systemically administered corticosteroids are secreted into breast milk in quantities not likely to have a deleterious effect on the infant. Nevertheless, caution should be exercised when topical corticosteroids are administered to a nursing woman.

Pediatric use: Safety and effectiveness in children have not been established.

Adverse Reactions: Adverse reactions include increased intraocular pressure which may be associated with optic nerve damage and defects in the visual fields; posterior subcapsular cataract formation; secondary ocular infections from fungi or viruses liberated from ocular tissues; and perforation of the globe when used in conditions where there is thinning of the cornea or sclera. Systemic side effects may occur rarely with extensive use of topical steroids.

Overdosage: Overdosage will not ordinarily cause acute problems. If accidentally ingested, drink fluids to dilute.

Dosage and Administration: Shake well before using. Instill one to two drops into the conjunctival sac two to four times daily. During the initial 24 to 48 hours, the dosing frequency may be safely increased if necessary. Care should be taken not to discontinue therapy prematurely.

Note: Keep this and all medications out of the reach of children.

How Supplied: PRED MILD® (prednisolone acetate) 0.12% sterile ophthalmic suspension is supplied in plastic dropper bottles in the following sizes:

5 mL—NDC 11980-174-05
10 mL—NDC 11980-174-10

Note: Store at controlled room temperature 15°-30°C (59°-86°F). Protect from freezing.

Caution: Federal (U.S.A.) law prohibits dispensing without prescription.

Allergan America, Hormiguerous, Puerto Rico 00660

PROPINE® ℞
(dipivefrin HCl)
ophthalmic solution, USP, 0.1% sterile with C CAP® Compliance Cap B.I.D.

Description: PROPINE® contains dipivefrin hydrochloride in a sterile, isotonic solution. Dipivefrin HCl is a white, crystalline powder, freely soluble in water.

Empirical Formula: $C_{19}H_{29}O_5N \cdot HCl$

Chemical Name: (±)-3,4-Dihydroxy-α-[(methylamino)methyl]benzyl alcohol 3,4-dipivalate hydrochloride.

Contains:
Dipivefrin HCl* 0.1%
with: benzalkonium chloride 0.005%; edetate disodium; sodium chloride; hydrochloric acid to adjust pH; and purified water.
*Licensed under U.S. Patent Nos. 3,839,584 and 3,809,714.

Clinical Pharmacology: PROPINE® (dipivefrin HCl) is a member of a class of drugs known as prodrugs. Prodrugs are usually not active in themselves and require biotransformation to the parent compound before therapeutic activity is seen. These modifications are undertaken to enhance absorption, decrease side effects and enhance stability and comfort, thus making the parent compound a more useful drug. Enhanced absorption makes the prodrug a more efficient delivery system for the parent drug because less drug will be needed to produce the desired therapeutic response.
PROPINE® is a prodrug of epinephrine formed by the diesterification of epinephrine and pivalic acid. The addition of pivaloyl groups to the epinephrine molecule enhances its lipophilic character and, as a consequence, its penetration into the anterior chamber.
PROPINE® is converted to epinephrine inside the human eye by enzyme hydrolysis. The liberated epinephrine, an adrenergic agonist, appears to exert its action by decreasing aqueous production and by enhancing outflow facility. The PROPINE® prodrug delivery system is a more efficient way of delivering the therapeutic effects of epinephrine, with fewer side effects than are associated with conventional epinephrine therapy.
The onset of action with one drop of PROPINE® occurs about 30 minutes after treatment, with maximum effect seen at about one hour.
Using a prodrug means that less drug is needed for therapeutic effect since absorption is enhanced with the prodrug. PROPINE® at 0.1% dipivefrin was judged less irritating than a 1% solution of epinephrine hydrochloride or bitartrate. In addition, only 8 of 455 patients (1.8%) treated with PROPINE® reported discomfort due to photophobia, glare or light sensitivity.

Indications: PROPINE® (dipivefrin HCl) is indicated as initial therapy for the control of intraocular pressure in chronic open-angle glaucoma. Patients responding inadequately to other antiglaucoma therapy may respond to addition of PROPINE®.
In controlled and open-label studies of glaucoma, PROPINE® demonstrated a statistically significant intraocular pressure-lowering effect. Patients using PROPINE® twice daily in studies with mean durations of 76–146 days experienced mean pressure reductions ranging from 20–24%.
Therapeutic response to PROPINE® twice daily is somewhat less than 2% epinephrine twice daily. Controlled studies showed statistically significant differences in lowering of intraocular pressure between PROPINE® and 2% epinephrine. In controlled studies in patients with a history of epinephrine intolerance, only 3% of patients treated with PROPINE® exhibited intolerance, while 55% of those treated with epinephrine again developed an intolerance.
Therapeutic response to PROPINE® twice daily therapy is comparable to 2% pilocarpine 4 times daily. In controlled clinical studies comparing PROPINE® and 2% pilocarpine, there were no statistically significant differences in the maintenance of IOP levels for the two medications. PROPINE® does not produce miosis or accommodative spasm which cholinergic agents are known to produce. The blurred vision and night blindness often associated with miotic agents are not present with PROPINE® therapy. Patients with cataracts avoid the inability to see around lenticular opacities caused by constricted pupil.

Contraindications: PROPINE® should not be used in patients with narrow angles since any dilation of the pupil may predispose the patient to an attack of angle-closure glaucoma. This product is contraindicated in patients who are hypersensitive to any of its components.

Precautions:
Aphakic Patients. Macular edema has been shown to occur in up to 30% of aphakic patients treated with epinephrine. Discontinuation of epinephrine generally results in reversal of the maculopathy.
Pregnancy: Pregnancy Category B. Reproduction studies have been performed in rats and rabbits at daily oral doses up to 10 mg/kg body weight (5 mg/kg in teratogenicity studies), and have revealed no evidence of impaired fertility or harm to the fetus due to dipivefrin HCl. There are, however, no adequate and well-controlled studies in pregnant women. Because animal reproduction studies are not always predictive of human response, this drug should be used during pregnancy only if clearly needed.
Nursing Mothers. It is not known whether this drug is excreted in human milk. Because many drugs are excreted in human milk, caution should be exercised when PROPINE® is administered to a nursing woman.
Usage in Children. Clinical studies for safety and efficacy in children have not been done.
Animal Studies. Rabbit studies indicated a dose-related incidence of meibomian gland retention cysts following topical administration of both dipivefrin hydrochloride and epinephrine.

Adverse Reactions:
Cardiovascular Effects. Tachycardia, arrhythmias and hypertension have been reported with ocular administration of epinephrine.
Local Effects. The most frequent side effects reported with PROPINE® alone were injection in 6.5% of patients and burning and stinging in 6%. Follicular conjunctivitis, mydriasis and allergic reactions to PROPINE® have been reported infrequently. Epinephrine therapy can lead to adrenochrome deposits in the conjunctiva and cornea.

Dosage and Administration:
Initial Glaucoma Therapy. The usual dosage of PROPINE® is one drop in the eye(s) every 12 hours.
Replacement with PROPINE®. When patients are being transferred to PROPINE® from antiglaucoma agents other than epinephrine, on the first day continue the previous medication and add one drop of PROPINE® in each eye every 12 hours. On the following day, discontinue the previously used antiglaucoma agent and continue with PROPINE®.
In transferring patients from conventional epinephrine therapy to PROPINE®, simply discontinue the epinephrine medication and institute the PROPINE® regimen.
Addition of PROPINE®. When patients on other antiglaucoma agents require additional therapy, add one drop of PROPINE® every 12 hours.
Concomitant Therapy. For difficult to control patients, the addition of PROPINE® to other agents such as pilocarpine, carbachol, echothiophate iodide or acetazolamide has been shown to be effective.
Note: Not for injection.

How Supplied: PROPINE® (dipivefrin HCl) ophthalmic solution, USP, 0.1%, is supplied sterile in plastic dropper bottles as follows:
C CAP® Compliance Cap B.I.D. (twice daily)
5 mL—NDC 11980-260-25
10 mL—NDC 11980-260-20
15 mL—NDC 11980-260-21

Note: Store in tight, light-resistant containers.

Caution: Federal (U.S.A.) law prohibits dispensing without prescription.

C CAP® Compliance Cap Patient Instructions
Instructions for use:
1. On the first usage, make sure the number "1" appears in the window. If not, click the cap to the right station.
2. Remove the cap and apply medication.
3. Replace the cap. Hold the C CAP® between your thumb and forefinger. Now rotate the bottle until the cap clicks to the next station.
4. When it's time to take your next dose, repeat steps 2 and 3.

Important Notes: Don't try to catch up on missed doses by applying more than one dose at a time.
Each time you replace the cap, turn it until you hear the click.
The number in the window specifies your *next* dosage.

Shown in Product Identification Guide, page 103

Alza Pharmaceuticals
950 PAGE MILL ROAD
PO BOX 10950
PALO ALTO, CA 94303-0802

OCUSERT® Pilo-20 ℞
[*ok "u-sert*]
(pilocarpine)
Ocular Therapeutic System
20 μg/hr. for one week
and
OCUSERT® Pilo-40 ℞
(pilocarpine)
Ocular Therapeutic System
40 μg/hr. for one week

Description: OCUSERT® pilocarpine system is an elliptically shaped unit designed for continuous release of pilocarpine following placement in the cul-de-sac of the eye. Clinical evaluation in appropriate patients has demonstrated therapeutic efficacy of the system in the eye for one week. Two strengths are available, Pilo-20 and Pilo-40.
OCUSERT® systems contain a core reservoir consisting of pilocarpine and alginic acid. Pilocarpine is designated chemically as 2 (3H)-Furanone,3-ethyldihydro-4(1-methyl-1H-

Continued on next page

Alza—Cont.

imidazol-5-yl) methyl]-, (3S-cis)-and has the following structural formula:

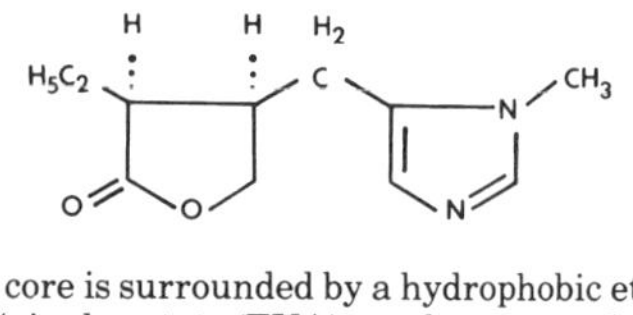

The core is surrounded by a hydrophobic ethylene/vinyl acetate (EVA) copolymer membrane which controls the diffusion of pilocarpine from the OCUSERT® system into the eye. The Pilo-40 membrane contains di(2-ethylhexyl) phthalate, which increases the rate of diffusion of pilocarpine across the EVA membrane. Of the total content of pilocarpine in the Pilo-20 or Pilo-40 system (5 mg or 11 mg, respectively), a portion serves as the thermodynamic diffusional energy source to release the drug and remains in the unit at the end of the week's use. The alginic acid component of the core is not released from the system. The readily visible white margin around the system contains titanium dioxide. The Pilo-20 system is 5.7 × 13.4 mm on its axes and 0.3 mm thick; the Pilo-40 system is 5.5 × 13 mm on its axes and 0.5 mm thick.

Release Rate Concept: With the OCUSERT® system form of therapy, the particular strength is described by the rated release, the mean release rate of drug from the system over seven days, in micrograms per hour. To cover the range of drug therapy needed to control the increased intraocular pressure associated with the glaucomas, two rated releases of pilocarpine from the OCUSERT® system are available, 20 and 40 micrograms per hour, for one week.

During the first few hours of the seven day time course, the release rate is higher than that prevailing over the remainder of the one-week period. The system releases drug at three times the rated value in the first hours and drops to the rated value in approximately six hours. A total of 0.3 mg to 0.7 mg pilocarpine (Pilo-20 or Pilo-40, respectively) is released during this initial six-hour period (one drop of 2% pilocarpine ophthalmic solution contains 1 mg pilocarpine). During the remainder of the seven day period the release rate is within ±20% of the rated value.

Clinical Pharmacology: Pilocarpine is released from the OCUSERT® system as soon as it is placed in contact with the conjunctival surfaces. Pilocarpine is a direct acting parasympathomimetic drug which produces pupillary constriction, stimulates the ciliary muscle, and increases aqueous humor outflow facility. Because of its action on ciliary muscle, pilocarpine induces transient myopia, generally more pronounced in younger patients. In association with the increase in outflow facility, there is a decrease in intraocular pressure.

Preclinical Results: The levels of ^{14}C- pilocarpine in the ocular tissues of rabbits following OCUSERT® system and eyedrop administration have been determined. The OCUSERT® system produces constant low pilocarpine levels in the ciliary body and iris. Following ^{14}C-pilocarpine eyedrop treatment, the initial levels of pilocarpine in the cornea, aqueous humor, ciliary body and iris are 3 to 5 times higher than the corresponding levels with the OCUSERT® system, declining over the next six hours to approximately the tissue concentrations maintained by the OCUSERT® system. In contrast, in the conjunctiva, lens, and vitreous the ^{14}C-pilocarpine concentrations remain consistently high from eyedrops and do not return to the constant low levels maintained by the OCUSERT® system. Pilocarpine does not accumulate in ocular tissues during OCUSERT® system use. These studies in rabbits have not been done in humans.

Clinical Results: The ocular hypotensive effect of both the Pilo-20 and Pilo-40 systems is fully developed within 1½ to 2 hours after placement in the cul-de-sac. A satisfactory ocular hypotensive response is maintained around-the-clock. Intraocular pressure reduction for an entire week is achieved with the OCUSERT® system from either 3.4 mg or 6.7 mg pilocarpine (20 or 40 μg/hour times 24 hours/day times 7 days, respectively), as compared with 28 mg administered as a 2% ophthalmic solution four times a day.

During the first several hours after insertion of an OCUSERT® pilocarpine system into the conjunctival cul-de-sac, induced myopia may occur. In contrast to the fluctuating and high levels of induced myopia typical of pilocarpine administration by eyedrop, the amount of induced myopia with OCUSERT® systems decreases after the first several hours to a low baseline level, approximately 0.5 diopters or less, which persists for the therapeutic life of the OCUSERT® system. Pilocarpine-induced miosis approximately parallels the induced myopia.

Of the 302 patients who used the OCUSERT® system in clinical studies for more than two weeks, 229 (75%) preferred it to previously used pilocarpine eyedrops. This percentage increased with further wearing experience.

Indications and Usage: OCUSERT® pilocarpine system is indicated for control of elevated intraocular pressure in pilocarpine responsive patients. Clinical studies have demonstrated OCUSERT® system efficacy in certain glaucomatous patients.

The patient should be instructed on the use of the OCUSERT® system and should read the package insert instructions for use. The patient should demonstrate to the ophthalmologist his ability to place, adjust and remove the units.

Concurrent Therapy: OCUSERT® systems have been used concomitantly with various ophthalmic medications. The release rate of pilocarpine from the OCUSERT® system is not influenced by carbonic anhydrase inhibitors, epinephrine or timolol ophthalmic solutions, fluorescein, or anesthetic, antibiotic, or anti-inflammatory steroid ophthalmic solutions. Systemic reactions consistent with an increased rate of absorption from the eye of an autonomic drug, such as epinephrine, have been observed. The occurrence of mild bulbar conjunctival edema, which is frequently present with epinephrine ophthalmic solutions, is not influenced by the OCUSERT® pilocarpine system.

Contraindications: OCUSERT® pilocarpine system is contraindicated where pupillary constriction is undesirable, such as for glaucomas associated with acute inflammatory disease of the anterior segment of the eye, and glaucomas occurring or persisting after extracapsular cataract extraction where posterior synechiae may occur.

Warnings: Patients with acute infectious conjunctivitis or keratitis should be given special consideration and evaluation prior to the use of the OCUSERT® pilocarpine system.

Damaged or deformed systems should not be placed or retained in the eye. Systems believed to be associated with an unexpected increase in drug action should be removed and replaced with a new system.

Precautions:

General

OCUSERT® pilocarpine system safety in retinal detachment patients and in patients with filtration blebs has not been established. The conjunctival erythema and edema associated with epinephrine ophthalmic solutions are not substantially altered by concomitant OCUSERT® pilocarpine system therapy. The use of pilocarpine drops should be considered when intense miosis is desired in certain ocular conditions.

Drug Interactions

Although ophthalmic solutions have been used effectively in conjunction with the OCUSERT® system, systemic reactions consistent with an increased rate of absorption from the eye of an autonomic drug, such as epinephrine, have been observed. In rare instances, reactions of this type can be severe.

Carcinogenesis, Mutagenesis, Impairment of Fertility

No long-term carcinogenicity and reproduction studies in animals have been conducted with the OCUSERT® system.

Pregnancy Category C

Although the use of the OCUSERT® pilocarpine system has not been reported to have adverse effect on pregnancy, the safety of its use in pregnant women has not been absolutely established. While systemic absorption of pilocarpine from the OCUSERT® system is highly unlikely, pregnant women should use it only if clearly needed.

Nursing Mothers

It is not known whether pilocarpine is excreted in human milk. Because many drugs are excreted in human milk, caution should be exercised when the OCUSERT® system is used by a nursing woman.

Pediatric Use

Safety and effectiveness in children have not been established.

Adverse Reactions: Ciliary spasm is encountered with pilocarpine usage but is not a contraindication to continued therapy unless the induced myopia is debilitating to the patient. Irritation from pilocarpine has been infrequently encountered and may require cessation of therapy depending on the judgement of the physician. True allergic reactions are uncommon but require discontinuation of therapy should they occur. Corneal abrasion and visual impairment have been reported with use of the OCUSERT® System.

Although withdrawal of the peripheral iris from the anterior chamber angle by miosis may reduce the tendency for narrow angle closure, miotics can occasionally precipitate angle closure by increasing the resistance to aqueous flow from posterior to anterior chamber. Miotic agents may also cause retinal detachment; thus, care should be exercised with all miotic therapy especially in young myopic patients.

Some patients may notice signs of conjunctival irritation, including mild erythema with or without a slight increase in mucous secretion when they first use OCUSERT® pilocarpine systems. These symptoms tend to lessen or disappear after the first week of therapy. In rare instances a sudden increase in pilocarpine effects has been reported during system use.

Dosage and Administration:

Initiation of Therapy: A patient whose intraocular pressure has been controlled by 1% or 2% pilocarpine eyedrop solution has a higher probability of pressure control with the Pilo-20 system than a patient who has used a higher strength pilocarpine solution and might require Pilo-40 therapy. However, there is no direct correlation between the OCUSERT® system (Pilo-20 or Pilo-40) and the strength of pilocarpine eyedrop solutions required to achieve a given level of pressure lowering. The OCUSERT® system reduces the amount of drug necessary to achieve adequate medical control; therefore, therapy may be started with the OCUSERT® Pilo-20 system irrespective of the strength of pilocarpine solution the patient previously required. Because of the patient's age, family history, and disease status or progression, however, the ophthalmologist may elect to begin therapy with the Pilo-40. The patient should then return during the first week of therapy for evaluation of his intraocu-

lar pressure, and as often therafter as the ophthalmologist deems necessary.
If the pressure is satisfactorily reduced with the OCUSERT® Pilo-20 system the patient should continue its use, replacing each unit every 7 days. If the physician desires intraocular pressure reduction greater than that achieved by the Pilo-20 system, the patient should be transferred to the Pilo-40 system. If necessary, an epinephrine ophthalmic solution or a carbonic anhydrase inhibitor may be used concurrently with OCUSERT® system.
After a satisfactory therapeutic regimen has been established with the OCUSERT® pilocarpine system, the frequency of follow-up should be determined by the ophthalmologist according to the status of the patient's disease process.
Placement and Removal of the OCUSERT® System: The OCUSERT® system is readily placed in the eye by the patient, according to patient instructions provided in the package. The instructions also describe procedures for removal of the system. It is strongly recommended that the patient's ability to manage the placement and removal of the system be reviewed at the first patient visit after initiation of therapy.
Since the pilocarpine-induced myopia from the OCUSERT® systems may occur during the first several hours of therapy (average of 1.4 diopters in a group of young subjects), the patient should be advised to place the system into the conjunctial cul-de-sac at bedtime. By morning the induced myopia is at a stable level (about 0.5 diopters or less in young subjects).
Sanitary Handling: Patients should be instructed to wash their hands thoroughly with soap and water before touching or manipulating the OCUSERT® system. In the event a displaced unit contacts unclean surfaces, rinsing with cool tap water before replacing is advisable. Obviously bacteriologically contaminated units should be discarded and replaced with a fresh unit.
OCUSERT® System Retention in the Eye: During the initial adaptation period, the OCUSERT® unit may slip out of the conjunctival cul-de-sac onto the cheek. The patient is usually aware of such movement and can replace the unit without difficulty.
In those patients in whom retention of the OCUSERT® unit is a problem, superior cul-de-sac placement is often more desirable. The OCUSERT® unit can be manipulated from the lower to the upper conjunctival cul-de-sac by a gentle digital massage through the lid, a technique readily learned by the patient. If possible the unit should be moved before sleep to the upper conjunctival cul-de-sac for best retention. Should the unit slip out of the conjunctival cul-de-sac during sleep, its ocular hypotensive effect following loss continues for a period of time comparable to that following instillation of eyedrops. The patient should be instructed to check for the presence of the OCUSERT® unit before retiring at night and upon arising.
How Supplied: OCUSERT® Pilo-20 and Pilo-40 systems are available in packages containing eight individual sterile systems.
Storage and Handling: Store under refrigeration (36°–46°F).
Caution: ***Federal law prohibits dispensing without prescription.***
ALZA Corp.,
Palo Alto, CA 94304
Printed in USA, 1991

Refer to contents page
for information on
Instruments and Equipment

Ayerst Laboratories

Division of American Home Products Corporation
685 THIRD AVE.
NEW YORK, NY 10017-4071

As a result of a merger of Wyeth Laboratories and Ayerst Laboratories, all prescription products formerly of Ayerst are products of Wyeth-Ayerst Laboratories. All nonprescription products formerly of Ayerst are products of Whitehall Laboratories.

Bausch & Lomb Personal Products Division

1400 N GOODMAN ST., PO BOX 450
ROCHESTER, NY 14692-0450

ALLERGY DROPS — OTC

Lubricant/Redness Reliever Eye Drops

Description: Bausch & Lomb Allergy Drops is a sterile lubricating eye drop that relieves minor irritation caused by allergens—pollen, dust, animal hair, air pollutants, and other common eye irritants. It relieves redness and keeps on working to protect eyes against further irritation.
Ingredients: Polyethylene glycol 300 (0.2%), naphazoline hydrochloride (0.012%). Also contains: boric acid, disodium edetate, purified water, sodium borate, sodium chloride; preserved with benzalkonium chloride (0.01%).
Indications: Relieves redness of the eye due to minor eye irritations. For the temporary relief of burning and irritation due to dryness of the eye and for use as a protectant against further irritation, or to relieve dryness of the eye.
Warnings: To avoid contamination, do not touch tip of container to any surface. Replace cap after using. If solution changes color or becomes cloudy, do not use. If you experience eye pain, changes in vision, continued redness or irritation of the eye, or if the condition worsens or persists for more than 72 hours, discontinue use and consult a doctor. If you have glaucoma, do not use this product except under the advice and supervision of a doctor. Overuse of this product may produce increased redness of the eye.
Keep this and all medication out of the reach of children. In case of accidental ingestion seek professional assistance or contact a Poison Control Center immediately.
Store at room temperature.
REMOVE CONTACT LENSES BEFORE USING.
Directions: Instill 1 or 2 drops in the affected eye(s) up to four times daily.
How Supplied: In plastic bottles of 0.5 fl oz.

Shown in Product Identification Guide, page 103

MAXIMUM STRENGTH ALLERGY DROPS — OTC

Lubricant/Redness Reliever Eye Drops

Description: Bausch & Lomb Maximum Strength Allergy Drops' fast-acting formula contains the highest concentration of naphazoline available without a prescription to provide even greater redness relief. It provides fast relief from the irritation caused by allergens such as pollen, dust, pet hair, air pollutants, and other common eye irritants. Maximum Strength Allergy Drops' dual-action formula also contains a lubricant to relieve eyes from the itching, burning, and irritation that allergies often cause. And it keeps on working to protect against further irritation.
Ingredients: Hydroxypropyl methylcellulose 0.5%, and naphazoline hydrochloride 0.03%. Also contains boric acid, edetate disodium, purified water, sodium borate, sodium chloride; preserved with benzalkonium chloride 0.01%.
Indications: For the termporary relief of discomfort due to minor irritations of the eye or to exposure to wind or sun. For use as a lubricant to prevent further irritation or to relieve dryness of the eye. Also relieves redness of the eye due to minor eye irritations.
Warnings: To avoid contamination, do not touch tip of container to any surface. Replace cap after using. If solution changes color or becomes cloudy, do not use. If you experience eye pain, changes in vision, continued redness or irritation of the eye, or if the condition worsens or persists for more than 72 hours, discontinue use and consult doctor. If you have glaucoma, do not use this product except under the advice and supervision of a doctor. Overuse of this product may produce increased redness of the eye.
Keep this and all medication out of the reach of children. In case of accidental ingestion, seek professional assistance or contact a Poison Control Center immediately.
Store at room temperature.
REMOVE CONTACT LENSES BEFORE USING.
Directions: Instill 1 or 2 drops in the affected eye(s) up to four times daily.
How Supplied: In plastic bottles of 0.5 fl. oz.

Shown in Product Identification Guide, page 103

DRY EYE THERAPY® — OTC

Lubricating Eye Drops
Preservative Free

Description: Bausch & Lomb Dry Eye Therapy is a preservative free treatment that, like natural tears, contains a lubricant and four essential nutrients: calcium, zinc, potassium, and magnesium. It provides soothing relief for dry eyes.
Ingredients: Glycerin 0.3%, with: calcium chloride, magnesium chloride, purified water, potassium chloride, sodium chloride, sodium citrate, sodium phosphate, and zinc chloride.
Indications: For the temporary relief of burning and irritation due to dryness of the eye and for use as a lubricant to prevent further irritation or to relieve dryness of the eye. For the temporary relief of discomfort due to minor irritations of the eye or to exposure to wind or sun.
Warnings: To avoid contamination, do not touch tip of container to any surface. Do not re-use. Once opened, discard. If you experience eye pain, changes in vision, continued redness or irritation of the eye, or if the condition worsens or persists for more than 72 hours, discontinue use and consult a doctor. If solution changes color or becomes cloudy, do not use. Use only if single-use container is intact.
Keep this and all drugs out of the reach of children.
Store at room temperature.
Directions:
- Make sure single-use container is intact before use.
- Separate one container from the strip of four.
- Open the single-use container by completely twisting off the top tab.
- Place thumb and forefinger on the center of the bubble.
- Gently squeeze 1 to 2 drops in the affected eye(s).
- After placing the drops in eye(s), throw away the container. Do not re-use.

Continued on next page

Bausch & Lomb—Cont.

Dry Eye Therapy may be used as often as needed.
How Supplied: 32 sterile, single-use containers, each 0.01 fl. oz. now more squeezable container.

Shown in Product Identification Guide, page 103

DUOLUBE® OTC
Sterile Lubricant Eye Ointment
Preservative-free

Description: Bausch & Lomb Duolube provides long lasting relief for dry eyes and contains protective lubricants.
Ingredients: White petrolatum 80% and mineral oil 20%. Contains no preservatives.
Indications: For use as a lubricant to prevent further irritation or to relieve dryness of the eye.
Warnings: To avoid contamination, do not touch tip of container to any surface. Replace cap after using. If you experience eye pain, changes in vision, continued redness, irritation of the eye, or if the condition worsens or persists for more than 72 hours, discontinue use and consult a doctor. (Keep out of reach of children.) **Not for use with contact lenses.**
DO NOT USE IF BOTTOM RIDGE OF CAP IS EXPOSED PRIOR TO INITIAL USE.
Store at room temperature.
Directions: Pull down the lower lid of the affected eye and apply a small amount (one-fourth inch) of Duolube ointment to the inside of the eyelid.
How Supplied: In ⅛-oz (NDC 10119-020-13) tube.

Shown in Product Identification Guide, page 103

BAUSCH & LOMB® EYE WASH OTC
Sterile Isotonic Buffered Solution

Description: Bausch & Lomb Eye Wash is a sterile, isotonic solution that contains boric acid, purified water, sodium borate and sodium chloride; preserved with disodium edetate 0.025% and sorbic acid 0.1%. CONTAINS NO THIMEROSAL (MERCURY).
Indications: For cleansing the eye to help relieve irritation, burning, stinging and itching by removing loose, foreign material, air pollutants (smog or pollen) or chlorinated water.
Warnings: To avoid contamination, do not touch tip of container to any surface. Replace cap after using. If you experience eye pain, changes in vision, continued redness or irritation of the eye, or if the condition worsens or persists, consult a doctor. Obtain immediate medical treatment for all open wounds in or near the eyes. If solution changes color or becomes cloudy, do not use.
Use only as directed. If you experience any chemical burns, consult a doctor immediately. Keep this and all drugs out of the reach of children.
Directions: Without Eye Cup—Flush the affected eye as needed, controlling the rate of flow of solution by pressure on the bottle.
Directions: With Eye Cup—Rinse cup with BAUSCH & LOMB® Eye Wash immediately before and after each use. Avoid contamination of rim and inside surfaces of cup. Fill cup one-half full with BAUSCH & LOMB Eye Wash. Apply cup tightly to the affected eye to prevent spillage and tilt head backward. Open eyelids wide and rotate eyeball to thoroughly wash the eye.
NOTE: Enclosed eye cup is sterile if packaging intact.
How Supplied: In plastic dropper bottles of 4 fl oz, packaged with sterile eye cup.

Shown in Product Identification Guide, page 103

MOISTURE DROPS® OTC
Artificial Tears
Lubricant Eye Drops

Description: Bausch & Lomb Moisture Drops Artificial Tears quickly provides soothing relief to dry, itchy, burning, irritated eyes. Its unique triple-action formula keeps on working, so your eyes stay moist, healthy, protected against further irritation. And unlike some eye drops, Moisture Drops can be used as often as needed.
Ingredients: Hydroxypropyl methylcellulose (0.5%), povidone (0.1%) and glycerin (0.2%). Also contains: boric acid, edetate disodium, potassium chloride, sodium borate, sodium chloride; preserved with benzalkonium chloride (0.01%).
Indications: For the temporary relief of burning and irritation due to dryness of the eye and for use as a protectant against further irritation, or to relieve dryness of the eye.
Warnings: To avoid contamination, do not touch tip of container to any surface. Replace cap after using. If solution changes color or becomes cloudy, do not use. If you experience eye pain, changes in vision, continued redness or irritation of the eye, or if the condition worsens or persists for more than 72 hours, discontinue use and consult a doctor.
Keep this and all drugs out of the reach of children.
REMOVE CONTACT LENSES BEFORE USING.
Directions: Instill 1 or 2 drops in the affected eye(s) as needed.
Store at room temperature.
How Supplied: In plastic bottles of 0.5 and 1.0 fl oz.

Shown in Product Identification Guide, page 103

Bausch & Lomb Pharmaceutical Division

8500 HIDDEN RIVER PARKWAY
TAMPA, FL 33637

NDC 24208	PRODUCT	
-825-55	**ATROPINE SULFATE OPHTHALMIC OINTMENT, 1%-STERILE** 3.5 gram tubes	℞
-750-	**ATROPINE SULFATE OPHTHALMIC SOLUTION, 1%-STERILE** 5mL: -60 15mL: -06	℞
*280-99	**BIO-COR®** (formerly **BIO-COR® 12 HR**) Collagen Corneal Shield	℞
*281-99	**BIO-COR® II** (formerly **BIO-COR® 24 HR**) Collagen Corneal Shield	℞
*282-99	**BIO-COR® EXT** (formerly **BIO-COR® 72 HR**) Collagen Corneal Sheild	℞
-640-55	**DEXAMETHASONE SODIUM PHOSPHATE OPHTHALMIC OINTMENT, 0.05%, USP-STERILE** 3.5 gram tubes	℞
-720-02	**DEXAMETHASONE SODIUM PHOSPHATE OPHTHALMIC SOLUTION, 0.1%, USP-STERILE** 5mL	℞
-796-35	**DEXASPORIN® OINTMENT** Neomycin and Polymyxin B Sulfates and Dexamethasone 0.1% Ophthalmic Ointment-Sterile 3.5 gram tubes	℞
-740-	**PHENYLEPHRINE HYDROCHLORIDE OPHTHALMIC SOLUTION, 2.5%-STERILE** 2mL: -59 5mL: -02 15mL: -06	℞
-505-	**LEVOBUNOLOL HYDROCHLORIDE OPHTHALMIC SOLUTION USP, 0.5%** 5mL: -05 10mL: -10 15 mL: -15	℞
-545-	**LEVOBUNOLOL HYDROCHLORIDE OPHTHALMIC USP, 0.25%** 5mL: -05 10mL: -10	℞
-580-	**GENTAMICIN SOLUTION** Gentamicin Sulfate Ophthalmic Solution-Sterile USP 5mL: -60 15mL: -64	℞
725-06	**NAFAZAIR® SOLUTION** (Naphazoline Hydrochloride Ophthalmic Solution, 0.1%) 15mL	℞
-585-	**TROPICAMIDE OPHTHALMIC SOLUTION, USP 1%-STERILE** 2mL: -59 15mL: -64	℞
-590-64	**TROPICAMIDE OPHTHALMIC SOLUTION, USP 0.5%-STERILE** 15mL	℞
-279-15	**OPCON® SOLUTION** Naphazoline Hydrochloride Ophthalmic Solution, 0.1% USP-Sterile 15mL	℞
-278-05	**MUROCOLL® 2 SOLUTION** Phenylephrine Hydrochloride 10% and Scopolamine Hydrobromide 0.3% Ophthalmic Solution 5 mL	℞
-280-15	**MUROCEL® SOLUTION** Methylcellulose 1% Lubricant Ophthalmic Solution 15 mL	OTC
-955-60	**NEODEXAIR® SOLUTION** Neomycin Sulfate and Dexamethasone Sodium Phosphate Ophthalmic Solution-Sterile 5mL	℞
-782-35	**OCUTRICIN® OINTMENT** Neomycin and Polymyxin B Sulfates and Bacitracin Zinc Ophthalmic Ointment-Sterile 3.5 gram tubes	℞
-786-35	**NEOTRICIN™ HC OINTMENT** Neomycin and Polymyxin B Sulfates, Bacitracin Zinc, and Hydrocortisone Acetate Ophthalmic Ointment-Sterile 3.5 gram tubes	℞
-735-	**PENTOLAIR® SOLUTION** Cyclopentolate Hydrochloride Ophthalmic Solution, 1%, USP -Sterile 2mL: -01 15mL: -06	℞
-806-15	**PILOSTAT® 0.5% SOLUTION** Pilocarpine Hydrochloride Ophthalmic Solution, 0.5%-Sterile 15mL	℞

-676- **PILOSTAT® 1% SOLUTION** ℞
Pilocarpine Hydrochloride
Ophthalmic Solution,
1%-Sterile
15mL: -15
TWIN PACK 2×15 mL: -30

-681- **PILOSTAT® 2% SOLUTION** ℞
Pilocarpine Hydrochloride
Ophthalmic Solution,
2%-Sterile
15mL: -15
TWIN PACK 2×15 mL: -30

-811-15 **PILOSTAT® 3% SOLUTION** ℞
Pilocarpine Hydrochloride
Ophthalmic Solution,
3%-Sterile
15mL

-686- **PILOSTAT® 4% SOLUTION** ℞
Pilocarpine Hydrochloride
Ophthalmic Solution,
4%-Sterile
15mL: -15
TWIN PACK 2×15 mL: -30

-821-15 **PILOSTAT® 6% SOLUTION** ℞
Pilocarpine Hydrochloride
Ophthalmic Solution,
6%-Sterile
15mL

-771-35 **SULFACETAMIDE SODIUM OPHTHALMIC OINTMENT, USP 10%-STERILE** ℞
3.5 gram tubes

-670 **SULFACETAMIDE SODIUM OPHTHALMIC SOLUTION, USP 10%-STERILE** ℞
2mL: -59
15mL: -04

-290-05 **TOBRAMYCIN OPHTHALMIC SOLUTION USP, 0.3%** ℞
5mL

-920-64 **TETRACAINE HYDRO-CHLORIDE OPHTHALMIC SOLUTION 0.5%-STERILE** ℞
15mL

-275- **OPTIPRANOLOL® SOLUTION** ℞
Metipranolol 0.3%
Ophthalmic Solution-Sterile
5 mL: -07
10 mL: -09

-276-15 **MURO 128® 2% SOLUTION** OTC
Sodium Chloride 2% Hypertonicity
Ophthalmic Solution-Sterile
15 mL

-277- **MURO 128® 5% SOLUTION** OTC
Sodium Chloride 5% Hypertonicity
Ophthalmic Solution-Sterile
15 mL -15
30 mL -30

-385 **MURO 128® 5% OINTMENT** OTC
Sodium Chloride 5% Hypertonicity
Ophthalmic Ointment-Sterile
3.5g -55
TWIN PACK 2× 3.5g: -56

NDC 57782	PRODUCT

-595-73 **EYE DROPS** OTC
Tetrahydrozoline Hydro-chloride Ophthalmic
Solution-Sterile
(15 mL)

-596-15 **EYE DROPS EXTRA** OTC
Tetrahydrozoline Hydrochloride
Ophthalmic Solution
15 mL

-597-15 **EYE DROPS AR** OTC
Tetrahydrozoline Hydrochloride
0.05% and Zinc Sulfate 0.25%
Ophthalmic Solution
15 mL

-835-80 **EYE WASH** OTC
Eye Irrigating Solution-Sterile
4 fl. oz. (120 mL)

-841-15 **LUBRITEARS® SOLUTION** OTC
Hydroxypropyl
Methylcellulose 2906,
Dextran 70
Lubricant Eye Drops-Sterile
15 mL

-481-35 **LUBRITEARS® OINTMENT** OTC
White petrolatum, Mineral Oil,
Lanolin Oil Lubricant Eye
Ointment-Sterile
3.5 gram tube

-755-15 **DRY EYES SOLUTION** OTC
Polyvinyl Alcohol
1.4% Lubricant Eye
Drops-Sterile
15 mL

-761-35 **DRY EYES OINTMENT** OTC
White Petrolatum,
Mineral Oil, Lanolin Oil
Lubricant Eye
Ointment-Sterile
3.5 gram tubes

*Product Number Only

MURO 128® 2% OTC

[*mŭ 'rō 128*]

Sodium Chloride Hypertonicity Ophthalmic Solution, 2%

MURO 128® 5% OTC

Sodium Chloride Hypertonicity Ophthalmic Solution, 5%

STERILE OPHTHALMIC SOLUTION

Description: Muro 128® 2% Solution is a sterile ophthalmic solution used to draw water out of the cornea of the eye.

Each mL Contains: ACTIVE: Sodium Chloride 2%; INACTIVES: Boric Acid, Hydroxypropyl Methylcellulose 2910, Propylene Glycol, Sodium Borate, Purified Water. Sodium Hydroxide and/or Hydrochloric Acid may be added to adjust pH.

PRESERVATIVES: Methylparaben 0.046%, Propylparaben 0.02%.

Description: Muro 128® 5% Solution is a sterile ophthalmic solution used to draw water out of the cornea of the eye.

Each mL Contains: ACTIVE: Sodium Chloride 5%; INACTIVES: Boric Acid, Hydroxypropyl Methylcellulose 2910, Propylene Glycol, Sodium Borate, Purified Water. Sodium Hydroxide and/or Hydrochloric Acid may be added to adjust pH.

PRESERVATIVES: Methylparaben 0.023%, Propylparaben 0.01%.

Indication: For the temporary relief of corneal edema.

Warnings: Do not use this product except under the advice and supervision of a doctor.

If you experience eye pain, changes in vision, continued redness or irritation of the eye, or if the condition worsens or persists, consult a doctor.

To avoid contamination of the product, do not touch the tip of the container to any surface. Replace cap after using.

This product may cause temporary burning and irritation on being instilled into the eye.

If the solution changes color or becomes cloudy, do not use.

In case of accidental ingestion, seek professional assistance or contact a Poison Control Center immediately.

Directions: Instill 1 or 2 drops in the affected eye(s) every 3 or 4 hours, or as directed by a doctor.

FOR OPHTHALMIC USE ONLY

How Supplied: Muro 128 2% Solution is supplied in plastic controlled drop tip bottle in the following size:

½ Fl. Oz. (15 mL) (NDC 24208-277-15)—Prod. No. AB15511

Muro 128 5% Solution is supplied in ½ Fl. Oz. (15 mL) or 1 Fl. Oz. (30 mL) plastic controlled dropper tip bottles.

15 mL [NDC 24208-277-15]—Prod. No. AB15611

30 mL [NDC 24208-277-30]—Prod. No. AB15616

DO NOT USE IF IMPRINTED NECKBAND IS NOT INTACT

Storage: Store between 15°–30°C (59°–86°F)

KEEP TIGHTLY CLOSED.

KEEP OUT OF REACH OF CHILDREN

Bausch & Lomb
Pharmaceutical Division
Tampa, FL 33637

MURO is a trademark of MURO Pharmaceutical, Inc.

MURO 128 2%–X050189 REV. 4/94-4D
MURO 128 5%–X050187 REV. 11/93-3K

Shown in Product Identification Guide, page 103

MURO 128® OINTMENT OTC

[*mŭ 'rō 128*]

Sodium Chloride Hypertonicity Ophthalmic Ointment, 5%

FOR CORNEAL EDEMA

STERILE OPHTHALMIC OINTMENT

Description: Muro 128® Ointment is a sterile ophthalmic ointment used to draw water out of the cornea of the eye.

Each Gram Contains: ACTIVE: Sodium Chloride, 5%; INACTIVES: Lanolin, Mineral Oil, White Petrolatum, Purified Water.

Indication: For the temporary relief of corneal edema.

Warnings: Do not use this product except under the advice and supervision of a doctor.

If you experience eye pain, changes in vision, continued redness or irritation of the eye, or if the condition worsens or persists, consult a doctor.

To avoid contamination of the product, do not touch the tip of the container to any surface. Replace cap after using.

This product may cause temporary burning and irritation on being instilled into the eye.

In case of accidental ingestion, seek professional assistance or contact a Poison Control Center immediately.

Directions: Pull down the lower lid of the affected eye(s) and apply a small amount (approximately ¼ inch) of the ointment to the inside of the eyelid every 3 or 4 hours, or as directed by a doctor.

FOR OPHTHALMIC USE ONLY

How Supplied: Muro 128® Ointment is supplied in a ⅛ oz. (3.5 g) tube.

[NDC 24208-385-55]—Prod. No. AB15834

TWIN PACK: 2×⅛ oz (2×3.5 g)

[NDC 24208-385-56]—Prod. No. AB15899

NOTE: Tubes are filled by weight (⅛ oz/3.5 g) not volume.

See Crimp of tube for Lot Number and Expiration Date.

DO NOT USE IF BOTTOM RIDGE OF TUBE CAP IS EXPOSED AND IMPRINTED SEAL ON BOX IS BROKEN OR MISSING.

KEEP OUT OF REACH OF CHILDREN.

Storage: Store between 15°–30°C (59°–86°F).

KEEP TIGHTLY CLOSED.

Bausch & Lomb
Pharmaceutical Division
Tampa, FL 33637

MURO is a trademark of MURO Pharmaceutical, Inc. X050196 REV.3/94-4C

Shown in Product Identification Guide, page 103

Continued on next page

Bausch & Lomb—Cont.

OPTIPRANOLOL® ℞
Metipranolol 0.3%
Sterile Ophthalmic Solution

Description: OPTIPRANOLOL® (metipranolol 0.3%) Sterile Ophthalmic Solution contains metipranolol, a non-selective beta-adrenergic receptor blocking agent. Metipranolol is a white, odorless, crystalline powder. The molecular weight is 309.40.
The empiric chemical formula of metipranolol is $C_{17}H_{27}NO_4$.
The chemical name of metipranolol is (±)-1-(4-Hydroxy-2, 3, 5-trimethylphenoxy)-3-(isopropylamino)-2-propanol-4-acetate.
The chemical structure of metipranolol is:

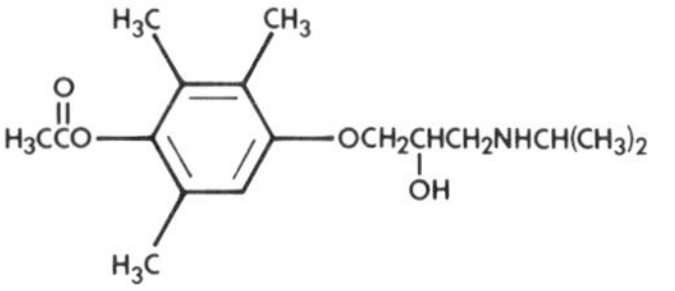

Each mL of OPTIPRANOLOL® contains 3 mg metipranolol. INACTIVES: povidone, glycerol, hydrochloric acid, sodium chloride, edetate disodium, and purified water. Sodium Hydroxide may be added to adjust pH. PRESERVATIVE: Benzalkonium chloride 0.004%.
Clinical Pharmacology: Metipranolol blocks beta and $beta_2$ (non-selective) adrenergic receptors. It does not have significant intrinsic sympathomimetic activity, and has only weak local anesthetic (membrane-stabilizing) and myocardial depressant activity.
Orally administered beta-adrenergic blocking agents reduce cardiac output in both healthy subjects and patients with heart disease. In patients with severe impairment of myocardial function, beta-adrenergic receptor antagonists may inhibit the sympathetic stimulatory effect necessary to maintain adequate cardiac output.
Beta-adrenergic receptor blockade in the bronchi and bronchioles may result in significantly increased airway resistance from unopposed para-sympathetic activity. Such an effect is potentially dangerous in patients with asthma or other bronchospastic conditions (see CONTRAINDICATIONS and WARNINGS).
OPTIPRANOLOL® Ophthalmic Solution, when applied topically in the eye, has the action of reducing elevated as well as normal intraocular pressure (IOP), whether or not accompanied by glaucoma. Elevated intraocular pressure is a major risk factor in the pathogenesis of glaucomatous visual field loss. The higher the level of intraocular pressure, the greater the likelihood of glaucomatous visual field loss and optic nerve damage.
The primary mechanism of the ocular hypotensive action of metipranolol is most likely due to a reduction in aqueous humor production. A slight increase in outflow may be an additional mechanism. OPTIPRANOLOL® Ophthalmic Solution reduces IOP with little or no effect on pupil size or accommodation.
Animal Pharmacology: In rabbits administered metipranolol in one eye at 2 to 4 fold increased concentrations, multi-focal interstitial nephritis was observed in male animals, and lympho-hystiocytic and heterophilic interstitial pneumonia was observed in female animals. The clinical relevance of these findings is unknown.
Indications and Usage: OPTIPRANOLOL® Ophthalmic Solution is indicated in the treatment of ocular conditions where lowering intraocular pressure is likely to be of therapeutic benefit; including patients with ocular hypertension, and patients with chronic open angle glaucoma.
In controlled studies of patients with intraocular pressure greater than 24 mmHg at baseline, OPTIPRANOLOL® Ophthalmic Solution reduced the average intraocular pressure approximately 20–26%.
The onset of action of OPTIPRANOLOL® Ophthalmic Solution, as measured by a reduction in intraocular pressure, occurs within 30 minutes after a single administration. The maximum effect occurs at about 2 hours. A reduction in intraocular pressure can be demonstrated 24 hours after a single dose. Clinical studies in patients with glaucoma treated for up to two years indicate that an intraocular pressure lowering effect is maintained.
In clinical trials, OPTIPRANOLOL® Ophthalmic Solution was safely used during concommitant therapy with pilocarpine, epinephrine or acetazolamide.
Contraindications: Hypersensitivity to any component of this product.
OPTIPRANOLOL® Ophthalmic Solution is contraindicated in patients with bronchial asthma or a history of bronchial asthma, or severe chronic obstructive pulmonary disease; symptomatic sinus bradycardia; greater than a first degree atrioventricular block; cardiogenic shock; or overt cardiac failure.
Warnings: As with other topically applied ophthalmic drugs, this drug may be absorbed systemically. Thus, the same adverse reactions found with systemic administration of beta-adrenergic blocking agents may occur with topical administration. For example, severe respiratory reactions and cardiac reactions, including death due to bronchospasm in patients with asthma, and rarely, death in association with cardiac failure, have been reported following topical application of beta-adrenergic blocking agents (see CONTRAINDICATIONS).
Since OPTIPRANOLOL® Ophthalmic Solution had a minor effect on heart rate and blood pressure in clinical studies, caution should be observed in treating patients with a history of cardiac failure. Treatment with OPTIPRANOLOL® Ophthalmic Solution should be discontinued at the first evidence of cardiac failure.
OPTIPRANOLOL® Ophthalmic Solution, or other beta-blockers, should not, in general, be administered to patients with chronic obstructive pulmonary disease (e.g., chronic bronchitis, emphysema) of mild or moderate severity (see CONTRAINDICATIONS). However, if the drug is necessary in such patients, then it should be administered with caution since it may block bronchodilation produced by endogenous and exogenous catecholamine stimulation of beta-receptors.
Precautions:
General: Because of potential effects of beta-adrenergic receptor blocking agents relative to blood pressure and pulse, these agents should be used with caution, in patients with cerebrovascular insufficiency. If signs or symptoms suggesting reduced cerebral blood flow develop following initiation of therapy with OPTIPRANOLOL® Ophthalmic Solution, alternative therapy should be considered.
Some authorities recommend gradual withdrawal of beta-adrenergic receptor blocking agents in patients undergoing elective surgery. If necessary during surgery, the effects of beta-adrenergic receptor blocking agents may be reversed by sufficient doses of such agonists as isoproterenol, dopamine, dobutamine or levarterenol.
While OPTIPRANOLOL® Ophthalmic Solution has demonstrated a low potential for systemic effect, it should be used with caution in patients with diabetes (especially labile diabetes) because of possible masking of signs and symptoms of acute hypoglycemia.
Beta-adrenergic receptor blocking agents may mask certain signs and symptoms of hyperthyroidism, and their abrupt withdrawal might precipitate a thyroid storm.
Beta-adrenergic blockade has been reported to potentiate muscle weakness consistent with certain myasthenic symptoms (e.g., diplopia, ptosis, and generalized weakness).
Risk of anaphylactic reaction: While taking beta-blockers, patients with a history of severe anaphylactic reaction to a variety of allergens may be more reactive to repeated challenge, either accidental, diagnostic, or therapeutic. Such patients may be unresponsive to the usual doses of epinephrine used to treat allergic reaction.
Drug Interactions: OPTIPRANOLOL® Ophthalmic Solution should be used with caution in patients who are receiving a beta-adrenergic blocking agent orally, because of the potential for additive effects on systemic beta-blockade. Close observation of the patient is recommended when a beta-blocker is administered to patients receiving catecholamine-depleting drugs such as reserpine, because of possible additive effects and the production of hypotension and/or bradycardia.
Caution should be used in the coadministration of beta-adrenergic receptor blocking agents, such as metipranolol, and oral or intravenous calcium channel antagonists, because of possible precipitation of left ventricular failure, and hypotension. In patients with impaired cardiac function, who are receiving calcium channel antagonists, coadministration should be avoided.
The concomitant use of beta-adrenergic receptor blocking agents with digitalis and calcium channel antagonists may have additive effects, prolonging arterioventricular conduction time.
Caution should be used in patients using concomitant adrenergic psychotropic drugs.
Ocular: In patients with angle-closure glaucoma, the immediate treatment objective is to re-open the angle by constriction of the pupil with a miotic agent. OPTIPRANOLOL® Ophthalmic Solution has little or no effect on the pupil, therefore, when it is used to reduce intraocular pressure in angle-closure glaucoma, it should be used only with concomitant administration of a miotic agent.
Carcinogenesis, Mutagenesis, Impairment of Fertility: Lifetime studies with metipranolol have been conducted in mice at oral doses of 5, 50 and 100 mg/kg/day and in rats at oral doses of up to 70 mg/kg/day. Metipranolol demonstrated no carcinogenic effect. In the mouse study, female animals receiving the low, but not the intermediate or high dose, had an increased number of pulmonary adenomas. The significance of this observation is unknown. In a variety of *in vitro* and *in vivo* bacterial and mammalian cell assays, metipranolol was nonmutagenic.
Reproduction and fertility studies of metipranolol in rats and mice showed no adverse effect on male fertility at oral doses of up to 50 mg/kg/day, and female fertility at oral doses of up to 25 mg/kg/day.
Pregnancy:
Pregnancy Category C. No drug related effects were reported for the segment II teratology study in fetal rats after administration, during organogenesis, to dams of up to 50 mg/kg/day. OPTIPRANOLOL® Ophthalmic Solution has been shown to increase fetal resorption, fetal death, and delayed development when administered orally to rabbits at 50 mg/kg during organogenesis.
There are no adequate and well-controlled studies in pregnant women. OPTIPRANOLOL® Ophthalmic Solution should be used during pregnancy only if the potential benefit justifies the potential risk to the fetus.
Nursing Mothers: It is not known whether OPTIPRANOLOL® Ophthalmic Solution is excreted in human milk. Because many drugs

are excreted in human milk, caution should be exercised when OPTIPRANOLOL® Ophthalmic Solution is administered to nursing women.

Pediatric Use: Safety and effectiveness in children have not been established.

Adverse Reactions: In clinical trials, the use of OPTIPRANOLOL® Ophthalmic Solution has been associated with transient local discomfort.

Other ocular adverse reactions, such as conjunctivitis, eyelid dermatitis, blepharitis, blurred vision, tearing, browache, abnormal vision, photophobia, and edema have been reported in small numbers of patients, either in U.S. clinical trials or from post-marketing experience in Europe.

Other systemic adverse reactions, such as allergic reaction, headache, asthenia, hypertension, myocardial infarct, atrial fibrillation, angina, palpitation, bradycardia, nausea, rhinitis, dyspnea, epistaxis, bronchitis, coughing, dizziness, anxiety, depression, somnolence, nervousness, arthritis, myalgia, and rash have also been reported in small numbers of patients.

Overdosage: No information is available on overdosage of OPTIPRANOLOL® Ophthalmic Solution in humans. The symptoms which might be expected with an overdose of a systemically administered beta-adrenergic receptor blocking agent are bradycardia, hypotension and acute cardiac failure.

Dosage and Administration: The recommended dose is one drop of OPTIPRANOLOL® Ophthalmic Solution in the affected eye(s) twice a day.

If the patient's IOP is not at a satisfactory level on this regimen, use of more frequent administration or a larger dose of OPTIPRANOLOL® Ophthalmic Solution is not known to be of benefit. Concomitant therapy to lower intraocular pressure can be instituted.

How Supplied: OPTIPRANOLOL® Ophthalmic Solution is supplied in white opaque, plastic ophthalmic bottle dispensers with a controlled drop tip and white plastic screw-top cap as follows:

2 mL: NDC 24208-275-03
5 mL: NDC 24208-275-07
10 mL: NDC 24208-275-09

Storage: Store at controlled room temperature, 15°-30°C (59°-86°F).

FOR OPHTHALMIC USE ONLY

CAUTION: Federal law prohibits dispensing without prescription.

Bausch & Lomb
Pharmaceutical Division
Tampa, FL 33637

X050164 REV. 8/92

Made in Germany

PB 262/1/2-10ml-US-D 1539

Shown in Product Identification Guide, page 103

PILOSTAT® ℞

Pilocarpine Hydrochloride
Ophthalmic Solution USP
STERILE OPHTHALMIC SOLUTION

Description: Pilocarpine Hydrochloride is a cholinergic prepared as a sterile topical ophthalmic solution. The active ingredient is represented by the chemical structural formula:

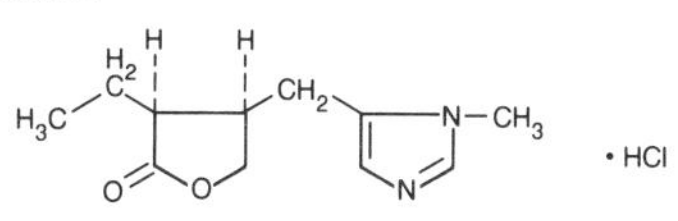

$C_{11}H_{16}N_2O_2 \cdot HCl$ Mol.Wt. 244.72

2 (3*H*)-Furanone, 3-ethyldihydro-4-[(1-methyl-1*H*-imidazol-5-yl)methyl]·monohydrochloride, [3*S*-*cis*]-

Pilocarpine HCl 0.5%

Each mL Contains: ACTIVE: Pilocarpine Hydrochloride 5 mg (0.5%); INACTIVES: Monobasic Sodium Phosphate, Hydroxypropyl Methylcellulose 2906, Sodium Chloride, Edetate Disodium, Dibasic Sodium Phosphate, Purified Water. Sodium Hydroxide and/or Hydrochloric Acid may be added to adjust pH (3.5–5.5). PRESERVATIVE: Benzalkonium Chloride 0.01%

Pilocarpine HCl 3%

Each mL Contains: ACTIVE: Pilocarpine Hydrochloride 30 mg (3%); INACTIVES: Monobasic Sodium Phosphate, Hydroxypropyl Methylcellulose 2906, Edetate Disodium, Purified Water. Sodium Hydroxide and/or Hydrochloric Acid may be added to adjust pH (3.5–5.5). PRESERVATIVE: Benzalkonium Chloride 0.01%

Pilocarpine HCl 1%
Pilocarpine HCl 2%
Pilocarpine HCl 6%

Each mL contains: ACTIVE: Pilocarpine Hydrochloride 10 mg (1%), 20 mg (2%) or 60 mg (6%); INACTIVES: Monobasic Sodium Phosphate, Hydroxypropyl Methylcellulose 2906, Edetate Disodium, Dibasic Sodium Phosphate, Purified Water. Sodium Hydroxide and/or Hydrochloric Acid may be added to adjust pH (3.5–5.5). PRESERVATIVE: Benzalkonium Chloride 0.01%

Pilocarpine HCl 4%

Each mL Contains: ACTIVE: Pilocarpine Hydrochloride 40 mg (4%); INACTIVES: Hydroxypropyl Methylcellulose 2906, Monobasic Sodium Phosphate, Edetate Disodium, Dibasic Sodium Phosphate, Purified Water. Sodium Hydroxide and/or Hydrochloric Acid may be added to adjust pH (3.5–5.5). PRESERVATIVE: Benzalkonium Chloride 0.01%

Clinical Pharmacology: The actions of pilocarpine hydrochloride are those of pilocarpine, a cholinergic substance. Its penetration, following topical application to the eye, results in parasympathomimetic reactions by responsive tissues.

Indications and Usage: Pilocarpine hydrochloride can be used in the medical management of glaucoma, especially open-angle glaucoma, in those cases in which the intraocular pressure can be controlled adequately by the topical administration of pilocarpine. In acute (closed-angle) glaucoma, pilocarpine hydrochloride may be used alone, or in combination with other cholinergic agents or carbonic anhydrase inhibitors, to relieve tension prior to emergency surgery.

Patients may be maintained on pilocarpine hydrochloride as long as intraocular pressure is controlled and there is no deterioration in the visual fields. The choice of concentration should be determined by the severity of the condition and the response of the patient. Pilocarpine hydrochloride is also indicated to counter the effects of cycloplegics and mydriatics following surgery or ophthalmoscopic examination.

Contraindications: Parasympathomimetics are contraindicated where miosis is undesirable such as acute iritis or pupillary block glaucoma.

This product is also contraindicated in persons hypersensitive to one or more of the components of this preparation.

Warnings: Not for internal use. To prevent contaminating the dropper tip and solution, care should be taken not to touch the eyelids or surrounding areas with the dropper tip of the bottle.

Precautions: This pilocarpine-induced miosis may cause difficulty in dark adaptation. The patient should exercise caution when involved in night driving or other hazardous activities in poor light.

Carcinogenesis, Mutagenesis, Impairment of Fertility: There have been no long-term studies done using pilocarpine in animals to evaluate carcinogenic potential.

Pregnancy Category C: Animal studies have not been conducted with pilocarpine. It is also not known whether pilocarpine can cause fetal harm when administered to a pregnant woman or can affect reproduction capacity. Pilocarpine should be given to a pregnant woman only if clearly needed.

Nursing Mothers: It is not known whether the drug is excreted in human milk. Because many drugs are excreted in human milk, caution should be exercised when pilocarpine is administered to a nursing woman.

Adverse Reactions:

OCULAR: Transient symptoms of stinging and burning may occur. Ciliary spasm, conjunctival vascular congestion, temporal or supraorbital headache, lacrimation and induced myopia may occur. This is especially true in younger individuals who have recently started administration. Reduced visual acuity in poor illumination is frequently experienced by older individuals and individuals with lens opacity. Miotic agents may also cause *retinal detachment;* thus, care should be exercised with all miotic therapy especially in young myopic patients. Lens opacity may occur with prolonged use of pilocarpine.

SYSTEMIC: Systemic reactions following topical administration, although extremely rare, have included hypertension, tachycardia, bronchiolar spasm, pulmonary edema, salivation, sweating, nausea, vomiting, and diarrhea.

Dosage and Administration: The initial dose is one or two drops in the affected eye(s). This may be repeated up to three or four times daily or as directed by a physician. The frequency of instillation and concentration of pilocarpine hydrochloride ophthalmic solution are determined by the severity of the glaucoma and miotic response of the patient. Individuals with heavily pigmented irides may require higher strengths.

During acute phases, the miotic must be instilled into the unaffected eye to prevent an attack of angle-closure glaucoma.

DO NOT USE IF IMPRINTED NECKBAND IS NOT INTACT.

How Supplied: Pilostat® (Pilocarpine Hydrochloride Ophthalmic Solution USP) is supplied in a plastic squeeze bottle with a controlled drop tip in the following strengths and sizes:

Pilostat® 0.5%
15 mL (NDC 24208-806-15)—Prod. No. AB02011

Pilostat® 1%
15 mL (NDC 24208-676-15)—Prod. No. AB02111
TWIN-PACK: 2 × 15 mL (NDC 24208-676-30) —AB02199

Pilostat® 2%
15 mL (NDC 24208-681-15)—Prod. No. AB02211
TWIN PACK: 2 ×15 mL (NDC 24208-681-30) —AB02299

Pilostat® 3%
15 mL (NDC 24208-811-15)—Prod. No. AB02311

Pilostat® 4%
15 mL (NDC 24208-686-15)—Prod. No. AB02411
TWIN PACK: 2 × 15 mL (NDC 24208-686-30) —AB02499

Pilostat® 6%
15 mL (NDC 24208-821-15)—Prod. No. AB02611

NOT FOR INJECTION
FOR OPHTHALMIC USE ONLY

Storage: Store between 15°-30°C (59°-86°F).

Continued on next page

Bausch & Lomb—Cont.

KEEP OUT OF REACH OF CHILDREN.
FOR OPHTHALMIC USE ONLY
CAUTION: Federal law prohibits dispensing without prescription.
Bausch & Lomb
Pharmaceutical Division
Tampa, FL 33637
© 1993 Bausch & Lomb Pharmaceuticals, Inc.
X050041 REV. 3/94-4C

Beiersdorf Inc.
P.O. BOX 5529
NORWALK, CT 06856-5529

COVERLET®
eye occlusor

Description: **Eye Occlusor Construction**
- Middle layer is light absorbing black for superior protection from direct and peripheral light penetration.
- The flexible backing fabric "breathes" for comfort and stretches for conformity
- Soft inner non absorbent, non-sterile pad cushions eye

Common Applications: Where light occlusion therapy is indicated, as in certain cases of strabismus, post-surgically or post-traumatically.
Indications: For light occlusion therapy or treatments where a non absorbent covering for the eye is necessary.
How Supplied:
[See table below.]
Colorful decals encourage good patching behavior and compliance*
Eye Occlusors are wrapped individually to provide protection against dust and dirt.
***Decals not to be used by children under 5 years old unless supervised by parent or adult.**
Coverlet is a registered trademark of Beiersdorf AG
®1994 Beiersdorf Inc.

Beiersdorf medical

Beiersdorf Inc Norwalk CT 06856-5529

COVERLET®

PRODUCT	LIST #	CASE CONTENTS	BOX CONTENTS	DESCRIPTION
Coverlet® Eye Occlusors	46429	12 boxes	20 Occlusors	Junior Size
	46430	12 boxes	20 Occlusors	Regular Size

Burroughs Wellcome Co.
3030 CORNWALLIS ROAD
RESEARCH TRIANGLE PARK, NC 27709

LITERATURE AVAILABLE: Folders, package inserts, and file cards.

CORTISPORIN® ℞
[*kor 'tĭ-spor "ĭn*]
OPHTHALMIC OINTMENT Sterile
(neomycin and polymyxin B sulfates, bacitracin zinc, and hydrocortisone ophthalmic ointment, USP)

Description: CORTISPORIN® Ophthalmic Ointment, (neomycin and polymyxin B sulfates, bacitracin zinc, and hydrocortisone ophthalmic ointment) is a sterile antimicrobial and anti-inflammatory ointment for ophthalmic use. Each gram contains: neomycin sulfate equivalent to 3.5 mg neomycin base, polymyxin B sulfate equivalent to 10,000 polymyxin B units, bacitracin zinc equivalent to 400 bacitracin units, hydrocortisone 10 mg (1%), and special white petrolatum, q.s.
Neomycin sulfate is the sulfate salt of neomycin B and C, which are produced by the growth of *Streptomyces fradiae* Waksman (Fam. Streptomycetaceae). It has a potency equivalent of not less than 600 μg of neomycin standard per mg, calculated on an anhydrous basis.
Polymyxin B sulfate is the sulfate salt of polymyxin B_1 and B_2, which are produced by the growth of *Bacillus polymyxa* (Prazmowski) Migula (Fam. Bacillaceae). It has a potency of not less than 6,000 polymyxin B units per mg, calculated on an anhydrous basis.
Bacitracin zinc is the zinc salt of bacitracin, a mixture of related cyclic polypeptides (mainly bacitracin A) produced by the growth of an organism of the *licheniformis* group of *Bacillus subtilis* var Tracy. It has a potency of not less than 40 bacitracin units per mg.
Hydrocortisone, 11β, 17, 21-trihydroxypregn-4-ene-3, 20-dione, is an anti-inflammatory hormone.
Clinical Pharmacology: Corticosteroids suppress the inflammatory response to a variety of agents and they probably delay or slow healing. Since corticosteroids may inhibit the body's defense mechanism against infection, concomitant antimicrobial drugs may be used when this inhibition is considered to be clinically significant in a particular case.
When a decision to administer both a corticosteroid and antimicrobials is made, the administration of such drugs in combination has the advantage of greater patient compliance and convenience, with the added assurance that the appropriate dosage of all drugs is administered. When each type of drug is in the same formulation, compatibility of ingredients is assured and the correct volume of drug is delivered and retained.
The relative potency of corticosteroids depends on the molecular structure, concentration, and release from the vehicle.
Microbiology: The anti-infective components in CORTISPORIN Ophthalmic Ointment are included to provide action against specific organisms susceptible to it. Neomycin sulfate and polymyxin B sulfate are active in vitro against susceptible strains of the following microorganisms: *Staphylococcus aureus*, streptococci including *Streptococcus pneumoniae, Escherichia coli, Haemophilus influenzae, Klebsiella/Enterobacter* species, *Neisseria* species, and *Pseudomonas aeruginosa*. This product does not provide adequate coverage against *Serratia marcescens* (see INDICATIONS AND USAGE).
Indications and Usage: CORTISPORIN Ophthalmic Ointment is indicated for steroid-responsive inflammatory ocular conditions for which a corticosteroid is indicated and where bacterial infection or a risk of bacterial infection exists.
Ocular corticosteroids are indicated in inflammatory conditions of the palpebral and bulbar conjunctiva, cornea, and anterior segment of the globe where the inherent risk of corticosteroid use in certain infective conjunctivitides is accepted to obtain a diminution in edema and inflammation. They are also indicated in chronic anterior uveitis and corneal injury from chemical, radiation, or thermal burns, or penetration of foreign bodies.
The use of a combination drug with an anti-infective component is indicated where the risk of infection is high or where there is an expectation that potentially dangerous numbers of bacteria will be present in the eye (see CLINICAL PHARMACOLOGY: Microbiology).
The particular anti-infective drugs in this product are active against the following common bacterial eye pathogens: *Staphylococcus aureus*, streptococci, including *Streptococcus pneumoniae, Escherichia coli, Haemophilus influenzae, Klebsiella-Enterobacter* species, *Neisseria* species and *Pseudomonas aeruginosa*.
The product does not provide adequate coverage against *Serratia marcescens*.
Contraindications: CORTISPORIN Ophthalmic Ointment is contraindicated in most viral diseases of the cornea and conjunctiva including: epithelial herpes simplex keratitis (dendritic keratitis) vaccinia and varicella, and also in mycobacterial infection of the eye and fungal diseases of ocular structures.
CORTISPORIN Ophthalmic Ointment is also contraindicated in individuals who have shown hypersensitivity to any of its components. Hypersensitivity to the antibiotic component occurs at a higher rate than for other components.
Warnings: NOT FOR INJECTION INTO THE EYE. CORTISPORIN Ophthalmic Ointment should never be directly introduced into the anterior chamber of the eye. Ophthalmic ointments may retard corneal wound healing. Prolonged use of corticosteriods may result in ocular hypertension and/or glaucoma, with damage to the optic nerve, defects in visual acuity and fields of vision, and in posterior subcapsular cataract formation.
Prolonged use may suppress the host response and thus increase the hazard of secondary ocular infections. In those diseases causing thinning of the cornea or sclera, perforations have been known to occur with the use of topical corticosteroids. In acute purulent conditions of the eye, corticosteroids may mask infection or enhance existing infection.
If these products are used for 10 days or longer, intraocular pressure should be routinely monitored even though it may be difficult in uncooperative patients. Corticosteroids should be used with caution in the presence of glaucoma.
The use of corticosteroids after cataract surgery may delay healing and increase the incidence of filtering blebs.
Use of ocular corticosteroids may prolong the course and may exacerbate the severity of many viral infections of the eye (including herpes simplex). Employment of corticosteroid medication in the treatment of herpes simplex requires great caution.
Topical antibiotics, particularly neomycin sulfate, may cause cutaneous sensitization. A precise incidence of hypersensitivity reactions (primarily skin rash) due to topical antibiotics is not known. The manifestations of sensitization to topical antibiotics are usually itching, reddening, and edema of the conjunctiva and eyelid. A sensitization reaction may manifest simply as a failure to heal. During long-term use of topical antibiotic products, periodic examination for such signs is advisable, and the patient should be told to discontinue the product if they are observed. Symptoms usually subside quickly on withdrawing the medication. Applications of products containing these ingredients should be avoided for the patient thereafter (See PRECAUTIONS: General).
Precautions:
General: The initial prescription and renewal of the medication order beyond 8 grams should be made by a physician only after examination of the patient with the aid of magnification, such as slit lamp biomicroscopy and, where appropriate, fluorescein staining. If signs and symptoms fail to improve after two days, the patient should be re-evaluated.
The possibility of fungal infections of the cornea should be considered after prolonged corticosteroid dosing. Fungal cultures should be taken when appropriate.

If this product is used for 10 days or longer, intraocular pressure should be monitored (see WARNINGS).

There have been reports of bacterial keratitis associated with the use of topical ophthalmic products in multiple-dose containers which have been inadvertently contaminated by patients, most of whom had a concurrent corneal disease or a disruption of the ocular epithelial surface (see PRECAUTIONS: Information for Patients).

Allergic cross-reactions may occur which could prevent the use of any or all of the following antibiotics for the treatment of future infections: kanamycin, paromomycin, streptomycin, and possibly gentamicin.

Information For Patients: Patients should be instructed to avoid allowing the tip of the dispensing container to contact the eye, eyelid, fingers, or any other surface. The use of this product by more than one person may spread infection.

Patients should be instructed that ocular products, if handled improperly, can become contaminated by common bacteria known to cause ocular infections. Serious damage to the eye and subsequent loss of vision may result from using contaminated products (see PRECAUTIONS: General).

If the condition persists or gets worse, or if a rash or allergic reaction develops, the patient should be advised to stop use and consult a physician. Do not use this product if you are allergic to any of the listed ingredients.

Keep tightly closed when not in use. Keep out of the reach of children.

Carcinogenesis, Mutagenesis, Impairment of Fertility: Long-term studies in animals to evaluate carcinogenic or mutagenic potential have not been conducted with polymyxin B sulfate or bacitracin. Treatment of cultured human lymphocytes in vitro with neomycin increased the frequency of chromosome aberrations at the highest concentrations (80 μg/mL) tested; however, the effects of neomycin on carcinogenesis and mutagenesis in humans are unknown.

Long-term studies in animals (rats, rabbits, mice) showed no evidence of carcinogenicity or mutagenicity attributable to oral administration of corticosteroids. Long-term animal studies have not been performed to evaluate the carcinogenic potential of topical corticosteroids. Studies to determine mutagenicity with hydrocortisone have revealed negative results. Polymyxin B has been reported to impair the motility of equine sperm, but its effects on male or female fertility are unknown. No adverse effects on male or female fertility, litter size, or survival were observed in rabbits given bacitracin zinc 100 gm/ton of diet. Long-term animal studies have not been performed to evaluate the effect on fertility of topical corticosteroids.

Pregnancy: *Teratogenic Effects:* Pregnancy Category C. Corticosteroids have been found to be teratogenic in rabbits when applied topically at concentrations of 0.5% on days 6 to 18 of gestation and in mice when applied topically at a concentration of 15% on days 10 to 13 of gestation. There are no adequate and well-controlled studies in pregnant women. CORTISPORIN Ophthalmic Ointment should be used during pregnancy only if the potential benefit justifies the potential risk to the fetus.

Nursing Mothers: It is not known whether topical administration of corticosteroids could result in sufficient systemic absorption to produce detectable quantities in human milk. Systemically administered corticosteroids appear in human milk and could suppress growth, interfere with endogenous corticosteroid production, or cause other untoward effects. Because of the potential for serious adverse reactions in nursing infants from CORTISPORIN Ophthalmic Ointment, a decision should be made whether to discontinue nursing or to discontinue the drug, taking into account the importance of the drug to the mother.

Pediatric Use: Safety and effectiveness in children have not been established.

Adverse Reactions: Adverse reactions have occurred with corticosteroid/anti-infective combination drugs which can be attributed to the corticosteroid component, the anti-infective component, or the combination. The exact incidence is not known.

Reactions occurring most often from the presence of the anti-infective ingredient are allergic sensitization reactions including itching, swelling, and conjunctival erythema (see WARNINGS). More serious hypersensitivity reactions, including anaphylaxis, have been reported rarely.

The reactions due to the corticosteroid component in decreasing order of frequency are: elevation of intraocular pressure (IOP) with possible development of glaucoma, and infrequent optic nerve damage; posterior subcapsular cataract formation; and delayed wound healing.

Secondary Infection: The development of secondary infection has occurred after use of combinations containing corticosteroids and antimicrobials. Fungal and viral infections of the cornea are particularly prone to develop coincidentally with long-term applications of a corticosteroid. The possibility of fungal invasion must be considered in any persistent corneal ulceration where corticosteroid treatment has been used.

Local irritation on instillation has also been reported.

Dosage and Administration: Apply the ointment in the affected eye every 3 or 4 hours, depending on the severity of the condition.

Not more than 8 grams should be prescribed initially and the prescription should not be refilled without further evaluation as outlined in PRECAUTIONS above.

How Supplied: Tube of ⅛ oz (3.5 g) with ophthalmic tip (NDC-0081-0197-86).

Caution: Federal law prohibits dispensing without a prescription.

Store at 15° to 25°C (59° to 77°F).

454967

Shown in Product Identification Guide, page 103

CORTISPORIN® ℞

[*kor 'tĭ spor "ĭn*]

Ophthalmic Suspension Sterile (neomycin and polymyxin B sulfates and hydrocortisone ophthalmic suspension, USP)

Description: CORTISPORIN® Ophthalmic Suspension (neomycin and polymyxin B sulfates and hydrocortisone ophthalmic suspension) is a sterile antimicrobial and anti-inflammatory suspension for ophthalmic use. Each mL contains: neomycin sulfate equivalent to 3.5 mg neomycin base, polymyxin B sulfate equivalent to 10,000 polymyxin B units, and hydrocortisone 10 mg (1%). The vehicle contains thimerosal 0.001% (added as a preservative) and the inactive ingredients cetyl alcohol, glyceryl monostearate, mineral oil, polyoxyl 40 stearate, propylene glycol, and Water for Injection. Sulfuric acid may be added to adjust pH.

Neomycin sulfate is the sulfate salt of neomycin B and C, which are produced by the growth of *Streptomyces fradiae* Waksman (Fam. Streptomycetaceae). It has a potency equivalent of not less than 600 μg of neomycin standard per mg, calculated on an anhydrous basis.

Polymyxin B sulfate is the sulfate salt of polymyxin B_1 and B_2, which are produced by the growth of *Bacillus polymyxa* (Prazmowski) Migula (Fam. Bacillaceae). It has a potency of not less than 6,000 polymyxin B units per mg, calculated on an anhydrous basis.

Hydrocortisone, 11β,17,21-trihydroxypregn-4-ene-3,20-dione, is an anti-inflammatory hormone.

Clinical Pharmacology: Corticosteroids suppress the inflammatory response to a variety of agents and they probably delay or slow healing. Since corticosteroids may inhibit the body's defense mechanism against infection, concomitant antimicrobial drugs may be used when this inhibition is considered to be clinically significant in a particular case.

When a decision to administer both a corticosteroid and antimicrobials is made, the administration of such drugs in combination has the advantage of greater patient compliance and convenience, with the added assurance that the appropriate dosage of all drugs is administered. When each type of drug is in the same formulation compatibility of ingredients is assured and the correct volume of drug is delivered and retained.

The relative potency of corticosteroids depends on the molecular structure, concentration, and release from the vehicle.

Microbiology: The anti-infective components in CORTISPORIN Ophthalmic Suspension are included to provide action against specific organisms susceptible to it. Neomycin sulfate and polymyxin B sulfate are active in vitro against susceptible strains of the following microorganisms: *Staphylococcus aureus, Escherichia coli, Haemophilus influenzae, Klebsiella/Enterobacter* species, *Neisseria* species, and *Pseudomonas aeruginosa.* The product does not provide adequate coverage against *Serratia marcescens* and streptococci, including *Streptococcus pneumoniae* (see INDICATIONS AND USAGE).

Indications and Usage: CORTISPORIN Ophthalmic Suspension is indicated for steroid-responsive inflammatory ocular conditions for which a corticosteroid is indicated and where bacterial infection or a risk of bacterial infection exists.

Ocular corticosteroids are indicated in inflammatory conditions of the palpebral and bulbar conjunctiva, cornea, and anterior segment of the globe where the inherent risk of corticosteroid use in certain infective conjunctivitides is accepted to obtain a diminution in edema and inflammation. They are also indicated in chronic anterior uveitis and corneal injury from chemical, radiation, or thermal burns, or penetration of foreign bodies.

The use of a combination drug with an anti-infective component is indicated where the risk of infection is high or where there is an expectation that potentially dangerous numbers of bacteria will be present in the eye (see CLINICAL PHARMACOLOGY: Microbiology).

The particular anti-infective drugs in this product are active against the following common bacterial eye pathogens: *Staphylococcus aureus, Escherichia coli, Haemophilus influenzae, Klebsiella/Enterobacter* species, *Neisseria* species, and *Pseudomonas aeruginosa.*

The product does not provide adequate coverage against *Serratia marcescens* and streptococci, including *Streptococcus pneumoniae.*

Contraindications: CORTISPORIN Ophthalmic Suspension is contraindicated in most viral diseases of the cornea and conjunctiva including: epithelial herpes simplex keratitis (dendritic keratitis), vaccinia, varicella, and also in mycobacterial infection of the eye and fungal diseases of ocular structures. CORTISPORIN Ophthalmic Suspension is also contraindicated in individuals who have shown hypersensitivity to any of its components. Hypersensitivity to the antibiotic component occurs at a higher rate than for other components.

Continued on next page

Burroughs Wellcome—Cont.

Warnings: NOT FOR INJECTION INTO THE EYE. CORTISPORIN Ophthalmic Suspension should never be directly introduced into the anterior chamber of the eye. Prolonged use of corticosteriods may result in ocular hypertension and/or glaucoma, with damage to the optic nerve, defects in visual acuity and fields of vision, and in posterior subcapsular cataract formation.
Prolonged use may suppress the host response and thus increase the hazard of secondary ocular infections. In those diseases causing thinning of the cornea or sclera, perforations have been known to occur with the use of topical corticosteroids. In acute purulent conditions of the eye, corticosteroids may mask infection or enhance existing infection.
If these products are used for 10 days or longer, intraocular pressure should be routinely monitored even though it may be difficult in uncooperative patients. Corticosteroids should be used with caution in the presence of glaucoma.
The use of corticosteroids after cataract surgery may delay healing and increase the incidence of filtering blebs.
Use of ocular corticosteroids may prolong the course and may exacerbate the severity of many viral infections of the eye (including herpes simplex). Employment of corticosteroid medication in the treatment of herpes simplex requires great caution.
Topical antibiotics, particularly neomycin sulfate, may cause cutaneous sensitization. A precise incidence of hypersensitivity reactions (primarily skin rash) due to topical antibiotics is not known. The manifestations of sensitization to topical antibiotics are usually itching, reddening, and edema of the conjunctiva and eyelid. A sensitization reaction may manifest simply as a failure to heal. During long-term use of topical antibiotic products, periodic examination for such signs is advisable, and the patient should be told to discontinue the product if they are observed. Symptoms usually subside quickly on withdrawing the medication. Application of products containing these ingredients should be avoided for the patient thereafter (see PRECAUTONS: General).

Precautions:

General: The initial prescription and renewal of the medication order beyond 20 milliliters should be made by a physician only after examination of the patient with the aid of magnification, such as slit lamp biomicroscopy and, where appropriate, fluorescein staining. If signs and symptoms fail to improve after two days, the patient should be re-evaluated.
The possibility of fungal infections of the cornea should be considered after prolonged corticosteroid dosing. Fungal cultures should be taken when appropriate.
If this product is used for 10 days or longer, intraocular pressure should be monitored (see WARNINGS).
There have been reports of bacterial keratitis associated with the use of topical ophthalmic products in multiple-dose containers which have been inadvertently contaminated by patients, most of whom had a concurrent corneal disease or a disruption of the ocular epithelial surface (see PRECAUTIONS: Information for Patients).
Allergic cross-reactions may occur which could prevent the use of any or all of the following antibiotics for the treatment of future infections: kanamycin, paromomycin, streptomycin, and possibly gentamicin.

Information for Patients: Patients should be instructed to avoid allowing the tip of the dispensing container to contact the eye, eyelid, fingers, or any other surface. The use of this product by more than one person may spread infection.
Patients should also be instructed that ocular products, if handled improperly, can become contaminated by common bacteria known to cause ocular infections. Serious damage to the eye and subsequent loss of vision may result from using contaminated products (see PRECAUTIONS: General).
If the condition persists or gets worse, or if a rash or allergic reaction develops, the patient should be advised to stop use and consult a physician. Do not use this product if you are allergic to any of the listed ingredients.
Keep tightly closed when not in use. Keep out of reach of children.

Carcinogenesis, Mutagenesis, Impairment of Fertility: Long-term studies in animals to evaluate carcinogenic or mutagenic potential have not been conducted with polymyxin B sulfate. Treatment of cultured human lymphocytes in vitro with neomycin increased the frequency of chromosome aberrations at the highest concentrations (80 μg/mL) tested; however, the effects of neomycin on carcinogenesis and mutagenesis in humans are unknown.
Long-term studies in animals (rats, rabbits, mice) showed no evidence of carcinogenicity or mutagenicity attributable to oral administration of corticosteroids. Long-term animal studies have not been performed to evaluate the carcinogenic potential of topical corticosteroids. Studies to determine mutagenicity with hydrocortisone have revealed negative results.
Polymyxin B has been reported to impair the motility of equine sperm, but its effects on male or female fertility are unknown. Long-term animal studies have not been performed to evaluate the effect on fertility of topical corticosteroids.

Pregnancy: ***Teratogenic Effects:*** Pregnancy Category C. Corticosteroids have been found to be teratogenic in rabbits when applied topically at concentrations of 0.5% on days 6 to 18 of gestation and in mice when applied topically at a concentration of 15% on days 10 to 13 of gestation. There are no adequate and well-controlled studies in pregnant women. CORTISPORIN Ophthalmic Suspension should be used during pregnancy only if the potential benefit justifies the potential risk to the fetus.

Nursing Mothers: It is not known whether topical administration of corticosteroids could result in sufficient systemic absorption to produce detectable quantities in human milk. Systemically administered corticosteroids appear in human milk and could suppress growth, interfere with endogenous corticosteroid production, or cause other untoward effects. Because of the potential for serious adverse reactions in nursing infants from CORTISPORIN Ophthalmic Suspension, a decision should be made whether to discontinue nursing or to discontinue the drug, taking into account the importance of the drug to the mother.

Pediatric Use: Safety and effectiveness in children have not been established.

Adverse Reactions: Adverse reactions have occurred with corticosteroid/anti-infective combination drugs which can be attributed to the corticosteroid component, the anti-infective component, or the combination. The exact incidence is not known.
Reactions occurring most often from the presence of the anti-infective ingredient are allergic sensitization reactions, including itching, swelling, and conjunctival erythema (see WARNINGS). More serious hypersensitivity reactions, including anaphylaxis, have been reported rarely.
The reactions due to the corticosteroid component in decreasing order of frequency are: elevation of intraocular pressure (IOP) with possible development of glaucoma, and infrequent optic nerve damage; posterior subcapsular cataract formation; and delayed wound healing.

Secondary Infection: The development of secondary infection has occurred after use of combinations containing corticosteroids and antimicrobials. Fungal and viral infections of the cornea are particularly prone to develop coincidentally with long-term applications of a corticosteroid. The possibility of fungal invasion must be considered in any persistent corneal ulceration where corticosteroid treatment has been used.
Local irritation on instillation has also been reported.

Dosage and Administration: One or two drops in the affected eye every 3 or 4 hours, depending on the severity of the condition. The suspension may be used more frequently if necessary.
Not more than 20 milliliters should be prescribed initially and the prescription should not be refilled without further evaluation as outlined in PRECAUTIONS above.

SHAKE WELL BEFORE USING.

How Supplied: Plastic DROP DOSE® dispenser bottle of 7.5 mL (NDC-0081-0193-02).

Caution: Federal law prohibits dispensing without a prescription.
Store at 15° to 25°C (59° to 77°F).

Shown in Product Identification Guide, page 103

NEOSPORIN® ℞

[*nē"ō-spor'ĭn*]

Ophthalmic Ointment Sterile
(neomycin and polymyxin B sulfates and bacitracin zinc ophthalmic ointment, USP)

Description: NEOSPORIN Ophthalmic Ointment (neomycin and polymyxin B sulfates and bacitracin zinc ophthalmic ointment) is a sterile antimicrobial ointment for ophthalmic use. Each gram contains: neomycin sulfate equivalent to 3.5 mg neomycin base, polymyxin B sulfate equivalent to 10,000 polymyxin B units, bacitracin zinc equivalent to 400 bacitracin units, and special white petrolatum, q.s.
Neomycin sulfate is the sulfate salt of neomycin B and C, which are produced by the growth of *Streptomyces fradiae* Waksman (Fam. Streptomycetaceae). It has a potency equivalent of not less than 600 μg of neomycin standard per mg, calculated on an anhydrous basis.
Polymyxin B sulfate is the sulfate salt of polymyxin B_1 and B_2 which are produced by the growth of *Bacillus polymyxa* (Prazmowski) Migula (Fam. Bacillaceae). It has a potency of not less than 6,000 polymyxin B units per mg, calculated on an anhydrous basis.
Bacitracin zinc is the zinc salt of bacitracin, a mixture of related cyclic polypeptides (mainly bacitracin A) produced by the growth of an organism of the *licheniformis* group of *Bacillus subtilis* var Tracy. It has a potency of not less than 40 bacitracin units per mg.

Clinical Pharmacology: A wide range of antibacterial action is provided by the overlapping spectra of neomycin, polymyxin B sulfate, and bacitracin.
Neomycin is bactericidal for many gram-positive and gram-negative organisms. It is an aminoglycoside antibiotic which inhibits protein synthesis by binding with ribosomal RNA and causing misreading of the bacterial genetic code.
Polymyxin B is bactericidal for a variety of gram-negative organisms. It increases the permeability of the bacterial cell membrane by interacting with the phospholipid components of the membrane.
Bacitracin is bactericidal for a variety of gram-positive and gram-negative organisms. It interferes with bacterial cell wall synthesis by inhibition of the regeneration of phospholipid receptors involved in peptidoglycan synthesis.

Microbiology: Neomycin sulfate, polymyxin B sulfate, and bacitracin zinc together are considered active against the following microorganisms: *Staphylococcus aureus*, streptococci including *Streptococcus pneumoniae*, *Escherichia coli*, *Haemophilus influenzae*, *Klebsiella/Enterobacter* species, *Neisseria* species and *Pseudomonas aeruginosa*. The product does not provide adequate coverage against *Serratia marcescens*.

Indications and Usage: NEOSPORIN Ophthalmic Ointment is indicated for the short-term topical treatment of superficial infections of the external eye and its adnexa caused by susceptible bacteria. Such infections encompass conjunctivitis, keratitis and keratoconjunctivitis, blepharitis and blepharoconjunctivitis.

Contraindications: NEOSPORIN Ophthalmic Ointment is contraindicated in individuals who have shown hypersensitivity to any of its components.

WARNINGS: NOT FOR INJECTION INTO THE EYE. NEOSPORIN Ophthalmic Ointment should never be directly introduced into the anterior chamber of the eye. Ophthalmic ointments may retard corneal wound healing.

Topical antibiotics, particularly neomycin sulfate, may cause cutaneous sensitization. A precise incidence of hypersensitivity reactions (primarily skin rash) due to topical antibiotics is not known. The manifestations of sensitization to topical antibiotics are usually itching, reddening, and edema of the conjunctiva and eyelid. A sensitization reaction may manifest simply as a failure to heal. During long-term use of topical antibiotic products, periodic examination for such signs is advisable, and the patient should be told to discontinue the product if they are observed. Symptoms usually subside quickly on withdrawing the medication. Application of products containing these ingredients should be avoided for the patient thereafter (see PRECAUTIONS: General).

Precautions:

General: As with other antibiotic preparations, prolonged use of NEOSPORIN Ophthalmic Ointment may result in overgrowth of nonsusceptible organisms including fungi. If superinfection occurs, appropriate measures should be initiated.

Bacterial resistance to NEOSPORIN Ophthalmic Ointment may also develop. If purulent discharge, inflammation, or pain becomes aggravated, the patient should discontinue use of the medication and consult a physician.

There have been reports of bacterial keratitis associated with the use of topical ophthalmic products in multiple-dose containers which have been inadvertently contaminated by patients, most of whom had a concurrent corneal disease or a disruption of the ocular epithelial surface (see PRECAUTIONS: Information for Patients).

Allergic cross-reactions may occur which could prevent the use of any or all of the following antibiotics for the treatment of future infections: kanamycin, paromomycin, streptomycin, and possibly gentamicin.

Information for Patients: Patients should be instructed to avoid allowing the tip of the dispensing container to contact the eye, eyelid, fingers, or any other surface. The use of this product by more than one person may spread infection.

Patients should also be instructed that ocular products, if handled improperly, can become contaminated by common bacteria known to cause ocular infections. Serious damage to the eye and subsequent loss of vision may result from using contaminated products (see PRECAUTIONS: General).

If the condition persists or gets worse, or if a rash or allergic reaction develops, the patient should be advised to stop use and consult a physician. Do not use this product if you are allergic to any of the listed ingredients.

Keep tightly closed when not in use. Keep out of reach of children.

Carcinogenesis, Mutagenesis, Impairment of Fertility: Long-term studies in animals to evaluate carcinogenic or mutagenic potential have not been conducted with polymyxin B sulfate or bacitracin. Treatment of cultured human lymphocytes in vitro with neomycin increased the frequency of chromosome aberrations at the highest concentration (80 μg/mL) tested; however, the effects of neomycin on carcinogenesis and mutagenesis in humans are unknown.

Polymyxin B has been reported to impair the motility of equine sperm, but its effects on male or female fertility are unknown. No adverse effects on male or female fertility, litter size or survival were observed in rabbits given bacitracin zinc 100 gm/ton of diet.

Pregnancy; ***Teratogenic Effects:*** Pregnancy Category C. Animal reproduction studies have not been conducted with neomycin sulfate, polymyxin B sulfate, or bacitracin. It is also not known whether NEOSPORIN Ophthalmic Ointment can cause fetal harm when administered to a pregnant woman or can affect reproduction capacity. NEOSPORIN Ophthalmic Ointment should be given to a pregnant woman only if clearly needed.

Nursing Mothers: It is not known whether this drug is excreted in human milk. Because many drugs are excreted in human milk, caution should be exercised when NEOSPORIN Ophthalmic Ointment is administered to a nursing woman.

Pediatric Use: Safety and effectiveness in children have not been established.

Adverse Reactions: Adverse reactions have occurred with the anti-infective components of NEOSPORIN Ophthalmic Ointment. The exact incidence is not known. Reactions occurring most often are allergic sensitization reactions including itching, swelling, and conjunctival erythema (see WARNINGS). More serious hypersensitivity reactions, including anaphylaxis, have been reported rarely.

Local irritation on instillation has also been reported.

Dosage and Administration: Apply the ointment every 3 or 4 hours for 7 to 10 days, depending on the severity of the infection.

How Supplied: Tube of ⅛ oz (3.5 g) with ophthalmic tip (NDC-0081-0732-86).

Caution: Federal law prohibits dispensing without a prescription.

Store at 15° to 25°C (59° to 77°F).

Shown in Product Identification Guide, page 103

NEOSPORIN® ℞

[nē″ō-spor′ĭn]

OPHTHALMIC SOLUTION Sterile (Polymyxin B Sulfate-Neomycin Sulfate-Gramicidin)

Description: Neosporin Ophthalmic Solution (polymyxin B sulfate-neomycin sulfate-gramicidin) is a sterile antimicrobial solution for ophthalmic use. Each ml contains: Aerosporin® (polymyxin B sulfate) 10,000 units, neomycin sulfate equivalent to 1.75 mg neomycin base and gramicidin 0.025 mg. The vehicle contains alcohol 0.5%, thimerosal 0.001% (added as a preservative) and the inactive ingredients propylene glycol, polyoxyethylene polyoxypropylene compound, sodium chloride and water for injection.

Polymyxin B sulfate is the sulfate salt of polymyxin B_1 and B_2 which are produced by the growth of *Bacillus polymyxa* (Prazmowski) Migula (Fam. Bacillaceae). It has a potency of not less than 6,000 polymyxin B units per mg, calculated on an anhydrous basis.

Neomycin sulfate is the sulfate salt of neomycin B and C, which are produced by the growth of *Streptomyces fradiae* Waksman (Fam. Streptomycetaceae). It has a potency equivalent of not less than 600 μg of neomycin standard per mg, calculated on an anhydrous basis.

Gramicidin (also called Gramicidin D) is a mixture of three pairs of antibacterial substances (Gramicidin A, B and C) produced by the growth of *Bacillus brevis* Dubos (Fam. Bacillaceae). It has a potency of not less than 900 μg of standard gramicidin per mg.

Clinical Pharmacology: A wide range of antibacterial action is provided by the overlapping spectra of polymyxin B sulfate, neomycin and gramicidin. The spectrum of action encompasses most bacterial pathogens capable of causing external infections of the eye and its adnexa.

Polymyxin B is bactericidal for a variety of gram-negative organisms. It increases the permeability of the bacterial cell membrane by interacting with the phospholipid components of the membrane.

Neomycin is bactericidal for many gram-positive and gram-negative organisms. It is an aminoglycoside antibiotic which inhibits protein synthesis by binding with ribosomal RNA and causing misreading of the bacterial genetic code.

Gramicidin is bactericidal for a variety of gram-positive organisms. It increases the permeability of the bacterial cell membrane to inorganic cations by forming a network of channels through the normal lipid bilayer of the membrane.

When used topically, polymyxin B, neomycin and gramicidin are rarely irritating, and absorption from the intact skin or mucous membrane is insignificant. The incidence of skin sensitization to this combination has been shown to be low on normal skin.[1,2] Since these antibiotics are seldom used systemically, the patient is spared sensitization to those antibiotics which might later be required systemically.

Microbiology: Polymyxin B sulfate, neomycin sulfate and gramicidin together are considered active against the following microorganisms: *Staphylococcus aureus*, streptococci, including *Streptococcus pneumoniae*, *Escherichia coli*, *Haemophilus influenzae*, *Klebsiella-Enterobacter* species, *Neisseria* species and *Pseudomonas aeruginosa*. The product does not provide adequate coverage against *Serratia marcescens*.

Indications and Usage: Neosporin Ophthalmic Solution is indicated in the short-term treatment of superficial external ocular infections caused by organisms susceptible to one or more of the antibiotics contained therein.

Contraindications: This product is contraindicated in those individuals who have shown hypersensitivity to any of its components.

Warnings: The manifestations of sensitization to neomycin are usually itching, reddening and edema of the conjunctiva and eyelid. It may be manifest simply as a failure to heal. During long-term use of neomycin-containing products, periodic examination for such signs is advisable, and the patient should be told to discontinue the product if they are observed. These symptoms subside quickly on withdrawing the medication. Neomycin-containing applications should be avoided for the patient thereafter.

Precautions:

General: As with other antibiotic preparations, prolonged use may result in overgrowth of nonsusceptible organisms including fungi. Appropriate measures should be taken if this occurs.

Allergic cross-reactions may occur which could prevent the use of any or all of the following antibiotics for the treatment of future infections: kanamycin, paromomycin, streptomycin, and possibly gentamicin.

Continued on next page

Burroughs Wellcome—Cont.

Information for Patients: If redness, irritation, swelling or pain persists or increases, discontinue use and contact your physician.

Avoid contaminating the applicator tip with material from the eye, fingers, or other source. This caution is necessary if the sterility of the drops is to be preserved.

Adverse Reactions: Neomycin Sulfate may cause cutaneous and conjunctival sensitization. A precise incidence of hypersensitivity reactions (primarily skin rash) due to topical neomycin is not known.

Dosage and Administration: The suggested dosage is one or two drops in the affected eye two to four times daily, or more frequently as required, for 7 to 10 days. In acute infections, initiate therapy with one or two drops every 15 to 30 minutes, reducing the frequency of instillation gradually as the infection is controlled.

How Supplied: Drop Dose® of 10 ml (plastic dispenser bottle) (NDC-0081-0728-69).

Store at 15°–25°C (59°–77°F) and protect from light.

References:

1. Leyden JJ, and Kligman AM. Contact Dermatitis to Neomycin Sulfate. *JAMA* 242(12):1276–1278, 1979.
2. Prystowsky SD, Allen AM, Smith RW, Nonomura JH, Odom RB and Akers WA. Allergic Contact Hypersensitivity to Nickel, Neomycin, Ethylenediamine, and Benzocaine. *Arch Dermatol* 115:959–962, 1979.

561834

Shown in Product Identification Guide, page 103

POLYSPORIN® ℞

[*pah "l ē-spor 'ĭn*]

OPHTHALMIC OINTMENT Sterile
(Polymyxin B-Bacitracin)

Description: Each gram contains Aerosporin® (Polymyxin B Sulfate) 10,000 units, bacitracin zinc 500 units, special white petrolatum qs.

Actions: Polymyxin B attacks gram-negative bacilli, including virtually all strains of *Pseudomonas aeruginosa* and *H influenzae* species. Bacitracin is active against most gram-positive bacilli and cocci, including hemolytic streptococci.

Indications: For the treatment of superficial ocular infections involving the conjunctiva and/or cornea caused by organisms susceptible to polymyxin B sulfate and bacitracin zinc.

Contraindications: This product is contraindicated in those individuals who have shown hypersensitivity to any of its components.

Warnings: Ophthalmic ointments may retard corneal healing.

Precautions: As with other antibiotic preparations, prolonged use may result in overgrowth of nonsusceptible organisms, including fungi. Appropriate measures should be taken if this occurs.

Dosage and Administration: Apply the ointment every 3 or 4 hours, depending on the severity of the infection.

How Supplied: Tube of ⅛ oz with ophthalmic tip (NDC 0081-0797-86). 575940

Shown in Product Identification Guide, page 104

VIROPTIC® ℞

[*vī-rŏp 'tĭk "*]

OPHTHALMIC SOLUTION, 1% Sterile
(Trifluridine)

Description: Viroptic is the brand name for trifluridine (also known as trifluorothymidine, F_3TdR, F_3T), an antiviral drug for topical treatment of epithelial keratitis caused by Herpes simplex virus. The chemical name of trifluridine is 2′-deoxy-5-(trifluoromethyl)uridine.

Viroptic sterile ophthalmic solution contains 1% trifluridine in an aqueous solution with acetic acid and sodium acetate (buffers), sodium chloride, and thimerosal 0.001% (added as a preservative).

Clinical Pharmacology: Trifluridine is a fluorinated pyrimidine nucleoside with *in vitro* and *in vivo* activity against Herpes simplex virus, types 1 and 2 and vacciniavirus. Some strains of Adenovirus are also inhibited *in vitro*.

Trifluridine interferes with DNA synthesis in cultured mammalian cells. However, its antiviral mechanism of action is not completely known.

In vitro perfusion studies on excised rabbit corneas have shown that trifluridine penetrates the intact cornea as evidenced by recovery of parental drug and its major metabolite, 5-carboxy-2′-deoxyuridine, on the endothelial side of the cornea. Absence of the corneal epithelium enhances the penetration of trifluridine approximately two-fold.

Intraocular penetration of trifluridine occurs after topical instillation of Viroptic into human eyes. Decreased corneal integrity or stromal or uveal inflammation may enhance the penetration of trifluridine into the aqueous humor. Unlike the results of ocular penetration of trifluridine *in vitro*, 5-carboxy-2′-deoxyuridine was not found in detectable concentrations within the aqueous humor of the human eye.

Systemic absorption of trifluridine following therapeutic dosing with Viroptic appears to be negligible. No detectable concentrations of trifluridine or 5-carboxy-2′-deoxyuridine were found in the sera of adult healthy normal subjects who had Viroptic instilled into their eyes seven times daily for 14 consecutive days.

Indications and Usage: Viroptic (Trifluridine) Ophthalmic Solution, 1% is indicated for the treatment of primary keratoconjunctivitis and recurrent epithelial keratitis due to Herpes simplex virus, types 1 and 2. Viroptic is also effective in the treatment of epithelial keratitis that has not responded clinically to the topical administration of idoxuridine or when ocular toxicity or hypersensitivity to idoxuridine has occurred. In a smaller number of patients found to be resistant to topical vidarabine, Viroptic was also effective.

The clinical efficacy of Viroptic in the treatment of stromal keratitis and uveitis due to Herpes simplex virus or ophthalmic infections caused by vacciniavirus and Adenovirus has not been established by well-controlled clinical trials. Viroptic has not been shown to be effective in the prophylaxis of Herpes simplex virus keratoconjunctivitis and epithelial keratitis by well-controlled clinical trials. Viroptic is not effective against bacterial, fungal or chlamydial infections of the cornea or nonviral trophic lesions.

During controlled multicenter clinical trials, 92 of 97 (95%) patients (78 of 81 with dendritic and 14 of 16 with geographic ulcers) responded to Viroptic therapy as evidenced by complete corneal re-epithelialization within the 14-day therapy period. In these controlled studies, 56 of 75 (75%) patients (49 of 58 with dendritic and 7 of 17 with geographic ulcers) responded to idoxuridine therapy. The mean time to corneal re-epithelialization for dendritic ulcers (6 days) and geographic ulcers (7 days) was similar for both therapies. In other clinical studies, Viroptic was evaluated in the treatment of Herpes simplex virus keratitis in patients who were unresponsive or intolerant to the topical administration of idoxuridine or vidarabine. Viroptic was effective in 138 of 150 (92%) patients (109 of 114 with dendritic and 29 of 36 with geographic ulcers) as evidenced by corneal re-epithelialization. The mean time to corneal re-epithelialization was 6 days for patients with dendritic ulcers and 12 days for patients with geographic ulcers.

Contraindications: Viroptic (Trifluridine) Ophthalmic Solution, 1%, is contraindicated for patients who develop hypersensitivity reactions or chemical intolerance to trifluridine.

Warnings: The recommended dosage and frequency of administration should not be exceeded (see DOSAGE AND ADMINISTRATION).

Precautions:

General: Viroptic (Trifluridine) Ophthalmic Solution, 1% should be prescribed only for patients who have a clinical diagnosis of herpetic keratitis.

Viroptic may cause mild local irritation of the conjunctiva and cornea when instilled but these effects are usually transient.

Although documented *in vitro* viral resistance to trifluridine has not been reported following multiple exposure to Viroptic, the possibility exists of viral resistance development.

Drug Interactions: The following drugs have been administered topically to the eye and concurrently with Viroptic in a limited number of patients without apparent evidence of adverse interaction: antibiotics—chloramphenicol, erythromycin, polymyxin B sulfate, bacitracin, gentamicin sulfate, tetracycline HCl, sodium sulfacetamide, neomycin sulfate; steroids—dexamethasone, dexamethasone sodium phosphate, prednisolone acetate, prednisolone sodium phosphate, hydrocortisone, fluorometholone; and other ophthalmic drugs—atropine sulfate, scopolamine hydrobromide, naphazoline hydrochloride, cyclopentolate hydrochloride, homatropine hydrobromide, pilocarpine, l-epinephrine hydrochloride, sodium chloride.

Carcinogenesis, Mutagenesis, Impairment of Fertility: ***Mutagenic Potential:*** Trifluridine has been shown to exert mutagenic, DNA-damaging and cell-transforming activities in various standard *in vitro* test systems, and clastogenic activity in *Vicia faba* cells. It did not induce chromosome aberrations in bone marrow cells of male or female rats following a single subcutaneous dose of 100 mg/kg, but was weakly positive in female, but not in male, rats following daily subcutaneous administration at 700 mg/kg/day for 5 days.

Although the significance of these test results is not clear or fully understood, there exists the possibility that mutagenic agents may cause genetic damage in humans.

Oncogenic Potential. Lifetime carcinogenicity bioassays in rats and mice given daily subcutaneous doses of trifluridine have been performed. Rats tested at 1.5, 7.5 and 15 mg/kg/day had increased incidences of adenocarcinomas of the intestinal tract and mammary glands, hemangiosarcomas of the spleen and liver, carcinosarcomas of the prostate gland and granulosa-thecal cell tumors of the ovary. Mice were tested at 1, 5 and 10 mg/kg/day; those given 10 mg/kg/day trifluridine had significantly increased incidences of adenocarcinomas of the intestinal tract and uterus. Those given 10 mg/kg/day also had a significantly increased incidence of testicular atrophy as compared to vehicle control mice.

Pregnancy: ***Teratogenic Effects:*** Pregnancy Category C. Trifluridine was not teratogenic at doses up to 5.0 mg/kg/day (23 times the estimated human exposure) when given subcutaneously to rats and rabbits. However, fetal toxicity consisting of delayed ossification of portions of the skeleton occurred at dose levels of 2.5 and 5.0 mg/kg/day in rats and at 2.5 mg/kg/day in rabbits. In addition, both 2.5 and 5.0 mg/kg/day produced fetal death and resorption in rabbits. In both rats and rabbits, 1.0 mg/kg/day (5 times the estimated human exposure) was a no-effect level. There were no teratogenic or fetotoxic effects after topical application of Viroptic Ophthalmic Solution 1% (approximately 5 times the estimated human exposure) to the eyes of rabbits on the 6th through the 18th days of pregnancy.[1] In a nonstandard test, trifluridine solution has been shown to be teratogenic when injected directly into the yolk sac of chicken eggs.[2] There are no adequate and well-controlled studies in pregnant women. Viroptic Ophthalmic Solution 1% should be used during pregnancy only if the potential benefit justifies the potential risk to the fetus.

Nursing Mothers: It is unlikely that trifluridine is excreted in human milk after ophthalmic instillation of Viroptic because of the relatively small dosage (≤ 5.0 mg/day), its dilution in body fluids and its extremely short half-life (approximately 12 minutes). The drug should not be prescribed for nursing mothers unless the potential benefits outweigh the potential risks.

Adverse Reactions: The most frequent adverse reactions reported during controlled clinical trials were mild, transient burning or stinging upon instillation (4.6%) and palpebral edema (2.8%). Other adverse reactions in decreasing order of reported frequency were superficial punctate keratopathy, epithelial keratopathy, hypersensitivity reaction, stromal edema, irritation, keratitis sicca, hyperemia, and increased intraocular pressure.

Overdosage: Overdosage by ocular instillation is unlikely because any excess solution should be quickly expelled from the conjunctival sac.

Acute overdosage by accidental oral ingestion of Viroptic has not occurred. However, should such ingestion occur, the 75 mg dosage of trifluridine in a 7.5 mL bottle of Viroptic is not likely to produce adverse effects. Single intravenous doses of 15–30 mg/kg/day in children and adults with neoplastic disease produce reversible bone marrow depression as the only potentially serious toxic effect and only after 3–5 courses of therapy.[3] The acute oral LD_{50} in the mouse and rat was 4379 mg/kg or higher.

Dosage and Administration: Instill one drop of Viroptic Ophthalmic Solution, 1% onto the cornea of the affected eye every two hours while awake for a maximum daily dosage of nine drops until the corneal ulcer has completely re-epithelialized. Following re-epithelialization, treatment for an additional seven days of one drop every four hours while awake for a minimum daily dosage of five drops is recommended.

If there are no signs of improvement after seven days of therapy or complete re-epithelialization has not occurred after 14 days of therapy, other forms of therapy should be considered. Continuous administration of Viroptic for periods exceeding 21 days should be avoided because of potential ocular toxicity.

How Supplied: Viroptic Ophthalmic Solution, 1% is supplied as a sterile ophthalmic solution in a plastic Drop Dose® dispenser bottle of 7.5 mL. (NDC 0081-0968-02)

Store under refrigeration 2° to 8°C (36° to 46°F).

Animal Pharmacology and Animal Toxicology: Corneal wound healing studies in rabbits showed that Viroptic did not significantly retard closure of epithelial wounds. However, mild toxic changes such as intracellular edema of the basal cell layer, mild thinning of the overlying epithelium and reduced strength of stromal wounds were observed.

Whereas instillation of Viroptic into rabbit eyes during a subchronic toxicity study produced some degree of corneal epithelial thinning, a 12-month chronic toxicity study in rabbits in which Viroptic was instilled into eyes in intermittent, multiple, full-therapy courses showed no drug-related changes in the cornea.

References:

1. Itoi M, Getter JW, Kaneko N, et al: Teratogenicities of ophthalmic drugs. I. Antiviral ophthalmic drugs. *Arch Ophthalmol* 1975;93:46–51.
2. Kury G, Crosby RJ: The teratogenic effect of 5-trifluoromethyl-2′-deoxyuridine in chicken embryos. *Toxicol Appl Pharmacol* 1967;11:72–80.
3. Ansfield FJ, Ramirez G: Phase I and II studies of 2′-deoxy-5-(trifluoromethyl)-uridine (NSC-75520). *Cancer Chemother Rep* 1971;55(pt 1):205–208.

643060

Shown in Product Identification Guide, page 104

CIBA Vision Ophthalmics

11460 JOHN'S CREEK PARKWAY
DULUTH, GA 30136

AQUASITE™ OTC

Lubricant Eye Drops
Preservative-Free Single-Use Containers
Multidose Bottle

Unlike other artificial tear drops, AquaSite is specially formulated with the patented DuraSite™ technology. AquaSite provides long lasting relief of eye discomfort due to minor irritations such as wind, sun, glare, dryness and computer screen exposure. Once instilled, AquaSite also acts as a protectant against further eye discomfort.

Instillation in the lower cul de sac ensures that AquaSite provides gradual, long-lasting relief.

Contains: Polyethylene glycol 400, 0.2%; Dextran 70, 0.1%; with DuraSite (polycarbophil, purified water, sodium chloride, edetate disodium, and sodium hydroxide to adjust the pH). AquaSite in the multidose bottle is the same formulation with sorbic acid 0.2% added as a preservative.

Indications: For the temporary relief of discomfort due to minor irritations of the eye from exposure to wind, sun or other irritants. For use as a protectant against further irritation or to relieve dryness of the eye.

Directions: Instill 1 or 2 drops in the lower cul de sac of the affected eye(s) as needed.

Warnings: If you experience eye pain, change in vision, continued redness or irritation of the eye, or if the condition worsens or persists for more than 72 hours, discontinue use and consult a doctor. To avoid contamination, do not touch tip of container to any surface. Do not use these products if you are allergic to any of their ingredients.

Keep this and all drugs out of the reach of children.

Preservative-Free: Do not reuse, Once opened, discard. If solution changes color or becomes cloudy, do not use.

Multidose Bottle: Replace cap after using.

How Supplied: AquaSite Lubricant Eye Drops Preservative-Free is supplied in sterile, disposable, single-use containers—NDC 58768-101-24. Use only if single-use container is intact.

AquaSite Lubricant Eye Drops Multidose Bottle is supplied in a dropper-tipped plastic squeeze bottle containing 15mL—NDC 58768-101-15. Do not use if safety seal around cap is broken or missing.

Storage: Store at controlled room temperature, 15°–30°C (59°–86°F).

Manufactured by Ciba Vision Sterile Manufacturing, Mississauga, Canada for Ciba Vision Ophthalmics®, Atlanta, Georgia 30136. AquaSite and DuraSite are trademarks of INSITE Vision™ Incorporated. U.S. Pat. Nos. 4,615,697; 4,983,392; 5,188,826; 5,225,196

EYE•SCRUB™ OTC

An extra gentle, hypoallergenic sterile eyelid cleanser

Cleanser Ingredients: Water for Injection USP, PEG-200 Glyceryl Tallowate, Disodium Laureth Sulfosuccinate, Cocamidopropylamine Oxide, PEG-78 Glyceryl Cocoate, Benzyl Alcohol and Disodium EDTA.

Ready to use, needs no diluting. For External Use Only. Do Not Use Directly In The Eye.

The Development of EYE•SCRUB™: Developed by a leading ophthalmologist and a pharmacist, EYE•SCRUB™ Sterile Eyelid Cleanser and EYE•SCRUB™ Cleansing Pads provide an easy to use system for daily eyelid hygiene. EYE•SCRUB™ Cleanser is a patented, extremely mild, nonirritating, hypoallergenic solution that is pH balanced for maximum comfort.

EYE•SCRUB™ Cleansing Pads are made from special, virtually lint-free non-shedding, soft fibers that do not leave foreign material around the eyes. Once the Pads are wetted with EYE•SCRUB™ Cleanser, a rich, microbubble lather is produced that is remarkably safe for daily eye-lid hygiene.

Preferred Cleansing Regimen

Directions for Use:

1. **The warm compress.** Apply a warm compress such as a washcloth soaked in very warm water to closed eyes for several minutes before cleansing. This is essential to loosen oily debris and scales and to soothe the area around the eye.
2. **The lather.** Wet, but do not saturate an EYE•SCRUB™ Cleansing Pad with EYE•SCRUB™ Cleanser, fold the pad over and rub between thumb and forefinger to work up a lather. (Premoistened Pads: Develop lather before opening by rubbing pouch. Open pouch and rub pad to develop more lather.) EYE•SCRUB™'s special formula creates a unique microbubble lather which helps gently loosen debris.
3. **The cleansing.** In front of a well illuminated mirror, expose the lower eyelid edge by pulling the skin down with your finger. Rub the pad several times along the lid at the base where the lashes grow out. Be careful not to rub the surface of the eye. Next, using your finger, pull the upper lid up towards the brow and away from the eye surface. Repeat the process on the upper lid edge at the base of the lashes, again being careful not to rub the eye surface. Close the eye and rub the pad vigorously across the eyelashes several times. Open the eye, discard the pad and leave the lather on the area you cleaned. Repeat the process on the other eye using a clean EYE•SCRUB™ Cleansing Pad.
4. **The rinse.** Thoroughly rinse both eyes with clean, warm water and pat dry.

How Supplied: EYE•SCRUB™ Sterile Eyelid Cleanser is available in a complete kit including a 4 oz bottle of solution and 60 cleansing pads. EYE•SCRUB™ is also available in a box of 30 individually packaged premoistened pads.

Alternative Cleansing Regimen

Directions for Use: A cotton tipped applicator may be used in place of EYE•SCRUB™ Cleansing Pads according to your eyecare professional's instructions or your personal preference. When using the cotton tipped applicator, place a few drops of EYE•SCRUB™ Sterile Eyelid Cleanser on the padding and keep massaging it with your fingers until a lather forms. Then follow procedure for Preferred Cleanser Regimen.

If your local pharamcy does not have EYE•SCRUB™, call and we will help you find a local source.

Continued on next page

CIBA Vision—Cont.

Manufactured for:
Ciba Vision Ophthalmics®
Atlanta, GA 30136
1-800-845-6585
EYE•SCRUB™ is a trademark of CV Ophthalmics Inc. Patented Formula

---

MZM™ ℞
METHAZOLAMIDE

Description: Methazolamide, a sulfonamide derivative, is a white crystalline powder, weakly acidic, and slightly soluble in water, alcohol and acetone. It is available as 25 mg and 50 mg tablets. The chemical name for methazolamide is *N*-[5-(aminosulfonyl)-3-methyl-1,3,4-thia-diazol-2(3*H*)-ylidene]-acetamide and it has the following structural formula:

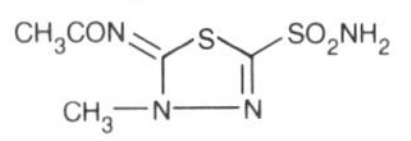

$C_5H_8N_4O_3S_2$ M.W. 238.26

Methazolamide tablets, USP contain 25 mg or 50 mg of methazolamide.

Inactive ingredients: croscarmellose, sodium, hydroxypropyl methylcellulose, lactose (hydrous), magnesium stearate, microcrystalline cellulose, and sodium lauryl sulfate.

Clinical Pharmacology: Methazolamide is a potent inhibitor of carbonic anhydrase.

Methazolamide is well absorbed from the gastrointestinal tract. Peak plasma concentrations are observed 1 to 2 hours after dosing. In a multiple-dose, pharmacokinetic study, administration of methazolamide 25 mg b.i.d., 50 mg b.i.d. and 100 mg b.i.d. demonstrated a linear relationship between plasma methazolamide levels and methazolamide dose. Peak plasma concentrations (C_{max}) for the 25 mg, 50 mg and 100 mg b.i.d. regimens were 2.5 mcg/mL, 5.1 mcg/mL and 10.7 mcg/mL, respectively. The area under the plasma concentration-time curves (AUC) were 1130 mcg-min/mL, 2571 mcg-min/mL and 5418 mcg-min/mL for the 25 mg, 50 mg and 100 mg dosage regimens, respectively.

Methazolamide is distributed throughout the body including the plasma, cerebrospinal fluid, aqueous humor of the eye, red blood cells, bile and extra-cellular fluid. The mean apparent volume of distribution (V_{area}/F) ranges from 17 to 23 L. Approximately 55% is bound to plasma proteins. The steady-state methazolamide red blood cell: plasma ratio varies with dose and was found to be 27:1, 16:1 and 10:1 following the administration of methazolamide 25 mg b.i.d., 50 mg b.i.d. and 100 mg b.i.d., respectively.

The mean steady-state plasma elimination half-life for methazolamide is approximately 14 hours. At steady-state approximately 25% of the dose is recovered unchanged in the urine over the dosing interval. Renal clearance accounts for 20 to 25% of the total clearance of drug. After repeated b.i.d.-t.i.d. dosing, methazolamide accumulates to steady-state concentrations in seven days.

Methazolamide's inhibitory action on carbonic anhydrase decreases the secretion of aqueous humor and results in a decrease in intraocular pressure. The onset of the decrease in intraocular pressure generally occurs within two to four hours, has a peak effect in six to eight hours, and a total duration of ten to eighteen hours.

Methazolamide is a sulfonamide derivative; however, it does not have any clinically significant antimicrobial properties. Although methazolamide achieves a high concentration in the cerebrospinal fluid, it is not considered an effective anticonvulsant.

Methazolamide has a weak and transient diuretic effect, therefore use results in an increase in urinary volume, with excretion of sodium, potassium and chloride. The drug should not be used as a diuretic. Inhibition of renal bicarbonate reabsorption produces an alkaline urine. Plasma bicarbonate decreases, and a relative, transient metabolic acidosis may occur due to a disequilibrium in carbon dioxide transport in the red cell. Urinary citrate excretion is decreased by approximately 40% after doses of 100 mg every 8 hours. Uric acid output has been shown to decrease 36% in the first 24 hour period.

Indications and Usage: Methazolamide is indicated in the treatment of ocular conditions where lowering intraocular pressure is likely to be of therapeutic benefit, such as chronic open-angle glaucoma, secondary glaucoma, and preoperatively in acute angle-closure glaucoma where lowering the intraocular pressure is desired before surgery.

Contraindications: Methazolamide therapy is contraindicated in situations in which sodium and/or potassium serum levels are depressed, in cases of marked kidney or liver disease or dysfunction, in adrenal gland failure, and in hyperchloremic acidosis. In patients with cirrhosis, use may precipitate the development of hepatic encephalopathy.

Long-term administration of methazolamide is contraindicated in patients with angle-closure glaucoma, since organic closure of the angle may occur in spite of lowered intraocular pressure.

Warnings: Fatalities have occurred, although rarely, due to severe reactions to sulfonamides including Stevens-Johnson syndrome, toxic epidermal necrolysis, fulminant hepatic necrosis, agranulocytosis, aplastic anemia, and other blood dyscrasias. Hypersensitivity reactions may recur when a sulfonamide is readministered, irrespective of the route of administration.

If hypersensitivity or other serious reactions occur, the use of this drug should be discontinued.

Caution is advised for patients receiving high-dose aspirin and methazolamide concomitantly, as anorexia, tachypnea, lethargy, coma and death have been reported with concommitant use of high-dose aspirin and carbonic anhydrase inhibitors.

Precautions:

General: Potassium excretion is increased initially upon administration of methazolamide and in patients with cirrhosis or hepatic insufficiency could precipitate a hepatic coma.

In patients with pulmonary obstruction or emphysema, where alveolar ventilation may be impaired methazolamide should be used with caution because it may precipitate or aggravate acidosis.

Information For Patients: Adverse reactions common to all sulfonamide derivatives may occur: anaphylaxis, fever, rash (including erythema multiforme, Stevens-Johnson syndrome, toxic epidermal necrolysis), crystalluria, renal calculus, bone marrow depression, thrombocytopenic purpura, hemolytic anemia, leukopenia, pancytopenia and agranulocytosis. Precaution is advised for early detection of such reactions and the drug should be discontinued and appropriate therapy instituted.

Caution is advised for patients receiving high-dose aspirin and methazolamide concomitantly.

Laboratory Tests: To monitor for hematologic reactions common to all sulfonamides, it is recommended that a baseline CBC and platelet count be obtained on patients prior to initiating methazolamide therapy and at regular intervals during therapy. If significant changes occur, early discontinuance and institution of appropriate therapy are important. Periodic monitoring of serum electrolytes is also recommended.

Drug Interactions: Methazolamide should be used with caution in patients on steroid therapy because of the potential for developing hypokalemia. Caution is advised for patients receiving high-dose aspirin and methazolamide concomitantly, as anorexia, tachypnea, lethargy, coma and death have been reported with concomitant use of high-dose aspirin and carbonic anhydrase inhibitors (see **WARNINGS**).

Carcinogenesis, Mutagenesis, Impairment of Fertility: Long-term studies in animals to evaluate methazolamide's carcinogenic potential and its effect on fertility have not been conducted. Methazolamide was not mutagenic in the Ames bacterial test.

Pregnancy: Teratogenic effects Pregnancy Category C. Methazolamide has been shown to be teratogenic (skeletal anomalies) in rats when given in doses approximately 40 times the human dose. There are no adequate and well controlled studies in pregnant women. Methazolamide should be used during pregnancy only if the potential benefit justifies the potential risk to the fetus.

Nursing Mothers: It is not known whether this drug is excreted in human milk. Because many drugs are excreted in human milk and because of the potential for serious adverse reactions in nursing infants from methazolamide, a decision should be made whether to discontinue nursing or to discontinue the drug, taking into account the importance of the drug to the mother.

Pediatric Use: The safety and effectiveness of methazolamide in children have not been established.

Adverse Reactions: Adverse reactions, occurring most often early in therapy, include paresthesias, particularly a "tingling" feeling in the extremities, hearing, dysfunction or tinnitus; fatigue; malaise; loss of appetite; taste alteration; gastrointestinal disturbances such as nausea, vomiting and diarrhea; polyuria; and occassional instances of drowsiness and confusion.

Metabolic acidosis and electrolyte imbalance may occur.

Transient myopia has been reported. This condition invariably subsides upon diminution or discontinuance of the medication.

Other occasional adverse reactions include urticaria, melena, hematuria, glycosuria, hepatic insufficiency, flaccid paralysis, photosensitivity; convulsions, and rarely, crystalluria and renal calculi. Also see **PRECAUTIONS**: **Information for Patients** for possible reactions common to sulfonamide derivatives. Fatalities have occurred, although rarely, due to severe reactions to sulfonamides including Stevens-Johnson syndrome, toxic epidermal necrolysis, fulminant hepatic necrosis, agranulocytosis, aplastic anemia, and other blood dyscrasias (see **WARNINGS**).

Overdosage: No data are available regarding methazolamide overdosage in humans as no cases of acute poisoning with this drug have been reported. Animal data suggest that even a high dose of methazolamide is nontoxic. No specific antidote is known. Treatment should be symptomatic and supportive.

Electrolyte imbalance, development of an acidotic state, and central nervous system effects might be expected to occur. Serum electrolyte levels (particularly potassium) and blood pH levels should be monitored.

Supportive measures may be required to restore electrolyte and pH balance.

Dosage and Administration: The effective therapeutic dose administered varies from 50 mg to 100 mg 2 or 3 times daily. The drug may be used concomitantly with miotic and osmotic agents.

How Supplied: Methazolamide tablets USP for oral administration are supplied as:
25 mg: Round, white, unscored tablets debossed GG 78 on one side and plain on the reverse side in bottles of 100. NDC 58768-106-01.
50 mg: Round, white scored tablets debossed GG 181 on one side and plain on the reverse side in bottles of 100. NDC 58768-116-01.
Store at controlled room temperature 15°–30°C (59°–86°F).
Dispense in a tight, light-resistant container.
Caution: Federal law prohibits dispensing without prescription.
Rev. 93-1E
Mfd. by: Geneva Pharmaceuticals, Inc. for
CIBAVision
Ophthalmics®
A Division of CIBA Vision Corporation
Atlanta, Georgia 30136

VOLTAREN OPHTHALMIC® ℞
(diclofenac sodium 0.1%)
Sterile Ophthalmic Solution

Description: Voltaren Ophthalmic (diclofenac sodium) 0.1% solution is a sterile, topical, nonsteroidal, anti-inflammatory product for ophthalmic use. Diclofenac sodium is designated chemically as 2-[(2,6-dichlorophenyl) amino] benzeneacetic acid, monosodium salt, with an empirical formula of $C_{14}H_{10}CL_2NO_2Na$. The structural formula of diclofenac sodium is

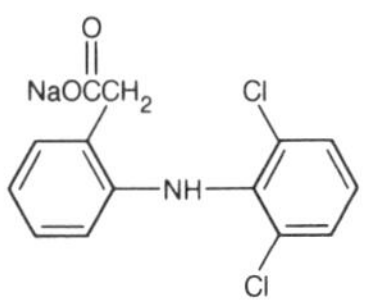

Voltaren Ophthalmic is available as a sterile solution, which contains diclofenac sodium 0.1% (1 mg/mL).
Inactive Ingredients. Boric acid, edetate disodium (1 mg/mL), polyoxyl 35 castor oil, purified water, sorbic acid (2 mg/mL), and tromethamine.
Diclofenac sodium is a faintly yellow-white to light-beige, slightly hygroscopic crystalline powder. It is freely soluble in methanol, sparingly soluble in water, very slightly soluble in acetonitrile, and insoluble in chloroform and in 0.1N hydrochloric acid. Its molecular weight is 318.14. Voltaren Ophthalmic 0.1% is an isoosmotic physiologically compatible solution with an osmolality of about 300 mOsmol/1000 g, buffered at approximately pH 7.2. Voltaren Ophthalmic solution has a faint characteristic odor of castor oil.
Clinical Pharmacology: Diclofenac sodium is one of a series of phenylacetic acids that have demonstrated anti-inflammatory and analgesic properties in pharmacological studies. It is thought to inhibit the enzyme cyclooxygenase, which is essential in the biosynthesis of prostaglandins.
Prostaglandins have been shown in many animal models to be mediators of certain kinds of intraocular inflammation. In studies performed in animal eyes, prostaglandins have been shown to produce disruption of the blood-aqueous humor barrier, vasodilation, increased vascular permeability, leukocytosis, and increased intraocular pressure. Prostaglandins also appear to play a role in the miotic response produced during ocular surgery by constricting the iris sphincter independently of cholinergic mechanisms. In clinical studies, Voltaren Ophthalmic has been shown to decrease the signs and symptoms of inflammation resulting from cataract surgery.
Results from clinical studies indicate that Voltaren Ophthalmic has no significant effect upon intraocular pressure; however, elevations in intraocular pressure may occur following cataract surgery.
Results from a bioavailability study established that plasma levels of diclofenac following ocular instillation of two drops of Voltaren Ophthalmic to each eye were below the limit of quantitation (10 ng/mL) over a 4-hour period. This study suggests that limited, if any, systemic absorption occurs with Voltaren Ophthalmic.
In two doubled-masked, controlled, efficacy studies of postoperative inflammation, a total of 206 cataract patients were treated with Voltaren Ophthalmic and 103 patients were treated with vehicle placebo. Voltaren Ophthalmic was statistically favored over vehicle placebo at all three visits over a 2-week period for the clinical assessments of inflammation (anterior chamber cells and flare, conjunctival erythema and ciliary flush). Patients who participated in two other trials were safely continued on Voltaren Ophthalmic for a period of up to 6 weeks.
In two separate, double-masked, comparative studies the effects of Voltaren Ophthalmic and prednisolone sodium phosphate 1% on the blood-aqueous humor barrier were examined by anterior chamber fluorophotometry at 1 week post surgery. One study compared 27 patients in the Voltaren Ophthalmic group with 32 patients in the prednisolone group, and the other compared 32 patients in the Voltaren Ophthalmic group with 35 pateints in the prednisolone group. Voltaren Ophthalmic was statistically more effective than prednisolone in expediting reestablishment of the blood-aqueous humor barrier disrupted by cataract extraction. However, the clinical benefit or harm in the reestablishment of the blood-aqueous barrier is unknown.
Voltaren Ophthalmic has been safely administered in conjunction with other ophthalmic medications such as antibiotics, beta blockers, carbonic anhydrase inhibitors, cycloplegics, and mydriatics.
Indications and Usage: Voltaren Ophthalmic is indicated for the treatment of postoperative inflammation in patients who have undergone cataract extraction.
Contraindications: Voltaren Ophthalmic is contraindicated in patients concurrently wearing soft contact lenses and in patients who are hypersensitive to any component of the medication. Patients wearing hydrogel soft contact lenses who have used Voltaren Ophthalmic concurrently have experienced ocular irritation manifested by redness and burning.
Warnings: There is the potential for cross-sensitivity to acetylsalicylic acid, phenylacetic acid derivatives, and other nonsteroidal anti-inflammatory agents. Therefore, caution should be used when treating individuals who have previously exhibited sensitivities to these drugs.
With some nonsteroidal anti-inflammatory drugs, there exists the potential for increased bleeding time due to interference with thrombocyte aggregation. There have been reports that ocularly applied nonsteroidal anti-inflammatory drugs may cause increased bleeding of ocular tissues (including hyphemas) in conjunction with ocular surgery.
Precautions:
General: It is recommended that Voltaren Ophthalmic be used with caution in surgical patients with known bleeding tendencies or who are receiving other medications that may prolong bleeding time.
Voltaren may slow or delay healing.
Carcinogenesis, Mutagenesis, Impairment of Fertility: Long-term carcinogenicity studies in rats given oral Voltaren up to 2 mg/kg/day (approximately the human oral dose) have revealed no significant increases in tumor incidence. There was a slight increase in benign rat mammary fibroadenomas in mid-dose females (high-dose females had excessive mortality) but the increase was not significant for this common rat tumor. A 2-year carcinogenicity study conducted in mice employing oral Voltaren up to 2 mg/kg/day did not reveal any oncogenic potential. Voltaren did not show mutagenic potential in various mutagenicity studies including the Ames test. Voltaren administered to male and female rats at 4 mg/kg/day did not affect fertility.
Pregnancy:
Teratogenic Effects:
Pregnancy Category B: Reproduction studies performed in mice at oral doses up to 5,000 times (20 mg/kg/day) and in rats and rabbits at oral doses up to 2,500 times (10 mg/kg/day) the human topical dose have revealed no evidence of teratogenicity due to Voltaren, despite the induction of maternal toxicity and fetal toxicity. In rats, maternally toxic doses were associated with dystocia, prolonged gestation, reduced fetal weights and growth, and reduced fetal survival. Voltaren has been shown to cross the placental barrier in mice and rats.
There are, however, no adequate and well-controlled studies in pregnant women. Because animal reproduction studies are not always predictive of human response, this drug should be used during pregnancy only if clearly needed.
Nonteratogenic Effects: Because of the known effects of prostaglandin-inhibiting drugs on the fetal cardiovascular system (closure of the ductus arteriosus), the use of Voltaren Ophthalmic during late pregnancy should be avoided.
Pediatric Use: Safety and effectiveness in children have not been established.
Adverse Reactions:
Ocular: Transient burning and stinging was reported in 15% of patients across all studies with the use of topical Voltaren Ophthalmic. In cataract studies, keratitis occurred in 28% of patients receiving Voltaren Ophthalmic; most of the cases of keratitis occurred prior to drug therapy. Elevated intraocular pressure was reported in 15% of patients receiving Voltaren Ophthalmic; most of these cases occurred post surgery and prior to drug administration.
Other ocular medical problems included anterior chamber reaction and ocular allergy.
Systemic: Nausea and vomiting occurred in 1% of patients receiving Voltaren Ophthalmic and in 0.5% of patients receiving vehicle alone. Viral infections occurred in $\leq 1\%$ of each of the Voltaren Ophthalmic and vehicle groups.
Overdosage: Overdosage will not ordinarily cause acute problems. If accidentally ingested, fluids should be taken to dilute the medication.
Dosage and Administration: One drop of Voltaren Ophthalmic should be applied to the affected eye four times daily beginning 24 hours after cataract surgery and continuing throughout the first 2 weeks of the postoperative period.
How Supplied: Voltaren Ophthalmic 0.1% (1 mg/mL) Sterile Solution is supplied in dropper-tip, plastic squeeze bottles in the following sizes:
Bottles of 2.5 mL ....NDC 58768-100-02
Bottles of 5 mL ....NDC 58768-100-05
Store between 59°–86°F (15°–30°C). Protect from light.
Dispense in original, unopened container only.
Dist. by:
CIBA Vision Ophthalmics®
A Division of Ciba Vision Corporation
Atlanta, Georgia 30136
Shown in Product Identification Guide, page 104

Escalon Ophthalmics, Inc.

MONTGOMERY KNOLL
182 TAMARACK CIRCLE
SKILLMAN, NJ 08558

BETADINE® 5% ℞
Sterile Ophthalmic
Prep Solution
providone-iodine 5%
(0.5% available iodine)

Description: Povidone-Iodine is a broad-spectrum microbicide with the chemical formulas: 2-pyrrolidinone, 1-ethenyl-, homopolymer, compound with iodine; 1-vinyl-2-pyrrolidinone polymer, compound with iodine.
The structural formula is as follows:

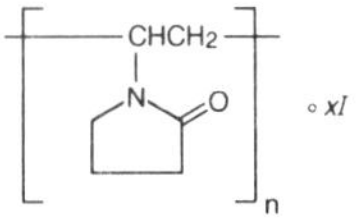

Betadine 5% Sterile Ophthalmic Prep Solution contains 5% povidone-iodine (0.5% available iodine) as a sterile solution stabilized by glycerin. Inactive Ingredients: Citric acid, Glycerin, Nonoxynol-9, Sodium chloride, Sodium hydroxide, and Sodium phosphate.

Clinical Pharmacology: A placebo-controlled study in 38 normal volunteers yielded data for 36 subjects who showed a mean $\log_{10}$ units in total aerobes at 10 minutes following prepping the skin with Betadine 5% Sterile Ophthalmic Prep Solution compared with reduction of 1.58 $\log_{10}$ units after prepping with vehicle free of the iodine complex. This placebo-controlled study indicates a mean $\log_{10}$ reduction by the iodine complex compared with the control solution of 1.47 $\log_{10}$ reduction at 10 minutes and 1.79 $\log_{10}$ units at 45 minutes. The base-line mean aerobic bacterial count was 7,586 organisms per square cm.

Indications and Usage: Betadine 5% Sterile Ophthalmic Prep Solution for the eye is indicated for prepping of the periocular region (lids, brow, and cheek) and irrigation of the ocular surface (cornea, conjunctiva, and palpebral fornices).

Contraindications: Do not use on individuals known to be sensitive to iodine.

Warnings: For external use only. NOT for intraocular injection or irrigation.

Precautions:

General: No studies are available in patients with thyroid disorders; therefore, caution is advised in using Betadine 5% Sterile Ophthalmic Prep Solution in these patients due to the possibility of iodine absorption.

Carcinogenesis, Mutagenesis, Impairment of Fertility: No long term studies in animals have been performed to evaluate the carcinogenic or mutagenic potential of povidone-iodine.

One report of the mutagenic potential of povidone-iodine indicated that it was positive in a modification of the Ames S. typhimurium model, but these results could not be reproduced by another researcher. Another test using mouse lymphoma and Balb/3T3 cells showed that povidone-iodine has no significant mutagenic or transformation capabilities. Other data indicated that it does not produce mutagenic effects in mice or hamsters according to the dominant lethal test, micronucleus test, and chromosome analysis.

Pregnancy Category C: Animal reproduction studies have not been conducted with Betadine 5% Sterile Ophthalmic Prep Solution. It is also not known whether Betadine 5% Sterile Ophthalmic Prep Solution can cause fetal harm when administered to a pregnant women or can affect reproductive capacity. Betadine 5% Sterile Ophthalmic Prep Solution should only be used on a pregnant woman if clearly needed.

Nursing Mothers: Because of the potential for serious adverse reactions in nursing infants from Betadine 5% Sterile Ophthalmic Prep Solution, a decision should be made to discontinue nursing or discontinue the drug, taking into account the importance of the drug to the mother.

Pediatric Use: Safety and effectiveness in children have not been established.

Adverse Reactions: There have been no reports from clinical trials of adverse reactions to Betadine 5% Sterile Ophthalmic Prep Solution; however, in occasional instances, local sensitivity has been exhibited by some individuals to Betadine Solution (povidone-iodine, 10%).

Dosage and Administration: While the inner surface and contents of the immediate container (i.e. bottle) are sterile, the outer surface of the bottle is not sterile. The use of the bottle in a sterile field should be avoided.

Betadine 5% Sterile Ophthalmic Prep Solution is used as follows:

1. **Twist clear overcap, piercing the blue container. Remove the overcap and gently squeeze entire contents of bottle into a sterile prep cup.**
2. **Saturate sterile cotton-tipped applicator to prep lashes and lid margins using one or more applicators per lid; repeat once.**
3. **Saturate sterile prep sponge or other suitable material to prep lids, brow and cheek in a circular ever-expanding fashion until the entire field is covered; repeat prep three (3) times.**
4. **While separating the lids, irrigate the cornea, conjunctiva and palpebral fornices with Betadine 5% Sterile Ophthalmic Prep Solution using a sterile bulb syringe.**
5. **After the Betadine 5% Sterile Ophthalmic Prep Solution has been left in contact for two minutes, sterile saline solution in a bulb syringe should be used to flush the residual prep solution from the cornea, conjunctiva, and the palpebral fornices.**

How Supplied: Betadine 5% Sterile Ophthalmic Prep Solution is packaged under sterile conditions and supplied in 1.7 fl. oz. (50 ml) form-seal plastic bottles (NDC#0034-0410-20). Twenty-four bottles are packed in each shipper.

Store at controlled room temperature 15-30°C (59-86°F).

Federal law prohibits dispensing without a prescription.

Manufactured for
The Purdue Frederick Company
Norwalk, CT 06856 by
PACO Pharmaceutical Services
Lakewood, NJ 08701.

Distributed by
Escalon® Ophthalmics, Inc.
182 Tamarack Circle
Skillman, NJ 08558
1-800-486-4848
December 4, 1991

Betadine is a registered trademark of The Purdue Frederick Company.
Escalon is a registered trademark of Escalon Ophthalmics, Inc.

Refer to contents page
for information on
Pharmaceutical Products.

Fisons Corporation

P.O. BOX 1766
ROCHESTER, NY 14603

ACULAR® ℞
(ketorolac tromethamine) 0.5%
Sterile Ophthalmic Solution

Description: ACULAR® (ketorolac tromethamine) is a member of the pyrrolo-pyrolle group of nonsteroidal anti-inflammatory drugs (NSAIDs) for ophthalmic use. Its chemical name is (±)-5-benzoyl-2, 3-dihydro-1*H*-pyrrolizine-1-carboxylic acid compound with 2-amino-2-(hydroxymethyl)-1,3-propanediol (1:1).

ACULAR® is supplied as a sterile isotonic aqueous 0.5% solution, with a pH of 7.4. ACULAR® is a racemic mixture of R-(+)- and S-(−)- ketorolac tromethamine. Ketorolac tromethamine may exist in three crystal forms. All forms are equally soluble in water. The pKa of ketorolac is 3.5. This white to off-white crystalline substance discolors on prolonged exposure to light. The molecular weight of ketorolac tromethamine is 376.41. Each mL of ACULAR® ophthalmic solution contains ketorolac tromethamine 0.5%, benzalkonium chloride 0.01%, edetate disodium 0.1%, octoxynol 40, sodium chloride, hydrochloric acid and/or sodium hydroxide to adjust the pH, and purified water. The osmolality of ACULAR® is 290 mOsmol/kg.

Animal Pharmacology: Ketorolac tromethamine prevented the development of increased intraocular pressure induced in rabbits with topically applied arachidonic acid. Ketorolac did not inhibit rabbit lens aldose reductase *in vitro.*

Ketorolac tromethamine ophthalmic solution did not enhance the spread of ocular infections induced in rabbits with *Candida albicans, Herpes simplex* virus type one, or *Pseudomonas aeruginosa.*

Clinical Pharmacology: Ketorolac tromethamine is a nonsteroidal anti-inflammatory drug which, when administered systemically, has demonstrated analgesic, anti-inflammatory and anti-pyretic activity. The mechanism of its action is thought to be due, in part, to its ability to inhibit prostaglandin biosynthesis. Ocular administration of ketorolac tromethamine reduces prostaglandin E_2 levels in aqueous humor. The mean concentration of PGE_2 was 80 pg/mL in the aqueous humor of eyes receiving vehicle and 28 pg/mL in the eyes receiving 0.5% ACULAR® ophthalmic solution. Ketorolac tromethamine given systemically does not cause pupil constriction.

Results from clinical studies indicate that ACULAR® ophthalmic solution has no significant effect upon intraocular pressure.

Two controlled clinical studies showed that ACULAR® ophthalmic solution was significantly more effective than its vehicle in relieving ocular itching caused by seasonal allergic conjunctivitis. Two drops (0.1 mL) of 0.5% ACULAR® ophthalmic solution instilled into the eyes of patients 12 hours and 1 hour prior to cataract extraction achieved measurable levels in 8 of 9 patients' eyes (mean ketorolac concentration 95 ng/mL aqueous humor, range 40 to 170 ng/mL).

One drop (0.05 mL) of 0.5% ACULAR® ophthalmic solution was instilled into one eye and one drop of vehicle into the other eye tid in 26 normal subjects. Only 5 of 26 subjects had a detectable amount of ketorolac in their plasma (range 10.7 to 22.5 ng/mL) at Day 10 during topical ocular treatment. When ketorolac tromethamine 10 mg is administered systemically every 6 hours, peak plasma levels at steady state are around 960 ng/mL. ACULAR® ophthalmic solution has been safely administered in conjunction with other ophthalmic medications, such as antibiotics, beta blockers, carbonic anhydrase inhibitors, cycloplegics, and mydriatics.

Indications and Usage: ACULAR® ophthalmic solution is indicated for the relief of ocular itching due to seasonal allergic conjunctivitis.

Contraindications: ACULAR® ophthalmic solution is contraindicated in patients while wearing soft contact lenses and in patients with previously demonstrated hypersensitivity to any of the ingredients in the formulation.

Warnings: There is the potential for cross-sensitivity to acetylsalicylic acid, phenylacetic acid derivatives, and other nonsteroidal anti-inflammatory agents. Therefore, caution should be used when treating individuals who have previously exhibited sensitivities to these drugs.

With some nonsteroidal anti-inflammatory drugs, there exists the potential for increased bleeding time due to interference with thrombocyte aggregation. There have been reports that ocularly applied nonsteroidal anti-inflammatory drugs may cause increased bleeding of ocular tissues (including hyphemas) in conjunction with ocular surgery.

Precautions: General: It is recommended that ACULAR® ophthalmic solution be used with caution in patients with known bleeding tendencies or who are receiving other medications which may prolong bleeding time.

Carcinogenesis, Mutagenesis, and Impairment of Fertility: An 18-month study in mice at oral doses of ketorolac tromethamine equal to the parenteral MRHD (Maximum Recommended Human Dose) and a 24-month study in rats at oral doses 2.5 times the parenteral MRHD, showed no evidence of tumorigenicity. Ketorolac tromethamine was not mutagenic in Ames test, unscheduled DNA synthesis and repair, and in forward mutation assays. Ketorolac did not cause chromosome breakage in the *in vivo* mouse micronucleus assay. At 1590 ug/mL (approximately 1000 times the average human plasma levels) and at higher concentrations, ketorolac tromethamine increased the incidence of chromosomal aberrations in Chinese hamster ovarian cells.

Impairment of fertility did not occur in male or female rats at oral doses of 9 mg/kg (53.1 mg/m^2) and 16 mg/kg (94.4 mg/m^2) respectively.

Pregnancy: Pregnancy Category C. Reproduction studies have been performed in rabbits, using daily oral doses at 3.6 mg/kg (42.35 mg/m^2) and in rats at 10 mg/kg (59 mg/m^2) during organogenesis. Results of these studies did not reveal evidence of teratogenicity to the fetus. Oral doses of ketorolac tromethamine at 1.5 mg/kg (8.8 mg/m^2), which was half of the human oral exposure, administered after gestation day 17 caused dystocia and higher pup mortality in rats. There are no adequate and well-controlled studies in pregnant women. Ketorolac tromethamine should be used during pregnancy only if the potential benefit justifies the potential risk to the fetus.

Nursing Mothers: Caution should be exercised when ACULAR® is administered to a nursing woman.

Pediatric Use: Safety and efficacy in children have not been established.

Adverse Reactions: In patients with allergic conjunctivitis, the most frequent adverse events reported with the use of ACULAR® ophthalmic solution have been transient stinging and burning on instillation. These events were reported by approximately 40% of patients treated with ACULAR® ophthalmic solution. In all development studies conducted, other adverse events reported during treatment with ACULAR® include ocular irritation (3%), allergic reactions (3%), superficial ocular infections (0.5%) and superficial keratitis (1%).

Dosage and Administration: The recommended dose of ACULAR® ophthalmic solution is one drop (0.25 mg) four times a day for relief of ocular itching due to seasonal allergic conjunctivitis. The efficacy of ACULAR® ophthalmic solution has not been established beyond one week of therapy.

How Supplied: ACULAR® (ketorolac tromethamine) ophthalmic solution is available for topical ophthalmic administration as a 0.5% sterile solution, and is supplied in a white opaque plastic bottle (5 mL fill) with a controlled dropper tip (NDC 0023-2181-05). Store at controlled room temperature 15–30°C (59–86°F) with protection from light.

CAUTION: Federal (U.S.A.) law prohibits dispensing without prescription.

U.S. Patent Nos. 4,089,969; 4,454,151; 5,110,493

©Allergan, Inc., Irvine, CA 92715, U.S.A.

ACULAR®, a registered trademark of Syntex (U.S.A.) Inc., is manufactured and distributed by Allergan, Inc. under license from its developer, Syntex (U.S.A.) Inc., Palo Alto, California, U.S.A.

ALLERGAN
Irvine, CA 92715

***FISONS* Pharmaceuticals**
Fisons Corporation
Rochester, NY 14623 U.S.A.

IOLAB Corporation Pharmaceuticals

500 IOLAB DRIVE
CLAREMONT, CA 91711

ATROPISOL® (atropine sulfate) 1% ℞
Sterile Ophthalmic Solution
How Supplied: 5mL, and 12×1mL DROPPERETTE®

IOCARE® Balanced Salt Solution ℞
Sterile Ophthalmic Solution
How Supplied: 36×15mL

DACRIOSE® OTC
Sterile Eye Irrigating Solution
How Supplied: 0.5, and 4 fl. oz.

DEXACIDIN® ℞
(Neomycin and Polymyxin B Sulfates and Dexamethasone, USP)
Sterile Ophthalmic Suspension
How Supplied: 5mL

DEXACIDIN® ℞
(Neomycin and Polymyxin B Sulfates and Dexamethasone, USP) Sterile Ophthalmic Ointment
Preservative Free and Lanolin Free
How Supplied: 3.5g

DROPPERETTES® Applicator—
Sterile Package

ATROPISOL® 1% (atropine sulfate) ℞
Sterile Ophthalmic Solution
How Supplied: 12×1mL DROPPERETTE®

Fluorescein Sodium 2% ℞
Sterile Ophthalmic Solution
How Supplied: 12×1mL DROPPERETTE®

Homatropine HBr ℞
Sterile Ophthalmic Solution, USP 5%
How Supplied: 12×1mL DROPPERETTE®

Phenylephrine HCl 10% (Rfg.) ℞
Sterile Ophthalmic Solution
How Supplied: 12×1mL DROPPERETTE®

PILOCAR® 1% (pilocarpine HCl) ℞
Sterile Ophthalmic Solution
How Supplied: 12×1mL DROPPERETTE®

PILOCAR® 2% (pilocarpine HCl) ℞
Sterile Ophthalmic Solution
How Supplied: 12×1mL DROPPERETTE®

PILOCAR® 4% (pilocarpine HCl) ℞
Sterile Ophthalmic Solution
How Supplied: 12×1mL DROPPERETTE®

SULF-10® (sulfacetamide sodium, USP) ℞
Sterile Ophthalmic Solution
How Supplied: 12×1mL DROPPERETTE®

Tetracaine HCl ½% ℞
Sterile Ophthalmic Solution
How Supplied: 12×1mL DROPPERETTE®

E-PILO-1® ℞
(epinephrine bitartrate 1%-pilocarpine HCl 1%)
Sterile Ophthalmic Solution
How Supplied: 10mL

E-PILO-2® ℞
(epinephrine bitartrate 1%-pilocarpine HCl 2%)
Sterile Ophthalmic Solution
How Supplied: 10mL

E-PILO-4® ℞
(epinephrine bitartrate 1%-pilocarpine HCl 4%)
Sterile Ophthalmic Solution
How Supplied: 10mL

E-PILO-6® ℞
(epinephrine bitartrate 1%-pilocarpine HCl 6%)
Sterile Ophthalmic Solution
How Supplied: 10mL

Eserine Sulfate (physostigmine sulfate) ℞
Sterile Ophthalmic Ointment, 0.25%
How Supplied: 3.5gm

FLUOR-OP® (Fluorometholone ℞
Sterile Ophthalmic Suspension, USP) 0.1%
How Supplied: 3, 5, 10 and 15mL

FUNDUSCEIN®-10 ℞
(fluorescein sodium) 10% Injection
How Supplied: 12×5mL amps

FUNDUSCEIN®-25 ℞
(fluorescein sodium) 25% Injection
How Supplied: 12×3mL amps

GENTACIDIN® (gentamicin sulfate ℞
sterile ophthalmic solution, USP)
How Supplied: 5mL

Gentamicin Sulfate ℞
Sterile Ophthalmic Ointment, USP
How Supplied: 3.5g

GLUCOSE-40 (liquid glucose) ℞
Sterile Ophthalmic Ointment
How Supplied: 3.5g

GONIOSOL®
(hydroxypropyl methylcellulose) 2.5% Diagnostic
Sterile Ophthalmic Solution
How Supplied: 15mL

Homatropine Hydrobromide ℞
Sterile Ophthalmic Solution, USP 5%
How Supplied: 5mL

HYPOTEARS® OTC
Sterile Lubricant Eye Drops
How Supplied: 0.5 and 1 fl. oz.

HYPOTEARS® PF OTC
Lubricant Eye Drops (Preservative Free)
How Supplied: 30 single-use vials per carton

HYPOTEARS® OTC
Sterile Bedtime Eye Lubricant
Preservative Free and Lanolin Free
How Supplied: 3.5g

Continued on next page

Information on IOLAB products listed on these pages is the full prescribing information from package inserts effective in June 1994. For information concerning all IOLAB products, please call 1-909-624-2020.

IOLAB Corporation—Cont.

INFLAMASE® MILD 1/8% ℞
(prednisolone sodium phosphate)
Sterile Ophthalmic Solution
How Supplied: 3, 5 and 10mL

INFLAMASE® FORTE 1% ℞
(prednisolone sodium phosphate)
Sterile Ophthalmic Solution
How Supplied: 3, 5, 10 and 15mL

LIVOSTIN™ 0.05% (levocabastine HCl ophthalmic suspension) 5 mL ℞

MIOCHOL®-E (acetylcholine chloride)
1:100 Intraocular with electrolyte diluent ℞
IOCARE®
Steri-Tags™
How Supplied: 2mL univial,

IOCARE® Steri-Tags™

MIOCHOL®-E System Pak™ ℞

Miochol-E (acetylcholine chloride) 1:100 Intraocular with electrolyte diluent 2mL univial
IOCARE® Steri-Tags™, 3mL B-D® Syringe 0.2 Micron DynaGard™ Filter

PILOCAR® (pilocarpine HCl) 1/2% ℞
Sterile Ophthalmic Solution
How Supplied: 15mL, Twin Pack (2×15mL)

PILOCAR® (pilocarpine HCl) 1% ℞
Sterile Ophthalmic Solution
How Supplied: 15mL, Twin Pack (2×15mL), DROPPERETTE® (12×1mL)

PILOCAR® (pilocarpine HCl) 2% ℞
Sterile Ophthalmic Solution
How Supplied: 15mL, Twin Pack (2×15mL), DROPPERETTE® (12×1mL)

PILOCAR® (pilocarpine HCl) 3% ℞
Sterile Ophthalmic Solution
How Supplied: 15mL, Twin Pack (2×15mL)

PILOCAR® (pilocarpine HCl) 4% ℞
Sterile Ophthalmic Solution
How Supplied: 15mL, Twin Pack (2×15mL), DROPPERETTE® (12×1mL)

PILOCAR® (pilocarpine HCl) 6% ℞
Sterile Ophthalmic Solution
How Supplied: 15mL, Twin Pack (2×15mL)

SULF-10® (sodium sulfacetamide ℞
sterile ophthalmic solution, USP)
How Supplied: 15mL, DROPPERETTE® (12×1mL)

TEARISOL® OTC
Sterile Lubricant Eye Drops
How Supplied: 0.5 fl. oz.

VASOCIDIN® ℞
(sulfacetamide sodium and prednisolone sodium phosphate sterile
ophthalmic solution, USP) 10%/0.25%
How Supplied: 5 and 10mL

VASOCIDIN® ℞
(sulfacetamide sodium-prednisolone acetate sterile ophthalmic ointment, USP) 10%/0.5%
Preservative Free and Lanolin Free
How Supplied: 3.5g

VASOCLEAR® OTC
Sterile Lubricant/Redness Reliever Eye Drop
How Supplied: 15mL

VASOCLEAR® A OTC
Sterile Astringent/Lubricant/Redness Reliever Eye Drops
How Supplied: 15mL

Vasocon-A ℞
(naphazoline HCl 0.05%-antazoline phosphate 0.5%)
Sterile Ophthalmic Solution
How Supplied: 15mL

Vasocon-Regular ℞
(naphazoline HCl 0.1%
Sterile Ophthalmic Solution, USP)
How Supplied: 15mL

VASOSULF® ℞
(sulfacetamide sodium 15%-phenylephrine hydrochloride 0.125%)
Sterile Ophthalmic Solution
How Supplied: 5 and 15mL

DEXACIDIN® ℞

[deks 'a-si-din]
(Neomycin and Polymyxin B Sulfates and Dexamethasone)
Ophthalmic Ointment

Description: DEXACIDIN Ophthalmic Ointment is a multidose, anti-infective steroid combination in a sterile topical ophthalmic ointment having the following composition:
Dexamethasone .... 1 mg/g
Neomycin .... 3.5 mg/g
(represented by neomycin sulfate)
Polymyxin B Sulfate .... 10,000 units/g
in a bland base containing white petrolatum and mineral oil.
The chemical name for dexamethasone is: Pregna-1,4-diene-3,20 dione,9-fluoro-11,17,21-trihydroxy-16-methyl-(11β, 16α)-, which has the following structure:

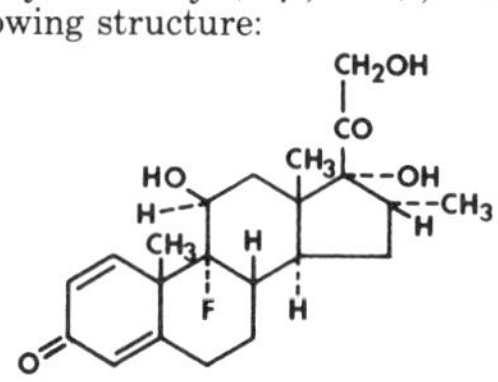

Clinical Pharmacology: Corticoids suppress the inflammatory response to a variety of agents and they probably delay or slow healing. Since corticoids may inhibit the body's defense mechanism against infection, a concomitant antimicrobial drug may be used when this inhibition is considered to be clinically significant in a particular case.
When a decision to administer both corticoid and an antimicrobial is made, the administration of such drugs in combination has the advantage of greater patient compliance and convenience, with the added assurance that the appropriate dosage of both drugs is administered, plus assured compatibility of ingredients when both types of drugs are in the same formulation and, particularly, that the correct volume of drug is delivered and retained.
The relative potency of corticosteroids depends on the molecular structure, concentration and release from the vehicle.

Indications and Usage: For steroid-responsive inflammatory ocular conditions for which a corticosteroid is indicated and where bacterial infection or a risk of bacterial ocular infection exists.
Ocular steroids are indicated in inflammatory conditions of the palpebral and bulbar conjunctiva, cornea, and anterior segment of the globe where the inherent risk of steroid use in certain infective conjunctivitides is accepted to obtain a diminution in edema and inflammation. They are also indicated in chronic anterior uveitis and corneal injury from chemical, radiation, thermal burns, or penetration of foreign bodies.
The use of a combination drug with anti-infective component is indicated where the risk of infection is high or where there is an expectation that potentially dangerous numbers of bacteria will be present in the eye.
The particular anti-infective drugs in this product are active against the following common bacterial eye pathogens: *Staphylococcus aureus, Escherichia coli, Haemophilus influenzae, Klebsiella/Enterobacter* species, *Neisseria* species, and *Pseudomonas aeruginosa.*
This product does not provide adequate coverage against: *Serratia marcescens* and Streptococci, including *Streptococcus pneumoniae.*

Contraindications: Epithelial herpes simplex keratitis (dendritic keratitis), vaccinia, varicella, and many other viral diseases of the cornea and conjunctiva. Mycobacterial infection of the eye. Fungal diseases of ocular structures. Hypersensitivity to a component of the medication. (Hypersensitivity to the antibiotic component occurs at a higher rate than for other components.)
The use of these combinations is always contraindicated after uncomplicated removal of a corneal foreign body.

Warnings: Prolonged use may result in glaucoma, with damage to the optic nerve, defects in visual acuity and fields of vision, and posterior subcapsular cataract formation. Prolonged use may suppress the host response and thus increase the hazard of secondary ocular infections. In those diseases causing thinning of the cornea or sclera, perforations have been known to occur with the use of topical steroids. In acute purulent conditions of the eye, steroids may mask infection or enhance existing infection. If these products are used for 10 days or longer, intraocular pressure should be routinely monitored even though it may be difficult in children and uncooperative patients.
Products containing neomycin sulfate may cause cutaneous sensitization.
Employment of steroid medication in the treatment of herpes simplex requires great caution.

Precautions: General: The initial prescription and renewal of the medication order beyond 8 g should be made by a physician only after examination of the patient with the aid of magnification, such as slit lamp biomicroscopy and, where appropriate, fluorescein staining.
The possibility of persistent fungal infections of the cornea should be considered after prolonged steroid dosing.
Information to the patient: To avoid contamination, do not touch tip of container to the eye, eyelid or any surface.

Adverse Reactions: Adverse reactions have occurred with steroid/anti-infective combination drugs which can be attributed to the steroid component, the anti-infective component, or the combination. Exact incidence figures are not available since no denominator of treated patients is available.
Reactions occurring most often from the presence of the anti-infective ingredient are allergic sensitizations. The reactions due to the steroid component in decreasing order of frequency are: elevation of intraocular pressure (IOP) with possible development of glaucoma, and infrequent optic nerve damage; posterior subcapsular cataract formation; and delayed wound healing.
Secondary Infection: The development of secondary infection has occurred after use of combinations containing steroids and antimicrobials. Fungal infections of the cornea are particularly prone to develop coincidentally with long-term applications of steroid. The possibility of fungal invasion must be considered in any persistent corneal ulceration where steroid treatment has been used.
Secondary bacterial ocular infection following suppression of host responses also occurs.

Dosage and Administration: DEXACIDIN Ophthalmic Ointment: Apply a small amount (about 1/2 inch) into the conjunctival sac(s) up to three or four times daily or apply at bedtime adjunctively with drops.
Not more than 8 g should be prescribed initially and the prescription should not be refilled without further evaluation as outlined in PRECAUTIONS above.

How Supplied: DEXACIDIN Ophthalmic Ointment: 3.5 g (1/8 oz.) tube. NDC 0058-2255-01.

Store at controlled room temperature 15° to 30°C (59°–86°F).
Caution: Federal (U.S.A.) law prohibits dispensing without prescription.
Manufactured by:
Altana Inc.
Melville, NY 11747
Manufactured for:
IOLAB®
A Johnson & Johnson Company
IOLAB Corporation **6081-E**
Claremont, California 91711
Revised: Oct. 1991

FLUOR-OP® ℞
(FLUOROMETHOLONE OPHTHALMIC SUSPENSION, USP) 0.1%

Description: Fluor-Op (fluorometholone ophthalmic suspension, USP) 0.1%, is a topical anti-inflammatory agent for ophthalmic use.
Chemical Name: 9-fluoro-11β, 17-dihydroxy-6α-methylpregna-1,4-diene-3,20-dione.
Contains:
Fluorometholone 0.1%
with: polyvinyl alcohol 1.4%; benzalkonium chloride 0.004%, edetate disodium; sodium chloride; sodium phosphate monobasic, monohydrate; sodium phosphate dibasic, anhydrous; polysorbate 80; sodium hydroxide to adjust the pH, and purified water.
Clinical Pharmacology: Corticosteroids inhibit the inflammatory response to a variety of inciting agents. They inhibit the edema, fibrin deposition, capillary dilation, leukocyte migration, phagocytic activity, capillary proliferation, fibroblast proliferation, deposition of collagen, and scar formation associated with inflammation.
No generally accepted explanation of steroid action is available. However, corticosteroids are thought to act by the induction of phospholipase A_2 inhibitory proteins, collectively called lipocortins. It is postulated that these proteins control the biosynthesis of potent mediators of inflammation such as prostaglandins and leukotrienes by inhibiting the release of their common precursor, arachidonic acid. Arachidonic acid is released from membrane phospholipids by phospholipase A_2.
Corticosteroids are capable of producing a rise in intraocular pressure. In clinical studies on patients' eyes treated with both dexamethasone and fluorometholone suspensions, fluorometholone demonstrated a lower propensity to increase intraocular pressure than did dexamethasone.
Indications and Usage: Fluor-Op is indicated for the treatment of corticosteroid-responsive inflammation of the palpebral and bulbar conjunctiva, cornea and anterior segment of the globe.
Contraindications: Fluor-Op is contraindicated in the following conditions:
Epithelial herpes simplex keratitis (dendritic keratitis), vaccinia, varicella and other viral diseases of the cornea and conjunctiva.
Tuberculosis of the eye.
Fungal diseases of the ocular structures.
Hypersensitivity to any ingredient of the medication.
Warnings: Corticosteroid medication in the treatment of patients with a history of herpes simplex keratitis (involving the stroma) requires great caution; frequent slit lamp microscopy is mandatory.
Prolonged use may result in elevation of IOP, with damage to the optic nerve, defects in visual acuity and fields of vision, and/or in posterior subcapsular cataract formation. It may also aid in the establishment of secondary ocular infections from fungi or viruses liberated from ocular tissues.
Various ocular diseases and long-term use of topical corticosteroids have been known to cause corneal and scleral thinning. Use of topical corticosteroids in the presence of thin corneal or scleral tissue may lead to perforation.
Acute purulent untreated infection of the eye may be masked or activity enhanced by presence of corticosteroid medication.
Precautions: General: As fungal infections of the cornea are particularly prone to develop coincidentally with long-term local corticosteroid applications, fungal invasion must be suspected in any persistent corneal ulceration where a corticosteroid has been used or is in use.
Intraocular pressure should be checked frequently.
Information to the Patient: To prevent contamination, care should be taken to avoid touching container tip to eyelids or to any other surface. Keep bottle tightly closed when not in use.
Carcinogenesis, mutagenesis, impairment of fertility: No studies have been conducted in animals or in humans to evalute the possibility of these effects with fluorometholone.
Pregnancy Category C: Fluorometholone has been shown to be teratogenic and embryocidal in rabbits when given in doses approximating the human dose and above. There are no adequate, well-controlled studies in pregnant women. Fluorometholone should be used during pregnancy only if the potential benefit outweighs the potential risk to the fetus.
Fluorometholone was ocularly applied to both eyes of pregnant rabbits at various dosage levels on days 6 to 18 of gestation. A significant dose-related increase in fetal abnormalities and in fetal loss was observed.
Nursing Mothers: It is not known whether topical administration of corticosteroids could result in sufficient systemic absorption to produce detectable quantities in breast milk, nevertheless, the physician should consider the patient discontinuing nursing while the drug is being administered.
Pediatric Use: Safety and effectiveness in children have not been established.
Adverse Reactions: Adverse reactions include, in decreasing order of frequency, elevation of intraocular pressure (IOP) with possible development of optic nerve damage; loss of visual acuity or defects in fields of vision; posterior subcapsular cataract formation; and delayed wound healing.
The following have also been reported after the use of topical corticosteroids: Secondary ocular infection from pathogens liberated from ocular tissues and, rarely, perforation of the globe when used in conditions where there is thinning of the cornea or scleral.
Dosage and Administration: Instill one drop into the conjunctival sac two to four times daily. During the initial 24 to 48 hours, the frequency of dosing may be safely increased if necessary. Care should be taken not to discontinue therapy prematurely.
How Supplied: Fluor-Op (fluorometholone ophthalmic suspension, USP) 0.1% is supplied in plastic dropper bottles in the following sizes:
3 mL NDC 0058-2358-03
5 mL NDC 0058-2358-05
10 mL NDC 0058-2358-10
15 mL NDC 0058-2358-15
Store at controlled room temperature 15°–30°C (59°–86°F).
Protect from freezing. Shake well before using. Keep bottle tightly closed when not in use.
Caution: Federal (U.S.A.) law prohibits dispensing without prescription.
IOLAB Corporation 6053-F
Claremont, California 91711
Revised: February 1992

GENTACIDIN® ℞
(Gentamicin Sulfate)
Ophthalmic Solution, USP, 0.3%
(Gentamicin Sulfate)
Ophthalmic Ointment, USP, 0.3%

Description: Gentamicin sulfate is a water-soluble antibiotic of the aminoglycoside group. GENTACIDIN Ophthalmic Solution is a sterile, aqueous solution buffered to approximately pH 7 for ophthalmic use. Each mL contains gentamicin sulfate, USP (equivalent to 3 mg gentamicin), dried sodium phosphate, monobasic sodium phosphate, sodium chloride, and purified water; preserved with benzalkonium chloride 0.1 mg/mL.
GENTACIDIN Ophthalmic Ointment is a sterile ointment, each gram containing gentamicin sulfate, USP (equivalent to 3.0 mg gentamicin) in a bland base of white petrolatum and mineral oil.
Gentamicin is obtained from cultures of *Micromonospora purpurea.* It is a mixture of the sulfate salts of gentamicin C_1, C_2, and C_{1a}. All three components appear to have similar antimicrobial activities. Gentamicin sulfate occurs as a white to buff powder and is soluble in water and insoluble in alcohol. The structure is as follows:

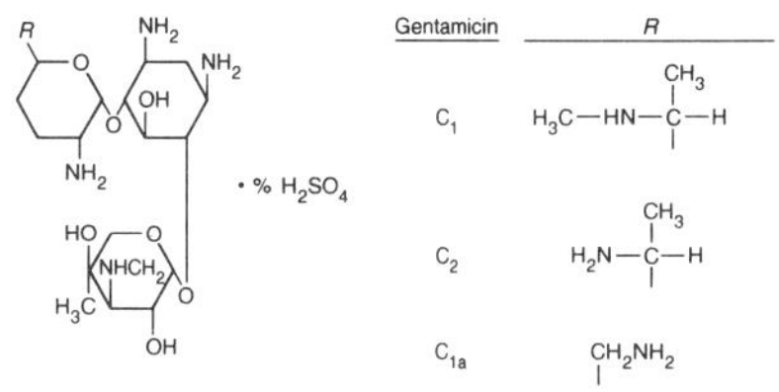

Clinical Pharmacology:
Microbiology: Gentamicin sulfate is active *in vitro* against many strains of the following microorganisms: *Staphylococcus aureus, Staphylococcus epidermidis, Streptococcus pyogenes, Streptococcus pneumoniae, Enterobacter aerogenes, Escherichia coli, Haemophilus influenzae, Klebsiella pneumoniae, Neisseria gonorrhoeae, Pseudomonas aeruginosa,* and *Serratia marcescens.*
Indications and Usage: GENTACIDIN Ophthalmic Solution and Ointment are indicated in the topical treatment of ocular bacterial infections including conjunctivitis, keratitis, keratoconjunctivitis, corneal ulcers, blepharitis, blepharoconjunctivitis, acute meibomianitis, and dacryocystitis, caused by susceptible strains of the following microorganisms: *Staphylococcus aureus, Staphylococcus epidermidis, Streptococcus pyogenes, Streptococcus pneumoniae, Enterobacter aerogenes, Escherichia coli. Haemophilus influenzae, Klebsiella pneumoniae, Neisseria gonorrhoeae, Pseudomonas aeruginosa,* and *Serratia marcescens.*
Contraindications: GENTACIDIN Ophthalmic Solution and Ointment are contraindicated in patients with known hypersensitivity to any of the components.
Warnings: NOT FOR INJECTION INTO THE EYE.
GENTACIDIN Ophthalmic Solution is not for injection. It should never be injected subconjunctivally, nor should it be directly introduced into the anterior chamber of the eye.
Precautions:
General: Prolonged use of topical antibiotics may give rise to overgrowth of nonsusceptible

Continued on next page

Information on IOLAB products listed on these pages is the full prescribing information from package inserts effective in June 1994. For information concerning all IOLAB products, please call 1-909-624-2020.

IOLAB Corporation—Cont.

organisms including fungi. Bacterial resistance to gentamicin may also develop. If purulent discharge, inflammation or pain becomes aggravated, the patient should discontinue use of the medication and consult a physician.
If irritation or hypersensitivity to any component of the drug develops, the patient should discontinue use of this preparation and appropriate therapy should be instituted.
Ophthalmic ointments may retard corneal healing.
Information for patients: To avoid contamination, do not touch tip of container to the eye, eyelid or any surface.
Carcinogenesis, mutagenesis, impairment of fertility: There are no published carcinogenicity or impairment of fertility studies on gentamicin. Aminoglycoside antibiotics have been found to be nonmutagenic.
Pregnancy: Pregnancy Category C. Gentamicin has been shown to depress body weights, kidney weights and median glomerular counts in newborn rats when administered systemically to pregnant rats in daily doses approximately 500 times the maximum recommended ophthalmic human dose. There are no adequate and well-controlled studies in pregnant women. Gentamicin should be used during pregnancy only if the potential benefit justifies the potential risk to the fetus.
Adverse Reactions: Bacterial and fungal corneal ulcers have developed during treatment with gentamicin ophthalmic preparations.
The most frequently reported adverse reactions are ocular burning and irritation upon drug instillation, non-specific conjunctivitis, conjunctival epithelial defects and conjunctival hyperemia.
Other adverse reactions which have occurred rarely are allergic reactions, thrombocytopenic purpura and hallucinations.
Dosage and Administration: GENTACIDIN Ophthalmic Solution: Instill one or two drops into affected eye every four hours. In severe infections, dosage may be increased to as much as two drops once every hour.
GENTACIDIN Ophthalmic Ointment: Apply a small amount (approximately ½ inch ribbon) of ointment to the affected eye two or three times a day.
How Supplied: GENTACIDIN Ophthalmic Solution, USP, 0.3%:
5 mL dropper-tip plastic squeeze bottles. (NDC 0058-2365-05).
GENTACIDIN Ophthalmic Ointment, USP, 0.3%:
3.5 g (⅛ oz.) sterile tube. (NDC 0058-2370-01).
To be dispensed only in original unopened container.
Store GENTACIDIN Ophthalmic Solution and Ointment between 2°–30°C (36°–86°F).
KEEP OUT OF THE REACH OF CHILDREN.
Caution: Federal (U.S.A.) law prohibits dispensing without prescription.
GENTACIDIN Ophthalmic Solution:
IOLAB Corporation
Claremont, California 91711
GENTACIDIN Ophthalmic Ointment:
Mfg. by:
Altana Inc.
Melville, NY 11747
Mfg. for:
IOLAB®
a Johnson&Johnson Company
IOLAB Corporation 6089-F
Claremont, California 91711
Revised: Apr. 1994

HYPOTEARS® LUBRICANT EYE DROPS OTC
HYPOTEARS® PF, Lubricant Eye Drops
HYPOTEARS® OINTMENT Bedtime Eye Lubricant

Description: HYPOTEARS Lubricant Eye Drops is a sterile, soothing hypotonic solution for use as an artificial tear and lubricant.
HYPOTEARS PF is a hypotonic and preservative-free solution, specially formulated to be a soothing artificial tear and lubricant.
HYPOTEARS Bedtime Eye Lubricant is preservative and lanolin-free.
Indications: For use as an ocular lubricant for the temporary relief of burning and irritation due to dryness of the eye or to exposure to wind or sun. Helps protect against further eye irritation.
Warnings: If you experience eye pain, changes in vision, continued redness or irritation of the eye, or if the condition worsens or persists for more than 72 hours, discontinue use and consult a doctor. To avoid contamination, do not touch tip of container to any surface. KEEP THIS AND ALL DRUGS OUT OF REACH OF CHILDREN. In case of accidental ingestion, seek professional assistance or contact a Poison Control Center immediately.
Eye Drops: Replace cap after using.
If solution of HYPOTEARS Eye Drops changes color or becomes cloudy, do not use. Do not use these products if you are allergic to any of their ingredients. Store at controlled room temperature 59°–86°F (15°–30°C).
PF: Use only if single-use container is intact. Use immediately after opening container. Do not store open container. Store at controlled room temperature 59°–86°F (15°–30°C).
Ointment: Store away from heat.
Directions:
Eye Drops: Instill 1 or 2 drops in the affected eye(s) as needed.
Ointment: Pull down the lower lid of the affected eye and apply a small amount (¼ inch) of ointment to the inside of the eyelid.
PF: To open, twist the top of the container. Apply 1–2 drop(s) in affected eye(s), as needed. Discard container immediately after use.
Contains:
Eye Drops: ACTIVE: Polyvinyl Alcohol 1% and polyethylene glycol 400 1%. Lipiden™ vehicle (dextrose, edetate disodium, and purified water); preserved with benzalkonium chloride. 0.1 mg/mL.
PF: Polyvinyl alcohol 1% and polyethylene glycol 400 1%. Lipiden™ vehicle (polyethylene glycol 400, dextrose, edetate disodium, and purified water).
Ointment: White petrolatum and light mineral oil.
How Supplied:
Eye Drops: 15 mL and 30 mL plastic squeeze bottle with dropper tip.
NDC 0058-0130-15
NDC 0058-0130-30
Eye Drops (PF): 30 convenient single-use containers, 0.02 fl. oz. each.
NDC 0058-0132-30
Ointment: ⅛ oz. (3.5 g) tube
NDC 0058-0131-01

INFLAMASE® MILD ⅛% ℞
[in 'fla-mās]
(prednisolone sodium phosphate)
Ophthalmic Solution

INFLAMASE® FORTE 1%
(prednisolone sodium phosphate)
Ophthalmic Solution

Description: INFLAMASE MILD and INFLAMASE FORTE (prednisolone sodium phosphate) ophthalmic solutions are sterile solutions for ophthalmic administration having the following compositions:

INFLAMASE MILD
Prednisolone Sodium Phosphate..1.25 mg/mL (adrenocortical steroid/anti-inflammatory) (equivalent to Prednisolone Phosphate 1.1 mg/mL)

INFLAMASE FORTE
Prednisolone Sodium Phosphate.....10 mg/mL (adrenocortical steroid/anti-inflammatory) (equivalent to Prednisolone Phosphate 9.1 mg/mL)

in buffered, isotonic solutions containing sodium biphosphate, sodium phosphate anhydrous, sodium chloride, edetate disodium and purified water; preserved with benzalkonium chloride, 0.1 mg/mL.
The chemical name for prednisolone sodium phosphate, $C_{21}H_{27}Na_2O_8P$, is Pregna-1,4-diene-3,20-dione,11,17-dihydroxy-21-(phosphonooxy)-,disodium salt,(11β)-, which has the following chemical structure:

Prednisolone Sodium Phosphate

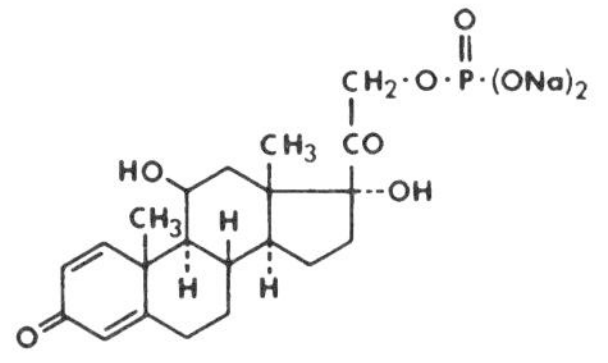

Clinical Pharmacology: Prednisolone sodium phosphate causes inhibition of the inflammatory response to inciting agents of a mechanical, chemical or immunological nature. No generally accepted explanation of this steroid property has been advanced.
Indications and Usage: INFLAMASE MILD and INFLAMASE FORTE Ophthalmic Solutions are indicated for the treatment of the following conditions: steroid responsive inflammatory conditions of the palpebral and bulbar conjunctiva, cornea, and anterior segment of the globe, such as allergic conjunctivitis, acne rosacea, superficial punctate keratitis, herpes zoster keratitis, iritis, cyclitis, selected infective conjunctivitis when the inherent hazard of steroid use is accepted to obtain an advisable diminution in edema and inflammation; corneal injury from chemical, radiation, or thermal burns, or penetration of foreign bodies.
INFLAMASE FORTE Ophthalmic Solution is recommended for moderate to severe inflammations, particularly when unusually rapid control is desired. In stubborn cases of anterior segment eye disease, systemic adrenocortical hormone therapy may be required. When the deeper ocular structures are involved, systemic therapy is necessary.
Contraindications: The use of these preparations is contraindicated in the presence of acute superficial herpes simplex keratitis, fungal diseases of ocular structures, acute infectious stages of vaccinia, varicella and most other viral diseases of the cornea and conjunctiva, tuberculosis of the eye and hypersensitivity to a component of this preparation.
The use of these preparations is always contraindicated after uncomplicated removal of a superficial corneal foreign body.
Warnings: Not for injection into the eye-for topical use only. Employment of steroid medication in the treatment of herpes simplex keratitis involving the stroma requires great caution; frequent slit-lamp microscopy is mandatory.
Prolonged use may result in elevated intraocular pressure and/or glaucoma, damage to the optic nerve, defects in visual acuity and fields of vision, posterior subcapsular cataract formation, or may result in secondary ocular infections. Viral, bacterial and fungal infections of the cornea may be exacerbated by the application of steroids. In those diseases causing thinning of the cornea or sclera, perforation has

been known to occur with the use of topical steroids. Acute purulent untreated infection of the eye may be masked or activity enhanced by the presence of steroid medication.
These drugs are not effective in mustard gas keratitis and Sjögren's keratoconjunctivitis. If irritation persists or develops, the patient should be advised to discontinue use and consult prescribing physician.
Precautions: General: As fungal infections of the cornea are particularly prone to develop coincidentally with long-term local steroid applications, fungus invasion must be suspected in any persistent corneal ulceration where a steroid has been used or is in use.
Intraocular pressure should be checked frequently.
Information for Patients: Do not touch dropper tip to any surface as this may contaminate the solution.
Pregnancy: Teratogenic Effects: Pregnancy Category C: Animal reproductive studies have not been conducted with prednisolone sodium phosphate. It is also not known whether prednisolone sodium phosphate can cause fetal harm when administered to a pregnant woman or can affect reproductive capacity. Prednisolone sodium phosphate should be given to a pregnant woman only if clearly needed.
The effect of prednisolone sodium phosphate on the later growth, development and functional maturation of the child is unknown.
Nursing Mothers: It is not known whether this drug is excreted in human milk. Because many drugs are excreted in human milk, caution should be exercised when prednisolone sodium phosphate is administered to a nursing woman.
Pediatric Use: Safety and effectiveness in children have not been established.
Adverse Reactions: The following adverse reactions have been reported: glaucoma with optic nerve damage, visual acuity and field defects, posterior subcapsular cataract formation, secondary ocular infections from pathogens including herpes simplex and fungi, and perforation of the globe.
Rarely, filtering blebs have been reported when topical steroids have been used following cataract surgery.
Rarely, stinging or burning may occur.
Dosage and Administration: Depending on the severity of inflammation, instill one or two drops of solution into the conjunctival sac up to every hour during the day and every two hours during night as necessary as initial therapy.
When a favorable response is observed, reduce dosage to one drop every four hours.
Later, further reduction in dosage to one drop three to four times daily may suffice to control symptoms.
The duration of treatment will vary with the type of lesion and may extend from a few days to several weeks, according to therapeutic responses. Relapses, more common in chronic active lesions than in self-limiting conditions, usually respond to retreatment.
How Supplied:
3 mL plastic squeeze bottle with dropper tip
INFLAMASE MILD..........NDC 0058-2875-03
1/8% (Prednisolone Sodium Phosphate)
INFLAMASE FORTE........NDC 0058-2877-03
1% (Prednisolone Sodium Phosphate)
5 mL plastic squeeze bottle with dropper tip
INFLAMASE MILD..........NDC 0058-2875-05
INFLAMASE FORTE........NDC 0058-2877-05
10 mL plastic squeeze bottle with dropper tip
INFLAMASE MILD..........NDC 0058-2875-10
INFLAMASE FORTE........NDC 0058-2877-10
15 mL plastic squeeze bottle with dropper tip
INFLAMASE FORTE........NDC 0058-2877-15
To be dispensed only in original, unopened container.
STORE AT CONTROLLED ROOM TEMPERATURE 15°–30°C (59°–86°F).
Protect from light. Keep out of reach of children.
Caution: Federal law prohibits dispensing without prescription.

LIVOSTIN™ ℞

0.05% (levocabastine hydrochloride ophthalmic suspension)

Description: LIVOSTIN™ 0.05% (levocabastine hydrochloride ophthalmic suspension) is a selective histamine H_1-receptor antagonist for topical ophthalmic use. Each mL contains 0.54 mg levocabastine hydrochloride equivalent to 0.5 mg levocabastine; 0.15 mg benzalkonium chloride; propylene glycol; polysorbate 80; dibasic sodium phosphate, anhydrous; monobasic sodium phosphate, monohydrate; disodium edetate; hydroxypropyl methylcellulose; and purified water. It has a pH of 6.0 to 8.0. The chemical name for levocabastine hydrochloride is (-)-*trans*-1-[*cis*-4-Cyano-4-(p-fluorophenyl)cyclohexyl]-3-methyl-4-phenylisonipecotic acid monohydrochloride, and is represented by the following chemical structure:

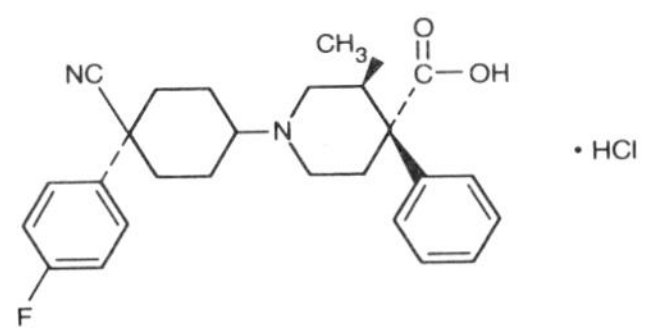

Clinical Pharmacology: Levocabastine is a potent, selective histamine H_1-antagonist.
Antigen challenge studies performed two and four hours after initial drug instillation indicated activity was maintained for at least two hours.
In an environmental study, LIVOSTIN™ 0.05% (levocabastine hydrochloride ophthalmic suspension) instilled four times daily was shown to be significantly more effective than its vehicle in reducing ocular itching associated with seasonal allergic conjunctivitis.
After instillation in the eye, levocabastine is systemically absorbed. However, the amount of systemically absorbed levocabastine after therapeutic ocular doses is low (mean plasma concentrations in the range of 1–2 ng/mL).
Indications and Usage: LIVOSTIN™ 0.05% (levocabastine hydrochloride ophthalmic suspension) is indicated for the temporary relief of the signs and symptoms of seasonal allergic conjunctivitis.
Contraindications: This product is contraindicated in persons with known or suspected hypersensitivity to any of its components. It should not be used while soft contact lenses are being worn.
Warning: For topical use only. Not for injection.
Precautions: Information for Patients: SHAKE WELL BEFORE USING. To prevent contaminating the dropper tip and suspension, care should be taken not to touch the eyelids or surrounding areas with the dropper tip of the bottle. Keep bottle tightly closed when not in use. Do not use if the suspension has discolored. Store at controlled room temperature. Protect from freezing.
Carcinogenesis, Mutagenesis, Impairment of Fertility: Levocabastine was not carcinogenic in male or female rats or in male mice when administered in the diet for up to 24 months. In female mice, levocabastine doses of 5,000 and 21,500 times the maximum recommended ocular human use level resulted in an increased incidence of pituitary gland adenoma and mammary gland adenocarcinoma possibly produced by increased prolactin levels. The clinical relevance of this finding is unknown with regard to the interspecies differences in prolactin physiology and the very low plasma concentrations of levocabastine following ocular administration.
Mutagenic potential was not demonstrated for levocabastine when tested in Ames' Salmonella Reversion test or in *Escherichia coli*, *Drosophila melanogaster*, a mouse Dominant Lethal Assay or in rat Micronucleus test.
In reproduction studies in rats, levocabastine showed no effects on fertility at oral doses of 20 mg/kg/day (8,300 times the maximum recommended human ocular dose).
Pregnancy: Teratogenic Effects: Pregnancy Category C. Levocabastine has been shown to be teratogenic (polydactyly) in rats when given in doses 16,500 times the maximum recommended human ocular dose. Teratogenicity (polydactyly, hydrocephaly, brachygnathia), embryotoxicity, and maternal toxicity were observed in rats at 66,000 times the maximum recommended ocular human dose. There are no adequate and well-controlled studies in pregnant women. Levocabastine should be used during pregnancy only if the potential benefit justifies the potential risk to the fetus.
Nursing Mothers: Based on determinations of levocabastine in breast milk after ophthalmic administration of the drug to one nursing woman, it was calculated that the daily dose of levocabastine in the infant was about 0.5 μg.
Pediatric Use: Safety and effectiveness in children below the age of 12 have not been established.
Adverse Reactions: The most frequent adverse experiences reported with the use of LIVOSTIN™ 0.05% (levocabastine hydrochloride ophthalmic suspension) were mild, transient stinging and burning (15%) and headache (5%).
Other adverse experiences which have been reported in approximately 1–3% of patients treated with LIVOSTIN™ were visual disturbances, dry mouth, fatigue, pharyngitis, eye pain/dryness, somnolence, red eyes, lacrimation/discharge, cough, nausea, rash/erythema, eyelid edema, and dyspnea.
Dosage and Administration: SHAKE WELL BEFORE USING. The usual dose is one drop instilled in affected eyes four times per day. Treatment may be continued for up to 2 weeks.
How Supplied: LIVOSTIN™ 0.05% (levocabastine hydrochloride ophthalmic suspension), 2.5 mL and 5 mL, is provided in white, polyethylene dropper tip squeeze bottles.
Keep tightly closed when not is use.
Do not use if the suspension has discolored.
Store at controlled room temperature 15° to 30°C (59° to 86°F).
Protect from freezing.
NDC 0058-2610-10 (10 mL)
NDC 0058-2610-05 (5.0 mL)
NDC 0058-2610-03 (2.5 mL)
Federal law prohibits dispensing without prescription.
Levocabastine hydrochloride is an original product of Janssen Pharmaceutica Inc.
Iolab
a Johnson & Johnson Company
IOLAB Corporation 6248-B
Claremont, California 91711
Revised: June 1994
Shown in Product Identification Guide, page 104

Continued on next page

Information on IOLAB products listed on these pages is the full prescribing information from package inserts effective in June 1994. For information concerning all IOLAB products, please call 1-909-624-2020.

IOLAB Corporation—Cont.

MIOCHOL®-E ℞
(Acetylcholine Chloride)
1:100 Intraocular
with Electrolyte Diluent

Description: MIOCHOL®-E (acetylcholine chloride) is a parasympathomimetic preparation for intraocular use packaged in a vial of two compartments; the lower chamber containing acetylcholine chloride 20 mg and mannitol 56 mg; the upper chamber containing 2 mL of a modified diluent of sodium chloride, potassium chloride, magnesium chloride hexahydrate, calcium chloride dihydrate and sterile water for injection.
The reconstituted liquid will be a sterile isotonic solution (275–330 milliosmoles/Kg) containing 20 mg acetylcholine chloride (1:100 solution) and 2.8% mannitol. The pH range is 5.0–8.2. Mannitol is used in the process of lyophilizing acetylcholine chloride, and is not considered an active ingredient.
The chemical name for acetylcholine chloride, $C_7H_{16}ClNO_2$, is Ethanaminium, 2-(acetyloxy)-*N,N,N*-trimethyl-, chloride and is represented by the following chemical structure:

$$CH_3\overset{O}{\overset{\|}{C}}O(CH_2)_2N^+(CH_3)_3\ Cl^-$$

Clinical Pharmacology: Acetylcholine is a naturally occurring neurohormone which mediates nerve impulse transmission at all cholinergic sites involving somatic and autonomic nerves. After release from the nerve ending, acetylcholine is rapidly inactivated by the enzyme acetylcholinesterase by hydrolysis to acetic acid and choline.
Direct application of acetylcholine to the iris will cause rapid miosis of short duration. Topical ocular instillation of acetylcholine to the intact eye causes no discernible response as cholinesterase destroys the molecule more rapidly than it can penetrate the cornea.
Indications and Usage: To obtain miosis of the iris in seconds after delivery of the lens in cataract surgery, in penetrating keratoplasty, iridectomy and other anterior segment surgery where rapid miosis may be required.
Contraindications: None known.
Warnings: DO NOT GAS STERILIZE. If blister or peelable backing is damaged or broken, sterility of the enclosed bottle cannot be assured. Open under aseptic conditions only.
Precautions: General: In the reconstitution of the solution, as described under Directions for Using Univial, if the center rubber plug seal in the univial does not go down or is down, do not use the vial.
If miosis is to be obtained quickly with MIOCHOL-E, anatomical hindrances to miosis, such as anterior or posterior synechiae, must be released, prior to administration of MIOCHOL-E. During cataract surgery, use MIOCHOL-E only after delivery of the lens.
Aqueous solutions of acetylcholine chloride are unstable. Prepare solution immediately before use. Do not use solution which is not clear and colorless. Discard any solution that has not been used.
Drug Interactions: Although clinical studies with acetylcholine chloride and animal studies with acetylcholine or carbachol revealed no interference, and there is no known pharmacological basis for an interaction, there have been reports that acetylcholine chloride and carbachol have been ineffective when used in patients treated with topical nonsteroidal anti-inflammatory agents.
Pediatric Use: Safety and effectiveness in children have not been established.
Adverse Reactions: Infrequent cases of corneal edema, corneal clouding, and corneal decompensation have been reported with the use of intraocular acetylcholine.
Adverse reactions have been reported rarely which are indicative of systemic absorption. These include bradycardia, hypotension, flushing, breathing difficulties and sweating.
Overdosage: Atropine sulfate (0.5 to 1 mg) should be given intramuscularly or intravenously and should be readily available to counteract possible overdosage. Epinephrine (0.1 to 1 mg subcutaneously) is also of value in overcoming severe cardiovascular or bronchoconstrictor responses.
Dosage and Administration: With a new needle of sturdy gauge, 18–20, draw all the solution into a dry, sterile syringe. Replace needle with a suitable atraumatic cannulae for intraocular irrigation.
The MIOCHOL-E solution is instilled into the anterior chamber before or after securing one or more sutures. Instillation should be gentle and parallel to the iris face and tangential to pupil border.
If there are no mechanical hindrances, the pupil starts to constrict in seconds and the peripheral iris is drawn away from the angle of the anterior chamber. Any anatomical hindrance to miosis must be released to permit the desired effect of the drug. In most cases, 0.5 to 2 mL produces satisfactory miosis.
In cataract surgery, use MICHOL-E only after delivery of the lens.
Aqueous solutions of acetylcholine chloride are unstable. Prepare solution immediately before use. Do not use solution which is not clear and colorless. Discard any solution that has not been used.

DIRECTIONS FOR USING THE UNIVIAL: STERILE UNLESS PACKAGE OPEN OR BROKEN

1. Inspect univial while inside unopened blister. Diluent must be in upper chamber.
2. Peel open blister.
3. Aseptically transfer univial to sterile field. Maintain sterility of outer container during preparation of solution.
4. Immediately before use, give plunger-stopper a quarter turn and press to force diluent and center plug into lower chamber.
5. Shake gently to dissolve drug.
6. Discard univial and any unused solution.

How Supplied:
Miochol-E with IOCARE® Steri-Tags™: **NDC** 0058-2772-52
One Miochol-E 2 mL sterile univial
One pack IOCARE Steri-Tags sterile labels
Miochol-E System Pak™: **NDC** 0058-2775-53
One Miochol-E 2 mL sterile univial
One pack IOCARE Steri-Tags sterile labels
One B-D® 3 mL sterile syringe
One Dynagard™ 0.2 micron sterile filter
Store at controlled room temperature 15°–30°C (59°–86°F).
KEEP FROM FREEZING
Caution: Federal law prohibits dispensing without prescription.
IOLAB®
a Johnson & Johnson Company
IOLAB Corporation 6245-A
Claremont, California 91711
Revised: April 1993
Shown in Product Identification Guide, page 104

PILOCAR® ℞
[*pī 'lō-car "*]
(pilocarpine hydrochloride)
Ophthalmic Solution

Description: PILOCAR® (pilocarpine hydrochloride) ophthalmic solution is a sterile solution for ophthalmic administration having the following composition:
Plastic Squeeze Bottle
Pilocarpine Hydrochloride ....5, 10, 20, 30, 40, or 60mg/mL
(cholinergic/parasympathomimetic)
in a buffered solution of boric acid, potassium chloride, hydroxypropylmethyl cellulose, sodium carbonate, edetate disodium and purified water, preserved with benzalkonium chloride.
Dropperettes® Applicator
Pilocarpine Hydrochloride ....10, 20 or 40mg/mL
(cholinergic/parasympathomimetic)
in an isotonic, buffered solution of boric acid, potassium chloride, sodium carbonate and purified water, preserved with benzalkonium chloride.
The chemical name is 2(3H)-Furanone, 3-ethyldihydro -4- [(1-methyl -1H- imidazol-5-yl) methyl]-, monohydrochloride, (3S-cis)-.
It has the following structure:

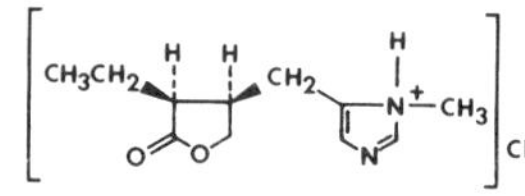

Clinical Pharmacology: Pilocarpine is a direct acting cholinergic (parasympathomimetic) agent causing pupillary constriction and reduction of intraocular pressure.
Indications and Usage: PILOCAR® ophthalmic solution is indicated for the treatment of primary open-angle glaucoma and also to lower intraocular pressure prior to surgery for acute angle-closure glaucoma. It may be used in combination with other miotics, beta adrenergic blocking agents, carbonic anhydrase inhibitors, hyperosmotic agents, or epinephrine.
Contraindications: When constriction is undesirable such as in acute iritis and in persons hypersensitive to one or more of the components of this preparation.
Precautions: The pilocarpine-induced miosis may cause difficulty in dark adaptation. The patient should exercise caution when involved in night driving or other hazardous activities in poor light.
Not for internal use. To prevent contaminating the dropper tip and solution, care should be taken not to touch the eyelids or surrounding areas with the dropper tip of the bottle.
Carcinogenesis, Mutagenesis, Impairment of Fertility: There have been no long-term studies done using pilocarpine in animals to evaluate carcinogenic potential.
Pregnancy: Pregnancy Category C. Animal reproduction studies have not been conducted with pilocarpine. It is also not known whether pilocarpine can cause fetal harm when administered to a pregnant woman or can affect reproduction capacity. Pilocarpine should be given to a pregnant woman only if clearly needed.
Nursing Mothers: It is not known whether this drug is excreted in human milk. Because many drugs are excreted in human milk, caution should be exercised when pilocarpine is administered to a nursing woman.
Adverse Reactions: Ocular: Ciliary spasm, conjunctival vascular congestion, temporal or supraorbital headache, lacrimation, and induced myopia may occur. This is especially true in younger individuals who have recently started administration. Reduced visual acuity in poor illumination is frequently experienced by older individuals and individuals with lens opacity. Miotic agents may also cause **retinal detachment**; thus, care should be exercised with all miotic therapy especially in young myopic patients. Lens opacity may occur with prolonged use of pilocarpine.
Systemic: Systemic reactions following topical administration, although extremely rare, have included hypertension, tachycardia, bronchiolar spasm, pulmonary edema, salivation, sweating, nausea, vomiting, and diarrhea.

Dosage and Administration: The initial dose is one or two drops. This may be repeated up to six times daily. The frequency of instillation and concentration of PILOCAR® ophthalmic solution are determined by the severity of the glaucoma and miotic response of the patient.

During acute phases, the miotic must be instilled into the unaffected eye to prevent an attack of angle-closure glaucoma.

How Supplied: 0.5%, 1%, 2%, 3%, 4%, and 6% solution: in 15mL plastic dropper-tip squeeze bottles.

0.5%, 1%, 2%, 3%, 4%, and 6% solution: in a Twin Pack of 2 × 15mL plastic dropper-tip squeeze bottles.

1%, 2%, and 4%: 1mL DROPPERETTES® Applicators package of 12.

Keep bottle tightly closed when not in use.

Caution: Federal law prohibits dispensing without prescription.

Shown in Product Identification Guide, page 104

VASOCIDIN® OPHTHALMIC OINTMENT ℞

[vas 'o-si-din]

(sulfacetamide sodium and prednisolone acetate)

Ophthalmic Ointment, USP

Description: VASOCIDIN is a sterile topical ophthalmic ointment combining an antibacterial and a corticosteroid which has the following composition:

Sulfacetamide Sodium .... 100 mg/g
(bacteriostatic antibacterial)
Prednisolone Acetate .... 5 mg/g
(corticosteroid/anti-inflammatory)

in a base containing white petrolatum and mineral oil.

The chemical name for sulfacetamide sodium is *N*-sulfanilylacetamide monosodium salt monohydrate.

The chemical name for prednisolone acetate is 11*β*, 17, 21-trihydroxypregna-1, 4-diene-3, 20-dione, 21-acetate.

They have the following chemical structures:

Sulfacetamide Sodium

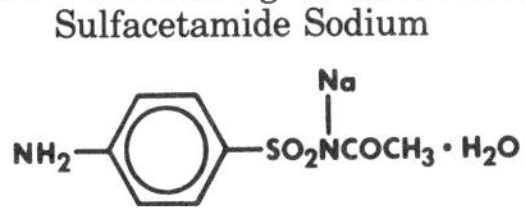

Prednisolone Acetate

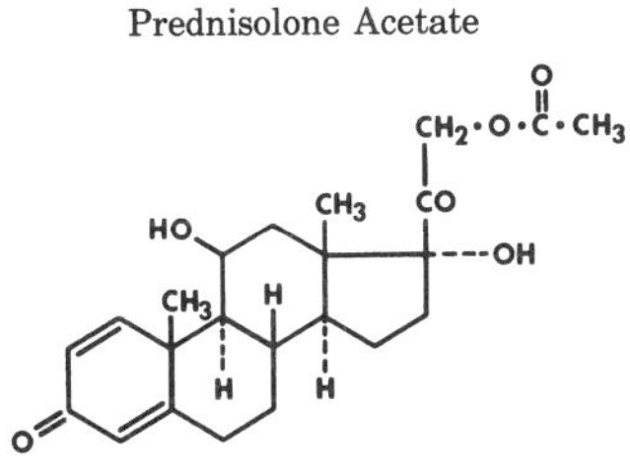

Clinical Pharmacology: Corticosteroids suppress the inflammatory response to a variety of agents and they probably delay or slow healing. Since corticosteroids may inhibit the body's defense mechanism against infection, a concomitant antibacterial drug may be used when this inhibition is considered to be clinically significant in a particular case.

When a decision to administer both a corticosteroid and an antibacterial is made, the administration of such drugs in combination has the advantage of greater patient compliance and convenience with the added assurance that the appropriate dosage of both drugs is administered, plus assured compatibility of ingredients when both types of drugs are in the same formulation and, particularly, that the correct volume of drug is delivered and retained.

The relative potency of corticosteroids depends on the molecular structure, concentration and release from the vehicle.

Microbiology: Sulfacetamide exerts a bacteriostatic effect against susceptible bacteria by restricting the synthesis of folic acid required for growth through competition with p-aminobenzoic acid.

Some strains of these bacteria may be resistant to sulfacetamide or resistant strains may emerge *in vivo.*

The anti-infective component in VASOCIDIN Ophthalmic Ointment is included to provide action against specific organisms susceptible to it. Sulfacetamide sodium is active *in vitro* against susceptible strains of the following microorganisms: *Escherichia coli, Staphylococcus aureus, Streptococcus pneumoniae, Streptococcus* (viridans group), *Haemophilus influenzae, Klebsiella/Enterobacter* species. This product does not provide adequate coverage against: *Neisseria* species, *Pseudomonas* species, *Serratia marcescens* (SEE INDICATIONS AND USAGE).

Indications and Usage: VASOCIDIN Ophthalmic Ointment is indicated for steroid-responsive inflammatory ocular conditions for which a corticosteroid is indicated and where superficial bacterial ocular infection or a risk of bacterial ocular infection exists.

Ocular corticosteroids are indicated in inflammatory conditions of the palpebral and bulbar conjunctiva, cornea, and anterior segment of the globe where the inherent risk of corticosteroid use in certain infective conjunctivitides is accepted to obtain diminution in edema and inflammation. They are also indicated in chronic anterior uveitis and corneal injury from chemical, radiation or thermal burns or penetration of foreign bodies.

The use of a combination drug with an anti-infective component is indicated where the risk of superficial ocular infection is high or where there is an expectation that potentially dangerous numbers of bacteria will be present in the eye.

The particular antibacterial drug in this product is active against the following common bacterial eye pathogens: *Escherichia coli, Staphylococcus aureus, Streptococcus pneumoniae, Streptococcus* (viridans group), *Haemophilus influenzae, Klebsiella* species, and *Enterobacter* species.

The product does not provide adequate coverage against: *Neisseria* species, *Pseudomonas* species, *Serratia marcescens.*

A significant percentage of staphylococcal isolates are completely resistant to sulfa drugs.

Contraindications: VASOCIDIN Ophthalmic Ointment is contraindicated in most viral diseases of the cornea and conjunctiva including epithelial herpes simplex keratitis (dendritic keratitis), vaccinia, and varicella, and also in mycobacterial infection of the eye and fungal diseases of ocular structures. VASOCIDIN is also contraindicated in individuals with known or suspected hypersensitivity to any of the ingredients of this preparation, to other sulfonamides and to other corticosteroids. (SEE WARNINGS.) (Hypersensitivity to the antimicrobial component occurs at a higher rate than for other components.)

Warnings: Prolonged use of corticosteroids may result in ocular hypertension/glaucoma with damage to the optic nerve, defects in visual acuity and fields of vision, and in posterior subcapsular cataract formation.

Acute anterior uveitis may occur in susceptible individuals, primarily Blacks.

Prolonged use of VASOCIDIN may suppress the host response and thus increase the hazard of secondary ocular infection. In those diseases causing thinning of the cornea or sclera, perforations have been known to occur with the use of topical corticosteroids. In acute purulent conditions of the eye, corticosteroids may mask infection or enhance existing infection.

If this product is used for 10 days or longer, intraocular pressure should be routinely monitored even though it may be difficult in children and uncooperative patients. Corticosteroids should be used with caution in the presence of glaucoma. Intraocular pressure should be checked frequently.

A significant percentage of staphylococcal isolates are completely resistant to sulfonamides.

The use of steroids after cataract surgery may delay healing and increase the incidence of filtering blebs.

The use of ocular corticosteroids may prolong the course and may exacerbate the severity of many viral infections of the eye (including herpes simplex). Employment of a corticosteroid medication in the treatment of herpes simplex requires great caution.

Topical steroids are not effective in mustard gas keratitis and Sjögren's keratoconjunctivitis.

Fatalities have occurred, although rarely, due to severe reactions to sulfonamides including Stevens-Johnson syndrome, toxic epidermal necrolysis, fulminant hepatic necrosis, agranulocytosis, aplastic anemia, and other blood dyscrasias. Sensitizations may recur when a sulfonamide is readministered, irrespective of the route of administration. If signs of hypersensitivity or other serious reactions occur, discontinue use of this preparation.

Cross-sensitivity among corticosteroids has been demonstrated (SEE ADVERSE REACTIONS).

Precautions: General: The initial prescription and renewal of the medication order beyond 8 g of VASOCIDIN Ophthalmic Ointment should be made by a physician only after examination of the patient with the aid of magnification, such as slit lamp biomicroscopy and, where appropriate, fluorescein staining. If signs and symptoms fail to improve after two days, the patient should be re-evaluated.

The possiblity of fungal infections of the cornea should be considered after prolonged corticosteroid dosing. Use with caution in patients with severe dry eye. Fungal cultures should be taken when appropriate.

The p-aminobenzoic acid present in purulent exudates competes with sulfonamides and can reduce their effectiveness.

Ophthalmic ointments may retard corneal healing.

Information for Patients: If inflammation or pain persists longer than 48 hours or becomes aggravated, the patient should be advised to discontinue use of the medication and consult a physician (SEE WARNINGS).

This product is sterile when packaged. To prevent contamination, care should be taken to avoid touching the tube tip to eyelids or to any other surface. The use of this tube by more than one person may spread infection. Keep tube tightly closed when not in use. Protect from light. Keep out of the reach of children.

Laboratory Tests: Eyelid cultures and tests to determine the susceptibility of organisms to sulfacetamide may be indicated if signs and symptoms persist or recur in spite of the recommended course of treatment with VASOCIDIN Ophthalmic Ointment.

Drug Interactions: VASOCIDIN Ophthalmic Ointment is incompatible with silver preparations. Local anesthetics related to p-aminoben-

Continued on next page

Information on IOLAB products listed on these pages is the full prescribing information from package inserts effective in June 1994. For information concerning all IOLAB products, please call 1-909-624-2020.

IOLAB Corporation—Cont.

zoic acid may antagonize the action of the sulfonamides.

Carcinogenesis, Mutagenesis, Impairment of Fertility: Prednisolone has been reported to be noncarcinogenic. Long-term animal studies for carcinogenic potential have not been performed with sulfacetamide.

One author detected chromosomal nondisjunction in the yeast *Saccharomyces cerevisiae* following application of sulfacetamide sodium. The signficance of this finding to topical ophthalmic use of sulfacetamide sodium in the human is unknown.

Mutagenic studies with prednisolone have been negative. Studies on reproduction and fertility have not been performed with sulfacetamide. A long-term chronic toxicity study in dogs showed that high oral doses of prednisolone prevented estrus. A decrease in fertility was seen in male and female rats that were mated following oral dosing with another glucocorticosteroid.

Pregnancy: Teratogenic Effects: Pregnancy Category C. Animal reproduction studies have not been conducted with sulfacetamide sodium. Prednisolone has been shown to be teratogenic in rabbits, hamsters, and mice. In mice, prednisolone has been shown to be teratogenic when given in doses 1 to 10 times the human ocular dose. Dexamethasone, hydrocortisone and prednisolone were ocularly applied to both eyes of pregnant mice five times per day on days 10 through 13 of gestation. A significant increase in the incidence of cleft palate was observed in the fetuses of the treated mice. There are no adequate well-controlled studies in pregnant women dosed with corticosteroids.

Kernicterus may be precipitated in infants by sulfonamides being given systemically during the third trimester of pregnancy. It is not known whether sulfacetamide sodium can cause fetal harm when administered to a pregnant woman or whether it can affect reproductive capacity.

VASOCIDIN Ophthalmic Ointment should be used during pregnancy only if the potential benefit justifies the potential risk to the fetus.

Nursing Mothers: It is not known whether topical administration of corticosteroids could result in sufficient systemic absorption to produce detectable quantities in human milk. Systemically administered corticosteroids appear in human milk and could suppress growth, interfere with endogenous corticosteroid production, or cause other untoward effects. Systemically administered sulfonamides are capable of producing kernicterus in infants of lactating women. Because of the potential for serious adverse reactions in nursing infants from VASOCIDIN, a decision should be made whether to discontinue nursing or to discontinue the medication.

Pediatric Use: Safety and effectiveness in children below the age of six have not been established.

Adverse Reactions: Adverse reactions have occurred with corticosteroid/antibacterial combination drugs which can be attributed to the corticosteroid component, the antibacterial component, or the combination. Exact incidence figures are not available since no denominator of treated patients is available.

Reactions occurring most often from the presence of the antibacterial ingredient are allergic sensitizations. Fatalities have occurred, although rarely, due to severe reactions to sulfonamides including Stevens-Johnson syndrome, toxic epidermal necrolysis, fulminant hepatic necrosis, agranulocytosis, aplastic anemia, and other blood dyscrasias (SEE WARNINGS).

Sulfacetamide sodium may cause local irritation.

The reactions due to the corticosteroid component in decreasing order of frequency are: elevation of intraocular pressure (IOP) with possible development of glaucoma and infrequent optic nerve damage, posterior subcapsular cataract formation, and delayed wound healing.

Although systemic effects are extremely uncommon, there have been rare occurrences of systemic hypercorticoidism after use of topical steroids.

Corticosteroid-containing preparations can also cause acute anterior uveitis or perforation of the globe. Mydriasis, loss of accommodation and ptosis have occasionally been reported following local use of corticosteroids.

Secondary Infection: The development of secondary infection has occurred after use of combinations containing corticosteroids and antibacterials. Fungal and viral infections of the cornea are particularly prone to develop coincidentally with long-term applications of corticosteroid. The possiblity of fungal invasion must be considered in any persistent corneal ulceration where corticosteroid treatment has been used.

Secondary bacterial ocular infection following suppression of host responses also occurs.

Dosage and Administration: VASOCIDIN Ophthalmic Ointment: A small amount, approximately 1/2 inch ribbon of ointment, should be applied in the conjunctival sac three or four times daily and once or twice at night. Not more than 8 g should be prescribed initially.

The dosing of VASOCIDIN may be reduced, but care should be taken not to discontinue therapy prematurely. In chronic conditions, withdrawal of treatment should be carried out by gradually decreasing the frequency of application

If signs and symptoms fail to improve after two days, the patient should be re-evaluated (SEE PRECAUTIONS).

How Supplied: VASOCIDIN Ophthalmic Ointment: 3.5 gm (1/8 oz) sterile tube. NDC 0058-3095-01

To be dispensed only in original, unopened container. Store at controlled room temperature 15°–30°C (59°–86°F).

KEEP OUT OF REACH OF CHILDREN.

Caution: Federal law prohibits dispensing without prescription.

Mfg. By:
Altana Inc.
Melville, NY 11747
Mfg. for:
IOLAB®
a Johnson & Johnson Company
IOLAB Corporation 6085-H
Claremont, California 91711

Revised: March 1992

VASOCIDIN® ℞

(sulfacetamide sodium-prednisolone sodium phosphate)
Ophthalmic Solution, USP

Description: VASOCIDIN is a sterile topical ophthalmic solution combining an anti-infective and an adrenocortical steroid having the following composition:

Sulfacetamide Sodium ....100 mg/mL
(bacteriostatic antibacterial)
Prednisolone Sodium Phosphate ..2.5 mg/mL
(equivalent to Prednisolone Phosphate 2.3 mg/mL)
(adrenocortical steroid/anti-inflammatory)

In a solution containing edetate disodium, poloxamer 407, boric acid, purified water, preserved with thimerosal 0.1 mg/mL. Hydrochloric acid and/or sodium hydroxide added to adjust pH.

The chemical name for sulfacetamide sodium is Acetamide, N-[(4-aminophenyl) sulfonyl]-, monosodium salt, monohydrate.

The chemical name for prednisolone sodium phosphate is 11β, 17, 21-trihydroxypregna-1,4-diene-3,20-dione, 21-(disodium phosphate).

They have the following chemical structures:

Sulfacetamide Sodium

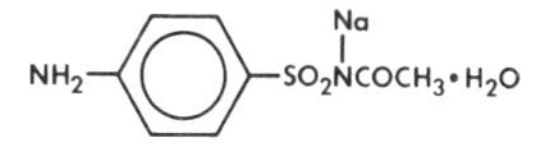

Prednisolone Sodium Phosphate

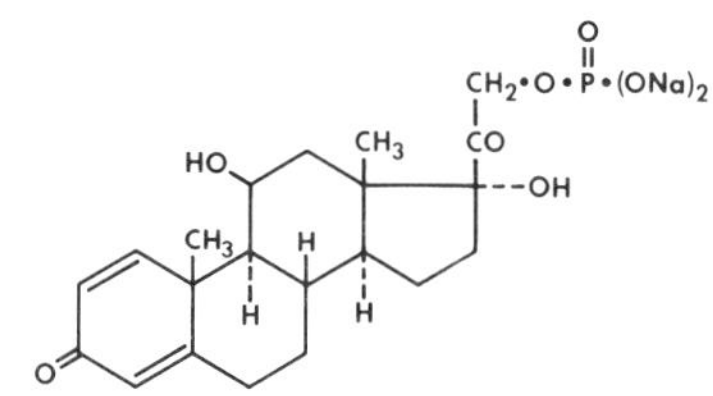

Clinical Pharmacology: Corticosteroids suppress the inflammatory response to a variety of agents and they probably delay or slow healing. Since corticosteroids may inhibit the body's defense mechanism against infection, a concomitant antimicrobial drug may be used when this inhibition is considered to be clinically significant in a particular case.

When a decision to administer both a corticoid and an antimicrobial is made, the administration of such drugs in combination has the advantage of greater patient compliance and convenience, with the added assurance that the appropriate dosage of both drugs is administered, plus assured compatibility of ingredients when both types of drugs are in the same formulation and, particularly, that the correct volume of drug is delivered and retained.

The relative potency of corticosteroids depends on the molecular structure, concentration, and release from the vehicle.

Microbiology: Sulfacetamide sodium exerts a bacteriostatic effect against susceptible bacteria by restricting the synthesis of folic acid required for growth through competition with p-aminobenzoic acid.

Some strains of bacteria may be resistant to sulfacetamide or resistant strains may emerge in vivo.

The anti-infective component in VASOCIDIN Ophthalmic Solution is included to provide action against specific organisms susceptible to it. Sulfacetamide sodium is active in-vitro against susceptible strains of the following microorganisms: *Escherichia coli, Staphylococcus aureus, Streptococcus pneumoniae, Streptococcus (viridans group), Haemophilus influenzae, Klebsiella* species, and *Enterobacter* species. SEE INDICATIONS AND USAGE SECTION BELOW.

Indications and Usage: VASOCIDIN is indicated for corticosteriod-responsive inflammatory ocular conditions for which a corticosteroid is indicated and where superficial bacterial ocular infection or a risk of bacterial ocular infection exists.

Ocular corticosteroids are indicated in inflammatory conditions of the palpebral and bulbar conjunctiva, cornea, and anterior segment of the globe where the inherent risk of corticosteroid use in certain infective conjunctivitides is accepted to obtain a diminution in edema and inflammation. They are also indicated in chronic anterior uveitis and corneal injury from chemical, radiation, or thermal burns or penetration of foreign bodies.

The use of a combination drug with an anti-infective component is indicated where the risk of superficial ocular infection is high or where there is an expectation that potentially dangerous numbers of bacteria will be present in the eye.

The particular anti-infective drug in this product is active against the following common bacterial eye pathogens: *Escherichia coli, Staphylococcus aureus, Streptococcus pneumoniae, Streptococcus (viridans group), Haemophilus influenzae, Klebsiella* species, and *Enterobacter* species.

This product does not provide adequate coverage against: *Neisseria* species, *Serratia marcescens.*

A significant percentage of staphylococcal isolates are completely resistant to sulfa drugs.

Contraindications: VASOCIDIN Ophthalmic Solution is contraindicated in most viral diseases of the cornea and conjunctiva including epithelial herpes simplex keratitis (dendritic keratitis), vaccinia, and varicella, and also in mycobacterial infection of the eye and fungal diseases of ocular structures. VASOCIDIN is also contraindicated in individuals with known or suspected hypersensitivity to any of the ingredients of this preparation, to other sulfonamides, or to other corticosteroids. (Hypersensitivity to the antimicrobial components occurs at a higher rate than for other components).

Warnings: NOT FOR INJECTION INTO THE EYE. Prolonged use of corticosteroids may result in ocular hypertension/glaucoma with damage to the optic nerve, defects in visual acuity and fields of vision, and in posterior subcapsular cataract formation.

Acute anterior uveitis may occur in susceptible individuals, primarily Blacks.

Prolonged use of VASOCIDIN may suppress the host response and thus increase the hazard of secondary ocular infections. In those diseases causing thinning of the cornea or sclera, perforations have been known to occur with the use of topical corticosteroids. In acute purulent conditions of the eye, corticosteroids may mask infection or enhance existing infection.

If this product is used for 10 days or longer, intraocular pressure should be routinely monitored even though it may be difficult in children and uncooperative patients. Corticosteroids should be used with caution in the presence of glaucoma. Intraocular pressure should be checked frequently.

The use of corticosteroids after cataract surgery may delay healing and increase the incidence of filtering blebs.

The use of ocular corticosteroids may prolong the course and may exacerbate the severity of many viral infections of the eye (including herpes simplex). Employment of corticosteroids medication in the treatment of herpes simplex requires great caution.

A significant percentage of staphylococcal isolates are completely resistant to sulfonamides.

Topical corticosteroids are not effective in mustard gas keratitis and Sjögren's keratoconjunctivitis.

Fatalities have occurred, although rarely, due to severe reactions to sulfonamides including Stevens-Johnson syndrome, toxic epidermal necrolysis, fulminant hepatic necrosis, agranulocytosis, aplastic anemia, and other blood dyscrasias. Sensitizations may recur when a sulfonamide is readministered irrespective of the route of administration. If signs of hypersensitivity or other serious reactions occur, discontinue use of this preparation. Cross-sensitivity among corticosteroids have been demonstrated (see ADVERSE REACTIONS).

Do not administer this product to patients who are sensitive/allergic to thimerosal or any other mercury-containing ingredient.

Precautions: General: The initial prescription and renewal of the medication order beyond 20 mL of VASOCIDIN Ophthalmic Solution should be made by a physician only after examination of the patient with the aid of magnification, such as slit-lamp biomicroscopy and, where appropriate, fluorescein staining. If signs and symptoms fail to improve after two days, the patient should return to the office for further evaluation.

The possibility of fungal infections of the cornea should be considered after prolonged corticosteroid dosing. Fungal cultures should be taken when appropriate.

The p-aminobenzoic acid present in purulent exudates competes with sulfonamides and can reduce their effectiveness.

Sulfonamide solutions darken on prolonged standing and exposure to heat and light. Do not use if solution has darkened. Yellowing does not affect activity.

Information to the Patient: If inflammation or pain persists longer than 48 hours or becomes aggravated, the patient should be advised to discontinue use of the medication and consult a physician.

This product is sterile when packaged. To prevent contamination, care should be taken to avoid touching dropper tip to eyelids or to any other surface. The use of this dispenser by more than one person may spread infection. Keep bottle tightly closed when not in use. Protect from light. Sulfonamide solutions darken on prolonged standing and exposure to heat and light. Do not use if solution has darkened. Yellowing does not affect activity. Keep out of the reach of children.

Laboratory Tests: Eyelid cultures and tests to determine the susceptibility of organisms to sulfacetamide may be indicated if signs and symptoms persist or recur in spite of the recommended course of treatment with VASOCIDIN Ophthalmic Solution.

Drug Interactions: VASOCIDIN Ophthalmic Solution is incompatible with silver preparations. Local anesthetics related to p-aminobenzoic acid may antagonize the action of the sulfonamides.

Carcinogenesis, Mutagenesis, and Impairment of Fertility: Prednisolone has been reported to be noncarcinogenic. Long-term animal studies for carcinogenic potential have not been performed with prednisolone or sulfacetamide. One author detected chromosomal nondisjunction in the yeast *Saccharomyces cerevisiae* following application of sulfacetamide sodium. The significance of this finding to the topical ophthalmic use of sulfacetamide sodium in the human is unknown.

Mutagenic studies with prednisolone have been negative. Studies on reproduction and fertility have not been performed with sulfacetamide. A long-term chronic toxicity study in dogs showed that high oral doses of prednisolone prevented estrus. A decrease in fertility was seen in male and female rats that were mated following oral dosing with another glucocorticosteroid.

Pregnancy: Teratogenic effects. Pregnancy Category C. Prednisolone has been shown to be teratogenic in rabbits, hamsters, and mice. In mice, prednisolone has been shown to be teratogenic when given in doses 1 to 10 times the human ocular dose. Dexamethasone, hydrocortisone and prednisolone were ocularly applied to both eyes of pregnant mice five times per day on days 10 through 13 of gestation. A significant increase in the incidence of cleft palate was observed in the fetuses of the treated mice. There are no adequate, well-controlled studies in pregnant women dosed with corticosteroids.

Kernicterus may be precipitated in infants by sulfonamides given systemically during the third trimester of pregnancy. It is not known whether sulfacetamide sodium can cause fetal harm when administered to a pregnant woman or whether it can affect reproductive capacity. VASOCIDIN Ophthalmic Solution should be used during pregnancy only if the potential benefit justifies the potential risk to the fetus.

Nursing Mothers: It is not known whether topical administration of corticosteroids could result in sufficient systemic absorption to produce detectable quantities in human milk. Systemically administered corticosteroids appear in human milk and could suppress growth, interfere with endogenous corticosteroid production, or cause other untoward effects. Systemically administered sulfonamides are capable of producing kernicterus in infants of lactating women. Because of the potential for serious adverse reactions in nursing infants from VASOCIDIN, a decision should be made whether to discontinue nursing or to discontinue the medication.

Pediatric Use: Safety and effectiveness in children below the age of six years have not been established.

Adverse Reactions: Adverse reactions have occurred with corticosteroids/anti-infective combination drugs which can be attributed to the corticosteroids component, the anti-infective component, or the combination. Exact incidence figures are not available since no denominator of treated patients is available.

Reactions occurring most often from the presence of the anti-infective ingredient are allergic sensitizations. Fatalities have occurred, although rarely, due to severe reactions to sulfonamides including Stevens-Johnson syndrome, toxic epidermal necrolysis, fulminant hepatic necrosis, agranulocytosis, aplastic anemia, and other blood dyscrasias (see WARNINGS).

Sulfacetamide sodium may cause local irritation.

The reactions due to the corticosteroid component in decreasing order of frequency are: elevation of intraocular pressure (IOP) with possible development of glaucoma, and infrequent optic nerve damage; posterior subcapsular cataract formation; and delayed wound healing.

Although systemic effects are extremely uncommon, there have been rare occurrences of systemic hypercorticoidism after use of topical corticosteroids.

Corticosteroid-containing preparations can also cause acute anterior uveitis or perforation of the globe. Mydriasis, loss of accommodation and ptosis have occasionally been reported following local use of corticosteroids.

Secondary Infection: The development of secondary infection has occurred after use of combinations containing corticosteroids and antimicrobials. Fungal and viral infections of the cornea are particularly prone to develop coincidentally with long-term applications of corticosteroid. The possibility of fungal invasion must be considered in any persistent corneal ulceration where corticosteroid treatment has been used.

Secondary bacterial ocular infection following suppression of host responses also occurs.

Dosage and Administration: Instill two drops of VASODICIN Ophthalmic Solution topically in the eye(s) every four hours.

Not more than 20 mL should be prescribed initially. If signs and symptoms fail to improve after two days, patients should be re-evaluated (see PRECAUTIONS).

Care should be taken not to discontinue therapy prematurely. In chronic conditions, withdrawal of treatment should be carried out by gradually decreasing the frequency of application.

How Supplied: VASOCIDIN Ophthalmic Solution: 5 mL NDC-0058-2887-05, and 10 mL

Continued on next page

Information on IOLAB products listed on these pages is the full prescribing information from package inserts effective in June 1994. For information concerning all IOLAB products, please call 1-909-624-2020.

IOLAB Corporation—Cont.

NDC-0058-2887-10 dropper-tip plastic squeeze bottles.
To be dispensed only in original, unopened container. Store at controlled room temperature, 15° to 30°C (59° to 86°F). Keep from freezing. PROTECT FROM LIGHT.
Sulfonamide solutions darken on prolonged standing and exposure to heat and light. Do not use if solution has darkened. Yellowing does not affect activity.
KEEP OUT OF REACH OF CHILDREN.
Caution: Federal law prohibits dispensing without prescription.

IOLAB®
a Johnson & Johnson Company
IOLAB Corporation 6032-J
Claremont, California 91711
Revised: January 1992

VASOCON-A® ℞

[vas"o-kon]
(naphazoline hydrochloride-antazoline phosphate)
Ophthalmic Solution

Description: VASOCON-A (naphazoline hydrochloride-antazoline phosphate) is a combination of an antihistamine and a vasoconstrictor prepared as a sterile solution for ophthalmic administration having the following composition:

Naphazoline Hydrochloride ..... 0.5 mg/mL
Antazoline Phosphate .... 5 mg/mL

in a solution containing polyethylene glycol 8000, sodium chloride, polyvinyl alcohol, edetate disodium and purified water, preserved with benzalkonium chloride (0.1 mg/mL). Sodium hydroxide and/or hydrochloric acid added to adjust pH when necessary. It has a pH of 5.5-6.3 and a tonicity of 280-350 mOsm/kg.
The chemical name for naphazoline hydrochloride is 1 H-imidazole,4,5-dihydro-2-(1-naphthalenyl-methyl)-,monohydrochloride.
The chemical name for antazoline phosphate is 1 H-imidazole-2-methanamine,4,5-dihydro-N-phenyl-N-(phenylmethyl)-,phosphate (1:1).
The active ingredients have the following chemical structures:

Naphazoline Hydrochloride

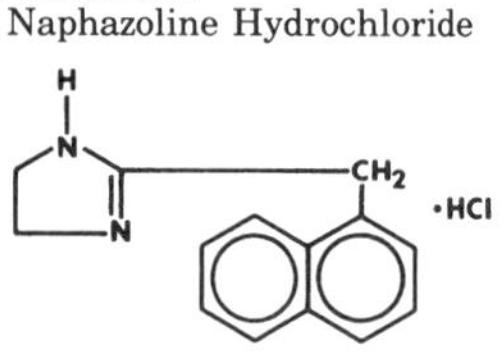

Antazoline Phosphate

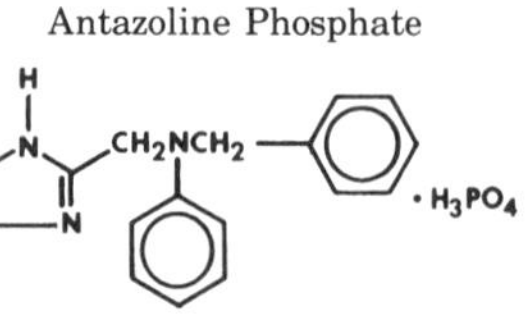

Clinical Pharmacology: VASOCON-A combines the effects of the antihistamine, antazoline, and the vasoconstrictor, naphazoline. Naphazoline hydrochloride is an alpha-sympathetic receptor agonist (sympathomimetic) producing vasoconstriction. Antazoline phosphate is an H_1-receptor antagonist producing antihistaminic effects.
Indications and Usage:
VASOCON-A Ophthalmic Solution is indicated for relief of signs and symptoms of allergic conjunctivitis.
Contraindications: Contraindicated in the presence of an anatomically narrow angle or in narrow angle glaucoma or in persons hypersensitive to one or more of the components of this preparation. VASOCON-A is contraindicated while soft contact lenses are being worn.
Warnings: Patients under therapy with monoamine oxidase (MAO) inhibitors may experience a severe hypertensive crisis if given a sympathomimetic drug. (See PRECAUTIONS)
Use of drugs in this pharmacologic class may cause CNS depression leading to unconsciousness and/or coma. Marked reduction in body temperature may occur in children, especially infants. Patients are advised not to wear contact lenses during treatment with VASOCON-A.
Precautions:
General: Use with caution in the presence of hypertension, cardiovascular abnormalities, hyperglycemia (diabetes), hyperthyroidism, ocular infection or injury and when other medications are being used.
Information to the patient: For topical use only. To prevent contaminating the dropper tip and solution, care should be taken not to touch the eyelids or surrounding areas with the dropper tip of the bottle. Keep bottle tightly closed when not in use. Protect from light. Do not use if the solution has darkened. Patients should be advised to discontinue the drug and consult a physician if relief is not obtained within 48 hours of therapy; if irritation, blurring or redness persists or increases; or if symptoms of systemic absorption occur, i.e., dizziness, headache, nausea, decrease in body temperature or drowsiness.
Overuse of this product may produce increased redness/irritation of the eyes.
Drug Interactions: Concurrent use of maprotiline or tricyclic antidepressants and naphazoline may potentiate the pressor effect of naphazoline. Patients under therapy with MAO inhibitors may experience a severe hypertensive crisis if given a sympathomimetic drug. (See WARNINGS)
Carcinogenesis, Mutagenesis, Impairment of Fertility: There have been no long-term studies done using naphazoline and/or antazoline in animals to evaluate carcinogenic or mutagenic potential.
Pregnancy: Pregnancy Category C. Animal reproduction studies have not been conducted with naphazoline and/or antazoline. It is also not known whether naphazoline and/or antazoline can cause fetal harm when administered to a pregnant woman or can affect reproduction capacity. VASOCON-A Ophthalmic Solution should be given to a pregnant woman only if clearly needed. There are no available data on the effect of the drug on later growth, development, and functional maturation of the child.
Nursing Mothers: It is not known whether naphazoline and/or antazoline are excreted in human milk. Because many drugs are excreted in human milk, caution should be exercised when these drugs are administered to a nursing woman.
Pediatric Use: Safety and effectiveness in children have not been established. (See WARNINGS)
Adverse Reactions:
Ocular: The most frequent complaint with the use of VASOCON-A Ophthalmic Solution is that of mild transient stinging/burning. Other adverse experiences that have been reported with naphazoline and/or antazoline include mydriasis, increased redness, irritation, blurring, punctate keratitis, lacrimation, increased intraocular pressure.
Systemic: Dizziness, headache, nausea, sweating, nervousness, drowsiness, weakness, hypertension, cardiac irregularities and hyperglycemia.
Dosage and Administration: Instill one to two drops in the conjunctival sac(s) every two hours as needed, but not to exceed four times per day.
How Supplied: VASOCON-A Ophthalmic Solution: 15 mL plastic dropper tip squeeze bottles. Keep tightly closed when not in use. Protect from light.
NDC 0058-2880-15
Do not store above 25°C (79°F).
Caution: Federal law prohibits dispensing without prescription.

VASOSULF® ℞

[vas"o-sulf]
(sulfacetamide sodium–phenylephrine hydrochloride)
Ophthalmic Solution

Description: VASOSULF (sulfacetamide sodium-phenylephrine hydrochloride) ophthalmic solution is a sterile solution for ophthalmic administration having the following composition:

Sulfacetamide Sodium 150mg/mL
(bacteriostatic antibacterial)
Phenylephrine Hydrochloride 1.25mg/mL
(sympathomimetic)

in a solution of mono and dibasic sodium phosphate, sodium thiosulfate, poloxamer 188 and purified water, preserved with methylparaben and propylparaben. Hydrochloric acid added to adjust pH when necessary.
The chemical name for sulfacetamide sodium is Acetamide, N-[(4-aminophenyl)sulfonyl]-, monosodium salt, monohydrate.
The chemical name for phenylephrine hydrochloride is Benzenemethanol, 3-hydroxy-α-[(methylamino)-methyl]-, hydrochloride (R)-.
They have the following chemical structures:

Sulfacetamide Sodium

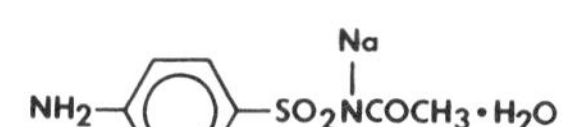

Phenylephrine Hydrochloride

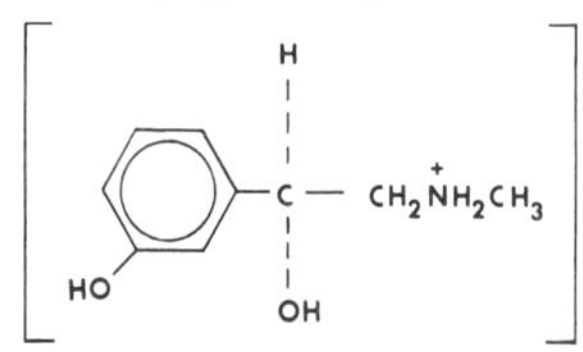

Clinical Pharmacology: Sulfacetamide sodium exerts a bacteriostatic effect against a wide range of gram-positive and gram-negative microorganisms by restricting through competition with p-aminobenzoic acid, the synthesis of folic acid which bacteria require for growth. Phenylephrine hydrochloride is an alpha sympathetic receptor agonist producing vasoconstriction.
Indications and Usage: VASOSULF ophthalmic solution is indicated for the treatment of conjunctivitis, corneal ulcer, and other superficial ocular infections due to susceptible microorganisms, and an adjunctive in systemic sulfonamide therapy of trachoma.
Contraindications: Contraindicated in persons hypersensitive to one or more of the components of this preparation.
Precautions: The solutions are incompatible with silver preparations. Local anesthetics related to p-aminobenzoic acid may antagonize the action of the sulfonamides. Bacteria initially sensitive to sulfonamides may acquire resistance to the drug. Nonsusceptible organisms, including fungi, may proliferate with the use of this preparation. Sulfonamides are inactivated by the p-aminobenzoic acid present in purulent exudates.
If signs of hypersensitivity or other untoward reactions occur, discontinue use of the preparation.

To prevent contaminating the dropper tip and solution, care should be taken not to touch the eyelids or surrounding area with the dropper tip of the bottle. Keep bottle tightly closed when not in use and protect from light. Do not use if the solution has darkened or contains a precipitate.
For topical use only.
Carcinogenesis, Mutagenesis, Impairment of Fertility: There have been no long-term studies done using sulfacetamide and/or phenylephrine in animals to evaluate carcinogenic potential.
Pregnancy: Pregnancy Category C. Animal reproduction studies have not been conducted with sulfacetamide and/or phenylephrine. It is also not known whether sulfacetamide and/or phenylephrine can cause fetal harm when administered to a pregnant woman or can affect reproduction capacity. Sulfacetamide and/or phenylephrine should be given to a pregnant woman only if clearly needed.
Nursing Mothers: It is not known whether these drugs are excreted in human milk. Because many drugs are excreted in human milk, caution should be exercised when sulfacetamide and/or phenylephrine is administered to a nursing woman.
Pediatric Use: Safety and effectiveness in children have not been established.
Adverse Reactions: Headache or browache, blurred vision, local irritation, burning, transient stinging, transient epithelial keratitis, and reactive hyperemia. Sensitization reactions to sulfacetamide sodium may occur, although rarely. Reactions occurring most often from the presence of the anti-infective ingredient are allergic sensitizations. Although hypersensitivity reactions to sulfacetamide sodium are rare, instances of Stevens-Johnson syndrome, systemic lupus erythematosus (in one case producing a fatal outcome), exfoliative dermatitis, toxic epidermal necrolysis, and photosensitivity have been reported following the use of sulfonamide preparations.
Dosage and Administration: Instill one or two drops into lower conjunctival sac every two or three hours during the day, less often at night.
How Supplied: 5mL and 15mL plastic dropper tip squeeze bottles.
NDC 0058-2883-05
NDC 0058-2883-15
Keep tightly closed when not in use. Protect from light.
Store at 15° to 30°C (59° to 86°F).
Caution: Federal law prohibits dispensing without prescription.

Lacrimedics, Inc.
190 N. ARROWHEAD AVE.
SUITE B
RIALTO, CALIFORNIA 92376-9908

COLLAGEN IMPLANTS

Description: Collagen implants, which dissolve in 4–7 days, provide temporary lacrimal occlusion by reducing tear drainage through partial blockage of the horizontal canaliculus.

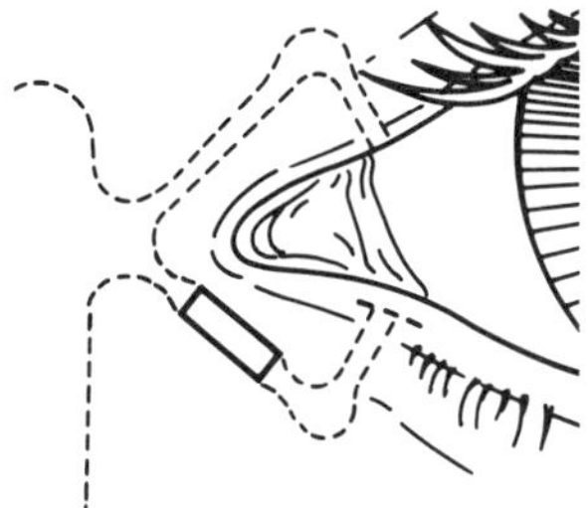

Collagen implants are used as a diagnostic aid to determine the potential effectiveness of long-term lacrimal occlusion (Lacrimal Efficiency Test™) or to provide temporary relief to patients requiring only **short-term treatment.** The implants are inserted using a jewelers forceps. Dilation of the punctum and use of a topical anesthetic is not usually required for insertion. When properly inserted, the implants will not fall out of the punctum or touch the eye at any time, and patients should have no discomfort from the implants. After insertion the implants will swell to nearly twice their original size.
For use as a short-term treatment (4–7 days), begin by taking a thorough patient history including primary and general symptoms (Symptoms Checklist available from Lacrimedics, Inc.) and perform an eye examination. Based upon the results, and the indications listed herein, insert one collagen implant through each of the four puncta. If two implants remain, consider inserting an additional implant through each of the inferior punctum of enhance the efficacy of the treatment.
For use in the Lacrimal Efficiency Test, follow the procedure previously stated and add a two-week follow-up visit. Patients experiencing symptomatic relief during the first week (4–7 days after insertion), whose symptoms return in the second week, indicates that the patient may benefit from long-term lacrimal occlusion using non-dissolvable Herrick Lacrimal Plugs™ (from Lacrimedics, Inc.).
Indications: Dissolvable collagen implants are indicated in patients experiencing dry eye symptoms such as: redness, burning, reflex tearing, itching or foreign body sensation.
Collagen implants may be used after eye surgery to prevent complications due to dry eye, to enhance the effect of ocular medications, and in patients experiencing dry eye-related contact lens discomfort. In each case, collagen implants provide only short-term occulsion.
By Diagnosis: Collagen implants may be used to provide short-term treatment for both dry eye syndrome and for dry eye component of any of the following ocular surface diseases (OSD) including: conjunctivitis, corneal ulcer, pterygium, blepharitis, keratitis, red lid margins, recurrent chalazion, recurrent corneal-erosion, filamentary keratitis, and other external eye diseases.
Contraindications: Tearing secondary to chronic dacryocystitis with mucopurulent discharge; allergy to bovine collagen; inflammation of the eye lid; and/or epiphora.
Patients experiencing epiphora should be evaluated for canalicular obstruction. If patients experience irritation, infection, or epiphora after a collagen implant has been inserted, saline irrigation or probing may be used to expel the implant through the lacrimal sac into the nose and throat.
Packaging and Product Parameters: One box of collagen implants contain 12 sterile packets. Each packet contains six implants made of bovine collagen.
Collagen implants are available in 0.2mm, 0.3mm, 0.4mm, 0.5mm and 0.6mm diameters, each approximately 1.75mm long. The most commonly used sizes are the 0.3mm and 0.4mm diameters.
Important Note: Read the *Practitioner Guide and Insertion Instructions* included in each box of collagen implants before using the product.

HERRICK LACRIMAL PLUG™

Description: The non-dissolvable Herrick Lacrimal Plug™ provides long-term lacrimal occlusion by reducing tear drainage through partial blockage of the horizontal canaliculus.

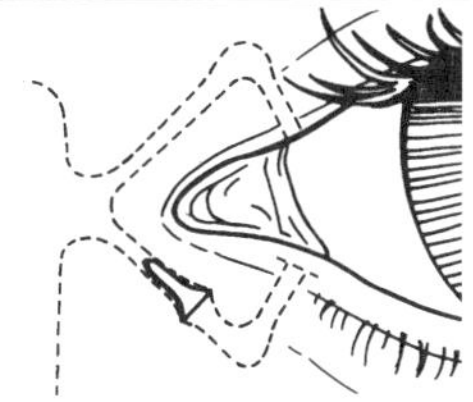

The Herrick Lacrimal Plug is easy to insert and well-tolerated by patients after placement. Dilation of the punctum and use of topical anesthetic is not usually required for insertion. When properly inserted, the Plug will not fall out of the punctum or touch the eye at any time.
When indicated, the Plug is typically inserted through the inferior puncta as a bilateral procedure. At this same time, dissolvable collagen implants can be inserted through the superior puncta to determine if it is necessary to occlude all four canaliculi.
Indications: Patients experiencing dry eye symptoms such as; redness, burning, reflex tearing, itching or foreign body sensation should first be tested using Collagen Implants For The Lacrimal Efficiency Test (available from Lacrimedics, Inc.)
The Herrick Lacrimal Plug is indicated for patients who respond favorably to the Lacrimal Efficiency Test.
When indicated, the Herrick Lacrimal Plug may also be used after eye surgery to prevent complications due to dry eye, to enhance the efficacy of ocular medications, and in patients experiencing dry eye-related contact lens problems.
By Diagnosis: The Herrick Lacrimal Plug may be used to treat dry eye syndrome and the dry eye component of any of the following ocular surface diseases (OSD): conjunctivitis, corneal ulcers, pterygium, blepharitis, keratitis, red lid margins, recurrent chalazion, recurrent corneal erosion, filamentary keratitis and other external eye diseases. In all cases, the Lacrimal Efficiency Test should be performed to determine the potential effectiveness of long-term lacrimal occlusion.
Contraindications: Tearing secondary to chronic dacryocystitis with mucopurulent discharge; inflammation of the eye lid; and/or epiphora.
Patients experiencing epiphora should be evaluated for canalicular obstruction. If patients experience irritation, infection, or epiphora after insertion, saline irrigation or probing may be used to expel the plug through the lacrimal sac into the nose and throat.
Packaging and Product Parameters: One box contains two Herrick Lacrimal Plugs. Each Plug is made of medical grade silicone and comes pre-mounted on a stilette to facilitate insertion. A sliding foam guide mounted on the stilette provides stability and facilitates insertion of the Plug.
The Herrick Lacrimal Plug is available in 0.3mm and 0.5mm shaft diameters. The collapsible bell on each Plug is approximately 0.8mm and 1.4mm in diameter respectively. The most commonly prescribed size is the 0.5mm diameter.
The size of the Herrick Lacrimal Plug used does not directly correspond with the size of the collagen implant used. A collagen implant swells to nearly twice its size following insertion.
Important Note: Read the *Practitioner Guide and Insertion Instructions* included in each box of Herrick Lacrimal Plugs before using the product.

Lederle Laboratories

A Division of American Cyanamid Co.
ONE CYANAMID PLAZA
WAYNE, NJ 07470

see Storz Ophthalmics, page 319

Merck & Co., Inc.

WEST POINT, PA 19486

CHIBROXIN® ℞

(Norfloxacin)
Sterile Ophthalmic Solution

Description

CHIBROXIN* (Norfloxacin) Ophthalmic Solution is a synthetic broad-spectrum antibacterial agent supplied as a sterile isotonic solution for topical ophthalmic use. Norfloxacin, a fluoroquinolone, is 1-ethyl-6-fluoro-1,4-dihydro-4-oxo-7-(1-piperazinyl) -3- quinolinecarboxylic acid. Its empirical formula is $C_{16}H_{18}FN_3O_3$ and the structural formula is:

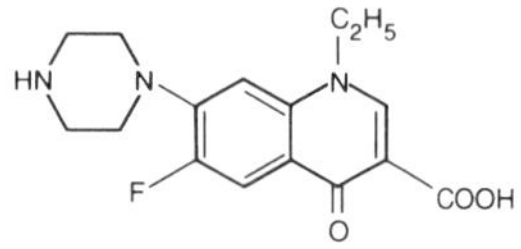

Norfloxacin is a white to pale yellow crystalline powder with a molecular weight of 319.34 and a melting point of about 221°C. It is freely soluble in glacial acetic acid and very slightly soluble in ethanol, methanol and water.
CHIBROXIN Ophthalmic Solution 0.3% is supplied as a sterile isotonic solution. Each mL contains 3 mg norfloxacin. Inactive ingredients: disodium edetate, sodium acetate, sodium chloride, hydrochloric acid (to adjust pH) and water for injection. Benzalkonium chloride 0.0025% is added as preservative. The pH of CHIBROXIN is approximately 5.2 and the osmolarity is approximately 285 m0smol/liter.
Norfloxacin, a fluoroquinolone, differs from quinolones by having a fluorine atom at the 6 position and a piperazine moiety at the 7 position.

*Registered trademark of MERCK & CO., INC.

Clinical Pharmacology

Microbiology

Norfloxacin has *in vitro* activity against a broad spectrum of gram-positive and gram-negative aerobic bacteria. The fluorine atom at the 6 position provides increased potency against gram-negative organisms and the piperazine moiety at the 7 position is responsible for anti-pseudomonal activity.
Norfloxacin inhibits bacterial deoxyribonucleic acid synthesis and is bactericidal. At the molecular level three specific events are attributed to CHIBROXIN in *E. coli* cells:
1) inhibition of the ATP-dependent DNA supercoiling reaction catalyzed by DNA gyrase;
2) inhibition of the relaxation of supercoiled DNA;
3) promotion of double-stranded DNA breakage.

There is generally no cross-resistance between norfloxacin and other classes of antibacterial agents. Therefore, norfloxacin generally demonstrates activity against indicated organisms resistant to some other antimicrobial agents. When such cross-resistance does occur, it is probably due to decreased entry of the drugs into the bacterial cells. Antagonism has been demonstrated *in vitro* between norfloxacin and nitrofurantoin.
Norfloxacin has been shown to be active against most strains of the following organisms both *in vitro* and clinically in ophthalmic infections (see INDICATIONS AND USAGE):
Gram-positive bacteria including:
Staphylococcus aureus
Staphylococcus epidermidis
Staphylococcus warnerii
Streptococcus pneumoniae
Gram-negative bacteria including:
Acinetobacter calcoaceticus
Aeromonas hydrophila
Haemophilus influenzae
Proteus mirabilis
Pseudomonas aeruginosa
Serratia marcescens

Norfloxacin has been shown to be active *in vitro* against most strains of the following organisms; however, *the clinical significance of these data in ophthalmic infections is unknown.*
Gram-positive bacteria:
Bacillus cereus
Enterococcus faecalis (formerly *Streptococcus faecalis*)
Staphylococcus saprophyticus
Gram-negative bacteria:
Citrobacter diversus
Citrobacter freundii
Edwardsiella tarda
Enterobacter aerogenes
Enterobacter cloacae
Escherichia coli
Hafnia alvei
Haemophilus aegyptius (Koch-Weeks bacillus)
Klebsiella oxytoca
Klebsiella pneumoniae
Klebsiella rhinoscleromatis
Morganella morganii
Neisseria gonorrhoeae
Proteus vulgaris
Providencia alcalifaciens
Providencia rettgeri
Providencia stuartii
Salmonella typhi
Vibrio cholerae
Vibrio parahemolyticus
Yersinia enterocolitica
Other:
Ureaplasma urealyticum

Norfloxacin is not active against obligate anaerobes.

Clinical Studies

Clinical studies were conducted comparing CHIBROXIN Ophthalmic Solution (n=152) with ophthalmic solutions of tobramycin, gentamicin, and chloramphenicol (n=158) in patients with conjunctivitis and positive bacterial cultures. After seven days of therapy with CHIBROXIN Ophthalmic Solution, 72 percent of patients were clinically cured. Of those cured, 85 percent had all their pathogens eradicated. Eradication was also achieved in 62 percent (23/37) of patients whose clinical outcome was not completely cured by day seven. These results were similar among all treatment groups.
Another clinical study compared CHIBROXIN Ophthalmic Solution with placebo in patients with conjunctivitis and positive bacterial cultures. Placebo in this study was the liquid vehicle for CHIBROXIN Ophthalmic Solution and contained the preservative. After five days of therapy, 64 percent (36/56) of patients on CHIBROXIN Ophthalmic Solution were clinically cured compared to 50 percent (23/46) of patients receiving placebo. Of those cured, 78 percent had all their pathogens eradicated. Eradication was also achieved in 50 percent (10/20) of patients whose clinical outcome was not completely cured. The response to CHIBROXIN Ophthalmic Solution was statistically significantly better than the response to placebo.

Indications and Usage

CHIBROXIN Ophthalmic Solution is indicated for the treatment of conjunctivitis when caused by susceptible strains of the following bacteria:
*Acinetobacter calcoaceticus**
*Aeromonas hydrophila**
Haemophilus influenzae
*Proteus mirabilis**
*Pseudomonas aeruginosa**
*Serratia marcescens**
Staphylococcus aureus
Staphylococcus epidermidis
*Staphylococcus warnerii**
Streptococcus pneumoniae

Appropriate monitoring of bacterial response to topical antibiotic therapy should accompany the use of CHIBROXIN Ophthalmic Solution.

*Efficacy for this organism was studied in fewer than 10 infections.

Contraindications

CHIBROXIN Ophthalmic Solution is contraindicated in patients with a history of hypersensitivity to norfloxacin, or the other members of the quinolone group of antibacterial agents or any other component of this medication.

Warnings

NOT FOR INJECTION INTO THE EYE.

Serious and occasionally fatal hypersensitivity (anaphylactoid or anaphylactic) reactions, some following the first dose, have been reported in patients receiving systemic quinolone therapy. Some reactions were accompanied by cardiovascular collapse, loss of consciousness, tingling, pharyngeal or facial edema, dyspnea, urticaria, and itching. Only a few patients had a history of hypersensitivity reactions. Serious anaphylactoid or anaphylactic reactions require immediate emergency treatment with epinephrine. Oxygen, intravenous steroids and airway management, including intubation, should be administered as indicated.

Precautions

General

As with other antibiotic preparations, prolonged use may result in overgrowth of nonsusceptible organisms, including fungi. If superinfection occurs, appropriate measures should be initiated. Whenever clinical judgment dictates, the patient should be examined with the aid of magnification, such as slit lamp biomicroscopy and, where appropriate, fluorescein staining.

Information For Patients

Patients should be instructed to avoid allowing the tip of the dispensing container to contact the eye or surrounding structures.
Patients should be advised that norfloxacin may be associated with hypersensitivity reactions, even following a single dose, and to discontinue the drug at the first sign of a skin rash or other allergic reaction.
Patients being treated for bacterial conjunctivitis generally should not wear contact lenses. However, if the physician considers the use of contact lenses appropriate, patients should be instructed to wait at least 15 minutes after instilling CHIBROXIN Ophthalmic Solution before inserting their lenses because the preservative in CHIBROXIN Ophthalmic Solution, benzalkonium chloride, may be absorbed by contact lenses.

Drug Interactions

Specific drug interaction studies have not been conducted with norfloxacin ophthalmic solution. However, the systemic administration of some quinolones has been shown to elevate plasma concentrations of theophylline, interfere with the metabolism of caffeine, and enhance the effects of the oral anticoagulant warfarin and its derivatives. Elevated serum levels of cyclosporine have been reported with concomitant use of cyclosporine with norfloxacin. Therefore, cyclosporine serum levels should be monitored and appropriate cyclosporine dosage adjustments made when these drugs are used concomitantly.

Carcinogenesis, Mutagenesis, Impairment of Fertility
No increase in neoplastic changes was observed with norfloxacin as compared to controls in a study in rats, lasting up to 96 weeks at doses eight to nine times the usual human oral dose*.
Norfloxacin was tested for mutagenic activity in a number of *in vivo* and *in vitro* tests. Norfloxacin had no mutagenic effect in the dominant lethal test in mice and did not cause chromosomal aberrations in hamsters or rats at doses 30 to 60 times and usual oral dose*. Norfloxacin had no mutagenic activity *in vitro* in the Ames microbial mutagen test, Chinese hamster fibroblasts and V-79 mammalian cell assay. Although norfloxacin was weakly positive in the Rec-assay for DNA repair, all other mutagenic assays were negative including a more sensitive test (V-79).
Norfloxacin did not adversely affect the fertility of male and female mice at oral doses up to 33 times the usual human oral dose*.
Pregnancy
Pregnancy Category C: Norfloxacin has been shown to produce embryonic loss in monkeys when given in doses 10 times the maximum human oral dose* (400 mg b.i.d.), with peak plasma levels that are two to three times those obtained in humans. There has been no evidence of a teratogenic effect in any of the animal species tested (rat, rabbit, mouse, monkey) at 6 to 50 times the human oral dose. There are no adequate and well-controlled studies in pregnant women. CHIBROXIN Ophthalmic Solution should be used during pregnancy only if the potential benefit justifies the potential risk to the fetus.
Nursing Mothers
It is not known whether norfloxacin is excreted in human milk following ocular administration. Because many drugs are excreted in human milk, and because of the potential for serious adverse reactions in nursing infants from norfloxacin, a decision should be made to discontinue nursing or to discontinue the drug, taking into account the importance of the drug to the mother (see ANIMAL PHARMACOLOGY).
Pediatric Use
Safety and effectiveness in infants below the age of one year have not been established.
Although quinolones including norfloxacin have been shown to cause arthropathy in immature animals after oral administration, topical ocular administration of other quinolones to immature animals has not shown any arthropathy and there is no evidence that the ophthalmic dosage form of those quinolones has any effects on the weight-bearing joints.

*All factors are based on a standard patient weight of 50 kg. The usual oral dose of norfloxacin is 800 mg daily. One drop of CHIBROXIN Ophthalmic Solution 0.3% contains about 1/6,666 of this dose (0.12 mg).

Adverse Reactions
In clinical trials, the most frequently reported drug-related adverse reaction was local burning or discomfort. Other drug-related adverse reactions were conjunctival hyperemia, chemosis, photophobia and a bitter taste following instillation.
Dosage and Administration
The recommended dose in adults and pediatric patients (one year and older) is one or two drops of CHIBROXIN Ophthalmic Solution applied topically to the affected eye(s) four times daily for up to seven days. Depending on the severity of the infection, the dosage for the first day of therapy may be one or two drops every two hours during the waking hours.
How Supplied
CHIBROXIN Ophthalmic Solution is a clear, colorless to light yellow solution.
No. 3526—CHIBROXIN Ophthalmic Solution 0.3% is supplied in a white, opaque, plastic OCUMETER* ophthalmic dispenser with a controlled drop tip as follows:
NDC 0006-3526-03, 5 mL.
Storage
Store CHIBROXIN Ophthalmic Solution at room temperature, 15°–30°C (59°–86°F). Protect from light.
Animal Pharmacology
The oral administration of single doses of norfloxacin, six times the recommended human oral dose**, caused lameness in immature dogs. Histologic examination of the weight-bearing joints of these dogs revealed permanent lesions of the cartilage. Related drugs also produced erosions of the cartilage in weight-bearing joints and other signs of arthropathy in immature animals of various species.

*Registered trademark of MERCK & CO., INC.
**All factors are based on a standard patient weight of 50 kg. The usual oral dose of norfloxacin is 800 mg daily. One drop of CHIBROXIN Ophthalmic Solution 0.3% contains about 1/6,666 of this dose (0.12 mg).

Additional Cautionary Information
Norfloxacin is available as an oral dosage form in addition to the ophthalmic dosage form. The following adverse effects, while they have not been reported with the ophthalmic dosage form, have been reported with the oral dosage form. However, it should be noted that the usual dosage of oral norfloxacin (800 mg/day) contains 6,666 times the amount in one drop of CHIBROXIN Ophthalmic Solution 0.3% (0.12 mg).
Convulsions have been reported in patients receiving oral norfloxacin. Convulsions, increased intracranial pressure, and toxic psychoses have been reported with other drugs in this class. Orally administered quinolones may also cause central nervous system (CNS) stimulation which may lead to tremors, restlessness, lightheadedness, confusion and hallucinations. If these reactions occur in patients receiving norfloxacin, the drug should be discontinued and appropriate measures instituted.
The effects of norfloxacin on brain function or on the electrical activity of the brain have not been tested. Therefore, as with all quinolones, norfloxacin should be used with caution in patients with known or suspected CNS disorders, such as severe cerebral arteriosclerosis, epilepsy, and other factors which predispose to seizures.
The following adverse effects have been reported with Tablets NOROXIN* (Norfloxacin). *Hypersensitivity Reactions:* Hypersensitivity reactions including anaphylactoid reactions, angioedema, dyspnea, vasculitis, urticaria, arthritis, arthralgia, myalgia; *Gastrointestinal:* Pseudomembranous colitis, hepatitis, jaundice, including cholestatic jaundice, pancreatitis; *Hematologic:* Neutropenia, leukopenia, thrombocytopenia; *Nervous System/Psychiatric:* CNS effects characterized as generalized seizures and myoclonus; neurological changes such as ataxia, diplopia and possible exacerbation of myasthenia gravis; psychic disturbances including psychotic reactions and confusion, depression; *Renal:* Interstitial nephritis, renal failure; *Skin:* Toxic epidermal necrolysis, Stevens-Johnson syndrome and erythema multiforme, exfoliative dermatitis, rash, photosensitivity; *Special Senses:* Transient hearing loss.
Abnormal laboratory values observed with oral norfloxacin included elevation of ALT (SGPT) and AST (SGOT), alkaline phosphatase, BUN, serum creatinine, and LDH.
Please consult the package circular for Tablets NOROXIN (Norfloxacin) for additional information concerning these and other adverse effects and other cautionary information.

*Registered trademark of MERCK & CO., INC.
DC 7679104 Issued June 1993

Shown in Product Identification Guide, page 104

DARANIDE® ℞
(Dichlorphenamide), U.S.P.
Tablets

Description
DARANIDE* (Dichlorphenamide) is an oral carbonic anhydrase inhibitor. Dichlorphenamide, a dichlorinated benzenedisulfonamide, is known chemically as 4,5-dichloro-1,3-benzenedisulfonamide. Its empirical formula is $C_6H_6Cl_2N_2O_4S_2$ and its structural formula is:

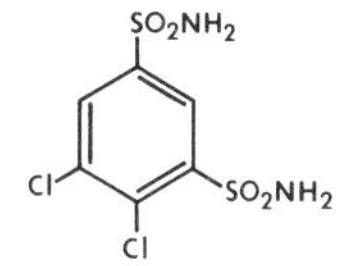

Dichlorphenamide is a white or practically white, crystalline compound with a molecular weight of 305.16. It is very slightly soluble in water but soluble in dilute solutions of sodium carbonate and sodium hydroxide. Dilute alkaline solutions of dichlorphenamide are stable at room temperature.
DARANIDE is supplied as tablets, for oral administration, each containing 50 mg dichlorphenamide. Inactive ingredients are D&C Yellow 10, lactose, magnesium stearate, and starch.

*Registered trademark of MERCK & CO., INC.

Clinical Pharmacology
Carbonic anhydrase inhibitors reduce intraocular pressure by partially suppressing the secretion of aqueous humor (inflow), although the mechanism by which they do this is not fully understood. Evidence suggests that HCO_3^- ions are produced in the ciliary body by hydration of carbon dioxide under the influence of carbonic anhydrase and diffuse into the posterior chamber with Na+ ions. The aqueous fluid contains more Na+ and HCO_3^- ions than does plasma and consequently is hypertonic. Water is attracted to the posterior chamber by osmosis. Systemic administration of a carbonic anhydrase inhibitor has been shown to inactivate carbonic anhydrase in the ciliary body of the rabbit's eye and to reduce the high concentration of HCO_3^- ions in ocular fluids.
As is the case with all carbonic anhydrase inhibitors, DARANIDE in high doses causes some decrease in renal blood flow and glomerular filtration rate.
In man, DARANIDE begins to act within an hour and maximal effect is observed in two to four hours. The lowered intraocular tension may be maintained for approximately 6 to 12 hours.
Indications and Usage
For adjunctive treatment of: chronic simple (open-angle) glaucoma, secondary glaucoma, and preoperatively in acute angle-closure glaucoma where delay of surgery is desired in order to lower intraocular pressure.

Continued on next page

Information on the Merck and Co., Inc. products listed on these pages is the full prescribing information from product circulars in effect August 31, 1994.

Merck and Co, Inc.—Cont.

Contraindications
DARANIDE is contraindicated in hepatic insufficiency, renal failure, adrenocortical insufficiency, hyperchloremic acidosis, or in conditions in which serum levels of sodium or potassium are depressed. DARANIDE should not be used in patients with severe pulmonary obstruction who are unable to increase their alveolar ventilation since their acidosis may be increased.
DARANIDE is contraindicated in patients who are hypersensitive to this product.

Precautions
General
Potassium excretion is increased by DARANIDE and hypokalemia may develop with brisk diuresis, when severe cirrhosis is present, or during concomitant use of steroids or ACTH. Interference with adequate oral electrolyte intake will also contribute to hypokalemia. Hypokalemia can sensitize or exaggerate the response of the heart to the toxic effects of digitalis (e.g., increased ventricular irritability). Hypokalemia may be avoided or treated by use of potassium supplements such as foods with a high potassium content. DARANIDE should be used with caution in patients with respiratory acidosis.
Drug Interactions
Caution is advised in patients receiving concomitant high-dose aspirin and carbonic anhydrase inhibitors, as anorexia, tachypnea, lethargy and coma have been rarely reported due to a possible drug interaction.
Carcinogenesis, Mutagenesis, Impairment of Fertility
Long-term studies in animals have not been performed to evaluate the effects upon fertility or carcinogenic potential of DARANIDE.
Pregnancy
Pregnancy Category C. Dichlorphenamide has been shown to be teratogenic in the rat (skeletal anomalies) when given in doses 100 times the human dose. There are no adequate and well-controlled studies in pregnant women. DARANIDE should not be used in women of childbearing age or in pregnancy, especially during the first trimester, unless the potential benefits outweigh the potential risks.
Nursing Mothers
It is not known whether dichlorphenamide is excreted in human milk. Because many drugs are excreted in human milk, caution should be exercised when dichlorphenamide is administered to a nursing woman.
Pediatric Use
Safety and effectiveness in children have not been established.

Adverse Reactions
Certain side effects characteristic of carbonic anhydrase inhibitors may occur with DARANIDE, particularly with increasing doses. The most common effects include gastrointestinal disturbances (anorexia, nausea, and vomiting), drowsiness and paresthesias.
Included in the listing which follows are some adverse reactions which have not been reported with DARANIDE. However, pharmacological similarities among the carbonic anhydrase inhibitors make it advisable to consider the following reactions when dichlorphenamide is administered. *Central Nervous System/ Psychiatric:* ataxia, tremor, tinnitus, headache, weakness, nervousness, globus hystericus, lassitude, depression, confusion, disorientation, dizziness; *Gastrointestinal:* constipation, hepatic insufficiency; *Metabolic:* loss of weight, metabolic acidosis, electrolyte imbalance (hypokalemia, hyperchloremia), hyperuricemia; *Hypersensitivity:* skin eruptions, pruritus, fever; *Hematologic:* leukopenia, agranulocytosis, thrombocytopenia; *Genitourinary:* urinary frequency, renal colic, renal calculi, phosphaturia.

Overdosage
The oral LD_{50} of DARANIDE is 1710 and 2600 mg/kg in the mouse and rat respectively.
Symptoms of overdosage or toxicity may include drowsiness, anorexia, nausea, vomiting, dizziness, paresthesias, ataxia, tremor and tinnitus.
In the event of overdosage, induce emesis or perform gastric lavage. The electrolyte disturbance most likely to be encountered from overdosage is hyperchloremic acidosis that may respond to bicarbonate administration. Potassium supplementation may be required. The patient should be carefully observed and given supportive treatment.

Dosage and Administration
DARANIDE is usually given in conjunction with topical ocular hypotensive agents. In acute angle-closure glaucoma, it may be used together with miotics and osmotic agents in an attempt to reduce intraocular tension rapidly. If this is not quickly relieved, surgery may be mandatory.
Dosage must be adjusted carefully to meet the requirements of the individual patient. A priming dose of 100 to 200 mg of DARANIDE (2 to 4 tablets) is suggested for adults, followed by 100 mg (2 tablets) every 12 hours until the desired response has been obtained. The recommended maintenance dosage for adults is 25 to 50 mg (½ to 1 tablet) once to three times daily.

How Supplied
No. 3256—Tablets DARANIDE, 50 mg each, are yellow, round, scored, compressed tablets, coded MSD 49. They are supplied as follows:
NDC 0006-0049-68 bottles of 100.
A.H.F.S. Category: 52:10
DC 7412517 Issued November 1986

Shown in Product Identification Guide, page 104

DECADRON® Phosphate ℞
(Dexamethasone Sodium Phosphate), U.S.P.
0.05% Dexamethasone Phosphate Equivalent
Sterile Ophthalmic Ointment

Description
Dexamethasone sodium phosphate is 9-fluoro-11β, 17-dihydroxy-16α-methyl-21-(phosphonooxy)pregna-1,4-diene-3,20-dione disodium salt. Its empirical formula is $C_{22}H_{28}FNa_2O_8P$ and its structural formula is:

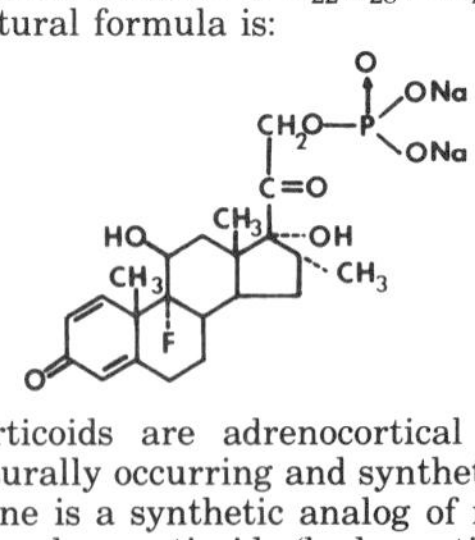

Glucocorticoids are adrenocortical steroids, both naturally occurring and synthetic. Dexamethasone is a synthetic analog of naturally occurring glucocorticoids (hydrocortisone and cortisone). Dexamethasone sodium phosphate is a water soluble, inorganic ester of dexamethasone. Its molecular weight is 516.41.
Sterile Ophthalmic Ointment DECADRON* Phosphate (Dexamethasone Sodium Phosphate) is a topical steroid ointment containing dexamethasone sodium phosphate equivalent to 0.5 mg (0.05%) dexamethasone phosphate in each gram. Inactive ingredients: white petrolatum and mineral oil.
Dexamethasone sodium phosphate is an inorganic ester of dexamethasone.

*Registered trademark of MERCK & CO., INC.

Clinical Pharmacology
Dexamethasone sodium phosphate suppresses the inflammatory response to a variety of agents and it probably delays or slows healing. No generally accepted explanation of these steroid properties have been advanced.

Indications and Usage
For the treatment of the following conditions:
Steroid responsive inflammatory conditions of the palpebral and bulbar conjunctiva, cornea, and anterior segment of the globe, such as allergic conjunctivitis, acne rosacea, superficial punctate keratitis, herpes zoster keratitis, iritis, cyclitis, selected infective conjunctivitis when the inherent hazard of steroid use is accepted to obtain an advisable diminution in edema and inflammation; corneal injury from chemical or thermal burns, or penetration of foreign bodies.

Contraindications
Epithelial herpes simplex keratitis (dendritic keratitis).
Acute infectious stages of vaccinia, varicella, and many other viral diseases of the cornea and conjunctiva.
Mycobacterial infection of the eye.
Fungal diseases of ocular structures.
Hypersensitivity to a component of the medication.

Warnings
Prolonged use may result in ocular hypertension and/or glaucoma, with damage to the optic nerve, defects in visual acuity and fields of vision, and posterior subcapsular cataract formation. Prolonged use may suppress the host response and thus increase the hazard of secondary ocular infections. In those diseases causing thinning of the cornea or sclera, perforations have been known to occur with the use of topical corticosteroids. In acute purulent conditions of the eye, corticosteroids may mask infection or enhance existing infection. If these products are used for 10 days or longer, intraocular pressure should be routinely monitored even though it may be difficult in children and uncooperative patients.
Employment of corticosteroid medication in the treatment of herpes simplex other than epithelial herpes simplex keratitis, in which it is contraindicated, requires great caution; periodic slit-lamp microscopy is essential.

Precautions
General
The possibility of persistent fungal infections of the cornea should be considered after prolonged corticosteroid dosing.
There have been reports of bacterial keratitis associated with the use of multiple dose containers of topical ophthalmic products. These containers had been inadvertently contaminated by patients who, in most cases, had a concurrent corneal disease or a disruption of the ocular epithelial surface. (See PRECAUTIONS, *Information for Patients.*)
Information for Patients
Patients should be instructed to avoid allowing the tip of the dispensing container to contact the eye or surrounding structures.
Patients should also be instructed that ocular preparations, if handled improperly, can become contaminated by common bacteria known to cause ocular infections. Serious damage to the eye and subsequent loss of vision may result from using contaminated preparations. (See PRECAUTIONS, *General.*)
Patients should also be advised that if they develop an intercurrent ocular condition (e.g., trauma, ocular surgery or infection), they should immediately seek their physician's advice concerning the continued use of the present multidose container.
Carcinogenesis, Mutagenesis, Impairment of Fertility
Long-term animal studies have not been performed to evaluate the carcinogenic potential

or the effect on fertility of Ophthalmic Ointment DECADRON Phosphate.

Pregnancy

Pregnancy Category C. Dexamethasone has been shown to be teratogenic in mice and rabbits following topical ophthalmic application in multiples of the therapeutic dose.

In the mouse, corticosteroids produce fetal resorptions and a specific abnormality, cleft palate. In the rabbit, corticosteroids have produced fetal resorptions and multiple abnormalities involving the head, ears, limbs, palate, etc.

There are no adequate or well-controlled studies in pregnant women. Ophthalmic Ointment DECADRON Phosphate should be used during pregnancy only if the potential benefit to the mother justifies the potential risk to the embryo or fetus. Infants born of mothers who have received substantial doses of corticosteroids during pregnancy should be observed carefully for signs of hypoadrenalism.

Nursing Mothers

Topically applied steroids are absorbed systemically. Therefore, because of the potential for serious adverse reactions in nursing infants from dexamethasone sodium phosphate, a decision should be made whether to discontinue nursing or discontinue the drug, taking into account the importance of the drug to the mother.

Pediatric Use

Safety and effectiveness in children have not been established.

Adverse Reactions

Glaucoma with optic nerve damage, visual acuity and field defects, posterior subcapsular cataract formation, secondary ocular infection from pathogens including herpes simplex, perforation of the globe.

Rarely, filtering blebs have been reported when topical steroids have been used following cataract surgery.

Rarely, stinging or burning may occur.

Dosage and Administration

The duration of treatment will vary with the type of lesion and may extend from a few days to several weeks, according to therapeutic response. Relapses, more common in chronic active lesions than in self-limited conditions, usually respond to retreatment.

Apply a thin coating of ointment three or four times a day. When a favorable response is observed, reduce the number of daily applications to two, and later to one a day as a maintenance dose if this is sufficient to control symptoms.

Ophthalmic Ointment DECADRON Phosphate is particularly convenient when an eye pad is used. It may also be the preparation of choice for patients in whom therapeutic benefit depends on prolonged contact of the active ingredients with ocular tissues.

How Supplied

No. 7615—0.05% Sterile Ophthalmic Ointment DECADRON Phosphate is a clear unctuous ointment and is supplied as follows:

NDC 0006-7615-04 in 3.5 g tubes
(6505-00-961-5508 0.05% 3.5 g).
DC 7612331 Issued October 1993
Shown in Product Identification Guide, page 104

DECADRON® Phosphate ℞
(Dexamethasone Sodium Phosphate), U.S.P.
0.1% Dexamethasone Phosphate Equivalent
Sterile Ophthalmic Solution

Description

Dexamethasone sodium phosphate is 9-fluoro-11β, 17-dihydroxy-16α-methyl-21-(phosphonooxy)pregna-1,4-diene-3,20-dione disodium salt. Its empirical formula is $C_{22}H_{28}FNa_2O_8P$ and its structural formula is:

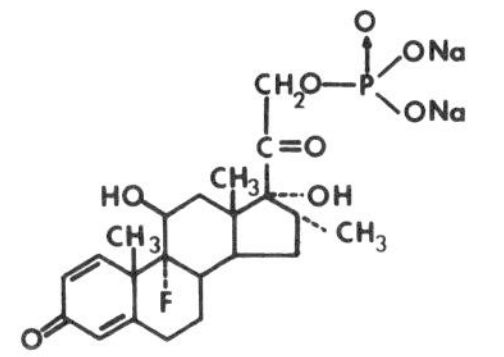

Glucocorticoids are adrenocortical steroids, both naturally occurring and synthetic. Dexamethasone is a synthetic analog of naturally occurring glucocorticoids (hydrocortisone and cortisone). Dexamethasone sodium phosphate is a water soluble, inorganic ester of dexamethasone. It is approximately three thousand times more soluble in water at 25°C than hydrocortisone. Its molecular weight is 516.41.

Ophthalmic Solution DECADRON* Phosphate (Dexamethasone Sodium Phosphate) in the 5 mL OCUMETER* ophthalmic dispenser is a topical steroid solution containing dexamethasone sodium phosphate equivalent to 1 mg (0.1%) dexamethasone phosphate in each milliliter of buffered solution. Inactive ingredients: creatinine, sodium citrate, sodium borate, polysorbate 80, disodium edetate, hydrochloric acid to adjust pH, and water for injection. Sodium bisulfite 0.1%, phenylethanol 0.25% and benzalkonium chloride 0.02% added as preservatives.

---

*Registered trademark of MERCK & CO., INC.

Clinical Pharmacology

Dexamethasone sodium phosphate suppresses the inflammatory response to a variety of agents and it probably delays or slows healing. No generally accepted explanation of these steroid properties has been advanced.

Indications and Usage

For the treatment of the following conditions:

Ophthalmic:

Steroid responsive inflammatory conditions of the palpebral and bulbar conjunctiva, cornea, and anterior segment of the globe, such as allergic conjunctivitis, acne rosacea, superficial punctate keratitis, herpes zoster keratitis, iritis, cyclitis, selected infective conjunctivitis when the inherent hazard of steroid use is accepted to obtain an advisable diminution in edema and inflammation; corneal injury from chemical or thermal burns, or penetration of foreign bodies.

Otic:

Steroid responsive inflammatory conditions of the external auditory meatus, such as allergic otitis externa, selected purulent and nonpurulent infective otitis externa when the hazard of steroid use is accepted to obtain an advisable diminution in edema and inflammation.

Contraindications

Epithelial herpes simplex keratitis (dendritic keratitis).

Acute infectious stages of vaccinia, varicella, and many other viral diseases of the cornea and conjunctiva.

Mycobacterial infection of the eye.

Fungal diseases of ocular or auricular structures.

Hypersensitivity to any component of this product, including sulfites (see WARNINGS).

Perforation of a drum membrane.

Warnings

Prolonged use may result in ocular hypertension and/or glaucoma, with damage to the optic nerve, defects in visual acuity and fields of vision, and posterior subcapsular cataract formation. Prolonged use may suppress the host response and thus increase the hazard of secondary ocular infections. In those diseases causing thinning of the cornea or sclera, perforations have been known to occur with the use of topical corticosteroids. In acute purulent conditions of the eye or ear, corticosteroids may mask infection or enhance existing infection. If these products are used for 10 days or longer, intraocular pressure should be routinely monitored even though it may be difficult in children and uncooperative patients.

Employment of corticosteroid medication in the treatment of herpes simplex other than epithelial herpes simplex keratitis, in which it is contraindicated, requires great caution; periodic slit-lamp microscopy is essential.

Ophthalmic Solution DECADRON Phosphate contains sodium bisulfite, a sulfite that may cause allergic-type reactions including anaphylactic symptoms and life-threatening or less severe asthmatic episodes in certain susceptible people. The overall prevalence of sulfite sensitivity in the general population is unknown and probably low. Sulfite sensitivity is seen more frequently in asthmatic than in nonasthmatic people.

Precautions

General

The possibility of persistent fungal infections of the cornea should be considered after prolonged corticosteroid dosing.

There have been reports of bacterial keratitis associated with the use of multiple dose containers of topical ophthalmic products. These containers had been inadvertently contaminated by patients who, in most cases, had a concurrent corneal disease or a disruption of the ocular epithelial surface. (See PRECAUTIONS, *Information for Patients.*)

Information for Patients

Patients should be instructed to avoid allowing the tip of the dispensing container to contact the eye or surrounding structures.

Patients should also be instructed that ocular solutions, if handled improperly, can become contaminated by common bacteria known to cause ocular infections. Serious damage to the eye and subsequent loss of vision may result from using contaminated solutions. (See PRECAUTIONS, *General.*)

Patients should also be advised that if they develop an intercurrent ocular condition (e.g., trauma, ocular surgery or infection), they should immediately seek their physician's advice concerning the continued use of the present multidose container.

One of the preservatives in Ophthalmic Solution DECADRON Phosphate, benzalkonium chloride, may be absorbed by soft contact lenses. Patients wearing soft contact lenses should be instructed to wait at least 15 minutes after instilling Ophthalmic Solution DECADRON Phosphate before they insert their lenses.

Carcinogenesis, Mutagenesis, Impairment of Fertility

Long-term animal studies have not been performed to evaluate the carcinogenic potential or the effect on fertility of Ophthalmic Solution DECADRON Phosphate.

Pregnancy

Pregnancy Category C. Dexamethasone has been shown to be teratogenic in mice and rabbits following topical ophthalmic application in multiples of the therapeutic dose.

In the mouse, corticosteroids produce fetal resorptions and a specific abnormality, cleft palate. In the rabbit, corticosteroids have produced fetal resorptions and multiple abnormalities involving the head, ears, limbs, palate, etc.

Continued on next page

Information on the Merck and Co., Inc. products listed on these pages is the full prescribing information from product circulars in effect August 31, 1994.

Merck and Co, Inc.—Cont.

There are no adequate or well-controlled studies in pregnant women. Ophthalmic Solution DECADRON Phosphate should be used during pregnancy only if the potential benefit to the mother justifies the potential risk to the embryo or fetus. Infants born of mothers who have received substantial doses of corticosteroids during pregnancy should be observed carefully for signs of hypoadrenalism.

Nursing Mothers

Topically applied steroids are absorbed systemically. Therefore, because of the potential for serious adverse reactions in nursing infants from dexamethasone sodium phosphate, a decision should be made whether to discontinue nursing or discontinue the drug, taking into account the importance of the drug to the mother.

Pediatric Use

Safety and effectiveness in children have not been established.

Adverse Reactions

Glaucoma with optic nerve damage, visual acuity and field defects, posterior subcapsular cataract formation, secondary ocular infection from pathogens including herpes simplex, perforation of the globe.

Rarely, filtering blebs have been reported when topical steroids have been used following cataract surgery.

Rarely, stinging or burning may occur.

Dosage and Administration

The duration of treatment will vary with the type of lesion and may extend from a few days to several weeks, according to therapeutic response. Relapses, more common in chronic active lesions than in self-limited conditions, usually respond to retreatment.

Eye—Instill one or two drops of solution into the conjunctival sac every hour during the day and every two hours during the night as initial therapy. When a favorable response is observed, reduce dosage to one drop every four hours. Later, further reduction in dosage to one drop three or four times daily may suffice to control symptoms.

Ear—Clean the aural canal thoroughly and sponge dry. Instill the solution directly into the aural canal. A suggested initial dosage is three or four drops two or three times a day. When a favorable response is obtained, reduce dosage gradually and eventually discontinue.

If preferred, the aural canal may be packed with a gauze wick saturated with solution. Keep the wick moist with the preparation and remove from the ear after 12 to 24 hours. Treatment may be repeated as often as necessary at the discretion of the physician.

How Supplied

Sterile Ophthalmic Solution DECADRON Phosphate is a clear, colorless to pale yellow solution.

No. 7643—Ophthalmic Solution DECADRON Phosphate is supplied as follows:

NDC 0006-7643-03 in 5 mL white, opaque, plastic OCUMETER ophthalmic dispenser with a controlled drop tip.

(6505-00-007-4536 0.1% 5 mL)

DC 7261521 Issued October 1993

Shown in Product Identification Guide, page 104

FLOROPRYL® ℞

(Isoflurophate), U.S.P.
Sterile Ophthalmic Ointment
For Topical Application into the Conjunctival Sac Only

Description

FLOROPRYL* (Isoflurophate) is available as 0.025% sterile ophthalmic ointment in polyethylene mineral oil gel. Isoflurophate has a molecular weight of 184.15 and is known chemically as bis (1-methylethyl) phosphorofluoridate. Its empirical formula is $C_6H_{14}FO_3P$ and its structural formula is:

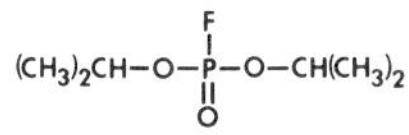

*Registered trademark of MERCK & CO., INC.

Clinical Pharmacology

FLOROPRYL is a cholinesterase inhibitor with sustained activity. Application to the eye produces intense miosis and ciliary muscle contraction due to inhibition of cholinesterase, allowing acetylcholine to accumulate at sites of cholinergic transmission.

FLOROPRYL *irreversibly* inactivates cholinesterase. Thus, following use of FLOROPRYL in the eye, cholinesterase must be either regenerated or supplied from depots elsewhere in the body before ophthalmic action dependent on cholinesterase returns.

If given systemically in sufficient amounts, FLOROPRYL reduces plasma cholinesterase to zero. However, when applied locally to the eye, plasma cholinesterase is usually reduced only slightly.

Indications and Usage

Open-angle glaucoma (FLOROPRYL should be used in glaucoma only when shorter-acting miotics have proved inadequate.)

Conditions obstructing aqueous outflow, such as synechial formation, that are amenable to miotic therapy

Following iridectomy

Accommodative esotropia (accommodative convergent strabismus)

Contraindications

Hypersensitivity to any component of this product.

Because of the toxicity of cholinesterase inhibitors in general, FLOROPRYL is contraindicated in women who are or who may become pregnant. If this drug is used during pregnancy, or if the patient becomes pregnant while taking this drug, the patient should be apprised of the potential hazard to the fetus.

Because miotics may aggravate inflammation, FLOROPRYL should not be used in active uveal inflammation and/or glaucoma associated with iridocyclitis.

Warnings

In patients receiving cholinesterase inhibitors such as FLOROPRYL, succinylcholine should be administered with extreme caution before and during general anesthesia because of possible respiratory and cardiovascular collapse.

Because of possible adverse additive effects, FLOROPRYL should be administered only with extreme caution to patients with myasthenia gravis who are receiving systemic anticholinesterase therapy; conversely, extreme caution should be exercised in the use of an anticholinesterase drug for the treatment of myasthenia gravis patients who are already undergoing topical therapy with cholinesterase inhibitors.

Precautions

General

FLOROPRYL should be used with caution in patients with chronic angle-closure (narrow-angle) glaucoma or in patients with narrow angles, because of the possibility of producing pupillary block and increasing angle blockage. Gonioscopy is recommended prior to medication with FLOROPRYL.

When an intraocular inflammatory process is present, the intensity and persistence of miosis and ciliary muscle contraction that result from anticholinesterase therapy require abstention from, or cautious use of, FLOROPRYL.

Systemic effects are infrequent when FLOROPRYL is applied carefully. The hands should be washed immediately following application. Discontinue FLOROPRYL if salivation, urinary incontinence, diarrhea, profuse sweating, muscle weakness, respiratory difficulties, shock, or cardiac irregularities occur.

Persons receiving cholinesterase inhibitors who are exposed to organophosphate-type insecticides and pesticides (gardeners, organophosphate plant or warehouse workers, farmers, residents of communities which are undergoing insecticide spraying or dusting, etc.) should be warned of the added systemic effects possible from absorption through the respiratory tract or skin. Wearing of respiratory masks, frequent washing, and clothing changes may be advisable.

Anticholinesterase drugs should be used with extreme caution, if at all, in patients with marked vagotonia, bronchial asthma, spastic gastrointestinal disturbances, peptic ulcer, pronounced bradycardia and hypotension, recent myocardial infarction, epilepsy, parkinsonism, and other disorders that may respond adversely to vagotonic effects.

After long-term use of FLOROPRYL, dilation of blood vessels and resulting greater permeability increase the possibility of hyphema during ophthalmic surgery. Therefore, this drug should be discontinued before surgery.

Despite observance of all precautions and the use of only the recommended dose, there is some evidence that repeated administration may cause depression of the concentration of cholinesterase in the serum and erythrocytes, with resultant systemic effects.

There have been reports of bacterial keratitis associated with the use of multiple dose containers of topical ophthalmic products. These containers had been inadvertently contaminated by patients who, in most cases, had a concurrent corneal disease or a disruption of the ocular epithelial surface. (See PRECAUTIONS, *Information for Patients.*)

Information for Patients

Patients should be instructed to avoid allowing the tip of the dispensing container to contact the eye or surrounding structures.

Patients should also be instructed that ocular preparations, if handled improperly, can become contaminated by common bacteria known to cause ocular infections. Serious damage to the eye and subsequent loss of vision may result from using contaminated preparations. (See PRECAUTIONS, *General.*)

Patients should also be advised that if they develop an intercurrent ocular condition (e.g., trauma, ocular surgery or infection), they should immediately seek their physician's advice concerning the continued use of the present multidose container.

Drug Interactions

See WARNINGS regarding possible drug interactions of FLOROPRYL with succinylcholine or with other anticholinesterase agents.

Carcinogenesis, Mutagenesis, Impairment of Fertility

Long-term studies in animals have not been performed to evaluate the effects of FLOROPRYL on fertility or carcinogenic potential.

Pregnancy

Pregnancy Category X: See CONTRAINDICATIONS.

Nursing Mothers

It is not known whether this drug is excreted in human milk. Because of the potential for serious adverse reactions in nursing infants from FLOROPRYL, a decision should be made whether to discontinue nursing or to discontinue the drug, taking into account the importance of the drug to the mother.

Pediatric Use

The occurrence of iris cysts is more frequent in children. (See ADVERSE REACTIONS and DOSAGE AND ADMINISTRATION.)

Extreme caution should be exercised in children receiving FLOROPRYL who may require general anesthesia (see WARNINGS).

Since FLOROPRYL is a potent cholinesterase inhibitor it should be kept out of the reach of children.

Adverse Reactions

Stinging, burning, lacrimation, lid muscle twitching, conjunctival and ciliary redness, brow ache, headache, and induced myopia with visual blurring may occur.

As with all miotic therapy, retinal detachment has been reported occasionally.

Activation of latent iritis or uveitis may occur.

Iris cysts may form, enlarge, and obscure vision. Occurrence is more frequent in children. The iris cyst usually shrinks upon discontinuance of the miotic. Rarely, the cyst may rupture or break free into the aqueous. Frequent examination for this occurrence is advised.

Prolonged use may cause conjunctival thickening and obstruction of nasolacrimal canals.

Systemic effects, which occur rarely, are suggestive of increased cholinergic activity. Such effects may include nausea, vomiting, abdominal cramps, diarrhea, urinary incontinence, salivation, sweating, difficulty in breathing, bradycardia, or cardiac irregularities. Medical management of systemic effects may be indicated (see TREATMENT OF ADVERSE EFFECTS).

Lens opacities have been reported in patients on miotic therapy. Routine slit-lamp examinations, including the lens, should accompany prolonged use.

Paradoxical increase in intraocular pressure may follow anticholinesterase application. This may be alleviated by pupil-dilating medication.

Treatment of Adverse Effects

If FLOROPRYL is taken systemically by accident, or if systemic effects occur after topical application in the eye or from accidental skin contact, atropine sulfate in a dose (for adults) of 0.4 to 0.6 mg or more should be given parenterally (intravenously if necessary). The recommended dosage of atropine in infants and children up to 12 years of age is 0.01 mg/kg repeated every two hours as needed until the desired effect is obtained, or adverse effects of atropine preclude further usage. The maximum single dose should not exceed 0.4 mg.

The use of much larger doses of atropine in treating anticholinesterase intoxication in adults has been reported in the literature. Initially 2 to 6 mg may be given followed by 2 mg every hour or more often, as long as muscarinic effects continue. The greater possibility of atropinization with large doses, particularly in sensitive individuals, should be borne in mind.

Pralidoxime* chloride has been reported to be useful in treatment of systemic effects due to cholinesterase inhibitors. However, its use is recommended in addition to and not as a substitute for atropine.

A short-acting barbiturate is indicated if convulsions occur that are not entirely relieved by atropine. Barbiturate dosage should be carefully adjusted to avoid central respiratory depression. Marked weakness or paralysis of muscles of respiration should be treated promptly by artificial respiration and maintenance of a clear airway.

The oral LD_{50} of FLOROPRYL is 37 mg/kg in the mouse, 5–10 mg/kg in the rat, and 4–10 mg/kg in the rabbit.

---

*PROTOPAM® Chloride (Pralidoxime Chloride), Ayerst Laboratories.

Dosage and Administration

FLOROPRYL *is intended solely for topical use in the conjunctival sac.*

Isoflurophate hydrolyzes in the presence of water to form hydrofluoric acid. To prevent absorption of moisture and loss of potency, the ointment tube should be kept tightly closed; the tip of the tube should not be washed or allowed to touch the eyelid or other moist surface.

Whenever possible, FLOROPRYL should be applied at night before retiring to lessen blurring of vision. As it is an extremely potent drug, it should be used with great care and only by those familiar with its use and thoroughly indoctrinated in the technic of application.

The required dose is applied in the conjunctival sac, with the patient supine, care being taken not to touch the cornea with the tip of the tube. *Wash the hands immediately after administration.*

FLOROPRYL *should not be used more often than directed. Caution is necessary to avoid overdosage.*

Keep frequency of use to a minimum in all patients, but especially in children, to reduce the chance of iris cyst development (see ADVERSE REACTIONS). If tolerance develops, another miotic should be used. FLOROPRYL may be resumed later.

Glaucoma

For initial therapy ¼ inch strip of ophthalmic ointment FLOROPRYL 0.025 per cent is placed in the glaucomatous eye every 8 to 72 hours. A decrease in intraocular pressure should occur within a few hours. During this period, keep the patient under supervision and make tonometric examinations at least hourly for 3 or 4 hours to be sure that no immediate rise in pressure occurs (see ADVERSE REACTIONS).

Strabismus

Essentially equal visual acuity of both eyes is a prerequisite to successful treatment. For initial evaluation FLOROPRYL may be used as a diagnostic aid to determine if an accommodative factor exists. This is especially useful preoperatively in young children and in patients with normal hypermetropic refractive errors. Not more than ¼ inch strip of ointment is administered every night for 2 weeks. If the eyes become straighter, an accommodative factor is demonstrated. This technic may supplement or complement standard testing with atropine and trial with glasses for the accommodative factor.

In esotropia uncomplicated by amblyopia or anisometropia, ophthalmic ointment FLOROPRYL may be used in both eyes, not more than ¼ inch strip at a time every night for 2 weeks, as too severe a degree of miosis may interfere with vision. The dosage is then reduced from ¼ inch strip every other day to ¼ inch strip once a week for 2 months, after which the patient's status should be re-evaluated.

If benefit can not be maintained with a dosage interval of at least 48 hours, therapy with FLOROPRYL should be stopped. Frequency of administration and duration of maintenance therapy depend on how long the eyes remain straight without medication. Intervals between administration should be gradually increased to the greatest length compatible with good results. Therapy may need to be continued for many years in some patients; in others, it has been possible to discontinue therapy after several months.

How Supplied

No. 7742—Sterile ophthalmic ointment FLOROPRYL 0.025 per cent is an opaque white, smooth, unctuous ointment and is supplied as follows:

NDC 0006-7742-04 in a 3.5 g tube.

Storage

Protect from moisture, freezing and excessive heat.

A.H.F.S. Category: 52:20

DC 7413722 Issued December 1991

Shown in Product Identification Guide, page 104

HUMORSOL® ℞

(Demecarium Bromide), U.S.P.
Sterile Ophthalmic Solution
For Topical Application into the Conjunctival Sac Only

Description

Ophthalmic Solution HUMORSOL* (Demecarium Bromide) is a sterile solution supplied in two dosage strengths: 0.125 percent and 0.25 percent. The inactive ingredients are sodium chloride and water for injection; benzalkonium chloride 1:5000 is added as preservative.

Demecarium bromide is a quaternary ammonium compound with a molecular weight of 716.60. Its chemical name is 3,3′-[1,10-decanediylbis [(methylimino)carbonyloxy]] bis [*N,N,N*-trimethylbenzenaminium] dibromide. Its empirical formula is $C_{32}H_{52}Br_2N_4O_4$ and its structural formula is:

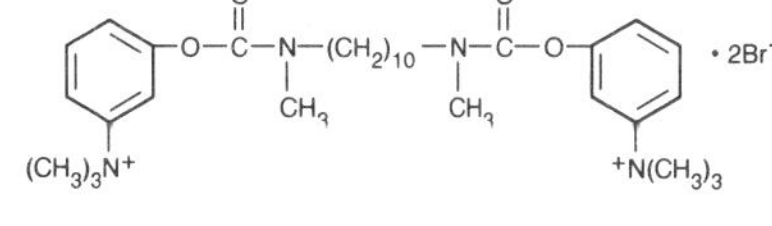

---

*Registered trademark of MERCK & CO., INC.

Clinical Pharmacology

HUMORSOL is a cholinesterase inhibitor with sustained activity. It acts mainly on true (erythrocyte) cholinesterase. Application of HUMORSOL to the eye produces intense miosis and ciliary muscle contraction due to inhibition of cholinesterase, allowing acetylcholine to accumulate at sites of cholinergic transmission. These effects are accompanied by increased capillary permeability of the ciliary body and iris, increased permeability of the blood-aqueous barrier, and vasodilation. Myopia may be induced or, if present, may be augmented by the increased refractive power of the lens that results from the accommodative effect of the drug. HUMORSOL indirectly produces some of the muscarinic and nicotinic effects of acetylcholine as quantities of the latter accumulate.

Indications and Usage

Open-angle glaucoma (HUMORSOL should be used in glaucoma only when shorter-acting miotics have proved inadequate).

Conditions obstructing aqueous outflow, such as synechial formation, that are amenable to miotic therapy

Following iridectomy

Accommodative esotropia (accommodative convergent strabismus)

Contraindications

Hypersensitivity to any component of this product.

Because of the toxicity of cholinesterase inhibitors in general, HUMORSOL is contraindicated in women who are or who may become pregnant. If this drug is used during pregnancy, or if the patient becomes pregnant while taking this drug, the patient should be apprised of the potential hazard to the fetus.

Because miotics may aggravate inflammation, HUMORSOL should not be used in active uveal inflammation and/or glaucoma associated with iridocyclitis.

Warnings

In patients receiving cholinesterase inhibitors such as HUMORSOL, succinylcholine should be administered with extreme caution before and during general anesthesia.

Because of possible adverse additive effects, HUMORSOL should be administered only

Continued on next page

Information on the Merck and Co., Inc. products listed on these pages is the full prescribing information from product circulars in effect August 31, 1994.

Merck and Co, Inc.—Cont.

with extreme caution to patients with myasthenia gravis who are receiving systemic anticholinesterase therapy; conversely, extreme caution should be exercised in the use of an anticholinesterase drug for the treatment of myasthenia gravis patients who are already undergoing topical therapy with cholinesterase inhibitors.

Precautions

General

Gonioscopy is recommended prior to medication with HUMORSOL.

HUMORSOL should be used with caution in patients with chronic angle-closure (narrow-angle) glaucoma or in patients with narrow angles, because of the possibility of producing pupillary block and increasing angle blockage.

When an intraocular inflammatory process is present, the intensity and persistence of miosis and ciliary muscle contraction that result from anticholinesterase therapy require abstention from, or cautious use of, HUMORSOL.

Systemic effects are infrequent when HUMORSOL is instilled carefully. Compression of the lacrimal duct for several seconds immediately following instillation minimizes drainage into the nasal chamber with its extensive absorption surface. Wash the hands immediately after instillation.

Discontinue HUMORSOL if salivation, urinary incontinence, diarrhea, profuse sweating, muscle weakness, respiratory difficulties, shock, or cardiac irregularities occur.

Persons receiving cholinesterase inhibitors who are exposed to organophosphate-type insecticides and pesticides (gardeners, organophosphate plant or warehouse workers, farmers, residents of communities which are undergoing insecticide spraying or dusting, etc.) should be warned of the added systemic effects possible from absorption through the respiratory tract or skin. Wearing of respiratory masks, frequent washing, and clothing changes may be advisable.

Anticholinesterase drugs should be used with extreme caution, if at all, in patients with marked vagotonia, bronchial asthma, spastic gastrointestinal disturbances, peptic ulcer, pronounced bradycardia and hypotension, recent myocardial infarction, epilepsy, parkinsonism, and other disorders that may respond adversely to vagotonic effects.

After long-term use of HUMORSOL, dilation of blood vessels and resulting greater permeability increase the possibility of hyphema during ophthalmic surgery. Therefore, this drug should be discontinued before surgery.

Despite observance of all precautions and the use of only the recommended dose, there is some evidence that repeated administration may cause depression of the concentration of cholinesterase in the serum and erythrocytes, with resultant systemic effects.

There have been reports of bacterial keratitis associated with the use of multiple dose containers of topical ophthalmic products. These containers had been inadvertently contaminated by patients who, in most cases, had a concurrent corneal disease or a disruption of the ocular epithelial surface. (See PRECAUTIONS, *Information for Patients.*)

Information for Patients

Patients should be instructed to avoid allowing the tip of the dispensing container to contact the eye or surrounding structures.

Patients should also be instructed that ocular solutions, if handled improperly, can become contaminated by common bacteria known to cause ocular infections. Serious damage to the eye and subsequent loss of vision may result from using contaminated solutions. (See PRECAUTIONS, *General.*)

Patients should also be advised that if they develop an intercurrent ocular condition (e.g., trauma, ocular surgery or infection), they should immediately seek their physician's advice concerning the continued use of the present multidose container.

The preservative in HUMORSOL, benzalkonium chloride, may be absorbed by soft contact lenses. Patients wearing soft contact lenses should be instructed to wait at least 15 minutes after instilling HUMORSOL before they insert their lenses.

Drug Interactions

See WARNINGS regarding possible drug interactions of HUMORSOL with succinylcholine or with other anticholinesterase agents.

Carcinogenesis, Mutagenesis, Impairment of Fertility

Long-term studies in animals have not been performed to evaluate the effects of HUMORSOL on fertility or carcinogenic potential.

Pregnancy

Pregnancy Category X: See CONTRAINDICATIONS.

Nursing Mothers

It is not known whether this drug is excreted in human milk. Because of the potential for serious adverse reactions in nursing infants from HUMORSOL, a decision should be made whether to discontinue nursing or to discontinue the drug, taking into account the importance of the drug to the mother.

Pediatric Use

The occurrence of iris cysts is more frequent in children. (See ADVERSE REACTIONS and DOSAGE AND ADMINISTRATION.)

Extreme caution should be exercised in children receiving HUMORSOL who may require general anesthesia (see WARNINGS).

Since HUMORSOL is a potent cholinesterase inhibitor it should be kept out of the reach of children.

Adverse Reactions

Stinging, burning, lacrimation, lid muscle twitching, conjunctival and ciliary redness, brow ache, headache, and induced myopia with visual blurring may occur.

Activation of latent iritis or uveitis may occur.

As with all miotic therapy, retinal detachment has been reported occasionally.

Iris cysts may form, enlarge, and obscure vision. Occurrence is more frequent in children. The iris cyst usually shrinks upon discontinuance of the miotic. Rarely, the cyst may rupture or break free into the aqueous. Frequent examination for this occurrence is advised.

Lens opacities have been reported in patients on miotic therapy. Routine slit-lamp examinations, including the lens, should accompany prolonged use.

Paradoxical increase in intraocular pressure may follow anticholinesterase instillation. This may be alleviated by pupil-dilating medication.

Prolonged use may cause conjunctival thickening and obstruction of nasolacrimal canals.

Systemic effects, which occur rarely, are suggestive of increased cholinergic activity. Such effects may include nausea, vomiting, abdominal cramps, diarrhea, urinary incontinence, salivation, sweating, difficulty in breathing, bradycardia, or cardiac irregularities. Medical management of systemic effects may be indicated (see TREATMENT OF ADVERSE EFFECTS).

Treatment of Adverse Effects

If HUMORSOL is taken systemically by accident, or if systemic effects occur after topical application in the eye or from accidental skin contact, administer atropine sulfate parenterally (intravenously if necessary) in a dose (for adults) of 0.4 to 0.6 mg or more. The recommended dosage of atropine in infants and children up to 12 years of age is 0.01 mg/kg repeated every two hours as needed until the desired effect is obtained, or adverse effects of atropine preclude further usage. The maximum single dose should not exceed 0.4 mg.

The use of much larger doses of atropine in treating anticholinesterase intoxication in adults has been reported in the literature. Initially 2 to 6 mg may be given followed by 2 mg every hour or more often, as long as muscarinic effects continue. The greater possibility of atropinization with large doses, particularly in sensitive individuals, should be borne in mind.

Pralidoxime* chloride has been reported to be useful in treating systemic effects due to cholinesterase inhibitors. However, its use is recommended in addition to and not as a substitute for atropine.

A short-acting barbiturate is indicated if convulsions occur that are not entirely relieved by atropine. Barbiturate dosage should be carefully adjusted to avoid central respiratory depression. Marked weakness or paralysis of muscles of respiration should be treated promptly by artificial respiration and maintenance of a clear airway.

The oral LD_{50} of HUMORSOL is 2.96 mg/kg in the mouse.

---

*PROTOPAM® Chloride (Pralidoxime Chloride), Ayerst Laboratories

Dosage and Administration

HUMORSOL *is intended solely for topical use in the conjunctival sac.*

As HUMORSOL is an extremely potent drug, the physician should thoroughly familiarize himself with its use and the technic of instillation.

The required dose is applied in the conjunctival sac, with the patient supine, care being taken not to touch the cornea with the tip of the OCUMETER* ophthalmic dispenser. *The patient or person administering the medication should apply continuous gentle pressure on the lacrimal duct with the index finger for several seconds immediately following instillation of the drops. This is to prevent drainage overflow of solution into the nasal and pharyngeal spaces, which might cause systemic absorption. Wash the hands immediately after administration.*

HUMORSOL *should not be used more often than directed. Caution is necessary to avoid overdosage.*

Initial titration and dosage adjustments with HUMORSOL must be individualized to obtain maximal therapeutic effect. The patient must be closely observed during the initial period. If the response is not adequate within the first 24 hours, other measures should be considered.

Keep frequency of use to a minimum in all patients, but especially in children, to reduce the chance of iris cyst development (see ADVERSE REACTIONS).

Glaucoma

For initial therapy with HUMORSOL (0.125 percent or 0.25 percent) place 1 drop (children) or 1 or 2 drops (adults) in the glaucomatous eye. A decrease in intraocular pressure should occur within a few hours. During this period, keep the patient under supervision and make tonometric examinations at least hourly for 3 or 4 hours to be sure that no immediate rise in pressure occurs (see ADVERSE REACTIONS).

Duration of effect varies with the individual. The usual dosage can vary from as much as 1 or 2 drops twice a day to as little as 1 or 2 drops twice a week. The 0.125 percent strength used twice a day usually results in smooth control of the physiologic diurnal variation in intraocular pressure. This is probably the preferred dosage for most wide (open) angle glaucoma patients.

Strabismus

Essentially equal visual acuity of both eyes is a prerequisite to the successful treatment of esotropia with HUMORSOL. For initial evaluation it may be used as a diagnostic aid to determine if an accommodative factor exists. This is especially useful preoperatively in young chil-

dren and in patients with normal hypermetropic refractive errors. One drop is given daily for 2 weeks, then 1 drop every 2 days for 2 to 3 weeks. If the eyes become straighter, an accommodative factor is demonstrated. This technic may supplement or complement standard testing with atropine and trial with glasses for the accommodative factor.
In esotropia uncomplicated by amblyopia or anisometropia, HUMORSOL may be instilled in both eyes, *not more than 1 drop at a time every day for 2 to 3 weeks*, as too severe a degree of miosis may interfere with vision. Then reduce the dosage to 1 drop every other day for 3 to 4 weeks and reevaluate the patient's status.
HUMORSOL may be continued in a dosage of 1 drop every 2 days to 1 drop twice a week. (The latter dosage may be maintained for several months.) Evaluate the patient's condition every 4 to 12 weeks. If improvement continues, change the schedule to 1 drop once a week and eventually to a trial without medication. However, if after 4 months, control of the condition still requires 1 drop every 2 days, therapy with HUMORSOL should be stopped.

*Registered trademark of MERCK & CO., INC.

How Supplied
Sterile Ophthalmic Solution HUMORSOL is a clear, colorless, aqueous solution and is supplied in a 5 mL white, opaque, plastic OCUMETER ophthalmic dispenser with a controlled-drop tip:
No. 3255—0.125 percent solution.
NDC 0006-3255-03.
No. 3267—0.25 percent solution.
NDC 0006-3267-03.
Storage
Protect from freezing and excessive heat.
DC 7414314 Issued May 1993

Shown in Product Identification Guide, page 104

LACRISERT® Sterile Ophthalmic Insert ℞
(Hydroxypropyl Cellulose), U.S.P.

Description: LACRISERT* (Hydroxypropyl Cellulose) is a sterile, translucent, rod-shaped, water soluble, ophthalmic insert made of hydroxypropyl cellulose, for administration into the inferior cul-de-sac of the eye.
The chemical name for hydroxypropyl cellulose is cellulose, 2-hydroxypropyl ether. It is an ether of cellulose in which hydroxypropyl groups ($-CH_2CHOHCH_3$) are attached to the hydroxyls present in the anhydroglucose rings of cellulose by ether linkages. A representative structure of the monomer is:

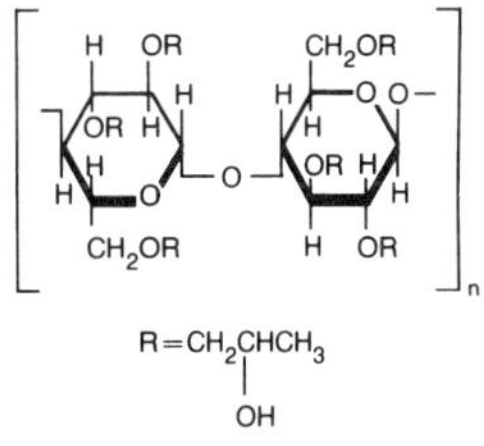

The molecular weight is typically 1×10^6.
Hydroxypropyl cellulose is an off-white, odorless, tasteless powder. It is soluble in water below 38°C, and in many polar organic solvents such as ethanol, propylene glycol, dioxane, methanol, isopropyl alcohol (95%), dimethyl sulfoxide, and dimethyl formamide.
Each LACRISERT is 5 mg of hydroxypropyl cellulose. LACRISERT contains no preservatives or other ingredients. It is about 1.27 mm in diameter by about 3.5 mm long.
LACRISERT is supplied in packages of 60 units, together with illustrated instructions and a special applicator for removing LACRISERT from the unit dose blister and inserting it into the eye. A spare applicator is included in each package.

*Registered trademark of MERCK & CO., INC.

Clinical Pharmacology
Pharmacodynamics
LACRISERT acts to stabilize and thicken the precorneal tear film and prolong the tear film breakup time which is usually accelerated in patients with dry eye states. LACRISERT also acts to lubricate and protect the eye.
LACRISERT usually reduces the signs and symptoms resulting from moderate to severe dry eye syndromes, such as conjunctival hyperemia, corneal and conjunctival staining with rose bengal, exudation, itching, burning, foreign body sensation, smarting, photophobia, dryness and blurred or cloudy vision. Progressive visual deterioration which occurs in some patients may be retarded, halted, or sometimes reversed.
In a multicenter crossover study the 5 mg LACRISERT administered once a day during the waking hours was compared to artificial tears used four or more times daily. There was a prolongation of tear film breakup time and a decrease in foreign body sensation associated with dry eye syndrome in patients during treatment with inserts as compared to artificial tears; these findings were statistically significantly different between the treatment groups. Improvement, as measured by amelioration of symptoms, by slit lamp examination and by rose bengal staining of the cornea and conjunctiva, was greater in most patients with moderate to severe symptoms during treatment with LACRISERT. Patient comfort was usually better with LACRISERT than with artificial tears solution, and most patients preferred LACRISERT.
In most patients treated with LACRISERT for over one year, improvement was observed as evidenced by amelioration of symptoms generally associated with keratoconjunctivitis sicca such as burning, tearing, foreign body sensation, itching, photophobia and blurred or cloudy vision.
During studies in healthy volunteers, a thickened precorneal tear film was usually observed through the slit-lamp while LACRISERT was present in the conjunctival sac.
Pharmacokinetics and Metabolism
Hydroxypropyl cellulose is a physiologically inert substance. In a study of rats fed hydroxypropyl cellulose or unmodified cellulose at levels up to 5% of their diet, it was found that the two were biologically equivalent in that neither was metabolized.
Studies conducted in rats fed ^{14}C -labeled hydroxypropyl cellulose demonstrated that when orally administered, hydroxypropyl cellulose is not absorbed from the gastrointestinal tract and is quantitatively excreted in the feces.
Dissolution studies in rabbits showed that hydroxypropyl cellulose inserts became softer within 1 hour after they were placed in the conjunctival sac. Most of the inserts dissolved completely in 14 to 18 hours; with a single exception, all had disappeared by 24 hours after insertion. Similar dissolution of the inserts was observed during prolonged administration (up to 54 weeks).
Indications and Usage: LACRISERT is indicated in patients with moderate to severe dry eye syndromes, including keratoconjunctivitis sicca. LACRISERT is indicated especially in patients who remain symptomatic after an adequate trial of therapy with artifical tear solutions.
LACRISERT is also indicated for patients with:
Exposure keratitis
Decreased corneal sensitivity
Recurrent corneal erosions
Contraindications: LACRISERT is contraindicated in patients who are hypersensitive to hydroxypropyl cellulose.
Warnings: Instructions for inserting and removing LACRISERT should be carefully followed.
Precautions
General
If improperly placed, LACRISERT may result in corneal abrasion (see DOSAGE AND ADMINISTRATION).
Information for Patients
Patients should be advised to follow the instructions for using LACRISERT which accompany the package.
Because this product may produce transient blurring of vision, patients should be instructed to exercise caution when operating hazardous machinery or driving a motor vehicle.
Drug Interactions
Application of hydroxypropyl cellulose inserts to the eyes of unanesthetized rabbits immediately prior to or two hours before instilling pilocarpine, proparacaine HCl (0.5%), or phenylephrine (5%) did not markedly alter the magnitude and/or duration of the miotic, local corneal anesthetic, or mydriatic activity, respectively, of these agents.
Under various treatment schedules, the antiinflammatory effect of ocularly instilled dexamethasone (0.1%) in unanesthetized rabbits with primary uveitis was not affected by the presence of hydroxypropyl cellulose inserts.
Carcinogenesis, Mutagenesis,
Impairment of Fertility
Feeding of hydroxypropyl cellulose to rats at levels up to 5% of their diet produced no gross or histopathologic changes or other deleterious effects.
Adverse Reactions: The following adverse reactions have been reported in patients treated with LACRISERT, but were in most instances mild and transient:
Transient blurring of vision
(See PRECAUTIONS)
Ocular discomfort or irritation
Matting or stickiness of eyelashes
Photophobia
Hypersensitivity
Edema of the eyelids
Hyperemia
Dosage and Administration: One LACRISERT ophthalmic insert in each eye once daily is usually sufficient to relieve the symptoms associated with moderate to severe dry eye syndromes. Individual patients may require more flexibility in the use of LACRISERT; some patients may require twice daily use for optimal results.
Clinical experience with LACRISERT indicates that in some patients several weeks may be required before satisfactory improvement of symptoms is achieved.
LACRISERT is inserted into the inferior cul-de-sac of the eye beneath the base of the tarsus, not in apposition to the cornea, nor beneath the eyelid at the level of the tarsal plate. If not properly positioned, it will be expelled into the interpalpebral fissure, and may cause symptoms of a foreign body. Illustrated instructions are included in each package. While in the licensed practitioner's office, the patient should read the instructions, then practice insertion

Continued on next page

Information on the Merck and Co., Inc. products listed on these pages is the full prescribing information from product circulars in effect August 31, 1994.

Merck and Co, Inc.—Cont.

and removal of LACRISERT until proficiency is achieved.
NOTE: Occasionally LACRISERT is inadvertently expelled from the eye, especially in patients with shallow conjunctival fornices. The patient should be cautioned against rubbing the eye(s) containing LACRISERT, especially upon awakening, so as not to dislodge or expel the insert. If required, another LACRISERT ophthalmic insert may be inserted. If experience indicates that transient blurred vision develops in an individual patient, the patient may want to remove LACRISERT a few hours after insertion to avoid this. Another LACRISERT ophthalmic insert may be inserted if needed.
If LACRISERT causes worsening of symptoms, the patient should be instructed to inspect the conjunctival sac to make certain LACRISERT is in the proper location, deep in the inferior cul-de-sac of the eye beneath the base of the tarsus. If these symptoms persist, LACRISERT should be removed and the patient should contact the practitioner.

How Supplied
No. 3380—LACRISERT, a sterile, translucent, rod-shaped, water soluble, ophthalmic insert made of hydroxypropyl cellulose, 5 mg, is supplied as follows:
NDC 0006-3380-60 in packages containing 60 unit doses, two reusable applicators and a storage container
(6505-01-153-4360, 5 mg 60's.)
Storage
Store below 30°C (86°F).
DC 7415108 Issued August 1989

Shown in Product Identification Guide, page 104

NEODECADRON® ℞
(Neomycin Sulfate-Dexamethasone Sodium Phosphate), U.S.P.
Sterile Ophthalmic Ointment

Description
Sterile ophthalmic ointment NEODECADRON* (Neomycin Sulfate-Dexamethasone Sodium Phosphate) is a topical corticosteroid-antibiotic ointment for use in certain disorders of the anterior segment of the eye.
Ophthalmic ointment NEODECADRON contains in each gram: dexamethasone sodium phosphate equivalent to 0.5 mg (0.05%) dexamethasone phosphate and neomycin sulfate equivalent to 3.5 mg neomycin base. Inactive ingredients: white petrolatum and mineral oil.
Dexamethasone sodium phosphate is an inorganic ester of dexamethasone. Its empirical formula is $C_{22}H_{28}FNa_2O_8P$.
Neomycin sulfate is the sulfate salt of neomycin, an antibacterial substance produced by the growth of *Streptomyces fradiae* Waksman (Fam. Streptomycetaceae).

*Registered trademark of MERCK & CO., INC.

Clinical Pharmacology
Dexamethasone sodium phosphate, a corticosteroid, suppresses the inflammatory response to a variety of agents, and it probably delays or slows healing. Since corticosteroids may inhibit the body's defense mechanism against infection, a concomitant antimicrobial drug may be used when this inhibition is considered to be clinically significant in a particular case.
Neomycin sulfate, the anti-infective component in the combination, is included to provide action against specific organisms susceptible to it. Neomycin sulfate is considered active mainly against gram-negative organisms, except *Bacteroides* spp. and *Pseudomonas aeruginosa*, which are resistant. Gram-positive organisms except for *Staphylococcus aureus* are usually resistant.
When a decision to administer both a corticosteroid and an antimicrobial is made, the administration of such drugs in combination has the advantage of greater patient compliance and convenience, with the added assurance that the appropriate dosage of both drugs is administered, plus assured compatibility of ingredient when both types of drug are in the same formulation and, particularly, that the correct volume of drug is delivered and retained.
The relative potency of corticosteroids depends on the molecular structure, concentration, and release from the vehicle.

Indications and Usage
For steroid-responsive inflammatory ocular conditions for which a corticosteroid is indicated and where bacterial infection or a risk of bacterial ocular infection exists.
Ocular steroids are indicated in inflammatory conditions of the palpebral and bulbar conjunctiva, cornea, and anterior segment of the globe where the inherent risk of steroid use in certain infective conjunctivitides is accepted to obtain a diminution in edema and inflammation. They are also indicated in chronic anterior uveitis and corneal injury from chemical, radiation, or thermal burns, or penetration of foreign bodies.
The use of a combination drug with an anti-infective component is indicated where the risk of infection is high or where there is an expectation that potentially dangerous numbers of bacteria will be present in the eye.
The particular anti-infective drug in this product is active against the following common bacterial eye pathogens:
Staphylococcus aureus
Escherichia coli
Haemophilus influenzae
Klebsiella/Enterobacter species
Neisseria species
The product does not provide adequate coverage against:
Pseudomonas aeruginosa
Serratia marcescens
Streptococci, including *Streptococcus pneumoniae*

Contraindications
Epithelial herpes simplex keratitis (dendritic keratitis), acute infectious stages of vaccinia, varicella, and many other viral diseases of the cornea and conjunctiva. Mycobacterial infection of the eye. Fungal diseases of ocular structures. Hypersensitivity to a component of the medication (hypersensitivity to the antibiotic component occurs at a higher rate than for other components).
The use of these combinations is always contraindicated after uncomplicated removal of a corneal foreign body.

Warnings
Prolonged use may result in glaucoma, with damage to the optic nerve, defects in visual acuity and fields of vision, and posterior subcapsular cataract formation. Prolonged use may suppress the host response and thus increase the hazard of secondary ocular infections. In those diseases causing thinning of the cornea or sclera, perforations have been known to occur with the use of topical corticosteroids. In acute purulent conditions of the eye, corticosteroids may mask infection or enhance existing infection. If these products are used for 10 days or longer, intraocular pressure should be routinely monitored even though it may be difficult in children and uncooperative patients.
Employment of corticosteroid medication in the treatment of herpes simplex requires great caution: periodic slit-lamp microscopy is recommended.
Any substance (e.g., neomycin sulfate) may occasionally cause cutaneous sensitization. If any reaction indicating such sensitivity is observed, discontinue use.

Precautions
The initial prescriptions and renewal of the medication order beyond 8 grams should be made by a physician only after examination of the patient with the aid of magnification, such as slit-lamp biomicroscopy and, where appropriate, fluorescein staining.
The possibility of persistent fungal infections of the cornea should be considered after prolonged corticosteroid dosing.
Usage in Pregnancy
Safety of intensive or protracted use of topical corticosteroids during pregnancy has not been substantiated.

Adverse Reactions
Adverse reactions have occurred with corticosteroid/anti-infective combination drugs which can be attributed to the corticosteroid component, the anti-infective component, or the combination. Exact incidence figures are not available since no denominator of treated patients is available.
Reactions occurring most often from the presence of the anti-infective ingredient are allergic sensitizations. The reactions due to the corticosteroid component in decreasing order of frequency are: elevation of intraocular pressure (IOP) with possible development of glaucoma, and infrequent optic nerve damage; posterior subcapsular cataract formation; and delayed wound healing.
Secondary Infection: The development of secondary infection has occurred after use of combinations containing corticosteroids and antimicrobials. Fungal infections of the cornea are particularly prone to develop coincidentally with long-term applications of corticosteroid. The possibility of fungal invasion must be considered in any persistent corneal ulceration where corticosteroid treatment has been used. Secondary bacterial ocular infection following suppression of host responses also occurs.

Dosage and Administration
The duration of treatment will vary with the type of lesion and may extend from a few days to several weeks, according to therapeutic response. Relapses, more common in chronic active lesions than in self-limited conditions, usually respond to retreatment.
Apply a thin coating of ophthalmic ointment NEODECADRON three or four times a day. When a favorable response is observed, reduce the number of daily applications to two, and later to one a day as maintenance dose if this is sufficient to control symptoms.
Not more than 8 grams should be prescribed initially and the prescription should not be refilled without further evaluation as outlined in PRECAUTIONS above.
Ophthalmic ointment NEODECADRON is particularly convenient when an eye pad is used. It may also be the preparation of choice for patients in whom therapeutic benefit depends on prolonged contact of the active ingredients with ocular tissues.

How Supplied
No. 7617—Sterile Ophthalmic Ointment NEODECADRON is a clear, unctuous ointment, and is supplied as follows:
NDC 0006-7617-04 in 3.5 g tubes
(6505-00-823-7956 0.05% 3.5 g)
DC 7612625 Issued October 1993
Shown in Product Identification Guide, page 104

NEODECADRON® ℞
(Neomycin Sulfate-Dexamethasone Sodium Phosphate), U.S.P.
Sterile Ophthalmic Solution

Description
Ophthalmic solution NEODECADRON* (Neomycin Sulfate-Dexamethasone Sodium Phosphate) is a topical corticosteroid-antibiotic solution for use in certain disorders of the anterior segment of the eye.
Each milliliter of buffered ophthalmic solution NEODECADRON in the OCUMETER* ophthalmic dispenser contains: dexamethasone sodium phosphate equivalent to 1 mg (0.1%) dexamethasone phosphate, and neomycin sulfate equivalent to 3.5 mg neomycin base. Inactive ingredients: creatinine, sodium citrate, sodium borate, polysorbate 80, disodium edetate, hydrochloric acid to adjust pH to 6.6–7.2, and water for injection. Benzalkonium chloride 0.02% and sodium bisulfite 0.1% added as preservatives.
Dexamethasone sodium phosphate is a water soluble, inorganic ester of dexamethasone. Its empirical formula is $C_{22}H_{28}FNa_2O_8P$. It is approximately three thousand times more soluble in water at 25°C than hydrocortisone.
Neomycin sulfate is the sulfate salt of neomycin, an antibacterial substance produced by the growth of *Streptomyces fradiae* Waksman (Fam. Streptomycetaceae).

*Registered trademark of MERCK & CO., INC.

Clinical Pharmacology
Dexamethasone sodium phosphate, a corticosteroid, suppresses the inflammatory response to a variety of agents, and it probably delays or slows healing. Since corticosteroids may inhibit the body's defense mechanism against infection, a concomitant antimicrobial drug may be used when this inhibition is considered to be clinically significant in a particular case.
Neomycin sulfate, the anti-infective component in the combination, is included to provide action against specific organisms susceptible to it. Neomycin sulfate is considered active mainly against gram-negative organisms, except *Bacteroides* spp. and *Pseudomonas aeruginosa,* which are resistant. Gram-positive organisms except for *Staphylococcus aureus* are usually resistant.
When a decision to administer both a corticosteroid and an anti-microbial is made, the administration of such drugs in combination has the advantage of greater patient compliance and convenience, with the added assurance that the appropriate dosage of both drugs is administered, plus assured compatibility of ingredients when both types of drug are in the same formulation and, particularly, that the correct volume of drug is delivered and retained.
The relative potency of corticosteroids depends on the molecular structure, concentration, and release from the vehicle.

Indications and Usage
For steroid-responsive inflammatory ocular conditions for which a corticosteroid is indicated and where bacterial infection or a risk of bacterial ocular infection exists.
Ocular steroids are indicated in inflammatory conditions of the palpebral and bulbar conjunctiva, cornea, and anterior segment of the globe where the inherent risk of steroid use in certain infective conjunctivitides is accepted to obtain a diminution in edema and inflammation. They are also indicated in chronic anterior uveitis and corneal injury from chemical, radiation, or thermal burns, or penetration of foreign bodies.
The use of a combination drug with an anti-infective component is indicated where the risk of infection is high or where there is an expectation that potentially dangerous numbers of bacteria will be present in the eye.
The particular anti-infective drug in this product is active against the following common bacterial eye pathogens:
Staphylococcus aureus
Escherichia coli
Haemophilus influenzae
Klebsiella/Enterobacter species
Neisseria species
The product does not provide adequate coverage against:
Pseudomonas aeruginosa
Serratia marcescens
Streptococci, including *Streptococcus pneumoniae*

Contraindications
Epithelial herpes simplex keratitis (dendritic keratitis), acute infectious stages of vaccinia, varicella, and many other viral diseases of the cornea and conjunctiva. Mycobacterial infection of the eye. Fungal diseases of ocular structures. Hypersensitivity to any component of this product, including sulfites (see WARNINGS). (Hypersensitivity to the antibiotic component occurs at a higher rate than for other components.)
The use of these combinations is always contraindicated after uncomplicated removal of a corneal foreign body.

Warnings
Prolonged use may result in glaucoma, with damage to the optic nerve, defects in visual acuity and fields of vision, and posterior subcapsular cataract formation. Prolonged use may suppress the host response and thus increase the hazard of secondary ocular infections. In those diseases causing thinning of the cornea or sclera, perforations have been known to occur with the use of topical corticosteroids. In acute purulent conditions of the eye, corticosteroids may mask infection or enhance existing infection. If these products are used for 10 days or longer, intraocular pressure should be routinely monitored even though it may be difficult in children and uncooperative patients.
Employment of corticosteroid medication in the treatment of herpes simplex requires great caution: periodic slit-lamp microscopy is recommended.
Any substance (e.g., neomycin sulfate) may occasionally cause cutaneous sensitization. If any reaction indicating such sensitivity is observed, discontinue use.
Ophthalmic Solution NEODECADRON contains sodium bisulfite, a sulfite that may cause allergic-type reactions including anaphylactic symptoms and life-threatening or less severe asthmatic episodes in certain susceptible people. The overall prevalence of sulfite sensitivity in the general population is unknown and probably low. Sulfite sensitivity is seen more frequently in asthmatic than in nonasthmatic people.

Precautions
The initial prescription and renewal of the medication order beyond 20 milliliters should be made by a physician only after examination of the patient with the aid of magnification, such as slit-lamp biomicroscopy and, where appropriate, fluorescein staining.
The possibility of persistent fungal infections of the cornea should be considered after prolonged corticosteroid dosing.
Information for Patients
One of the preservatives in Ophthalmic Solution NEODECADRON, benzalkonium chloride, may be absorbed by soft contact lenses. Patients wearing soft contact lenses should be instructed to wait at least 15 minutes after instilling Ophthalmic Solution NEODECADRON before they insert their lenses.
Usage in Pregnancy
Safety of intensive or protracted use of topical corticosteroids during pregnancy has not been substantiated.

Adverse Reactions
Adverse reactions have occurred with corticosteroid/anti-infective combination drugs which can be attributed to the corticosteroid component, the anti-infective component, the combination, or any other component of the product. Exact incidence figures are not available since no denominator of treated patients is available.
Reactions occurring most often from the presence of the anti-infective ingredient are allergic sensitizations. The reactions due to the corticosteroid component in decreasing order of frequency are: elevation of intraocular pressure (IOP) with possible development of glaucoma, and infrequent optic nerve damage; posterior subcapsular cataract formation; and delayed wound healing.
Secondary Infection: The development of secondary infection has occurred after use of combinations containing corticosteroids and antimicrobials. Fungal infections of the cornea are particularly prone to develop coincidentally with long-term applications of corticosteroid. The possibility of fungal invasion must be considered in any persistent corneal ulceration where corticosteroid treatment has been used. Secondary bacterial ocular infection following suppression of host responses also occurs.

Dosage and Administration
The duration of treatment will vary with the type of lesion and may extend from a few days to several weeks, according to therapeutic response. Relapses, more common in chronic active lesions than in self-limited conditions, usually respond to retreatment.
Instill one or two drops of ophthalmic solution NEODECADRON into the conjunctival sac every hour during the day and every two hours during the night as initial therapy. When a favorable response is observed, reduce dosage to one drop every four hours. Later, further reduction in dosage to one drop three or four times daily may suffice to control symptoms.
Not more than 20 milliliters should be prescribed initially and the prescription should not be refilled without further evaluation as outlined in PRECAUTIONS above.

How Supplied
Sterile ophthalmic solution NEODECADRON is a clear, colorless to pale yellow solution.
No. 7639—Ophthalmic solution NEODECADRON is supplied as follows:
NDC 0006-7639-03 in 5 mL white opaque, plastic OCUMETER ophthalmic dispenser with a controlled drop tip.
(6505-01-039-4352 0.1% 5 mL).

DC 7261323 Issued October 1993
Shown in Product Identification Guide, page 104

TIMOPTIC® ℞
(Timolol Maleate), U.S.P.
Sterile Ophthalmic Solution

Description
TIMOPTIC* (Timolol Maleate) Ophthalmic Solution is a non-selective beta-adrenergic receptor blocking agent. Its chemical name is (*S*)-1-[(1,1-dimethylethyl)amino]-3-[[4-(4-morpholinyl)-1,2,5-thiadiazol-3-yl]oxy]-2-propanol (*Z*)-2-butenedioate (1:1) salt. Timolol maleate possesses an asymmetric carbon atom in its structure and is provided as the levo isomer. The nominal optical rotation of timolol maleate is:

Continued on next page

Information on the Merck and Co., Inc. products listed on these pages is the full prescribing information from product circulars in effect August 31, 1994.

Merck and Co, Inc.—Cont.

$[\alpha]^{25^\circ}_{405\,nm}$ in 0.1N HCl (C = 5%) = −12.2°.

Its empirical formula is $C_{13}H_{24}N_4O_3S \cdot C_4H_4O_4$ and its structural formula is:

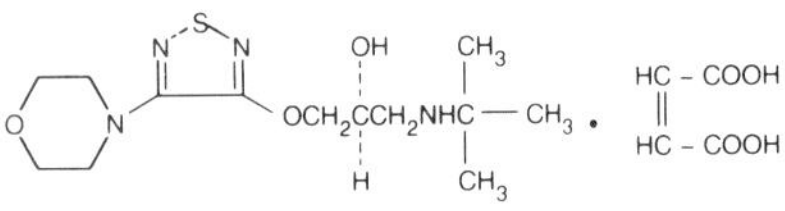

Timolol maleate has a molecular weight of 432.49. It is a white, odorless, crystalline powder which is soluble in water, methanol, and alcohol. TIMOPTIC is stable at room temperature.

TIMOPTIC Ophthalmic Solution is supplied as a sterile, isotonic, buffered, aqueous solution of timolol maleate in two dosage strengths: Each mL of TIMOPTIC 0.25% contains 2.5 mg of timolol (3.4 mg of timolol maleate). Each mL of TIMOPTIC 0.5% contains 5.0 mg of timolol (6.8 mg of timolol maleate). Inactive ingredients: monobasic and dibasic sodium phosphate, sodium hydroxide to adjust pH, and water for injection. Benzalkonium chloride 0.01% is added as preservative.

---

*Registered trademark of MERCK & CO., INC.

Clinical Pharmacology

Timolol maleate is a $beta_1$ and $beta_2$ (non-selective) adrenergic receptor blocking agent that does not have significant intrinsic sympathomimetic, direct myocardial depressant, or local anesthetic (membrane-stabilizing) activity.

Beta-adrenergic receptor blockade reduces cardiac output in both healthy subjects and patients with heart disease. In patients with severe impairment of myocardial function beta-adrenergic receptor blockade may inhibit the stimulatory effect of the sympathetic nervous system necessary to maintain adequate cardiac function.

Beta-adrenergic receptor blockade in the bronchi and bronchioles results in increased airway resistance from unopposed para-sympathetic activity. Such an effect in patients with asthma or other bronchospastic conditions is potentially dangerous.

TIMOPTIC Ophthalmic Solution, when applied topically in the eye, has the action of reducing elevated as well as normal intraocular pressure, whether or not accompanied by glaucoma. Elevated intraocular pressure is a major risk factor in the pathogenesis of glaucomatous visual field loss. The higher the level of intraocular pressure, the greater the likelihood of glaucomatous visual field loss and optic nerve damage.

The onset of reduction in intraocular pressure following administration of TIMOPTIC can usually be detected within one-half hour after a single dose. The maximum effect usually occurs in one to two hours and significant lowering of intraocular pressure can be maintained for periods as long as 24 hours with a single dose. Repeated observations over a period of one year indicate that the intraocular pressure-lowering effect of TIMOPTIC is well maintained.

The precise mechanism of the ocular hypotensive action of TIMOPTIC is not clearly established at this time. Tonography and fluorophotometry studies in man suggest that its predominant action may be related to reduced aqueous formation. However, in some studies a slight increase in outflow facility was also observed. Unlike miotics, TIMOPTIC reduces intraocular pressure with little or no effect on accommodation or pupil size. Thus, changes in visual acuity due to increased accommodation are uncommon, and dim or blurred vision and night blindness produced by miotics are not evident. In addition, in patients with cataracts the inability to see around lenticular opacities when the pupil is constricted is avoided.

In the clinical studies which are reported below, ocular pressure reductions to less than 22 mmHg were used as a reasonable reference point to allow comparisons between treatments. Reduction of ocular pressure to just below 22 mmHg may not be optimal for all patients; therapy should be individualized.

In controlled multiclinic studies in patients with untreated intraocular pressures of 22 mmHg or greater, TIMOPTIC 0.25 percent or 0.5 percent administered twice a day produced a greater reduction in intraocular pressure than 1, 2, 3, or 4 percent pilocarpine solution administered four times a day or 0.5, 1, or 2 percent epinephrine hydrochloride solution administered twice a day.

In the multiclinic studies comparing TIMOPTIC with pilocarpine, 61 percent of patients treated with TIMOPTIC had intraocular pressure reduced to less than 22 mmHg compared to 32 percent of patients treated with pilocarpine. For patients completing these studies, the mean reduction in pressure at the end of the study from pretreatment was 30.7 percent for patients treated with TIMOPTIC and 21.7 percent for patients treated with pilocarpine.

In the multiclinic studies comparing TIMOPTIC with epinephrine, 69 percent of patients treated with TIMOPTIC had intraocular pressure reduced to less than 22 mmHg compared to 42 percent of patients treated with epinephrine. For patients completing these studies, the mean reduction in pressure at the end of the study from pretreatment was 33.2 percent for patients treated with TIMOPTIC and 28.1 percent for patients treated with epinephrine.

In these studies, TIMOPTIC was generally well tolerated and produced fewer and less severe side effects than either pilocarpine or epinephrine. A slight reduction of resting heart rate in some patients receiving TIMOPTIC (mean reduction 2.9 beats/minute standard deviation 10.2) was observed.

TIMOPTIC has also been used in patients with glaucoma wearing conventional (PMMA) hard contact lenses, and has generally been well tolerated. TIMOPTIC has not been studied in patients wearing lenses made with materials other than PMMA. (See PRECAUTIONS, *Information for Patients.*)

Indications and Usage

Timoptic Ophthalmic Solution is indicated in the treatment of elevated intraocular pressure in patients with ocular hypertension or open-angle glaucoma.

Clinical trials have shown that in patients who respond inadequately to multiple antiglaucoma drug therapy the addition of TIMOPTIC may produce a further reduction of intraocular pressure.

Contraindications

TIMOPTIC is contraindicated in patients with bronchial asthma or with a history of bronchial asthma, or severe chronic obstructive pulmonary disease (see WARNINGS); sinus bradycardia; second and third degree atrioventricular block; overt cardiac failure (see WARNINGS); cardiogenic shock; hypersensitivity to any component of this product.

Warnings

As with other topically applied ophthalmic drugs, this drug may be absorbed systemically.

The same adverse reactions found with systemic administration of beta-adrenergic blocking agents may occur with topical administration. For example, severe respiratory reactions and cardiac reactions, including death due to bronchospasm in patients with asthma, and rarely death in association with cardiac failure, have been reported following administration of TIMOPTIC (Timolol Maleate) (see CONTRAINDICATIONS).

Cardiac Failure

Sympathetic stimulation may be essential for support of the circulation in individuals with diminished myocardial contractility, and its inhibition by beta-adrenergic receptor blockade may precipitate more severe failure.

In Patients Without a History of Cardiac Failure continued depression of the myocardium with beta-blocking agents over a period of time can, in some cases, lead to cardiac failure. At the first sign or symptom of cardiac failure TIMOPTIC should be discontinued.

Obstructive Pulmonary Disease

PATIENTS WITH CHRONIC OBSTRUCTIVE PULMONARY DISEASE (e.g., CHRONIC BRONCHITIS, EMPHYSEMA) OF MILD OR MODERATE SEVERITY, BRONCHOSPASTIC DISEASE OR A HISTORY OF BRONCHOSPASTIC DISEASE (OTHER THAN BRONCHIAL ASTHMA OR A HISTORY OF BRONCHIAL ASTHMA, IN WHICH 'TIMOPTIC' IS CONTRAINDICATED, see CONTRAINDICATIONS), SHOULD IN GENERAL NOT RECEIVE BETA BLOCKERS, INCLUDING 'TIMOPTIC'. However, if TIMOPTIC is necessary in such patients, then the drug should be administered with caution since it may block bronchodilation produced by endogenous and exogenous catecholamine stimulation of $beta_2$ receptors.

Major Surgery

The necessity or desirability of withdrawal of beta-adrenergic blocking agents prior to major surgery is controversial. Beta-adrenergic receptor blockade impairs the ability of the heart to respond to beta-adrenergically mediated reflex stimuli. This may augment the risk of general anesthesia in surgical procedures. Some patients receiving beta-adrenergic receptor blocking agents have been subject to protracted severe hypotension during anesthesia. Difficulty in restarting and maintaining the heartbeat has also been reported. For these reasons, in patients undergoing elective surgery, some authorities recommend gradual withdrawal of beta-adrenergic receptor blocking agents.

If necessary during surgery, the effects of beta-adrenergic blocking agents may be reversed by sufficient doses of such agonists as isoproterenol, dopamine, dobutamine or levarterenol (see OVERDOSAGE).

Diabetes Mellitus

Beta-adrenergic blocking agents should be administered with caution in patients subject to spontaneous hypoglycemia or to diabetic patients (especially those with labile diabetes) who are receiving insulin or oral hypoglycemic agents. Beta-adrenergic receptor blocking agents may mask the signs and symptoms of acute hypoglycemia.

Thyrotoxicosis

Beta-adrenergic blocking agents may mask certain clinical signs (e.g., tachycardia) of hyperthyroidism. Patients suspected of developing thyrotoxicosis should be managed carefully to avoid abrupt withdrawal of beta-adrenergic blocking agents which might precipitate a thyroid storm.

Precautions

General

Patients who are receiving a beta-adrenergic blocking agent orally and TIMOPTIC should be observed for a potential additive effect either on the intraocular pressure or on the known systemic effects of beta blockade.

Patients should not receive two topical ophthalmic beta-adrenergic blocking agents concurrently (see DOSAGE AND ADMINISTRATION).

Because of potential effects of beta-adrenergic blocking agents relative to blood pressure and pulse, these agents should be used with caution in patients with cerebrovascular insufficiency. If signs or symptoms suggesting reduced cerebral blood flow develop following initiation of therapy with TIMOPTIC, alternative therapy should be considered.

There have been reports of bacterial keratitis associated with the use of multiple dose containers of topical ophthalmic products. These containers had been inadvertently contaminated by patients who, in most cases, had a concurrent corneal disease or a disruption of the ocular epithelial surface. (See PRECAUTIONS, *Information for Patients.*)

In patients with angle-closure glaucoma, the immediate objective of treatment is to reopen the angle. This requires constricting the pupil with a miotic. TIMOPTIC has little or no effect on the pupil. When TIMOPTIC is used to reduce elevated intraocular pressure in angle-closure glaucoma, it should be used with a miotic and not alone.

As with the use of other antiglaucoma drugs, diminished responsiveness to TIMOPTIC after prolonged therapy has been reported in some patients. However, in one long-term study in which 96 patients have been followed for at least 3 years, no significant difference in mean intraocular pressure has been observed after initial stabilization.

Muscle Weakness: Beta-adrenergic blockade has been reported to potentiate muscle weakness consistent with certain myasthenic symptoms (e.g., diplopia, ptosis, and generalized weakness). Timolol has been reported rarely to increase muscle weakness in some patients with myasthenia gravis or myasthenic symptoms.

Information for Patients

Patients should be instructed to avoid allowing the tip of the dispensing container to contact the eye or surrounding structures.

Patients should also be instructed that ocular solutions, if handled improperly, can become contaminated by common bacteria known to cause ocular infections. Serious damage to the eye and subsequent loss of vision may result from using contaminated solutions. (See PRECAUTIONS, *General.*)

Patients should also be advised that if they develop an intercurrent ocular condition (e.g., trauma, ocular surgery or infection), they should immediately seek their physician's advice concerning the continued use of the present multidose container.

The preservative in TIMOPTIC, benzalkonium chloride, may be absorbed by soft contact lenses. Patients wearing soft contact lenses should be instructed to wait at least 15 minutes after instilling TIMOPTIC before they insert their lenses.

Drug Interactions

Although TIMOPTIC used alone has little or no effect on pupil size, mydriasis resulting from concomitant therapy with TIMOPTIC and epinephrine has been reported occasionally.

Close observation of the patient is recommended when a beta blocker is administered to patients receiving catecholamine-depleting drugs such as reserpine, because of possible additive effects and the production of hypotension and/or marked bradycardia, which may produce vertigo, syncope, or postural hypotension.

Caution should be used in the coadministration of beta-adrenergic blocking agents, such as TIMOPTIC, and oral or intravenous calcium antagonists, because of possible atrioventricular conduction disturbances, left ventricular failure, and hypotension. In patients with impaired cardiac function, coadministration should be avoided.

The concomitant use of beta-adrenergic blocking agents with digitalis and calcium antagonists may have additive effects in prolonging atrioventricular conduction time.

Risk from Anaphylactic Reaction: While taking beta-blockers, patients with a history of atopy or a history of severe anaphylactic reaction to a variety of allergens may be more reactive to repeated accidental, diagnostic, or therapeutic challenge with such allergens. Such patients may be unresponsive to the usual doses of epinephrine used to treat anaphylactic reactions.

Animal Studies

No adverse ocular effects were observed in rabbits and dogs administered TIMOPTIC topically in studies lasting one and two years respectively.

Carcinogenesis, Mutagenesis, Impairment of Fertility

In a two-year oral study of timolol maleate in rats, there was a statistically significant increase in the incidence of adrenal pheochromocytomas in male rats administered 300 mg/kg/day (250 times* the maximum recommended daily human oral dose†). Similar differences were not observed in rats administered oral doses equivalent to approximately 20 or 80 times* the maximum recommended daily human oral dose.

In a lifetime oral study in mice, there were statistically significant increases in the incidence of benign and malignant pulmonary tumors, benign uterine polyps and mammary adenocarcinoma in female mice at 500 mg/kg/day, (approximately 400 times* the maximum recommended daily human oral dose†), but not at 5 or 50 mg/kg/day. In a subsequent study in female mice, in which post-mortem examinations were limited to uterus and lungs, a statistically significant increase in the incidence of pulmonary tumors was again observed at 500 mg/kg/day.

The increased occurrence of mammary adenocarcinoma was associated with elevations in serum prolactin which occurred in female mice administered timolol at 500 mg/kg, but not at doses of 5 or 50 mg/kg/day. An increased incidence of mammary adenocarcinomas in rodents has been associated with administration of several other therapeutic agents which elevate serum prolactin, but no correlation between serum prolactin levels and mammary tumors has been established in man. Furthermore, in adult human female subjects who received oral dosages of up to 60 mg of timolol maleate, the maximum recommended daily human oral dosage, there were no clinically meaningful changes in serum prolactin.

Timolol maleate was devoid of mutagenic potential when evaluated *in vivo* (mouse) in the micronucleus test and cytogenetic assay (doses up to 800 mg/kg) and *in vitro* in a neoplastic cell transformation assay (up to 100 μg/mL). In Ames tests the highest concentrations of timolol employed, 5000 or 10,000 μg/plate, were associated with statistically significant elevations of revertants observed with tester strain TA100 (in seven replicate assays), but not in the remaining three strains. In the assays with tester strain TA100, no consistent dose response relationship was observed, nor did the ratio of test to control revertants reach 2. A ratio of 2 is usually considered the criterion for a positive Ames test.

Reproduction and fertility studies in rats showed no adverse effect on male or female fertility at doses up to 125 times* the maximum recommended daily human oral dose.

---

* Based on patient weight of 50 kg

† The maximum recommended daily oral dose is 60 mg of timolol. One drop of TIMOPTIC 0.5% contains about 1/300 of this dose which is about 0.2 mg.

Pregnancy

Pregnancy Category C. Teratogenicity studies with timolol in mice and rabbits at doses up to 50 mg/kg/day (approximately 40 times* the maximum recommended daily human oral dose†) showed no evidence of fetalmalformations. Although delayed fetal ossification was observed at this dose in rats, there were no adverse effects on postnatal development of offspring. Doses of 1000 mg/kg/day (approximately 830 times* the maximum recommended daily human oral dose†) were maternotoxic in mice and resulted in an increased number of fetal resorptions. Increased fetal resorptions were also seen in rabbits at doses of approximately 40 times* the maximum recommended daily human oral dose, in this case without apparent maternotoxicity. There are no adequate andwell-controlled studies in pregnant women. TIMOPTIC should beused during pregnancy only if the potential benefit justifies the potential risk to the fetus.

---

* Based on patient weight of 50 kg

† The maximum recommended daily oral dose is 60 mg of timolol. One drop of TIMOPTIC 0.5% contains about 1/300 of this dose which is about 0.2 mg

Nursing Mothers

Timolol maleate has been detected in human milk following oral and ophthalmic drug administration. Because of the potential for serious adverse reactions from TIMOPTIC in nursing infants, a decision should be made whether to discontinue nursing or to discontinue the drug, taking into account the importance of the drug to the mother.

Pediatric Use

Safety and effectiveness in children have not been established by adequate and well-controlled studies.

Adverse Reactions

The following adverse reactions have been reported either in clinical trials of up to 3 years duration prior to release in 1978 or since the drug has been marketed:

BODY AS A WHOLE

Headache, asthenia/fatigue, chest pain.

CARDIOVASCULAR

Bradycardia, arrhythmia, hypotension, syncope, heart block, cerebral vascular accident, cerebral ischemia, cardiac failure, palpitation, cardiac arrest.

DIGESTIVE

Nausea, diarrhea.

IMMUNOLOGIC

Systemic lupus erythematosus.

NERVOUS SYSTEM/PSYCHIATRIC

Dizziness, depression, increase in signs and symptoms of myasthenia gravis, paresthesia.

SKIN

Hypersensitivity, including localized and generalized rash; urticaria, alopecia.

RESPIRATORY

Bronchospasm (predominantly in patients with pre-existing bronchospastic disease), respiratory failure, dyspnea, nasal congestion, cough.

ENDOCRINE

Masked symptoms of hypoglycemia in diabetic patients (see WARNINGS).

SPECIAL SENSES

Signs and symptoms of ocular irritation, including conjunctivitis, blepharitis, keratitis, blepharoptosis, decreased corneal sensitivity, visual disturbances including refractive changes (due to withdrawal of miotic therapy in some cases), diplopia, ptosis.

Causal Relationship Unknown: The following adverse effects have been reported, and a causal relationship to therapy with TIMOPTIC has not been established: *Cardiovascular:* Hypertension, pulmonary edema, worsening of angina pectoris; *Digestive:* Dyspepsia, anorexia, dry mouth; *Nervous System/Psychiatric:* Behavioral changes including confusion, hallu-

Continued on next page

Information on the Merck and Co., Inc. products listed on these pages is the full prescribing information from product circulars in effect August 31, 1994.

Merck and Co, Inc.—Cont.

cinations, anxiety, disorientation, nervousness, somnolence, and other psychic disturbances; *Special Senses:* Aphakic cystoid macular edema; *Urogenital:* Retroperitoneal fibrosis, impotence.

The following additional adverse effects have been reported in clinical experience with oral timolol maleate, and may be considered potential effects of ophthalmic timolol maleate: *Body as a Whole:* Extremity pain, decreased exercise tolerance, weight loss; *Cardiovascular:* Edema, worsening of arterial insufficiency, Raynaud's phenomenon, vasodilatation; *Digestive:* Gastrointestinal pain, hepatomegaly, vomiting; *Hematologic:* Nonthrombocytopenic purpura; *Endocrine:* Hyperglycemia, hypoglycemia; *Skin:* Pruritus, skin irritation, increased pigmentation, sweating, cold hands and feet; *Musculoskeletal:* Arthralgia, claudication; *Nervous System/Psychiatric:* Vertigo, local weakness, decreased libido, nightmares, insomnia, diminished concentration; *Respiratory:* Rales, bronchial obstruction; *Special Senses:* Tinnitus, dry eyes; *Urogenital:* Urination difficulties.

Potential Adverse Effects: In addition, a variety of adverse effects have been reported with other beta-adrenergic blocking agents and may be considered potential effects of ophthalmic timolol maleate: *Digestive:* Mesenteric arterial thrombosis, ischemic colitis; *Hematologic:* Agranulocytosis, thrombocytopenic purpura; *Nervous System:* Reversible mental depression progressing to catatonia; an acute reversible syndrome characterized by disorientation for time and place, short-term memory loss, emotional lability, slightly clouded sensorium, and decreased performance on neuropsychometrics; *Allergic:* Erythematous rash, fever combined with aching and sore throat, laryngospasm with respiratory distress; *Urogenital:* Peyronie's disease.

There have been reports of a syndrome comprising psoriasiform skin rash, conjunctivitis sicca, otitis and sclerosing serositis attributed to the beta-adrenergic receptor blocking agent, practolol. This syndrome has not been reported with timolol maleate.

Overdosage

There have been reports of inadvertent overdosage with TIMOPTIC Ophthalmic Solution resulting in systemic effects such as dizziness, headache, shortness of breath, bradycardia, bronchospasm, and cardiac arrest.

Overdosage has been reported with Tablets BLOCADREN* (Timolol Maleate). A 30 year old female ingested 650 mg of BLOCADREN (maximum recommended oral daily dose is 60 mg) and experienced second and third degree heart block. She recovered without treatment but approximately two months later developed irregular heartbeat, hypertension, dizziness, tinnitus, faintness, increased pulse rate, and borderline first degree heart block.

The oral LD_{50} of the drug is 1190 and 900 mg/kg in female mice and female rats, respectively.

An *in vitro* hemodialysis study, using ^{14}C timolol added to human plasma or whole blood, showed that timolol was readily dialyzed from these fluids; however, a study of patients with renal failure showed that timolol did not dialyze readily.

The most common signs and symptoms to be expected with overdosage with administration of a systemic beta-adrenergic receptor blocking agent are symptomatic bradycardia, hypotension, bronchospasm, and acute cardiac failure. The following therapeutic measures should be considered:

(1) *Gastric lavage:* If ingested.

(2) *Symptomatic bradycardia:* Use atropine sulfate intravenously in a dosage of 0.25 mg to 2 mg to induce vagal blockade. If bradycardia persists, intravenous isoproterenol hydrochloride should be administered cautiously. In refractory cases the use of a transvenous cardiac pacemaker may be considered.

(3) *Hypotension:* Use sympathomimetic pressor drug therapy, such as dopamine, dobutamine or levarterenol. In refractory cases the use of glucagon hydrochloride has been reported to be useful.

(4) *Bronchospasm:* Use isoproterenol hydrochloride. Additional therapy with aminophylline may be considered.

(5) *Acute cardiac failure:* Conventional therapy with digitalis, diuretics, and oxygen should be instituted immediately. In refractory cases the use of intravenous aminophylline is suggested. This may be followed if necessary by glucagon hydrochloride which has been reported to be useful.

(6) *Heart block (second or third degree):* Use isoproterenol hydrochloride or a transvenous cardiac pacemaker.

---

*Registered trademark of MERCK & CO., INC.

Dosage and Administration

TIMOPTIC Ophthalmic Solution is available in concentrations of 0.25 and 0.5 percent. The usual starting dose is one drop of 0.25 percent TIMOPTIC in the affected eye(s) twice a day. If the clinical response is not adequate, the dosage may be changed to one drop of 0.5 percent solution in the affected eye(s) twice a day.

Since in some patients the pressure-lowering response to TIMOPTIC may require a few weeks to stabilize, evaluation should include a determination of intraocular pressure after approximately 4 weeks of treatment with TIMOPTIC.

If the intraocular pressure is maintained at satisfactory levels, the dosage schedule may be changed to one drop once a day in the affected eye(s). Because of diurnal variations in intraocular pressure, satisfactory response to the once-a-day dose is best determined by measuring the intraocular pressure at different times during the day.

Dosages above one drop of 0.5 percent TIMOPTIC twice a day generally have not been shown to produce further reduction in intraocular pressure. If the patient's intraocular pressure is still not at a satisfactory level on this regimen, concomitant therapy with pilocarpine and other miotics, and/or epinephrine, and/or systemically administered carbonic anhydrase inhibitors, such as acetazolamide, can be instituted.

When a patient is transferred from another topical ophthalmic beta-adrenergic blocking agent, that agent should be discontinued after proper dosing on one day and treatment with TIMOPTIC started on the following day with 1 drop of 0.25 percent TIMOPTIC in the affected eye(s) twice a day. The dose may be increased to one drop of 0.5 percent TIMOPTIC twice a day if the clinical response is not adequate.

When a patient is transferred from a single antiglaucoma agent, other than a topical ophthalmic beta-adrenergic blocking agent, continue the agent already being used and add one drop of 0.25 percent TIMOPTIC in the affected eye(s) twice a day. On the following day, discontinue the previously used antiglaucoma agent completely and continue with TIMOPTIC. If a higher dosage of TIMOPTIC is required, substitute one drop of 0.5 percent solution in the affected eye(s) twice a day.

When a patient is transferred from several concomitantly administered antiglaucoma agents, individualization is required. If any of the agents is an ophthalmic beta-adrenergic blocker, it should be discontinued before starting TIMOPTIC. Additional adjustments should involve one agent at a time and usually should be made at intervals of not less than one week. A recommended approach is to continue the agents being used and to add one drop of 0.25 percent TIMOPTIC in the affected eye(s) twice a day. On the following day, discontinue one of the other antiglaucoma agents. The remaining antiglaucoma agents may be decreased or discontinued according to the patient's response to treatment. If a higher dosage of TIMOPTIC is required, substitute one drop of 0.5 percent solution in the affected eye(s) twice a day. The physician may be able to discontinue some or all of the other antiglaucoma agents.

How Supplied

Sterile Ophthalmic Solution TIMOPTIC is a clear, colorless to light yellow solution.

No. 3366—TIMOPTIC Ophthalmic Solution, 0.25% timolol equivalent, is supplied in a white, opaque, plastic OCUMETER* ophthalmic dispenser with a controlled drop tip as follows:

NDC 0006-3366-32, 2.5 mL
NDC 0006-3366-03, 5 mL
(6505-01-069-6518, 0.25% 5 mL)
NDC 0006-3366-10, 10 mL
(6505-01-093-5458, 0.25% 10 mL)
NDC 0006-3366-12, 15 mL.

No. 3367—TIMOPTIC Ophthalmic Solution, 0.5% timolol equivalent, is supplied in a white, opaque, plastic OCUMETER ophthalmic dispenser with a controlled drop tip as follows:

NDC 0006-3367-32, 2.5 mL
NDC 0006-3367-03, 5 mL
(6505-01-069-6519, 0.5% 5 mL)
NDC 0006-3367-10, 10 mL
(6505-01-092-0422, 0.5% 10 mL)
NDC 0006-3367-12, 15 mL.

---

*Registered trademark of MERCK & CO., INC.

Storage

Protect from light. Store at room temperature.

DC 7115434 Issued November 1993

Shown in Product Identification Guide, page 105

TIMOPTIC® ℞
(Timolol Maleate)
in OCUDOSE® (Dispenser), U.S.P.
Preservative-Free Sterile Ophthalmic Solution in a Sterile Ophthalmic Unit Dose Dispenser

Description

Timolol maleate is a non-selective beta-adrenergic receptor blocking agent. Its chemical name is (*S*)-1-[(1,1-dimethylethyl)amino]-3-[[4-(4-morpholinyl)-1,2,5-thiadiazol-3-yl]oxy]-2-propanol (*Z*)-2-butenedioate (1:1) salt. Timolol maleate possesses an asymmetric carbon atom in its structure and is provided as the levo isomer. The nominal optical rotation of timolol maleate is

$$[\alpha]^{25°}_{405\ nm} \text{ in 0.1N HCl } (C = 5\%) = -12.2°.$$

Its empirical formula is $C_{13}H_{24}N_4O_3S \cdot C_4H_4O_4$ and its structural formula is:

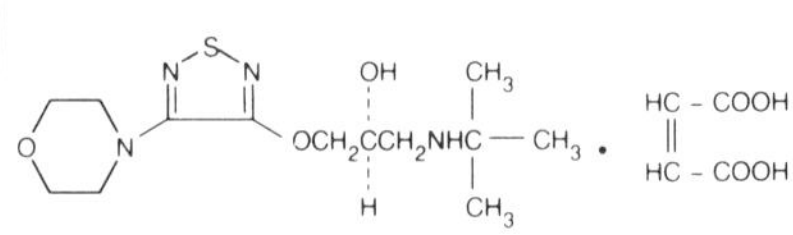

Timolol maleate has a molecular weight of 432.49. It is a white, odorless, crystalline powder which is soluble in water, methanol, and alcohol. Timolol maleate is stable at room temperature.

Timolol maleate ophthalmic solution is supplied in two formulations: Ophthalmic Solution TIMOPTIC* (Timolol Maleate), which contains the preservative, benzalkonium chloride; and Ophthalmic Solution TIMOPTIC*

(Timolol Maleate), the preservative-free formulation.

Preservative-free Ophthalmic Solution TIMOPTIC is supplied in OCUDOSE*, a unit dose container as a sterile, isotonic, buffered, aqueous solution of timolol maleate in two dosage strengths: Each mL of Preservative-free TIMOPTIC in OCUDOSE 0.25% contains 2.5 mg of timolol (3.4 mg of timolol maleate). Each mL of Preservative-free TIMOPTIC in OCUDOSE 0.5% contains 5.0 mg of timolol (6.8 mg of timolol maleate). Inactive ingredients: monobasic and dibasic sodium phosphate, sodium hydroxide to adjust pH, and water for injection.

*Registered trademark of MERCK & CO., INC.

Clinical Pharmacology

Timolol maleate is a $beta_1$ and $beta_2$ (non-selective) adrenergic receptor blocking agent that does not have significant intrinsic sympathomimetic, direct myocardial depressant, or local anesthetic (membrane-stabilizing) activity.

Beta-adrenergic receptor blockade reduces cardiac output in both healthy subjects and patients with heart disease. In patients with severe impairment of myocardial function beta-adrenergic receptor blockade may inhibit the stimulatory effect of the sympathetic nervous system necessary to maintain adequate cardiac function.

Beta-adrenergic receptor blockade in the bronchi and bronchioles results in increased airway resistance from unopposed parasympathetic activity. Such an effect in patients with asthma or other bronchospastic conditions is potentially dangerous.

TIMOPTIC (Timolol Maleate), when applied topically in the eye, has the action of reducing elevated as well as normal intraocular pressure, whether or not accompanied by glaucoma. Elevated intraocular pressure is a major risk factor in the pathogenesis of glaucomatous visual field loss. The higher the level of intraocular pressure, the greater the likelihood of glaucomatous visual field loss and optic nerve damage.

The onset of reduction in intraocular pressure following administration of TIMOPTIC (Timolol Maleate) can usually be detected within one-half hour after a single dose. The maximum effect usually occurs in one to two hours and significant lowering of intraocular pressure can be maintained for periods as long as 24 hours with a single dose. Repeated observations over a period of one year indicate that the intraocular pressure-lowering effect of TIMOPTIC (Timolol Maleate) is well maintained.

The precise mechanism of the ocular hypotensive action of TIMOPTIC (Timolol Maleate) is not clearly established at this time. Tonography and fluorophotometry studies in man suggest that its predominant action may be related to reduced aqueous formation. However, in some studies a slight increase in outflow facility was also observed. Unlike miotics, TIMOPTIC (Timolol Maleate) reduces intraocular pressure with little or no effect on accommodation or pupil size. Thus, changes in visual acuity due to increased accommodation are uncommon, and dim or blurred vision and night blindness produced by miotics are not evident. In addition, in patients with cataracts the inability to see around lenticular opacities when the pupil is constricted is avoided.

Clinical studies have shown that the mean percent reductions in intraocular pressure with Preservative-free TIMOPTIC and TIMOPTIC (Timolol Maleate) were similar. Preservative-free TIMOPTIC was generally well tolerated.

In the clinical studies which are reported below, ocular pressure reductions to less than 22 mmHg were used as a reasonable reference point to allow comparisons between treatments. Reduction of ocular pressure to just below 22 mmHg may not be optimal for all patients; therapy should be individualized.

In controlled multiclinic studies in patients with untreated intraocular pressures of 22 mmHg or greater, TIMOPTIC (Timolol Maleate) 0.25 percent or 0.5 percent administered twice a day produced a greater reduction in intraocular pressure than 1, 2, 3, or 4 percent pilocarpine solution administered four times a day or 0.5, 1, or 2 percent epinephrine hydrochloride solution administered twice a day.

In the multiclinic studies comparing TIMOPTIC (Timolol Maleate) with pilocarpine, 61 percent of patients treated with TIMOPTIC (Timolol Maleate) had intraocular pressure reduced to less than 22 mmHg compared to 32 percent of patients treated with pilocarpine. For patients completing these studies, the mean reduction in pressure at the end of the study from pretreatment was 30.7 percent for patients treated with TIMOPTIC (Timolol Maleate) and 21.7 percent for patients treated with pilocarpine.

In the multiclinic studies comparing TIMOPTIC (Timolol Maleate) with epinephrine, 69 percent of patients treated with TIMOPTIC (Timolol Maleate) had intraocular pressure reduced to less than 22 mmHg compared to 42 percent of patients treated with epinephrine. For patients completing these studies, the mean reduction in pressure at the end of the study from pretreatment was 33.2 percent for patients treated with TIMOPTIC (Timolol Maleate) and 28.1 percent for patients treated with epinephrine.

In these studies, TIMOPTIC (Timolol Maleate) was generally well tolerated and produced fewer and less severe side effects than either pilocarpine or epinephrine. A slight reduction of resting heart rate in some patients receiving TIMOPTIC (Timolol Maleate) (mean reduction 2.9 beats/minute standard deviation 10.2) was observed.

TIMOPTIC (Timolol Maleate) has also been used in patients with glaucoma wearing conventional (PMMA) hard contact lenses, and has generally been well tolerated. TIMOPTIC (Timolol Maleate) has not been studied in patients wearing lenses made with materials other than PMMA.

Indications and Usage

Preservative-free TIMOPTIC in OCUDOSE is indicated in the treatment of elevated intraocular pressure in patients with ocular hypertension or open-angle glaucoma.

Preservative-free TIMOPTIC in OCUDOSE may be used when a patient is sensitive to the preservative in TIMOPTIC (Timolol Maleate), benzalkonium chloride, or when use of a preservative-free topical medication is advisable.

Clinical trials have shown that in patients who respond inadequately to multiple antiglaucoma drug therapy the addition of TIMOPTIC (Timolol Maleate) may produce a further reduction of intraocular pressure.

Contraindications

Preservative-free TIMOPTIC in OCUDOSE is contraindicated in patients with bronchial asthma or with a history of bronchial asthma, or severe chronic obstructive pulmonary disease (see WARNINGS); sinus bradycardia; second and third degree atrioventricular block; overt cardiac failure (see WARNINGS); cardiogenic shock; hypersensitivity to any component of this product.

Warnings

As with other topically applied ophthalmic drugs, this drug may be absorbed systemically. **The same adverse reactions found with systemic administration of beta-adrenergic blocking agents may occur with topical administration. For example, severe respiratory reactions and cardiac reactions, including death due to bronchospasm in patients with asthma, and rarely death in association with cardiac failure, have been reported following administration of TIMOPTIC (Timolol Maleate) (see CONTRAINDICATIONS).**

Cardiac Failure

Sympathetic stimulation may be essential for support of the circulation in individuals with diminished myocardial contractility, and its inhibition by beta-adrenergic receptor blockade may precipitate more severe failure.

In Patients Without a History of Cardiac Failure continued depression of the myocardium with beta-blocking agents over a period of time can, in some cases, lead to cardiac failure. At the first sign or symptom of cardiac failure Preservative-free TIMOPTIC in OCUDOSE should be discontinued.

Obstructive Pulmonary Disease

PATIENTS WITH CHRONIC OBSTRUCTIVE PULMONARY DISEASE (e.g., CHRONIC BRONCHITIS, EMPHYSEMA) OF MILD OR MODERATE SEVERITY, BRONCHOSPASTIC DISEASE OR A HISTORY OF BRONCHOSPASTIC DISEASE (OTHER THAN BRONCHIAL ASTHMA OR A HISTORY OF BRONCHIAL ASTHMA, IN WHICH 'Preservative-free TIMOPTIC in OCUDOSE' IS CONTRAINDICATED, see CONTRAINDICATIONS), SHOULD IN GENERAL NOT RECEIVE BETA BLOCKERS, INCLUDING 'Preservative-free TIMOPTIC in OCUDOSE'. However, if Preservative-free TIMOPTIC in OCUDOSE is necessary in such patients, then the drug should be administered with caution since it may block bronchodilation produced by endogenous and exogenous catecholamine stimulation of $beta_2$ receptors.

Major Surgery

The necessity or desirability of withdrawal of beta-adrenergic blocking agents prior to major surgery is controversial. Beta-adrenergic receptor blockade impairs the ability of the heart to respond to beta-adrenergically mediated reflex stimuli. This may augment the risk of general anesthesia in surgical procedures. Some patients receiving beta-adrenergic receptor blocking agents have been subject to protracted severe hypotension during anesthesia. Difficulty in restarting and maintaining the heartbeat has also been reported. For these reasons, in patients undergoing elective surgery, some authorities recommend gradual withdrawal of beta-adrenergic receptor blocking agents.

If necessary during surgery, the effects of beta-adrenergic blocking agents may be reversed by sufficient doses of such agonists as isoproterenol, dopamine, dobutamine or levarterenol (see OVERDOSAGE).

Diabetes Mellitus

Beta-adrenergic blocking agents should be administered with caution in patients subject to spontaneous hypoglycemia or to diabetic patients (especially those with labile diabetes) who are receiving insulin or oral hypoglycemic agents. Beta-adrenergic receptor blocking agents may mask the signs and symptoms of acute hypoglycemia.

Thyrotoxicosis

Beta-adrenergic blocking agents may mask certain clinical signs (e.g., tachycardia) of hyperthyroidism. Patients suspected of developing thyrotoxicosis should be managed carefully to avoid abrupt withdrawal of beta-adrenergic blocking agents which might precipitate a thyroid storm.

Precautions

General

Patients who are receiving a beta-adrenergic blocking agent orally and Preservative-free

Continued on next page

Information on the Merck and Co., Inc. products listed on these pages is the full prescribing information from product circulars in effect August 31, 1994.

Merck and Co, Inc.—Cont.

TIMOPTIC in OCUDOSE should be observed for a potential additive effect either on the intraocular pressure or on the known systemic effects of beta blockade.

Patients should not receive two topical ophthalmic beta-adrenergic blocking agents concurrently (see DOSAGE AND ADMINISTRATION).

Because of potential effects of beta-adrenergic blocking agents relative to blood pressure and pulse, these agents should be used with caution in patients with cerebrovascular insufficiency. If signs or symptoms suggesting reduced cerebral blood flow develop following initiation of therapy with Preservative-free TIMOPTIC in OCUDOSE, alternative therapy should be considered.

Muscle Weakness: Beta-adrenergic blockade has been reported to potentiate muscle weakness consistent with certain myasthenic symptoms (e.g., diplopia, ptosis, and generalized weakness). Timolol has been reported rarely to increase muscle weakness in some patients with myasthenia gravis or myasthenic symptoms.

In patients with angle-closure glaucoma, the immediate objective of treatment is to reopen the angle. This requires constricting the pupil with a miotic. TIMOPTIC (Timolol Maleate) has little or no effect on the pupil. When Preservative-free TIMOPTIC in OCUDOSE is used to reduce elevated intraocular pressure in angle-closure glaucoma, it should be used with a miotic and not alone.

As with the use of other antiglaucoma drugs, diminished responsiveness to TIMOPTIC (Timolol Maleate) after prolonged therapy has been reported in some patients. However, in one long-term study in which 96 patients have been followed for at least 3 years, no significant difference in mean intraocular pressure has been observed after initial stabilization.

Information for Patients

Patients should be instructed about the use of Preservative-free TIMOPTIC in OCUDOSE.

Since sterility cannot be maintained after the individual unit is opened, patients should be instructed to use the product immediately after opening, and to discard the individual unit and any remaining contents immediately after use.

Drug Interactions

Although TIMOPTIC (Timolol Maleate) used alone has little or no effect on pupil size, mydriasis resulting from concomitant therapy with TIMOPTIC (Timolol Maleate) and epinephrine has been reported occasionally.

Close observation of the patient is recommended when a beta blocker is administered to patients receiving catecholamine-depleting drugs such as reserpine, because of possible additive effects and the production of hypotension and/or marked bradycardia, which may produce vertigo, syncope, or postural hypotension.

Caution should be used in the coadministration of beta-adrenergic blocking agents, such as Preservative-free TIMOPTIC in OCUDOSE, and oral or intravenous calcium antagonists, because of possible atrioventricular conduction disturbances, left ventricular failure, and hypotension. In patients with impaired cardiac function, coadministration should be avoided.

The concomitant use of beta-adrenergic blocking agents with digitalis and calcium antagonists may have additive effects in prolonging atrioventricular conduction time.

Risk from Anaphylactic Reaction: While taking beta-blockers, patients with a history of atopy or a history of severe anaphylactic reaction to a variety of allergens may be more reactive to repeated accidental, diagnostic, or therapeutic challenge with such allergens. Such patients may be unresponsive to the usual doses of epinephrine used to treat anaphylactic reactions.

Animal Studies

No adverse ocular effects were observed in rabbits and dogs administered TIMOPTIC (Timolol Maleate) topically in studies lasting one and two years respectively.

Carcinogenesis, Mutagenesis, Impairment of Fertility

In a two-year oral study of timolol maleate in rats, there was a statistically significant increase in the incidence of adrenal pheochromocytomas in male rats administered 300 mg/kg/day (250 times* the maximum recommended daily human oral dose†). Similar differences were not observed in rats administered oral doses equivalent to approximately 20 or 80 times* the maximum recommended daily human oral dose.

In a lifetime oral study in mice, there were statistically significant increases in the incidence of benign and malignant pulmonary tumors, benign uterine polyps and mammary adenocarcinoma in female mice at 500 mg/kg/day (approximately 400 times* the maximum recommended daily human oral dose†) but not at 5 or 50 mg/kg/day. In a subsequent study in female mice, in which post-mortem examinations were limited to uterus and lungs, a statistically significant increase in the incidence of pulmonary tumors was again observed at 500 mg/kg/day.

The increased occurrence of mammary adenocarcinoma was associated with elevations in serum prolactin which occurred in female mice administered timolol at 500 mg/kg, but not at doses of 5 or 50 mg/kg/day. An increased incidence of mammary adenocarcinomas in rodents has been associated with administration of several other therapeutic agents which elevate serum prolactin, but no correlation between serum prolactin levels and mammary tumors has been established in man. Furthermore, in adult human female subjects who received oral dosages of up to 60 mg of timolol maleate, the maximum recommended daily human oral dosage, there were no clinically meaningful changes in serum prolactin.

Timolol maleate was devoid of mutagenic potential when evaluated *in vivo* (mouse) in the micronucleus test and cytogenetic assay (doses up to 800 mg/kg) and *in vitro* in a neoplastic cell transformation assay (up to 100 μg/mL). In Ames tests the highest concentrations of timolol employed, 5000 or 10,000 μg/plate, were associated with statistically significant elevations of revertants observed with tester strain TA 100 (in seven replicate assays), but not in the remaining three strains. In the assays with tester strain TA 100, no consistent dose response relationship was observed, nor did the ratio of test to control revertants reach 2. A ratio of 2 is usually considered the criterion for a positive Ames test.

Reproduction and fertility studies in rats showed no adverse effect on male or female fertility at doses up to 125 times* the maximum recommended daily human oral dose.

*Based on patient weight of 50 kg

†The maximum recommended daily oral dose is 60 mg of timolol. One drop of Preservative-free TIMOPTIC in OCUDOSE 0.5% contains about 1/300 of this dose which is about 0.2 mg.

Pregnancy

Pregnancy Category C. Teratogenicity studies with timolol in mice, rats and rabbits at doses up to 50 mg/kg/day (approximately 40 times* the maximum recommended daily human oral dose†) showed no evidence of fetal malformations. Although delayed fetal ossification was observed at this dose in rats, there were no adverse effects on postnatal development of offspring. Doses of 1000 mg/kg/day (approximately 830 times* the maximum recommended daily human oral dose†) were maternotoxic in mice and resulted in an increased number of fetal resorptions. Increased fetal resorptions were also seen in rabbits at doses of approximately 40 times* the maximum recommended daily human oral dose, in this case without apparent maternotoxicity. There are no adequate and well-controlled studies in pregnant women. Preservative-free TIMOPTIC in OCUDOSE should be used during pregnancy only if the potential benefit justifies the potential risk to the fetus.

*Based on patient weight of 50 kg

†The maximum recommended daily oral dose is 60 mg of timolol. One drop of Preservative-free TIMOPTIC in OCUDOSE 0.5% contains about 1/300 of this dose which is about 0.2 mg.

Nursing Mothers

Timolol maleate has been detected in human milk following oral and ophthalmic drug administration. Because of the potential for serious adverse reactions from timolol in nursing infants, a decision should be made whether to discontinue nursing or to discontinue the drug, taking into account the importance of the drug to the mother.

Pediatric Use

Safety and effectiveness in children have not been established by adequate and well-controlled studies.

Adverse Reactions

The following adverse reactions have been reported with TIMOPTIC (Timolol Maleate), either in clinical trials of up to 3 years duration prior to release in 1978 or since the drug has been marketed, and may be expected to occur with Preservative-free TIMOPTIC.

BODY AS A WHOLE

Headache, asthenia/fatigue, chest pain.

CARDIOVASCULAR

Bradycardia, arrhythmia, hypotension, syncope, heart block, cerebral vascular accident, cerebral ischemia, cardiac failure, palpitation, cardiac arrest.

DIGESTIVE

Nausea, diarrhea.

IMMUNOLOGIC

Systemic lupus erythematosus.

NERVOUS SYSTEM/PSYCHIATRIC

Dizziness, depression, increase in signs and symptoms of myasthenia gravis, paresthesia.

SKIN

Hypersensitivity, including localized and generalized rash; urticaria, alopecia.

RESPIRATORY

Bronchospasm (predominantly in patients with pre-existing bronchospastic disease), respiratory failure, dyspnea, nasal congestion, cough.

ENDOCRINE

Masked symptoms of hypoglycemia in diabetic patients (see WARNINGS).

SPECIAL SENSES

Signs and symptoms of ocular irritation, including conjunctivitis, blepharitis, keratitis, blepharoptosis, decreased corneal sensitivity, visual disturbances including refractive changes (due to withdrawal of miotic therapy in some cases), diplopia, ptosis.

Causal Relationship Unknown: The following adverse effects have been reported, and a causal relationship to therapy with ophthalmic timolol maleate has not been established: *Cardiovascular:* Hypertension, pulmonary edema, worsening of angina pectoris; *Digestive:* Dyspepsia, anorexia, dry mouth; *Nervous System/Psychiatric:* Behavioral changes including confusion, hallucinations, anxiety, disorientation, nervousness, somnolence, and other psychic disturbances; *Special Senses:* Aphakic cystoid macular edema; *Urogenital:* Retroperitoneal fibrosis, impotence.

The following additional adverse effects have been reported in clinical experience with oral timolol maleate, and may be considered potential effects of ophthalmic timolol maleate: *Body as a Whole:* Extremity pain, decreased exercise tolerance, weight loss; *Cardiovascular:* Edema, worsening of arterial insufficiency, Raynaud's phenomenon, vasodilatation; *Digestive:* Gastrointestinal pain, hepatomegaly, vomiting; *Hematologic:* Nonthrombocytopenic purpura; *Endocrine:* Hyperglycemia, hypoglycemia; *Skin:* Pruritus, skin irritation, increased pigmentation, sweating, cold hands and feet; *Musculoskeletal:* Arthralgia, claudication; *Nervous System/Psychiatric:* Vertigo, local weakness, decreased libido, nightmares, insomnia, diminished concentration; *Respiratory:* Rales, bronchial obstruction; *Special Senses:* Tinnitus, dry eyes; *Urogenital:* Urination difficulties.

Potential Adverse Effects: In addition, a variety of adverse effects have been reported with other beta-adrenergic blocking agents and may be considered potential effects of ophthalmic timolol maleate: *Digestive:* Mesenteric arterial thrombosis, ischemic colitis; *Hematologic:* Agranulocytosis, thrombocytopenic purpura; *Nervous System:* Reversible mental depression progressing to catatonia; an acute reversible syndrome characterized by disorientation for time and place, short-term memory loss, emotional lability, slightly clouded sensorium, and decreased performance on neuropsychometrics; *Allergic:* Erythematous rash, fever combined with aching and sore throat, laryngospasm with respiratory distress; *Urogenital:* Peyronie's disease.

There have been reports of a syndrome comprising psoriasiform skin rash, conjunctivitis sicca, otitis and sclerosing serositis attributed to the beta-adrenergic receptor blocking agent, practolol. This syndrome has not been reported with timolol maleate.

Overdosage

There have been reports of inadvertent overdosage with Ophthalmic Solution TIMOPTIC (Timolol Maleate) resulting in systemic effects such as dizziness, headache, shortness of breath, bradycardia, bronchospasm, and cardiac arrest.

Overdosage has been reported with Tablets BLOCADREN* (Timolol Maleate). A 30 year old female ingested 650 mg of BLOCADREN (maximum recommended oral daily dose is 60 mg) and experienced second and third degree heart block. She recovered without treatment but approximately two months later developed irregular heart beat, hypertension, dizziness, tinnitus, faintness, increased pulse rate, and borderline first degree heart block.

The oral LD_{50} of timolol maleate is 1190 and 900 mg/kg in female mice and female rats, respectively.

An *in vitro* hemodialysis study, using ^{14}C timolol added to human plasma or whole blood, showed that timolol was readily dialyzed from these fluids; however, a study of patients with renal failure showed that timolol did not dialyze readily.

The most common signs and symptoms to be expected with overdosage with administration of a systemic beta-adrenergic receptor blocking agent are symptomatic bradycardia, hypotension, bronchospasm, and acute cardiac failure. The following additional therapeutic measures should be considered:

(1) *Gastric lavage:* If ingested.

(2) *Symptomatic bradycardia:* Use atropine sulfate intravenously in a dosage of 0.25 mg to 2 mg to induce vagal blockade. If bradycardia persists, intravenous isoproterenol hydrochloride should be administered cautiously. In refractory cases the use of a transvenous cardiac pacemaker may be considered.

(3) *Hypotension:* Use sympathomimetic pressor drug therapy, such as dopamine, dobutamine or levarterenol. In refractory cases the use of glucagon hydrochloride has been reported to be useful.

(4) *Bronchospasm:* Use isoproterenol hydrochloride. Additional therapy with aminophylline may be considered.

(5) *Acute cardiac failure:* Conventional therapy with digitalis, diuretics, and oxygen should be instituted immediately. In refractory cases the use of intravenous aminophylline is suggested. This may be followed if necessary by glucagon hydrochloride which has been reported to be useful.

(6) *Heart block (second or third degree):* Use isoproterenol hydrochloride or a transvenous cardiac pacemaker.

---

* Registered trademark of MERCK & CO., INC.

Dosage and Administration

Preservative-free TIMOPTIC in OCUDOSE is a sterile solution that does not contain a preservative. The solution from one individual unit is to be used immediately after opening for administration to one or both eyes. Since sterility cannot be guaranteed after the individual unit is opened, the remaining contents should be discarded immediately after administration.

Preservative-free TIMOPTIC in OCUDOSE is available in concentrations of 0.25 and 0.5 percent. The usual starting dose is one drop of 0.25 percent Preservative-free TIMOPTIC in OCUDOSE in the affected eye(s) administered twice a day. Apply enough gentle pressure on the individual container to obtain a single drop of solution. If the clinical response is not adequate, the dosage may be changed to one drop of 0.5 percent solution in the affected eye(s) administered twice a day.

Since in some patients the pressure-lowering response to Preservative-free TIMOPTIC in OCUDOSE may require a few weeks to stabilize, evaluation should include a determination of intraocular pressure after approximately 4 weeks of treatment with Preservative-free TIMOPTIC in OCUDOSE.

If the intraocular pressure is maintained at satisfactory levels, the dosage schedule may be changed to one drop once a day in the affected eye(s). Because of diurnal variations in intraocular pressure, satisfactory response to the once-a-day dose is best determined by measuring the intraocular pressure at different times during the day.

Dosages above one drop of 0.5 percent TIMOPTIC (Timolol Maleate) twice a day generally have not been shown to produce further reduction in intraocular pressure. If the patient's intraocular pressure is not at a satisfactory level during treatment with Preservative-free TIMOPTIC in OCUDOSE 0.5 percent, concomitant therapy with pilocarpine and other miotics, and/or epinephrine, and/or systemically administered carbonic anhydrase inhibitors, such as acetazolamide, can be instituted taking into consideration that the preparation(s) used concomitantly may contain one or more preservatives.

When a patient is transferred from another topical ophthalmic beta-adrenergic blocking agent, that agent should be discontinued after proper dosing on one day and treatment with Preservative-free TIMOPTIC in OCUDOSE started on the following day with 1 drop of 0.25 percent Preservative-free TIMOPTIC in OCUDOSE in the affected eye(s) twice a day. The dose may be increased to one drop of 0.5 percent Preservative-free TIMOPTIC in OCUDOSE twice a day if the clinical response is not adequate.

When a patient is transferred from a single antiglaucoma agent, other than a topical ophthalmic beta-adrenergic blocking agent, continue the agent already being used and add one drop of 0.25 percent Preservative-free TIMOPTIC in OCUDOSE in the affected eye(s) twice a day. On the following day, discontinue the previously used antiglaucoma agent completely and continue with Preservative-free TIMOPTIC in OCUDOSE. If a higher dosage of Preservative-free TIMOPTIC in OCUDOSE is required, substitute one drop of 0.5 percent solution in the affected eye(s) twice a day.

When a patient is transferred from several concomitantly administered antiglaucoma agents, individualization is required. If any of the agents is an ophthalmic beta-adrenergic blocker, it should be discontinued before starting Preservative-free TIMOPTIC in OCUDOSE. Additional adjustments should involve one agent at a time and usually should be made at intervals of not less than one week. A recommended approach is to continue the agents being used and to add one drop of 0.25 percent Preservative-free TIMOPTIC in OCUDOSE in the affected eye(s) twice a day. On the following day, discontinue one of the other antiglaucoma agents. The remaining antiglaucoma agents may be decreased or discontinued according to the patient's response to treatment. If a higher dosage of Preservative-free TIMOPTIC in OCUDOSE is required, substitute one drop of 0.5 percent solution in the affected eye(s) twice a day. The physician may be able to discontinue some or all of the other antiglaucoma agents.

How Supplied

Preservative-free Sterile Ophthalmic Solution TIMOPTIC in OCUDOSE is a clear, colorless to light yellow solution.

No. 3542—Preservative-free TIMOPTIC, 0.25% timolol equivalent, is supplied in OCUDOSE, a clear polyethylene unit dose container. Each individual unit contains 0.45 mL of solution, and is available in a foil laminate overwrapped pouch as follows:

NDC 0006-3542-60; 60 Individual Unit Doses (6505-01-316-8791, 0.25% 60 Individual Unit Doses).

No. 3543—Preservative-free TIMOPTIC, 0.5% timolol equivalent, is supplied in OCUDOSE, a clear polyethylene unit dose container. Each individual unit contains 0.45 mL of solution, and is available in a foil laminate overwrapped pouch as follows:

NDC 0006-3543-60; 60 Individual Unit Doses (6505-01-284-5154, 0.5% 60 Individual Unit Doses).

Storage

Store Preservative-free TIMOPTIC in OCUDOSE at room temperature.

Because evaporation can occur through the unprotected polyethylene unit dose container and prolonged exposure to direct light can modify the product, the unit dose container should be kept in the protective foil overwrap and used within one month after the foil package has been opened.

DC 7475309 Issued November 1993

Shown in Product Identification Guide, page 105

TIMOPTIC-XE™ ℞

Sterile Ophthalmic Gel Forming Solution (Timolol Maleate Ophthalmic Gel Forming Solution)

Description

TIMOPTIC-XE* (timolol maleate ophthalmic gel forming solution) is a non-selective beta-adrenergic receptor blocking agent. Its chemi-

Continued on next page

Information on the Merck and Co., Inc. products listed on these pages is the full prescribing information from product circulars in effect August 31, 1994.

Merck and Co, Inc.—Cont.

cal name is (-)-1-(*tert*-butyl-amino)-3-[(4-morpholino-1,2,5-thiadiazol-3-yl)oxy]-2-propanol maleate (1:1) (salt). Timolol maleate possesses an asymmetric carbon atom in its structure and is provided as the levo-isomer. The nominal optical rotation of timolol maleate is:

$[\alpha]^{25°}_{405\ nm}$ in 0.1N HCl (C=5%) = −12.2°.

Its molecular formula is $C_{13}H_{24}N_4O_3S \cdot C_4H_4O_4$ and its structural formula is:

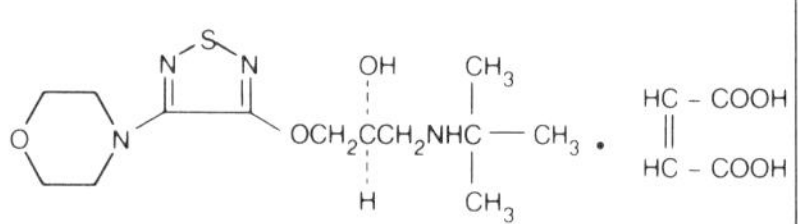

Timolol maleate has a molecular weight of 432.49. It is a white, odorless, crystalline powder which is soluble in water, methanol, and alcohol.

TIMOPTIC-XE Sterile Ophthalmic Gel Forming Solution is supplied as a sterile, isotonic, buffered, aqueous solution of timolol maleate in two dosage strengths. Each mL of TIMOPTIC-XE 0.25% contains 2.5 mg of timolol (3.4 mg of timolol maleate). Each mL of TIMOPTIC-XE 0.5% contains 5.0 mg of timolol (6.8 mg of timolol maleate). Inactive ingredients: GELRITE** gellan gum, tromethamine, mannitol, and water for injection. Preservative: benzododecinium bromide 0.012%.

GELRITE is a purified anionic heteropolysaccharide derived from gellan gum. An aqueous solution of GELRITE, in the presence of a cation, has the ability to gel. Upon contact with the precorneal tear film, TIMOPTIC-XE forms a gel that is subsequently removed by the flow of tears.

* Trademark of MERCK & CO., INC., Whitehouse Station, NJ, U.S.A.

** Registered trademark of MERCK & CO., INC., Whitehouse Station, NJ, U.S.A.

Clinical Pharmacology

Mechanism of Action

Timolol maleate is a $beta_1$ and $beta_2$ (non-selective) adrenergic receptor blocking agent that does not have significant intrinsic sympathomimetic, direct myocardial depressant, or local anesthetic (membrane-stabilizing) activity.

TIMOPTIC-XE, when applied topically on the eye, has the action of reducing elevated, as well as normal intraocular pressure, whether or not accompanied by glaucoma. Elevated intraocular pressure is a major risk factor in the pathogenesis of glaucomatous visual field loss and optic nerve damage.

The precise mechanism of the ocular hypotensive action of TIMOPTIC-XE is not clearly established at this time. Tonography and fluorophotometry studies of TIMOPTIC** (timolol maleate ophthalmic solution) in man suggest that its predominant action may be related to reduced aqueous formation. However, in some studies, a slight increase in outflow facility was also observed.

Beta-adrenergic receptor blockade reduces cardiac output in both healthy subjects and patients with heart disease. In patients with severe impairment of myocardial function beta-adrenergic receptor blockade may inhibit the stimulatory effect of the sympathetic nervous system necessary to maintain adequate cardiac function.

Beta-adrenergic receptor blockade in the bronchi and bronchioles results in increased airway resistance from unopposed parasympathetic activity. Such an effect in patients with asthma or other bronchospastic conditions is potentially dangerous.

Pharmacokinetics

In a study of plasma drug concentration in six subjects, the systemic exposure to timolol was determined following once daily administration of TIMOPTIC-XE 0.5% in the morning. The mean peak plasma concentration following this morning dose was 0.28 ng/mL.

Clinical Studies

In controlled, double-masked, multicenter clinical studies, comparing TIMOPTIC-XE 0.25% to TIMOPTIC 0.25% and TIMOPTIC-XE 0.5% to TIMOPTIC 0.5%, TIMOPTIC-XE administered once a day was shown to be equally effective in lowering intraocular pressure as the equivalent concentration of TIMOPTIC administered twice a day. The effect of timolol in lowering intraocular pressure was evident for 24 hours with a single dose of TIMOPTIC-XE. Repeated observations over a period of six months indicate that the intraocular pressure-lowering effect of TIMOPTIC-XE was consistent. The results from the largest U.S. and international clinical trials comparing TIMOPTIC-XE 0.5% to TIMOPTIC 0.5% are shown in Figure 1.

Figure 1

Mean IOP and Std Deviation (mm Hg) by Treatment Group

U.S. Study

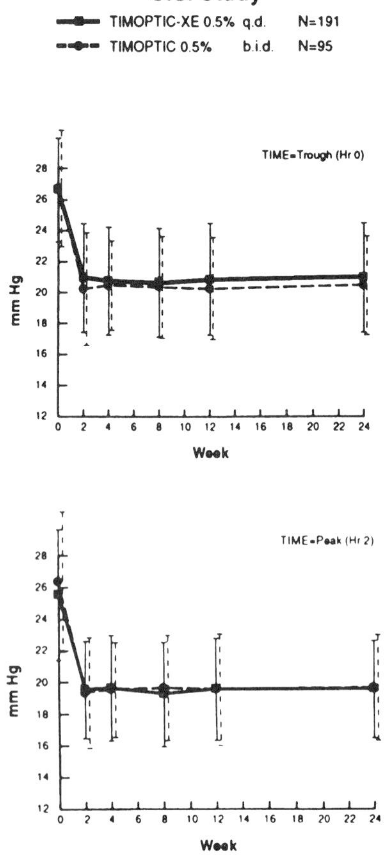

[See Figures at top of next column.]

TIMOPTIC-XE administered once daily had a safety profile similar to that of an equivalent concentration of TIMOPTIC administered

International Study

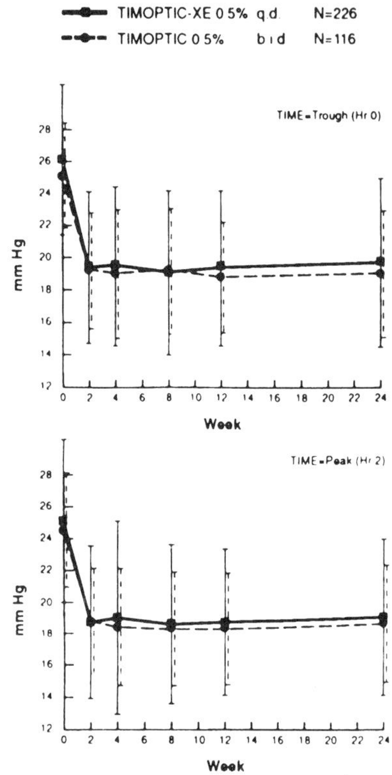

twice daily. Due to the physical characteristics of the formulation, there was a higher incidence of transient blurred vision in patients administered TIMOPTIC-XE. A slight reduction in resting heart rate was observed in some patients receiving TIMOPTIC-XE 0.5% (mean reduction 24 hours post-dose 0.8 beats/minute, mean reduction 2 hours post-dose 3.8 beats/minute). (See **ADVERSE REACTIONS.**)

TIMOPTIC-XE has not been studied in patients wearing contact lenses.

** Registered trademark of MERCK & CO., INC., Whitehouse Station, NJ, U.S.A.

Indications and Usage

TIMOPTIC-XE Sterile Ophthalmic Gel Forming Solution is indicated in the treatment of elevated intraocular pressure in patients with ocular hypertension or open-angle glaucoma.

Contraindications

TIMOPTIC-XE is contraindicated in patients with bronchial asthma or with (1) a history of bronchial asthma or severe chronic obstructive pulmonary disease (see **WARNINGS**); (2) sinus bradycardia; (3) second or third degree atrioventricular block; (4) overt cardiac failure (see **WARNINGS**); (5) cardiogenic shock; or (6) hypersensitivity to any component of this product.

Warnings

As with many topically applied ophthalmic drugs, this drug is absorbed systemically.

The same adverse reactions found with systemic administration of beta-adrenergic blocking agents may occur with topical ophthalmic administration. For example, severe respiratory reactions and cardiac reactions, including death due to bronchospasm in patients with asthma, and rarely death in association with cardiac failure, have been reported following systemic or ophthalmic administration of timolol maleate. (See CONTRAINDICATIONS.)

Cardiac Failure
Sympathetic stimulation may be essential for support of the circulation in individuals with diminished myocardial contractility, and its inhibition by beta-adrenergic receptor blockade may precipitate more severe failure.
In Patients Without a History of Cardiac Failure, continued depression of the myocardium with beta-blocking agents over a period of time can, in some cases, lead to cardiac failure. At the first sign or symptom of cardiac failure, TIMOPTIC-XE should be discontinued.
Obstructive Pulmonary Disease
Patients with chronic obstructive pulmonary disease (e.g., chronic bronchitis, emphysema) of mild or moderate severity, bronchospastic disease, or a history of bronchospastic disease (other than bronchial asthma or a history of bronchial asthma, in which TIMOPTIC-XE is contraindicated [see **CONTRAINDICATIONS**]) should, in general, not receive beta-blockers, including TIMOPTIC-XE.
Major Surgery
The necessity or desirability of withdrawal of beta-adrenergic blocking agents prior to major surgery is controversial. Beta-adrenergic receptor blockade impairs the ability of the heart to respond to beta-adrenergically mediated reflex stimuli. This may augment the risk of general anesthesia in surgical procedures. Some patients receiving beta-adrenergic receptor blocking agents have experienced protracted, severe hypotension during anesthesia. Difficulty in restarting and maintaining the heartbeat has also been reported. For these reasons, in patients undergoing elective surgery, some authorities recommend gradual withdrawal of beta-adrenergic receptor blocking agents.
If necessary during surgery, the effects of beta-adrenergic blocking agents may be reversed by sufficient doses of adrenergic agonists.
Diabetes Mellitus
Beta-adrenergic blocking agents should be administered with caution in patients subject to spontaneous hypoglycemia or to diabetic patients (especially those with labile diabetes) who are receiving insulin or oral hypoglycemic agents. Beta-adrenergic receptor blocking agents may mask the signs and symptoms of acute hypoglycemia.
Thyrotoxicosis
Beta-adrenergic blocking agents may mask certain clinical signs (e.g., tachycardia) of hyperthyroidism. Patients suspected of developing thyrotoxicosis should be managed carefully to avoid abrupt withdrawal of beta-adrenergic blocking agents that might precipitate a thyroid storm.

Precautions

General
Because of potential effects of beta-adrenergic blocking agents on blood pressure and pulse, these agents should be used with caution in patients with cerebrovascular insufficiency. If signs or symptoms suggesting reduced cerebral blood flow develop following initiation of therapy with TIMOPTIC-XE, alternative therapy should be considered.
There have been reports of bacterial keratitis associated with the use of multiple dose containers of topical ophthalmic products. These containers had been inadvertently contaminated by patients who, in most cases, had a concurrent corneal disease or a disruption of the ocular epithelial surface. (See **PRECAUTIONS,** *Information for Patients.*)
Angle-closure glaucoma: In patients with angle-closure glaucoma, the immediate objective of treatment is to reopen the angle. This may require constricting the pupil. Timolol maleate has little or no effect on the pupil. TIMOPTIC-XE should not be used alone in the treatment of angle-closure glaucoma.
Anaphylaxis: While taking beta-blockers, patients with a history of atopy or a history of severe anaphylactic reactions to a variety of allergens may be more reactive to repeated accidental, diagnostic, or therapeutic challenge with such allergens. Such patients may be unresponsive to the usual doses of epinephrine used to treat anaphylactic reactions.
Muscle Weakness: Beta-adrenergic blockade has been reported to potentiate muscle weakness consistent with certain myasthenic symptoms (e.g., diplopia, ptosis, and generalized weakness). Timolol has been reported rarely to increase muscle weakness in some patients with myasthenia gravis or myasthenic symptoms.
Information for Patients
Patients should be instructed to avoid allowing the tip of the dispensing container to contact the eye or surrounding structures.
Patients should also be instructed that ocular solutions, if handled improperly, can become contaminated by common bacteria known to cause ocular infections. Serious damage to the eye and subsequent loss of vision may result from using contaminated solutions. (See **PRECAUTIONS,** *General.*)
Patients should also be advised that if they develop an intercurrent ocular condition (e.g., trauma, ocular surgery, or infection), they should immediately seek their physician's advice concerning the continued use of the present multidose container.
Patients should be instructed to invert the closed container and shake once before each use. It is not necessary to shake the container more than once.
Patients requiring concomitant topical ophthalmic medications should be instructed to administer these at least 10 minutes before instilling TIMOPTIC-XE.
Patients with bronchial asthma, a history of bronchial asthma, severe chronic obstructive pulmonary disease, sinus bradycardia, second or third degree atrioventricular block, or cardiac failure should be advised not to take this product. (See **CONTRAINDICATIONS.**)
Drug Interactions
Beta-adrenergic blocking agents: Patients who are receiving a beta-adrenergic blocking agent orally and TIMOPTIC-XE should be observed for potential additive effects of beta-blockade, both systemic and on intraocular pressure. Patients should not usually receive two topical ophthalmic beta-adrenergic blocking agents concurrently.
Calcium antagonists: Caution should be used in the coadministration of beta-adrenergic blocking agents, such as TIMOPTIC-XE, and oral or intravenous calcium antagonists because of possible atrioventricular conduction disturbances, left ventricular failure, or hypotension. In patients with impaired cardiac function, coadministration should be avoided.
Catecholamine-depleting drugs: Close observation of the patient is recommended when a beta blocker is administered to patients receiving catecholamine-depleting drugs such as reserpine, because of possible additive effects and the production of hypotension and/or marked bradycardia, which may result in vertigo, syncope, or postural hypotension.
Digitalis and calcium antagonists: The concomitant use of beta-adrenergic blocking agents with digitalis and calcium antagonists may have additive effects in prolonging atrioventricular conduction time.
Injectable Epinephrine: (See **PRECAUTIONS,** *General, Anaphylaxis:*)
Carcinogenesis, Mutagenesis, Impairment of Fertility
In a two-year study of timolol maleate administered orally to rats, there was a statistically significant increase in the incidence of adrenal pheochromocytomas in male rats administered 300 mg/kg/day (approximately 42,000 times the systemic exposure following the maximum recommended human ophthalmic dose). Similar differences were not observed in rats administered oral doses equivalent to approximately 14,000 times the maximum recommended human ophthalmic dose.
In a lifetime oral study in mice, there were statistically significant increases in the incidence of benign and malignant pulmonary tumors, benign uterine polyps, and mammary adenocarcinomas in female mice at 500 mg/kg/day (approximately 71,000 times the systemic exposure following the maximum recommended human ophthalmic dose), but not at 5 or 50 mg/kg/day (approximately 700 or 7,000, respectively, times the systemic exposure following the maximum recommended human ophthalmic dose). In a subsequent study in female mice, in which post-mortem examinations were limited to the uterus and the lungs, a statistically significant increase in the incidence of pulmonary tumors was again observed at 500 mg/kg/day.
The increased occurrence of mammary adenocarcinomas was associated with elevations in serum prolactin, which occurred in female mice administered oral timolol at 500 mg/kg, but not at oral doses of 5 or 50 mg/kg/day. An increased incidence of mammary adenocarcinomas in rodents has been associated with administration of several other therapeutic agents that elevate serum prolactin, but no correlation between serum prolactin levels and mammary tumors has been established in humans. Furthermore, in adult human female subjects who received oral dosages of up to 60 mg of timolol maleate (the maximum recommended human oral dosage), there were no clinically meaningful changes in serum prolactin.
Timolol maleate was devoid of mutagenic potential when tested *in vivo* (mouse) in the micronucleus test and cytogenetic assay (doses up to 800 mg) and *in vitro* in a neoplastic cell transformation assay (up to 100 μg/mL). In Ames tests, the highest concentrations of timolol employed, 5,000 or 10,000 μg/plate, were associated with statistically significant elevations of revertants observed with tester strain TA100 (in seven replicate assays), but not in the remaining three strains. In the assays with tester strain TA100, no consistent dose response relationship was observed, and the ratio of test to control revertants did not reach 2. A ratio of 2 is usually considered the criterion for a positive Ames test.
Reproduction and fertility studies in rats demonstrated no adverse effect on male or female fertility at doses up to 21,000 times the systemic exposure following the maximum recommended human ophthalmic dose.
Pregnancy—Teratogenic effects:
Pregnancy Category C. Teratogenicity studies with timolol in mice and rabbits at oral doses up to 50 mg/kg/day (7,000 times the systemic exposure following the maximum recommended human ophthalmic dose) demonstrated no evidence of fetal malformations. Although delayed fetal ossification was observed at this dose in rats, there were no adverse effects on postnatal development of offspring. Doses of 1000 mg/kg/day (142,000 times the systemic exposure following the maximum recommended human ophthalmic dose) were maternotoxic in mice and resulted in an increased number of fetal resorptions. Increased fetal resorptions were also seen in rabbits at doses of 14,000 times the systemic exposure following the maximum recom-

Continued on next page

Information on the Merck and Co., Inc. products listed on these pages is the full prescribing information from product circulars in effect August 31, 1994.

Merck and Co, Inc.—Cont.

mended human ophthalmic dose, in this case without apparent maternotoxicity.

There are no adequate and well-controlled studies in pregnant women. TIMOPTIC-XE should be used during pregnancy only if the potential benefit justifies the potential risk to the fetus.

Nursing Mothers

Because of the potential for serious adverse reactions in nursing infants from timolol, a decision should be made whether to discontinue nursing or to discontinue the drug, taking into account the importance of the drug to the mother.

Pediatric Use

Safety and effectiveness in children have not been established.

Geriatric Use

Of the total number of patients in clinical studies of TIMOPTIC-XE, 46% were 65 years of age and over, while 14% were 75 years of age and over. No overall differences in effectiveness or safety were observed between these patients and younger patients, but greater sensitivity of some older individuals to the product cannot be ruled out.

Adverse Reactions

In clinical trials, transient blurred vision upon instillation of the drop was reported in approximately one in three patients (lasting from 30 seconds to 5 minutes). Less than 1% of patients discontinued from the studies due to blurred vision. The frequency of patients reporting burning and stinging upon instillation was comparable between TIMOPTIC-XE and TIMOPTIC (approximately one in eight patients).

Adverse experiences reported in 1–5% of patients were:

Ocular: Pain, conjunctivitis, discharge (e.g. crusting), foreign body sensation, itching and tearing;

Systemic: Headache, dizziness, and upper respiratory infections.

The following additional adverse experiences have been reported with the ocular administration of other timolol maleate formulations:

BODY AS A WHOLE

Asthenia, chest pain, fatigue.

CARDIOVASCULAR

Bradycardia, arrhythmia, hypotension, hypertension, syncope, heart block, cerebral vascular accident, cerebral ischemia, cardiac failure, worsening of angina pectoris, palpitation, cardiac arrest, pulmonary edema.

DIGESTIVE

Nausea, diarrhea, dyspepsia, anorexia, dry mouth.

NERVOUS SYSTEM/PSYCHIATRIC

Depression, increase in signs and symptoms of myasthenia gravis, paresthesia, behavioral changes including confusion, hallucinations, anxiety, disorientation, nervousness, somnolence and other psychic disturbances.

SKIN

Hypersensitivity, including localized and generalized rash; urticaria; alopecia.

RESPIRATORY

Bronchospasm (predominantly in patients with preexisting bronchospastic disease), respiratory failure, dyspnea, nasal congestion, cough.

ENDOCRINE

Masked symptoms of hypoglycemia in insulin-dependent diabetics (see **WARNINGS**).

SPECIAL SENSES

Signs and symptoms of ocular irritation, including blepharitis, keratitis, blepharoptosis, decreased corneal sensitivity, aphakic cystoid macular edema, and visual disturbances including refractive changes, diplopia, and ptosis.

UROGENITAL

Retroperitoneal fibrosis, impotence.

The following additional adverse effects have been reported in clinical experience with ORAL timolol maleate or other ORAL beta-blocking agents and may be considered potential effects of ophthalmic timolol maleate: *Allergic:* Erythematous rash, fever combined with aching and sore throat, laryngospasm with respiratory distress; *Body as a Whole:* Extremity pain, decreased exercise tolerance, weight loss; *Cardiovascular:* Edema, worsening of arterial insufficiency, Raynaud's phenomenon, vasodilatation; *Digestive:* Gastrointestinal pain, hepatomegaly, vomiting, mesenteric arterial thrombosis, ischemic colitis; *Hematologic:* Nonthrombocytopenic purpura, thrombocytopenic purpura, agranulocytosis; *Endocrine:* Hyperglycemia, hypoglycemia; *Skin:* Pruritus, skin irritation, increased pigmentation, sweating, cold hands and feet; *Musculoskeletal:* Arthralgia, claudication; *Nervous System/Psychiatric:* Vertigo, local weakness, decreased libido, nightmares, insomnia, diminished concentration, reversible mental depression progressing to catatonia, an acute reversible syndrome characterized by disorientation for time and place, short term memory loss, emotional lability, slightly clouded sensorium, and decreased performance on neuropsychometrics; *Respiratory:* Rales, bronchial obstruction; *Special Senses:* Tinnitus, dry eyes; *Urogenital:* Urination difficulties, Peyronie's disease.

Overdosage

No data are available in regard to human overdosage with or accidental oral ingestion of TIMOPTIC-XE.

Significant lethality was observed in female rats and female mice after a single oral dose of 900 and 1190 mg/kg (5310 and 3570 mg/m^2) of timolol, respectively.

An *in vitro* hemodialysis study, using ^{14}C timolol added to human plasma or whole blood, showed that timolol was readily dialyzed from these fluids; however, a study of patients with renal failure showed that timolol did not dialyze readily.

The most common signs and symptoms to be expected with overdosage with administration of a systemic beta-adrenergic receptor blocking agent are symptomatic bradycardia, hypotension, bronchospasm, and acute cardiac failure.

Dosage and Administration

Patients should be instructed to invert the closed container and shake once before each use. It is not necessary to shake the container more than once. Other topically applied ophthalmic medications should be administered at least 10 minutes before TIMOPTIC-XE. (See **PRECAUTIONS,** *Information for Patients.*)

TIMOPTIC-XE Sterile Ophthalmic Gel Forming Solution is available in concentrations of 0.25% and 0.5%. The dose is one drop of TIMOPTIC-XE (either 0.25% or 0.5%) in the affected eye(s) once a day.

Because in some patients the pressure-lowering response to TIMOPTIC-XE may require a few weeks to stabilize, evaluation should include a determination of intraocular pressure after approximately 4 weeks of treatment with TIMOPTIC-XE.

Dosages higher than one drop of 0.5% TIMOPTIC-XE once a day have not been studied. If the patient's intraocular pressure is still not at a satisfactory level on this regimen, concomitant therapy can be considered.

When patients have been switched from therapy with TIMOPTIC administered twice daily to TIMOPTIC-XE administered once daily, the ocular hypotensive effect has remained consistent.

How Supplied

TIMOPTIC-XE Sterile Ophthalmic Gel Forming Solution is a colorless to nearly colorless, slightly opalescent, and slightly viscous solution.

No. 3557—TIMOPTIC-XE Sterile Ophthalmic Gel Forming Solution, 0.25% timolol equivalent, is supplied in OCUMETER**, a white, opaque, plastic, ophthalmic dispenser with a controlled drop tip as follows:

NDC 0006-3557-32, 2.5 mL

NDC 0006-3557-03, 5 mL

NDC 0006-3557-91, 3 × 2.5 mL

No. 3558—TIMOPTIC-XE Sterile Ophthalmic Gel Forming Solution, 0.5% timolol equivalent, is supplied in OCUMETER, a white, opaque, plastic, ophthalmic dispenser with a controlled drop tip as follows:

NDC 0006-3558-32, 2.5 mL

NDC 0006-3558-03, 5 mL

NDC 0006-3558-91, 3 × 2.5 mL

Storage

Store between 15° and 25°C (59° and 77°F). **AVOID FREEZING.** Protect from light.

** Registered trademark of MERCK & CO., INC., Whitehouse Station, NJ, U.S.A.

7814401 Issued November 1993

Information on the Merck & Co. products listed on these pages is the full prescribing information from product circulars in effect August 31, 1994.

Shown in Product Identification Guide, page 105

Otsuka America Pharmaceutical, Inc.

1201 THIRD AVENUE, SUITE 5300
SEATTLE, WA 98101

OCUPRESS® OPHTHALMIC SOLUTION, 1% STERILE ℞

[*äk-yu-pres*]

(Carteolol Hydrochloride)

Description: Ocupress® (carteolol hydrochloride) Ophthalmic Solution, 1%, is a nonselective beta-adrenoceptor blocking agent for ophthalmic use.

The chemical name for carteolol hydrochloride is (±)-5-[3-[(1,1-dimethylethyl)amino]-2-hydroxypropoxy]-3,4-dihydro-2 (1H)-quinolinone monohydrochloride. The structural formula is as follows:

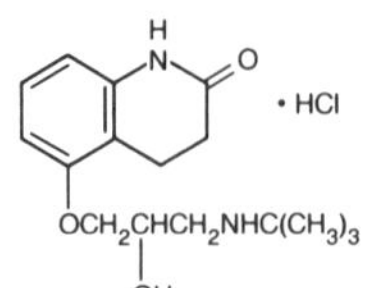

$C_{16}H_{24}N_2O_3 \cdot HCl$ **Mol. Wt. 328.84**

Each mL contains 10 mg carteolol hydrochloride and the inactive ingredients sodium chloride, monobasic and dibasic sodium phosphate, and Water for Injection USP. Benzalkonium chloride 0.05 mg (0.005%) is added as a preservative. The product has a pH range of 6.2 to 7.2.

Clinical Pharmacology: Carteolol HCl is a nonselective beta-adrenergic blocking agent with associated intrinsic sympathomimetic activity and without significant membrane-stabilizing activity.

Ocupress (carteolol HCl) reduces normal and elevated intraocular pressure (IOP) whether or not accompanied by glaucoma. The exact mechanism of the ocular hypotensive effect of beta-blockers has not been definitely demonstrated.

In general, beta-adrenergic blockers reduce cardiac output in patients in good and poor cardiovascular health. In patients with severe impairment of myocardial function, beta-blockers may inhibit the sympathetic stimulation necessary to maintain adequate cardiac function. Beta-adrenergic blockers may also increase airway resistance in the bronchi and bronchioles due to unopposed parasympathetic activity.

Given topically twice daily in controlled domestic clinical trials ranging from 1.5 to 3 months, Ocupress produced a median percent reduction of IOP 22% to 25%. No significant effects were noted on corneal sensitivity, tear secretion, or pupil size.

Indications and Usage: Ocupress Ophthalmic Solution, 1%, has been shown to be effective in lowering intraocular pressure and may be used in patients with chronic open-angle glaucoma and intraocular hypertension. It may be used alone or in combination with other intraocular pressure lowering medications.

Contraindications: Ocupress Ophthalmic Solution is contraindicated in those individuals with bronchial asthma or with a history of bronchial asthma, or severe chronic obstructive pulmonary disease (see WARNINGS); sinus bradycardia; second- and third-degree atrioventricular block; overt cardiac failure (see WARNINGS); cardiogenic shock; or hypersensitivity to any component of this product.

Warnings: Ocupress Ophthalmic Solution has not been detected in plasma following ocular instillation. However, as with other topically applied ophthalmic preparations, Ocupress may be absorbed systemically. The same adverse reactions found with systemic administration of beta-adrenergic blocking agents may occur with topical administration. For example, severe respiratory reactions and cardiac reactions, including death due to bronchospasm in patients with asthma, and rarely death in association with cardiac failure, have been reported with topical application of beta-adrenergic blocking agents (see CONTRAINDICATIONS).

Cardiac Failure: Sympathetic stimulation may be essential for support of the circulation in individuals with diminished myocardial contractility, and its inhibition by beta-adrenergic receptor blockade may precipitate more severe failure.

In Patients Without a History of Cardiac Failure: Continued depression of the myocardium with beta-blocking agents over a period of time can, in some cases, lead to cardiac failure. At the first sign or symptom or cardiac failure, Ocupress should be discontinued.

Non-allergic Bronchospasm: In patients with non-allergic bronchospasm or with a history of non-allergic bronchospasm (e.g., chronic bronchitis, emphysema), Ocupress should be administered with caution since it may block bronchodilation produced by endogenous and exogenous catecholamine stimulation of $beta_2$ receptors.

Major Surgery: The necessity or desirability of withdrawal of beta-adrenergic blocking agents prior to major surgery is controversial. Beta-adrenergic receptor blockade impairs the ability of the heart to respond to beta-adrenergically mediated reflex stimuli. This may augment the risk of general anesthesia in surgical procedures. Some patients receiving beta-adrenergic receptor blocking agents have been subject to protracted severe hypotension during anesthesia. For these reasons, in patients undergoing elective surgery, gradual withdrawal of beta-adrenergic receptor blocking agents may be appropriate.

If necessary during surgery, the effects of beta-adrenergic blocking agents may be reversed by sufficient doses of such agonists as isoproterenol, dopamine, dobutamine or levarterenol (see OVERDOSAGE).

Diabetes Mellitus: Beta-adrenergic blocking agents should be administered with caution in patients subject to spontaneous hypoglycemia or to diabetic patients (especially those with labile diabetes) who are receiving insulin or oral hypoglycemic agents. Beta-adrenergic receptor blocking agents may mask the signs and symptoms of acute hypoglycemia.

Thyrotoxicosis: Beta-adrenergic blocking agents may mask certain clinical signs (e.g., tachycardia) of hyperthyroidism. Patients suspected of developing thyrotoxicosis should be managed carefully to avoid abrupt withdrawal of beta-adrenergic blocking agents which might precipitate a thyroid storm.

Precautions: General: Ocupress Ophthalmic Solution should be used with caution in patients with known hypersensitivity to other beta-adrenoceptor blocking agents.

Use with caution in patients with known diminished pulmonary function.

In patients with angle-closure glaucoma, the immediate objective of treatment is to reopen the angle. This requires constricting the pupil with a miotic. Ocupress has little or no effect on the pupil. When Ocupress is used to reduce elevated intraocular pressure in angle-closure glaucoma, it should be used with a miotic and not alone.

Information to the Patient: For topical use only. To prevent contaminating the dropper tip and solution, care should be taken not to touch the eyelids or surrounding areas with the dropper tip of the bottle. Keep bottle tightly closed when not in use. Protect from light.

Risk from Anaphylactic Reaction: While taking beta-blockers, patients with a history of atopy or a history of severe anaphylactic reaction to a variety of allergens may be more reactive to repeated accidental, diagnostic, or therapeutic challenge with such allergens. Such patients may be unresponsive to the usual doses of epinephrine used to treat anaphylactic reactions.

Muscle Weakness: Beta-adrenergic blockade has been reported to potentiate muscle weakness consistent with certain myasthenic symptoms (e.g., diplopia, ptosis and generalized weakness).

Drug Interactions: Ocupress should be used with caution in patients who are receiving a beta-adrenergic blocking agent orally, because of the potential for additive effects on systemic beta-blockade.

Close observation of the patient is recommended when a beta-blocker is administered to patients receiving catecholamine-depleting drugs such as reserpine, because of possible additive effects and the production of hypotension and/or marked bradycardia, which may produce vertigo, syncope, or postural hypotension.

Carcinogenesis, Mutagenesis, Impairment of Fertility: Carteolol hydrochloride did not produce carcinogenic effects at doses up to 40 mg/kg/day in two-year oral rat and mouse studies. Tests of mutagenicity, including the Ames Test, recombinant (rec)-assay, *in vivo* cytogenetics and dominant lethal assay demonstrated no evidence for mutagenic potential. Fertility of male and female rats and male and female mice was unaffected by administration of carteolol hydrochloride dosages up to 150 mg/kg/day.

Pregnancy: Teratogenic Effects: Pregnancy Category C: Carteolol hydrochloride increased resorptions and decreased fetal weights in rabbits and rats at maternally toxic doses approximately 1052 and 5264 times the maximum recommended human oral dose (10 mg/70 kg/day), respectively. A dose-related increase in wavy ribs was noted in the developing rat fetus when pregnant females received daily doses of approximately 212 times the maximum recommended human oral dose. No such effects were noted in pregnant mice subjected to up to 1052 times the maximum recommended human oral dose. There are no adequate and well-controlled studies in pregnant women. Ocupress (carteolol hydrochloride) should be used during pregnancy only if the potential benefit justifies the potential risk to the fetus.

Nursing Mothers: It is not known whether this drug is excreted in human milk, although in animal studies carteolol has been shown to be excreted in breast milk. Caution should be exercised when Ocupress is administered to nursing mothers.

Pediatric Use: Safety and effectiveness in children have not been established.

Adverse Reactions: The following adverse reactions have been reported in clinical trials with Ocupress Ophthalmic Solution:

Ocular: Transient eye irritation, burning, tearing, conjunctival hyperemia and edema occurred in about 1 of 4 patients. Ocular symptoms including blurred and cloudy vision, photophobia, decreased night vision, and ptosis and ocular signs including blepharoconjunctivitis, abnormal corneal staining, and corneal sensitivity occurred occasionally.

Systemic: As is characteristic of nonselective adrenergic blocking agents, Ocupress may cause bradycardia and decreased blood pressure (see WARNINGS). The following systemic events have occasionally been reported with the use of Ocupress: cardiac arrhythmia, heart palpitation, dyspnea, asthenia, headache, dizziness, insomnia, sinusitis, and taste perversion.

The following additional adverse reactions have been reported with ophthalmic use of $beta_1$ and $beta_2$ (nonselective) adrenergic receptor blocking agents:

Body As a Whole: Headache

Cardiovascular: Arrhythmia, syncope, heart block, cerebral vascular accident, cerebral ischemia, congestive heart failure, palpitation (see WARNINGS)

Digestive: Nausea

Psychiatric: Depression

Skin: Hypersensitivity, including localized and generalized rash

Respiratory: Bronchospasm (predominantly in patients with pre-existing bronchospastic disease), respiratory failure (see WARNINGS)

Endocrine: Masked symptoms of hypoglycemia in insulin-dependent diabetics (see WARNINGS)

Special Senses: Signs and symptoms of keratitis, blepharoptosis, visual disturbances including refractive changes (due to withdrawal of miotic therapy in some cases), diplopia, ptosis

Other reactions associated with the oral use of nonselective adrenergic receptor blocking agents should be considered potential effects with ophthalmic use of these agents.

Overdosage: No specific information on emergency treatment of overdosage in humans is available. Should accidental ocular overdosage occur, flush eye(s) with water or normal saline. The most common effects expected with overdosage of a beta-adrenergic blocking agent are bradycardia, bronchospasm, congestive heart failure and hypotension.

In case of ingestion, treatment with Ocupress should be discontinued and gastric lavage considered. The patient should be closely observed and vital signs carefully monitored. The prolonged effects of carteolol must be considered when determining the duration of corrective therapy. On the basis of the pharmacologic profile, the following additional measures should be considered as appropriate:

Symptomatic Sinus Bradycardia or Heart Block: Administer atropine. If there is no response to vagal blockade, administer isoproterenol cautiously.

Continued on next page

Otsuka America—Cont.

Bronchospasm: Administer a $beta_2$-stimulating agent such as isoproterenol and/or a theophylline derivative.
Congestive Heart Failure: Administer diuretics and digitalis glycosides as necessary.
Hypotension: Administer vasopressors such as intravenous dopamine, epinephrine or norepinephrine bitartrate.
Dosage and Administration: The usual dose is one drop of Ocupress Ophthalmic Solution, 1%, in the affected eye(s) twice a day.
If the patient's IOP is not at a satisfactory level on this regimen, concomitant therapy with pilocarpine and other miotics, and/or epinephrine or dipivefrin, and/or systemically administered carbonic anhydrase inhibitors, such as acetazolamide, can be instituted.
How Supplied: Ocupress Ophthalmic Solution, 1%, is supplied as a sterile ophthalmic solution in plastic dispenser bottles of 5 mL (NDC 59148-001-01) and 10 mL (NDC 59148-001-02).
Store at 15° to 25°C (59° to 77°F) (room temperature) and protect from light.
Licensed under U.S. Patent Nos. 3910924 and 4309432.
Manufactured by Burroughs Wellcome Co. for
OTSUKA AMERICA
PHARMACEUTICAL, INC.
Rockville, MD 20850
Printed in U.S.A.
3026/03-92
Under license of Otsuka Pharmaceutical Co., Ltd.

Shown in Product Identification Guide, page 105

Parke-Davis
Division of Warner-Lambert Company
MORRIS PLAINS, NEW JERSEY 07950

CHLOROMYCETIN® ℞
[klo″ro-mi-se′tin]
HYDROCORTISONE OPHTHALMIC
(Chloramphenicol and Hydrocortisone Acetate for Suspension, USP)

> **WARNING**
> Bone marrow hypoplasia including aplastic anemia and death has been reported following the local application of chloramphenicol. Chloramphenicol should not be used when less potentially dangerous agents would be expected to provide effective treatment.

Description: Chloromycetin® Hydrocortisone Ophthalmic (Chloramphenicol and Hydrocortisone Acetate for Suspension, USP) is a sterile, buffered antibiotic/antiinflammatory dry mixture for suspension for ophthalmic administration. Each vial of Chloromycetin Hydrocortisone Ophthalmic contains 12.5 mg chloramphenicol and 25 mg hydrocortisone acetate with boric acid-sodium borate buffer, cholesterol, methylcellulose, sodium chloride, and Phemerol® (benzethonium chloride), 0.1 mg per ml, in the suspension when prepared as directed. A 5-mL vial of Sterile Distilled Water is included in each package for use as a diluent in the preparation of a suspension of Chloromycetin Hydrocortisone suitable for ophthalmic use.
The chemical names for chloramphenicol are:
(1) Acetamide,2,2-dichloro-N-[2-hydroxy-1-(hydroxymethyl)-2-(4-nitrophenyl) ethyl]-, and
(2) D-*threo*-(–)-2,2-Dichloro-N-[β-hydroxy-α-(hydroxymethyl)-*p*-nitrophenethyl] acetamide
Chloramphenicol has the following empirical and structural formulas:

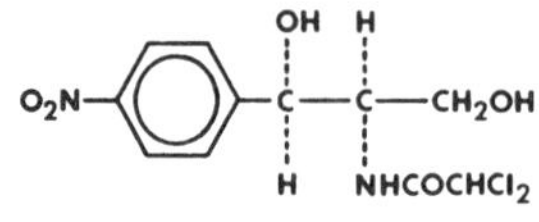

$C_{11}H_{12}Cl_2N_2O_5$ **Mol Wt 323.13**
The chemical names for hydrocortisone acetate are:
(1) Pregn-4-ene-3,20-dione,21-(acetyloxy)-11,17-dihydroxy-,(11β)-, and
(2) 17-Hydroxycorticosterone 21-acetate
Hydrocortisone acetate has the following empirical and structural formulas:

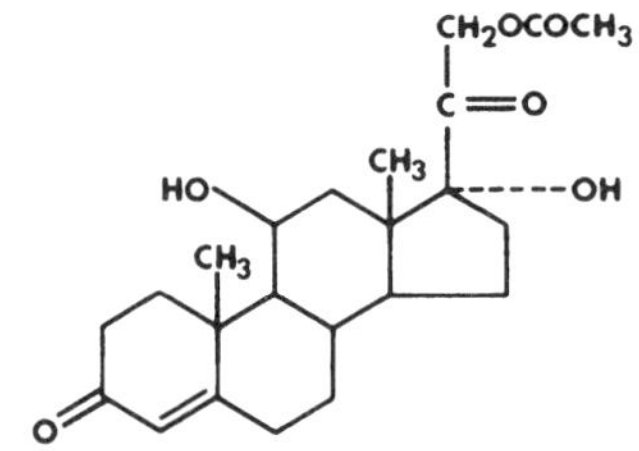

$C_{23}H_{32}O_6$ **Mol Wt 404.50**
Clinical Pharmacology: Corticoids suppress the inflammatory response to a variety of agents and they probably delay or slow healing. Since corticoids may inhibit the body's defense mechanism against infection, a concomitant antimicrobial drug may be used when this inhibition is considered to be clinically significant in a particular case.
The antiinfective component in this combination is included to provide action against specific organisms susceptible to it. Chloramphenicol is considered active against a wide spectrum of gram-negative and gram-positive organisms such as *Escherichia coli, Haemophilus influenzae, Staphylococcus aureus, Streptococcus hemolyticus,* and *Moraxella lacunata* (Morax-Axenfeld bacillus). Development of resistance to chloramphenicol can be regarded as minimal for staphylococci and many other species of bacteria. Chloramphenicol is primarily bacteriostatic and acts by inhibition of protein synthesis by interfering with the transfer of activated amino acids from soluble RNA to ribosomes. It has been noted that chloramphenicol is found in measurable amounts in the aqueous humor following local application to the eye.
When a decision to administer both a corticoid and an antimicrobial is made, the administration of such drugs in combination has the advantage of greater patient compliance and convenience, with the added assurance that the appropriate dosage of both drugs is administered, plus assured compatibility of ingredients when both types of drug are in the same formulation and, particularly, that the correct volume of drug is delivered and retained.
The relative potency of corticosteroids depends on the molecular structure, concentration, and release from the vehicle.
Indications and Usage: Chloramphenicol should be used only in those serious infections for which less potentially dangerous drugs are ineffective or contraindicated. Bacteriological studies should be performed to determine the causative organisms and their sensitivity to chloramphenicol (See Box Warning).
For steroid-responsive inflammatory ocular conditions for which a corticosteroid is indicated and where bacterial infection or a risk of bacterial ocular infection exists.
Ocular steroids are indicated in inflammatory conditions of the palpebral and bulbar conjunctiva, cornea, and anterior segment of the globe where the inherent risk of steroid use in certain infective conjunctivitides is accepted to obtain a diminution in edema and inflammation. They are also indicated in chronic anterior uveitis and corneal injury from chemical radiation, thermal burns, or penetration of foreign bodies.
The use of a combination drug with an antiinfective component is indicated where the risk of infection is high or where there is an expectation that potentially dangerous numbers of bacteria will be present in the eye.
The particular antiinfective drug in this product is active against the following common bacterial eye pathogens:
Staphylococcus aureus
Streptococci, including *Streptococcus pneumoniae*
Escherichia coli
Haemophilus influenzae
Klebsiella/Enterobacter species
Moraxella lacunata (Morax-Axenfeld bacillus)
Neisseria species
The product does not provide adequate coverage against:
Pseudomonas aeruginosa
Serratia marcescens
Contraindications: Epithelial herpes simplex keratitis (dendritic keratitis), vaccinia, varicella, and many other viral diseases of the cornea and conjunctiva. Mycobacterial infection of the eye. Fungal diseases of ocular structures. Hypersensitivity to a component of the medication. (Hypersensitivity to the antibiotic component occurs at a higher rate than for other components).
The use of these combinations is always contraindicated after uncomplicated removal of a corneal foreign body.
Warnings: SEE BOX WARNING
Prolonged use of steroids may result in glaucoma, with damage to the optic nerve, defects in visual acuity and fields of vision, and posterior subcapsular cataract formation. Prolonged use may suppress the host response and thus increase the hazard of secondary ocular infections. In those diseases causing thinning of the cornea or sclera, perforations have been known to occur with the use of topical steroids. In acute purulent conditions of the eye, steroids may mask infection or enhance existing infection. If these products are used for 10 days or longer, intraocular pressure should be routinely monitored even though it may be difficult in children and uncooperative patients.
Employment of steroid medication in the treatment of herpes simplex requires great caution.
Precautions: The initial prescription and renewal of the medication order beyond 20 milliliters should be made by a physician only after examination of the patient with the aid of magnification, such as slit lamp biomicroscopy and, where appropriate, fluorescein staining.
The possibility of persistent fungal infections of the cornea should be considered after prolonged steroid dosing.
The prolonged use of antibiotics may occasionally result in overgrowth of nonsusceptible organisms, including fungi. If new infections appear during medication, the drug should be discontinued and appropriate measures should be taken.
In all serious infections the topical use of chloramphenicol should be supplemented by appropriate systemic medication.
Adverse Reactions: Blood dyscrasias have been reported in association with the use of chloramphenicol. (See **Warnings**).
Adverse reactions have occurred with steroid/antiinfective combination drugs which can be attributed to the steroid component, the antiinfective component, or the combination. Exact incidence figures are not available since no denominator of treated patients is available.

Reactions occurring most often from the presence of the antiinfective ingredient are allergic sensitizations. The reactions due to the steroid component in decreasing order of frequency are: elevation of intraocular pressure (IOP) with possible development of glaucoma, and infrequent optic nerve damage; posterior subcapsular cataract formation; and delayed wound healing.

Secondary Infection: The development of secondary infection has occurred after use of combinations containing steroids and antimicrobials. Fungal infections of the cornea are particularly prone to develop coincidentally with long-term applications of steroid. The possibility of fungal invasion must be considered in any persistent corneal ulceration where steroid treatment has been used.

Secondary bacterial ocular infection following suppression of host responses also occurs.

Dosage and Administration: Two drops applied to the affected eye every three hours, or more frequently if deemed advisable by the prescribing physician. Administration should be continued day and night for the first 48 hours, after which the interval between applications may be increased. Treatment should be continued for at least 48 hours after the eye appears normal.

Directions for dispensing—Add 5 ml sterile distilled water to contents of vial under aseptic conditions. Shake to make uniform suspension. Place sterile dropper in vial. Each ml of suspension prepared as directed contains 2.5 mg Chloromycetin (chloramphenicol) and 5 mg Hydrocortisone Acetate.

Not more than 20 milliliters should be prescribed initially and the prescription should not be refilled without further evaluation as outlined in Precautions above.

How Supplied: N 0071-3228-36 Chloromycetin Hydrocortisone Ophthalmic (Chloramphenicol and Hydrocortisone Acetate for Suspension, USP) is supplied in a package containing dry ingredients in a 5 ml vial and also a vial containing 5 ml of Sterile Distilled Water for use as a diluent in preparation of the ophthalmic suspension. After dispensing, the product may be stored at room temperature for a period of not more than 10 days. A sterilized dropper-cap assembly for use with the vial is included in the package.

Chloromycetin, brand of chloramphenicol, Reg US Pat Off.

WARNING: Manufactured with CFC-12, a substance which harms public health and environment by destroying ozone in the upper atmosphere.

August 1993

PARKE DAVIS© 1993

Div. of Warner-Lambert Co./Morris Plains, NJ 07950 USA

3228G015

Shown in Product Identification Guide, page 105

CHLOROMYCETIN® ℞

[klo "ro-mi-se "tin]

OPHTHALMIC OINTMENT, 1%

(chloramphenicol ophthalmic ointment, USP)

> **WARNING:**
> Bone marrow hypoplasia including aplastic anemia and death has been reported following local application of chloramphenicol. Chloramphenicol should not be used when less potentially dangerous agents would be expected to provide effective treatment.

Description: Each gram of Chloromycetin Ophthalmic Ointment, 1%, contains 10 mg chloramphenicol in a special base of liquid petrolatum and polyethylene. It contains no preservatives. Sterile ointment.

The chemical names for chloramphenicol are:

(1) Acetamide,2,2-dichloro-*N*-[2-hydroxy-1-(hydroxymethyl)-2-(4-nitrophenyl) ethyl]-, and

(2) D-*threo*-(–)-2,2-Dichloro-*N*-[β-hydroxy-α-(hydroxymethyl)-*p*-nitrophenethyl] acetamide

Clinical Pharmacology: Chloramphenicol is a broad-spectrum antibiotic originally isolated from *Streptomyces venezuelae.* It is primarily bacteriostatic and acts by inhibition of protein synthesis by interfering with the transfer of activated amino acids from soluble RNA to ribosomes. It has been noted that chloramphenicol is found in measurable amounts in the aqueous humor following local application to the eye. Development of resistance to chloramphenicol can be regarded as minimal for staphylococci and many other species of bacteria.

Indications and Usage: Chloramphenicol should be used only in those serious infections for which less potentially dangerous drugs are ineffective or contraindicated. Bacteriological studies should be performed to determine the causative organisms and their sensitivity to chloramphenicol (See Box Warning).

Chloromycetin (chloramphenicol) Ophthalmic Ointment, 1%, is indicated for the treatment of surface ocular infections involving the conjunctiva and/or cornea caused by chloramphenicol-susceptible organisms.

The particular antiinfective drug in this product is active against the following common bacterial eye pathogens:

Staphylococcus aureus

Streptococci, including *Streptococcus pneumoniae*

Escherichia coli

Haemophilus influenzae

Klebsiella/Enterobacter species

Moraxella lacunata (Morax-Axenfeld bacillus)

Neisseria species

The product does not provide adequate coverage against:

Pseudomonas aeruginosa

Serratia marcescens

Contraindications: This product is contraindicated in persons sensitive to any of its components.

Warnings: SEE BOX WARNING

Ophthalmic ointments may retard corneal wound healing.

Precautions: The prolonged use of antibiotics may occasionally result in overgrowth of nonsusceptible organisms, including fungi. If new infections appear during medication, the drug should be discontinued and appropriate measures should be taken.

In all serious infections the topical use of chloramphenicol should be supplemented by appropriate systemic medication.

Adverse Reactions: Allergic or inflammatory reactions due to individual hypersensitivity and occasional burning or stinging may occur with the use of Chloromycetin Ophthalmic Ointment. Blood dyscrasias have been reported in association with the use of chloramphenicol (See WARNINGS).

Dosage and Administration: A small amount of ointment placed in the lower conjunctival sac every three hours, or more frequently if deemed advisable by the prescribing physician. Administration should be continued day and night for the first 48 hours, after which the interval between applications may be increased. Treatment should be continued for at least 48 hours after the eye appears normal.

How Supplied:

N 0071-3070-07

Chloromycetin Ophthalmic Ointment, 1% (Chloramphenicol Ophthalmic Ointment, USP) is supplied, sterile, in ophthalmic ointment tubes of 3.5 grams.

Chloromycetin, brand of chloramphenicol, Reg US Pat Off

AHFS Category 52:04.04

WARNING: Manufactured with CFC-12, a substance which harms public health and environment by destroying ozone in the upper atmosphere.

August 1993

PARKE DAVIS© 1993

Div. of Warner Lambert Co / Morris Plains, NJ 07950 USA

3070G023

Shown in Product Identification Guide, page 105

CHLOROMYCETIN® OPHTHALMIC ℞

[klo "ro-mi-se "tin]

(Chloramphenical for Ophthalmic Solution, USP)

> **WARNING**
> Bone marrow hypoplasia including aplastic anemia and death has been reported following local application of chloramphenicol. Chloramphenicol should not be used when less potentially dangerous agents would be expected to provide effective treatment.

Description: Each vial of Chloromycetin Ophthalmic contains 25 mg of Chloromycetin (chloramphenicol) with boric acid-sodium borate buffer. Sodium hydroxide may have been added for adjustment of pH. A 15 ml bottle of Sterile Distilled Water is included in each package for use as a diluent in the preparation of a solution of Chloromycetin suitable for ophthalmic use. By varying the quantity of diluent used solutions ranging in strength from 0.16% to 0.5% may be prepared. Both the powder for solution and the diluent contain no preservatives. Sterile powder.

The chemical names for chloramphenicol are:

(1) Acetamide,2,2-dichloro-*N*-[2-hydroxy-1-(hydroxymethyl)-2-(4-nitrophenyl) ethyl]-, and

(2) D-*threo*-(–)-2,2-Dichloro-*N*-[β-hydroxy-α-(hydroxymethyl)-*p*-nitrophenethyl] acetamide

Chloramphenicol has the following empirical and structural formulas:

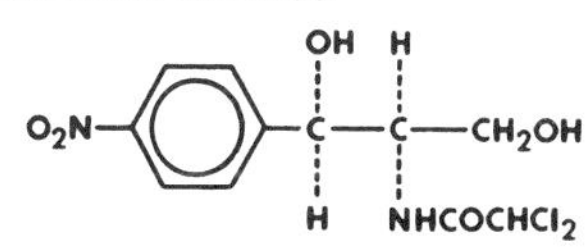

$C_{11}H_{12}Cl_2N_2O_5$ **Mol Wt 323.13**

Clinical Pharmacology: Chloramphenicol is a broad-spectrum antibiotic originally isolated from *Streptomyces venezuelae.* It is primarily bacteriostatic and acts by inhibition of protein synthesis by interfering with the transfer of activated amino acids from soluble RNA to ribosomes. It has been noted that chloramphenicol is found in measurable amounts in the aqueous humor following local application to the eye. Development of resistance to chloramphenicol can be regarded as minimal for

Continued on next page

The product information represents the package circular in effect June, 1994. Information on other Parke-Davis Products may be obtained by addressing PARKE-DAVIS, Division of Warner-Lambert Company, Morris Plains, New Jersey 07950

Parke-Davis—Cont.

staphylococci and many other species of bacteria.

Indications and Usage: Chloramphenicol should be used only in those serious infections for which less potentially dangerous drugs are ineffective or contraindicated. Bacteriological studies should be performed to determine the causative organisms and their sensitivity to chloramphenicol (See Box Warning).

Chloromycetin (chloramphenicol) Ophthalmic is indicated for the treatment of surface ocular infections involving the conjunctiva and/or cornea caused by chloramphenicol-susceptible organisms.

The particular antiinfective drug in this product is active against the following common bacterial eye pathogens:

Staphylococcus aureus
Streptococci, including *Streptococcus pneumoniae*
Escherichia coli
Haemophilus influenzae
Klebsiella/Enterobacter species
Moraxella lacunata (Morax-Axenfeld bacillus)
Neisseria species

The product does not provide adequate coverage against:

Pseudomonas aeruginosa
Serratia marcescens

Contraindications: This product is contraindicated in persons sensitive to any of its components.

Warnings: SEE BOX WARNING

Precautions: The prolonged use of antibiotics may occasionally result in overgrowth of nonsusceptible organisms, including fungi. If new infections appear during medication, the drug should be discontinued and appropriate measures should be taken.

In all serious infections the topical use of chloramphenicol should be supplemented by appropriate systemic medication.

Adverse Reactions: Blood dyscrasias have been reported in association with the use of chloramphenicol (See WARNINGS). Transient burning or stinging sensations may occur with use of Chloromycetin Ophthalmic Solution.

Dosage and Administration: Two drops applied to the affected eye every three hours, or more frequently if deemed advisable by the prescribing physician. Administration should be continued day and night for the first 48 hours, after which the interval between applications may be increased. Treatment should be continued for at least 48 hours after the eye appears normal.

Directions for dispensing—Prepare solution by adding sterile distilled water to the vial as follows:

Strength of solution desired	Add sterile distilled water
0.5%	5 ml
0.25%	10 ml
0.16%	15 ml

Solutions remain stable at room temperature for ten days.

How Supplied: N 0071-3213-35 Chloromycetin (chloramphenicol) Ophthalmic is supplied in a package containing dry ingredients in a 15 ml vial and also a vial containing 15 ml of Sterile Distilled Water for use as a diluent in preparing the solution for ophthalmic use. A sterilized dropper-cap assembly for use on the vial of solution is included in the package.

Store below 86°F (30°C).

Chloromycetin, brand of chloramphenicol. Reg US Pat Off

WARNING: Manufactured with CFC-12, a substance which harms public health and environment by destroying ozone in the upper atmosphere.

August 1993

PARKE DAVIS
Div. of Warner Lambert Co./ Morris Plains, NJ 07950 USA

3213G013

Shown in Product Identification Guide, page 105

OPHTHOCORT® ℞

[ŏf'thō-kort]

(Chloramphenicol, Polymyxin B Sulfate, and Hydrocortisone Acetate Ophthalmic Ointment, USP)

> **WARNING**
> Bone marrow hypoplasia including aplastic anemia and death has been reported following local application of chloramphenicol. Chloramphenicol should not be used when less potentially dangerous agents would be expected to provide effective treatment.

Description: Ophthocort® (Chloramphenicol, Polymyxin B Sulfate, and Hydrocortisone Acetate Ophthalmic Ointment, USP) is a sterile antibiotic/antiinflammatory ointment for ophthalmic administration. Each gram of Ophthocort contains 10 mg chloramphenicol, 10,000 units polymyxin B (as the sulfate), and 5 mg hydrocortisone acetate in a special base of liquid petrolatum and polyethylene. It contains no preservatives.

Clinical Pharmacology: Corticoids suppress the inflammatory response to a variety of agents and they probably delay or slow healing. Since corticoids may inhibit the body's defense mechanism against infection, a concomitant antimicrobial drug may be used when this inhibition is considered to be clinically significant in a particular case.

The antiinfective components in this combination are included to provide action against specific organisms susceptible to them. Chloramphenicol is considered active against a wide spectrum of gram-negative and gram-positive organisms such as *Escherichia coli, Haemophilus influenzae, Staphylococcus aureus, Streptococcus hemolyticus,* and *Moraxella lacunata* (Morax-Axenfeld bacillus). Development of resistance to chloramphenicol can be regarded as minimal for staphylococci and many other species of bacteria. Chloramphenicol is primarily bacteriostatic and acts by inhibition of protein synthesis by interfering with the transfer of activated amino acids from soluble RNA to ribosomes. It has been noted that chloramphenicol is found in measurable amounts in the aqueous humor following local application to the eye.

Polymyxin B sulfate has a bactericidal action against almost all gram-negative bacilli except the *Proteus* group. All gram-positive bacteria, fungi, and the gram-negative cocci, *Neisseria gonorrhoeae* and *N meningitidis,* are resistant.

When a decision to administer both a corticoid and an antimicrobial is made, the administration of such drugs in combination has the advantage of greater patient compliance and convenience, with the added assurance that the appropriate dosage of both drugs is administered, plus assured compatibility of ingredients when both types of drug are in the same formulation and, particularly, that the correct volume of drug is delivered and retained.

The relative potency of corticosteroids depends on the molecular structure, concentration, and release from the vehicle.

Indications and Usage: Chloramphenicol should be used only in those serious infections for which less potentially dangerous drugs are ineffective or contraindicated. Bacteriological studies should be performed to determine the causative organisms and their sensitivity to chloramphenicol (See Boxed Warning).

For steroid-responsive inflammatory ocular conditions for which a corticosteroid is indicated and where bacterial infection or a risk of bacterial ocular infection exists.

Ocular steroids are indicated in inflammatory conditions of the palpebral and bulbar conjunctiva, cornea, and anterior segment of the globe where the inherent risk of steroid use in certain infective conjunctivitides is accepted to obtain a diminution in edema and inflammation. They are also indicated in chronic anterior uveitis and corneal injury from chemical radiation, thermal burns, or penetration of foreign bodies.

The use of a combination drug with an antiinfective component is indicated where the risk of infection is high or where there is an expectation that potentially dangerous numbers of bacteria will be present in the eye.

The particular antiinfective drugs in this product are active against the following common bacterial eye pathogens:

Staphylococcus aureus
Streptococci, including *Streptococcus pneumoniae*
Escherichia coli
Hemophilus influenzae
Klebsiella/Enterobacter species
Neisseria species
Moraxella lacunata (Morax-Axenfeld bacillus)
Pseudomonas aeruginosa

The product does not provide adequate coverage against:

Serratia marcescens

Contraindications: Epithelial herpes simplex keratitis (dendritic keratitis), vaccinia, varicella, and many other viral diseases of the cornea and conjunctiva. Mycobacterial infection of the eye. Fungal diseases of ocular structures. Hypersensitivity to a component of the medication. (Hypersensitivity to the antibiotic component occurs at a higher rate than for other components.)

The use of these combinations is always contraindicated after uncomplicated removal of a corneal foreign body.

Warnings: SEE BOX WARNING

Prolonged use of steroids may result in glaucoma, with damage to the optic nerve, defects in visual acuity and fields of vision, and posterior subcapsular cataract formation. Prolonged use may suppress the host response and thus increase the hazard of secondary ocular infections. In those diseases causing thinning of the cornea or sclera, perforations have been known to occur with the use of topical steroids. In acute purulent conditions of the eye, steroids may mask infection or enhance existing infection. If these products are used for 10 days or longer, intraocular pressure should be routinely monitored even though it may be difficult in children and uncooperative patients.

Employment of steroid medication in the treatment of herpes simplex requires great caution.

Ophthalmic ointments may retard corneal wound healing.

Precautions: The initial prescription and renewal of the medication order beyond 8 grams should be made by a physician only after examination of the patient with the aid of magnification, such as slit lamp biomicroscopy and, where appropriate, fluorescein staining.

The possibility of persistent fungal infections of the cornea should be considered after prolonged steroid dosing.

The prolonged use of antibiotics may occasionally result in overgrowth of nonsusceptible organisms, including fungi. If new infections appear during medication, the drug should be discontinued and appropriate measures should be taken.

In all serious infections the topical use of chloramphenicol should be supplemented by appropriate systemic medication.

Adverse Reactions: There have been reports of punctate staining of the cornea following intensive treatment (every one to two hours during the waking day) of corneal ulcers with Ophthocort. In each reported case, the staining has disappeared after discontinuation of the medication.

Blood dyscrasias have been reported in association with the use of chloramphenicol. (See WARNINGS.)

Adverse reactions have occurred with steroid/antiinfective combination drugs which can be attributed to the steroid component, the antiinfective component, or the combination. Exact incidence figures are not available since no denominator of treated patients is available.

Reactions occurring most often from the presence of the antiinfective ingredient are allergic sensitizations. The reactions due to the steroid component in decreasing order of frequency are: elevation of intraocular pressure (IOP) with possible development of glaucoma, and infrequent optic nerve damage; posterior subcapsular cataract formation; and delayed wound healing.

Secondary Infection: The development of secondary infection has occurred after use of combinations containing steroids and antimicrobials. Fungal infections of the cornea are particularly prone to develop coincidentally with long-term applications of steroid. The possibility of fungal invasion must be considered in any persistent corneal ulceration where steroid treatment has been used.

Secondary bacterial ocular infection following suppression of host responses also occurs.

Dosage and Administration: Application of a small amount of ointment, placed in the lower conjunctival sac, is made to the affected eye every three hours, or more frequently if deemed advisable by the prescribing physician. Administration should be continued day and night for the first 48 hours, after which the interval between applications may be increased. Treatment should be continued for at least 48 hours after the eye appears normal.

Not more than 8 grams should be prescribed initially and the prescription should not be refilled without further evaluation as outlined in Precautions above.

How Supplied: N 0071-3079-07 Ophthocort (Chloramphenicol, Polymyxin B Sulfate, Hydrocortisone Acetate Ophthalmic Ointment, USP); Each gram of ointment contains 10 mg chloramphenicol, 10,000 units polymyxin B (as the sulfate), and 5 mg hydrocortisone acetate in a special base of liquid petrolatum and polyethylene. Supplied in 3.5 g tubes.

AHFS Category 52:04.04

WARNING: Manufactured with CFC-12, a substance which harms public health and environment by destroying ozone in the upper atmosphere.

July 1993

PARKE-DAVIS

Div. of Warner Lambert Co.

Morris Plains, NJ 07950 USA

3079G013

Shown in Product Identification Guide, page 105

VIRA-A® ℞

[*vī″rā-ā′*]

(Vidarabine Ophthalmic Ointment, USP) 3%

Description: VIRA-A is the trade name for vidarabine (also known as adenine arabinoside and Ara-A), an antiviral drug for the topical treatment of epithelial keratitis caused by Herpes simplex virus. The chemical name is 9-β-D-arabinofuranosyladenine. Each gram of the ophthalmic ointment contains 30 mg of vidarabine monohydrate equivalent to 28.11 mg of vidarabine in a sterile, inert, petrolatum base.

Clinical Pharmacology: VIRA-A is a purine nucleoside obtained from fermentation cultures of *Streptomyces antibioticus*. VIRA-A possesses *in vitro* and *in vivo* antiviral activity against Herpes simplex types 1 and 2, Varicella-Zoster, and Vaccinia viruses. Except for Rhabdovirus and Oncornavirus, VIRA-A does not display *in vitro* antiviral activity against other RNA or DNA viruses, including Adenovirus.

The antiviral mechanism of action has not been established. VIRA-A appears to interfere with the early steps of viral DNA synthesis. VIRA-A is rapidly deaminated to arabinosylhypoxanthine (Ara-Hx), the principal metabolite. Ara-Hx also possesses *in vitro* antiviral activity but this activity is less than that of VIRA-A. Because of the low solubility of VIRA-A, trace amounts of both VIRA-A and Ara-Hx can be detected in the aqueous humor only if there is an epithelial defect in the cornea. If the cornea is normal, only trace amounts of Ara-Hx can be recovered from the aqueous humor.

Systemic absorption of VIRA-A should not be expected to occur following ocular administration and swallowing lacrimal secretions. In laboratory animals, VIRA-A is rapidly deaminated in the gastrointestinal tract to Ara-Hx.

In contrast to topical idoxuridine, VIRA-A demonstrated less cellular toxicity in the regenerating corneal epithelium of the rabbit.

Indications and Usage: VIRA-A Ophthalmic Ointment, 3%, is indicated for the treatment of acute keratoconjunctivitis and recurrent epithelial keratitis due to Herpes simplex virus types 1 and 2. It is also effective in superficial keratitis caused by Herpes simplex virus which has not responded to topical idoxuridine or when toxic or hypersensitivity reactions to idoxuridine have occurred. The effectiveness of VIRA-A Ophthalmic Ointment, 3%, against stromal keratitis and uveitis due to Herpes simplex virus has not been established.

The clinical diagnosis of keratitis caused by Herpes simplex virus is usually established by the presence of typical dendritic or geographic lesions on slit-lamp examination.

In controlled and uncontrolled clinical trials, an average of seven and nine days of continuous VIRA-A Ophthalmic Ointment, 3%, therapy was required to achieve corneal re-epithelialization. In the controlled trials, 70 of 81 subjects (86%) re-epithelialized at the end of three weeks of therapy. In the uncontrolled trials, 101 of 142 subjects (71%) re-epithelialized at the end of three weeks. Seventy-five percent of the subjects in these uncontrolled trials had either not healed previously or had developed hypersensitivity to topical idoxuridine therapy.

The following topical antibiotics: gentamicin, erythromycin, chloramphenicol; or topical steroids: prednisolone or dexamethasone have been administered concurrently with VIRA-A Ophthalmic Ointment, 3%, without an increase in adverse reactions.

Contraindication: VIRA-A Ophthalmic Ointment, 3%, is contraindicated in patients who develop hypersensitivity reactions to it.

Warnings: Normally, corticosteroids alone are contraindicated in Herpes simplex virus infections of the eye. If VIRA-A Ophthalmic Ointment, 3%, is administered concurrently with topical corticosteroid therapy, corticosteroid-induced ocular side effects must be considered. These include corticosteroid-induced glaucoma or cataract formation and progression of a bacterial or viral infection.

VIRA-A is not effective against RNA virus or adenoviral ocular infections. It is also not effective against bacterial, fungal, or chlamydial infections of the cornea or nonviral trophic ulcers.

Although viral resistance to VIRA-A has not been observed, this possibility may exist.

Precautions:

General—The diagnosis of keratoconjunctivitis due to Herpes simplex virus should be established clinically prior to prescribing VIRA-A Ophthalmic Ointment, 3%.

Patients should be forewarned that VIRA-A Ophthalmic Ointment, 3%, like any ophthalmic ointment, may produce a temporary visual haze.

Carcinogenesis—Chronic parenteral (IM) studies of vidarabine have been conducted in mice and rats.

In the mouse study, there was a statistically significant increase in liver tumor incidence among the vidarabine-treated females. In the same study some vidarabine-treated male mice developed kidney neoplasia. No renal tumors were found in the vehicle-treated control mice or the vidarabine-treated female mice.

In the rat study, intestinal, testicular, and thyroid neoplasia occurred with greater frequency among the vidarabine-treated animals than in the vehicle-treated controls. The increases in thyroid adenoma incidence in the high dose (50 mg/kg) males and the low dose (30 mg/kg) females were statistically significant.

Hepatic megalocytosis, associated with vidarabine treatment, has been found in short- and long-term rodent (rat and mouse) studies. It is not clear whether or not this represents a preneoplastic change.

The recommended frequency and duration of administration should not be exceeded (See Dosage and Administration).

Mutagenesis—Results of *in vitro* experiments indicate that vidarabine can be incorporated into mammalian DNA and can induce mutation in mammalian cells (mouse L5178Y cell line). Thus far, *in vivo* studies have not been as conclusive, but there is some evidence (dominant lethal assay in mice) that vidarabine may be capable of producing mutagenic effects in male germ cells.

It has also been reported that vidarabine causes chromosome breaks and gaps when added to human leukocytes *in vitro*. While the significance of these effects in terms of mutagenicity is not fully understood, there is a well-known correlation between the ability of various agents to produce such effects and their ability to produce heritable genetic damage.

Pregnancy Category C—VIRA-A parenterally is teratogenic in rats and rabbits. Ten percent VIRA-A ointment applied to 10% of the body surface during organogenesis induced fetal abnormalities in rabbits. When 10% VIRA-A ointment was applied to 2% to 3% of the body surface of rabbits, no fetal abnormalities were found. This dose greatly exceeds the total recommended ophthalmic dose in humans. The possibility of embryonic or fetal damage in pregnant women receiving VIRA-A Ophthalmic Ointment, 3%, is remote. The topical ophthalmic dose is small, and the drug relatively insoluble. Its ocular penetration is very low. However, a safe dose for a human embryo or fetus has not been established. There are no adequate and well controlled studies in pregnant women. VIRA-A should be used during pregnancy only if the potential benefit justifies the potential risk to the fetus.

Continued on next page

The product information represents the package circular in effect June, 1994. Information on other Parke-Davis Products may be obtained by addressing PARKE-DAVIS, Division of Warner-Lambert Company, Morris Plains, New Jersey 07950

Parke-Davis—Cont.

Nursing Mothers—It is not known whether VIRA-A is secreted in human milk. Because many drugs are excreted in human milk and because of the potential for tumorigenicity shown for VIRA-A in animal studies, a decision should be made whether to discontinue nursing or to discontinue the drug, taking into account the importance of the drug to the mother. However, breast milk excretion is unlikely because VIRA-A is rapidly deaminated in the gastrointestinal tract.

Adverse Reactions: Lacrimation, foreign-body sensation, conjunctival injection, burning, irritation, superficial punctate keratitis, pain, photophobia, punctal occlusion, and sensitivity have been reported with VIRA-A Ophthalmic Ointment, 3%. The following have also been reported but appear disease-related: uveitis, stromal edema, secondary glaucoma, trophic defects, corneal vascularization, and hyphema.

Overdosage: Acute massive overdosage by oral ingestion of the ophthalmic ointment has not occurred. However, the rapid deamination to arabinosylhypoxanthine should preclude any difficulty. The oral LD_{50} for vidarabine is greater than 5020 mg/kg in mice and rats. No untoward effects should result from ingestion of the entire contents of a tube.

Overdosage by ocular instillation is unlikely because any excess should be quickly expelled from the conjunctival sac. Too frequent administration should be avoided.

Dosage and Administration: Administer approximately one half inch of VIRA-A Ophthalmic Ointment, 3%, into the lower conjunctival sac five times daily at three-hour intervals.

If there are no signs of improvement after 7 days, or complete re-epithelialization has not occurred by 21 days, other forms of therapy should be considered. Some severe cases may require longer treatment.

After re-epithelialization has occurred, treatment for an additional seven days at a reduced dosage (such as twice daily) is recommended in order to prevent recurrence.

How Supplied: N 0071-3677-07

VIRA-A Ophthalmic Ointment, 3%, is supplied sterile in ophthalmic ointment tubes of 3.5 g. The base is a 60:40 mixture of solid and liquid petrolatum.

WARNINGS: Manufactured with CFC-12, a substance which harms public health and environment by destroying ozone in the upper atmosphere.

August 1993

PARKE-DAVIS

Div. of Warner Lambert Co./ Morris Plains, NJ 07950 USA

3677G021

Shown in Product Identification Guide, page 105

The product information represents the package circular in effect June, 1994. Information on other Parke-Davis Products may be obtained by addressing PARKE-DAVIS, Division of Warner-Lambert Company, Morris Plains, New Jersey 07950

Refer to contents page for information on Contact Lenses.

Pfizer Consumer Health Care Group

Pfizer Inc
235 EAST 42nd ST.
NEW YORK, NY 10017

VISINE L. R.™ EYE DROPS
(oxymetazoline hydrochloride)

Description: Visine L. R. is a sterile, isotonic, buffered ophthalmic solution containing oxymetazoline hydrochloride 0.025%, boric acid, sodium borate, sodium chloride and water. It is preserved with benzalkonium chloride 0.01% and edetate disodium 0.1%.

Visine L. R. is produced by a process that assures sterility.

Indications: Visine L. R. is a decongestant ophthalmic solution designed for the relief of redness of the eye due to minor eye irritations. Visine L. R. is specially formulated to relieve redness of the eye in minutes with effective relief that lasts up to 6 hours.

Directions: *Adults and children 6 years of age and older*—Place 1 or 2 drops in the affected eye(s). This may be repeated as needed every 6 hours or as directed by a physician.

Warning: If you experience eye pain, changes in vision, continued redness or irritation of the eye, or if the condition worsens or persists for more than 72 hours, discontinue use and consult a physician. If you have glaucoma, do not use this product except under the advice and supervision of a physician. As with any medication, if you are pregnant seek the advice of a physician before using this product. Overuse of this product may produce increased redness of the eye. If solution changes color or becomes cloudy, do not use. To avoid contamination of this product, do not touch tip of container to any surface. Replace cap after using. Remove contact lenses before using this product.

Parents: Before using with children under 6 years of age, consult your physician. Keep this and all other medications out of the reach of children. In case of accidental ingestion, seek professional assistance or contact a poison control center immediately.

Caution: Should not be used if Visine-imprinted neckband on bottle is broken or missing.

Storage: Store between 2° and 30°C (36° and 86°F).

How Supplied: In 0.5 fl. oz. and 1 fl. oz. plastic dispenser bottle.

Shown in Product Identification Guide, page 105

VISINE MAXIMUM STRENGTH ALLERGY RELIEF®
Astringent/Redness Reliever Eye Drops

Description: Visine with allergy relief is a sterile, isotonic, buffered ophthalmic solution containing tetrahydrozoline hydrochloride 0.05%, zinc sulfate 0.25%, boric acid, sodium chloride, sodium citrate and purified water. It is preserved with benzalkonium chloride 0.01% and edetate disodium 0.1%. Visine with allergy relief is an ophthalmic solution combining the effects of the vasoconstrictor tetrahydrozoline hydrochloride with the astringent effects of zinc sulfate. The vasoconstrictor provides symptomatic relief of conjunctival edema and hyperemia secondary to minor irritation due to conditions such as dust and airborne pollutants as well as so-called nonspecific or catarrhal conjunctivitis, while zinc sulfate provides relief from burning and itching, symptoms often associated with hay fever, allergies, etc. Beneficial effects include amelioration of burning, irritation, pruritis, and removal of mucus from the eye. Relief is afforded by both ingredients, tetrahydrozoline hydrochloride and zinc sulfate.

Tetrahydrozoline hydrochloride is a sympathomimetic agent, which brings about decongestion by vasoconstriction. Reddened eyes are rapidly whitened by this effective vasoconstrictor, which limits the local vascular response by constricting the small blood vessels. The onset of vasoconstriction becomes apparent within minutes. Zinc sulfate is an ocular astringent which, by precipitating protein, helps to clear mucus from the outer surface of the eye.

The effectiveness of Visine with allergy relief in relieving conjunctival hyperemia and associated symptoms induced by allergies has been clinically demonstrated. In one double-blind study allergy sufferers experienced acute episodes of minor eye irritation. Visine with allergy relief produced statistically significant beneficial results versus a placebo of normal saline solution in relieving irritation of bulbar conjunctiva, irritation of palpebral conjunctiva, and mucous build-up. Treatment with Visine with allergy relief containing zinc sulfate also significantly improved burning and itching symptoms.

Indications: For temporary relief of discomfort and redness due to minor eye irritations.

Directions: Instill 1 to 2 drops in the affected eye(s) up to 4 times daily.

Warning: To avoid contamination, do not touch tip of container to any surface. Replace cap after using. If you experience eye pain, changes in vision, continued redness or irritation of the eye, or if the condition worsens or persists for more than 72 hours, discontinue use and consult a doctor. If you have glaucoma, do not use this product except under the advice and supervision of a doctor. Overuse of this product may produce increased redness of the eye. If solution changes color or becomes cloudy, do not use. Remove contact lenses before using.

Parents: Before using with children under 6 years of age, consult your physician. Keep this and all other drugs out of the reach of children. In case of accidental ingestion, seek professional assistance or contact a poison control center immediately.

How Supplied: In 0.5 fl. oz. and 1.0 fl. oz. plastic dispenser bottle.

Shown in Product Identification Guide, page 105

VISINE MOISTURIZING
Redness Reliever/Lubricant Eye Drops

Description: Visine Moisturizing is a sterile, isotonic, buffered ophthalmic solution containing tetrahydrozoline hydrochloride 0.05%, polyethylene glycol 400 1.0%, boric acid, sodium borate, sodium chloride and water. It is preserved with benzalkonium chloride 0.013% and edetate disodium 0.1%.

Visine Moisturizing is an ophthalmic solution combining the effects of the decongestant tetrahydrozoline hydrochloride with the demulcent effects of polyethylene glycol. It provides symptomatic relief of conjunctival edema and hyperemia secondary to ocular allergies, minor irritations and so-called nonspecific or catarrhal conjunctivitis. Tetrahydrozoline hydrochloride is a sympathomimetic agent, which brings about decongestion by vasoconstriction. Reddened eyes are rapidly whitened by this effective vasoconstrictor, which limits the local vascular response by constricting the small blood vessels. The onset of vasoconstriction becomes apparent within minutes. Additional effects include amelioration of burning, irritation, pruritus, soreness, and excessive lacrimation. Relief is afforded by polyethylene glycol.

Polyethylene glycol is an ophthalmic demulcent which has been shown to be effective for

the temporary relief of discomfort of minor irritations of the eye due to exposure to wind or sun. It is effective as a protectant and lubricant against further irritation or to relieve dryness of the eye.
The effectiveness of tetrahydrozoline hydrochloride in relieving conjunctival hyperemia and associated symptoms has been demonstrated by numerous clinicals, including several double-blind studies, involving more than 2000 subjects suffering from acute or chronic hyperemia induced by a variety of conditions. Visine Moisturizing is a product that combines the redness relieving effects of a vasoconstrictor and the soothing moisturizing and protective effects of a demulcent.
Indications: Relieves redness of the eye due to minor eye irritations. For use as a protectant against further irritation or to relieve dryness.
Directions: Instill 1 to 2 drops in the affected eye(s) up to 4 times daily.
Warning: To avoid contamination, do not touch tip of container to any surface. Replace cap after using. If you experience eye pain, changes in vision, continued redness or irritation of the eye, or if the condition worsens or persists for more than 72 hours, discontinue use and consult a doctor. If you have glaucoma, do not use this product except under the advice and supervision of a doctor. Overuse of this product may produce increased redness of the eye. If solution changes color or becomes cloudy, do not use. Remove contact lenses before using.
Parents: Before using with children under 6 years of age, consult your physician. Keep this and all other drugs out of the reach of children. In case of accidental ingestion, seek professional assistance or contact a poison control center immediately.
How Supplied: In 0.5 fl. oz. and 1.0 fl. oz. plastic dispenser bottle.
Shown in Product Identification Guide, page 105

VISINE® ORIGINAL
Tetrahydrozoline Hydrochloride
Redness Reliever Eye Drops

Description: Visine is a sterile, isotonic, buffered ophthalmic solution containing tetrahydrozoline hydrochloride 0.05%, boric acid, sodium borate, sodium chloride and water. It is preserved with benzalkonium chloride 0.01% and edetate disodium 0.1%. Visine is a decongestant ophthalmic solution designed to provide symptomatic relief of conjunctival edema and hyperemia secondary to minor irritations, due to conditions such as smoke, dust, other airborne pollutants, swimming etc. and so-called nonspecific or catarrhal conjunctivitis. Relief is afforded by tetrahydrozoline hydrochloride, a sympathomimetic agent, which brings about decongestion by vasoconstriction. Reddened eyes are rapidly whitened by this effective vasoconstrictor, which limits the local vascular response by constricting the small blood vessels. The onset of vasoconstriction becomes apparent within minutes.
The effectiveness of Visine in relieving conjunctival hyperemia has been demonstrated by numerous clinicals, including several double-blind studies, involving more than 2,000 subjects suffering from acute or chronic hyperemia induced by a variety of conditions. Visine was found to be efficacious in providing relief from conjunctival hyperemia.
Indications: Relieves redness of the eye due to minor eye irritations.
Directions: Instill 1 to 2 drops in the affected eye(s) up to four times daily.
Warning: To avoid contamination, do not touch tip of container to any surface. Replace cap after using. If you experience eye pain, changes in vision, continued redness or irritation of the eye, or if the condition worsens or persists for more than 72 hours, discontinue use and consult a doctor. If you have glaucoma, do not use this product except under the advice and supervision of a doctor. Overuse of this product may produce increased redness of the eye. If solution changes color or becomes cloudy, do not use. Remove contact lenses before using.
Parents: Before using with children under 6 years of age, consult your physician. Keep this and all other drugs out of the reach of children. In case of accidental ingestion, seek professional assistance or contact a poison control center immediately.
How Supplied: In 0.5 fl. oz., 0.75 fl. oz., and 1.0 fl. oz. plastic dispenser bottle and 0.5 fl. oz. plastic bottle with dropper.
Shown in Product Identification Guide, page 105

Pharmacia Inc. Ophthalmics
605 E. HUNTINGTON DRIVE
P.O. BOX 5036
MONROVIA, CA 91017-7136

HEALON® ℞
(sodium hyaluronate)

Description: Healon® is a sterile, nonpyrogenic, viscoelastic preparation of a highly purified, noninflammatory, high molecular weight fraction of sodium hyaluronate.
Healon® contains 10 mg/ml of sodium hyaluronate, dissolved in physiological sodium chloride phosphate buffer (pH 7.0–7.5). This high molecular weight polymer is made up of repeating disaccharide units of N-acetylglucosamine and sodium glucuronate linked by β 1–3 and β 1–4 glycosidic bonds.
Characteristics: Sodium hyaluronate is a physiological substance that is widely distributed in the extracellular matrix of connective tissues in both animals and man. For example, it is present in the vitreous and aqueous humor of the eye, the synovial fluid, the skin and the umbilical cord. Sodium hyaluronates prepared from various human and animal tissues are not chemically different from each other.
Healon® is a specific fraction of sodium hyaluronate developed as an ophthalmo-surgical aid for use in anterior segment and vitreous procedures. It is specific in that:
1. It has a high molecular weight;
2. It is reported to be nonantigenic[1,6];
3. It does not cause inflammatory[2] or foreign body reactions;
4. It has a high viscosity.

Furthermore, the 1% solution of Healon® is transparent, is reported to remain in the anterior chamber for less than 6 days[3] and protects corneal endothelial cells[4,5] and other ocular structures. Healon® does not interfere with epithelialization and normal wound healing.
Uses: Healon® is indicated for use as a surgical aid in cataract extraction (intra- and extracapsular), IOL implantation, corneal transplant, glaucoma filtration and retinal attachment surgery.
In surgical procedures in the anterior segment of the eye, instillation of Healon® serves to maintain a deep anterior chamber during surgery, allowing for efficient manipulation with less trauma to the corneal endothelium and other surrounding tissues.
Furthermore, its viscoelasticity helps to push back the vitreous face and prevent formation of a post-operative flat chamber.
In posterior segment surgery Healon® serves as a surgical aid to gently separate, maneuver and hold tissues. Healon® creates a clear field of vision thereby facilitating intra- and postoperative inspection of the retina and photocoagulation.
Contraindications: At present there are no known contraindications to the use of Healon® when used as recommended.
Precautions: Those normally associated with the surgical procedure being performed.
Overfilling the anterior or posterior segment of the eye with Healon® may cause increased intraocular pressure, glaucoma, or other ocular damage.
Postoperative intraocular pressure may also be elevated as a result of pre-existing glaucoma, compromised outflow, and by operative procedures and sequelae thereto, including enzymatic zonulysis, absence of an iridectomy, trauma to filtration structures, and by blood and lenticular remnants in the anterior chamber. Since the exact role of these factors is difficult to predict in any individual case, the following precautions are recommended:

- Don't overfill the eye chambers with Healon® (except in glaucoma surgery—see Application section).
- In posterior segment procedures in aphakic diabetic patients special care should be exercised to avoid using large amounts of Healon®.
- Remove some of the Healon® by irrigation and/or aspiration at the close of surgery (except in glaucoma surgery—see Application section).
- Carefully monitor intraocular pressure, especially during the immediate postoperative period. If significant rises are observed, treat with appropriate therapy.

Care should be taken to avoid trapping air bubbles behind Healon®.
Because Healon® is a highly purified fraction extracted from avian tissues and is known to contain minute amounts of protein, the physician should be aware of potential risks of the type that can occur with the injection of any biological material.
Because of reports of an occasional release of minute rubber particles, presumably formed when the diaphragm is punctured, the physician should be aware of this potential problem. Express a small amount of Healon® from the syringe prior to use and carefully examine the remainder as it is injected.
Avoid reuse of cannulas. If reuse becomes necessary, rinse cannula thoroughly with sterile distilled water.
Sporadic reports have been received indicating that Healon® may become "cloudy" or form a slight precipitate following instillation into the eye. The clinical significance of these reports, if any, is not known since the majority received to date do not indicate any harmful effects on ocular tissues. The physician should be aware of this phenomenon and, should it be observed, remove the cloudy or precipitated material by irrigation and/or aspiration.
In vitro laboratory studies suggest that this phenomenon may be related to interactions with certain concomitantly adminstered ophthalmic medications.
Use only if solution is clear.
Adverse Reactions: Healon® is extremely well tolerated after injection into human eyes. A transient rise of intraocular pressure postoperatively has been reported in some cases.
In posterior segment surgery intraocular pressure rises have been reported in some patients, especially in aphakic diabetics, after injection of large amount of Healon®.
Rarely, postoperative inflammatory reactions (iritis, hypopyon) as well as incidents of corneal edema and corneal decompensation have been reported. Their relationship to Healon® has not been established.

Continued on next page

Pharmacia Inc.—Cont.

Applications

Cataract surgery—IOL implantation

A sufficient amount of Healon® is slowly, and carefully introduced (using a cannula or needle) into the anterior chamber.

Injection of Healon® can be performed either before or after delivery of the lens. Injection prior to lens delivery will, however, have the additional advantage of protecting the corneal endothelium from possible damage arising from the removal of the cataractous lens[5]. Healon® may also be used to coat surgical instruments and the IOL prior to insertion.

Additional Healon® can be injected during surgery to replace any Healon® lost during surgical manipulation (see Precautions section).

Glaucoma filtration surgery

In conjunction with performing of the trabeculectomy, Healon® is injected slowly and carefully through a corneal paracentesis to reconstitute the anterior chamber. Further injection of Healon® can be continued allowing it to extrude into the subconjunctival filtration site and through and around the sutured outer scleral flap.

Corneal transplant surgery

After removal of the corneal button, the anterior chamber is filled with Healon®. The donor graft can then be placed on top of the bed of Healon® and sutured in place. Additional Healon® may be injected to replace the Healon® lost as a result of surgical manipulation (see Precautions section). Healon® has also been used in the anterior chamber of the donor eye prior to trepanation to protect the corneal endothelial cells of the graft[5].

Retinal attachment surgery

Healon® is slowly introduced into the vitreous cavity. By directing the injection, Healon® can be used to separate membranes (e.g., epiretinal membranes) away from the retina for safe excision and release of traction. Healon® also serves to maneuver tissues into the desired position, e.g., to gently push back a detached retina or unroll a retinal flap, and aids in holding the retina against the sclera for reattachment.

How Supplied: Healon® is a sterile, nonpyrogenic, viscoelastic preparation supplied in disposable glass syringes, delivering 0.85 ml, 0.55 ml or 0.4 ml sodium hyaluronate (10 mg/ml) dissolved in physiological sodium chloride-phosphate buffer (pH 7.0–7.5). Each ml of Healon® contains 10 mg of sodium hyaluronate, 8.5 mg sodium chloride, 0.28 mg of disodium hydrogen phosphate dihydrate, 0.04 mg of sodium dihydrogen phosphate hydrate and q.s. water for injection U.S.P. Healon® syringes are terminally sterilized and aseptically packaged.

A sterile single-use 27 G cannula is enclosed in the 0.4 ml, 0.55 ml and 0.85 ml boxes.

Refrigerated Healon® should be allowed to attain room temperature (approximately 30 minutes) prior to use.

For intraocular use.

Store at 2–8°C.

Protect from freezing.

Protect from light.

Caution: Federal law restricts this device to sale by or on the order of a physician.

References:

1. *Richter, W., Ryde, M. & Zetterström, O.:* Nonimmunogenicity of a purified sodium hyaluronate preparation in man.
Int Arch Appl Immun 59:45–48 (1979).
2. *Balazs, E. A.:* Ultrapure hyaluronic acid and the use thereof.
U.S. Patent 4,141,973 (1979).
3. *Balazs, E. A., Miller, D. & Stegmann, R.:* Viscosurgery and the use of Na-hyaluronate in intraocular lens implantation.
Lecture , Cannes, France (1979).
4. *Miller, D. & Stegmann, R.:* Use of Na-hyaluronate in anterior segment eye surgery.
Am Intra-Ocular Implant Soc J 6 (1980b) p 13–15.
5. *Pape, L. G. & Balazs, E. A.:* The use of sodium hyaluronate (Healon®) in human anterior segment surgery.
Ophthalmol 87 (1980) p 699–705.
6. *Richter, W.:* Non-immunogenicity of purified hyaluronic acid preparations tested by passive cutaneous anaphylaxis.
Int Arch All 47 (1974) p211–217.

MANUFACTURED BY

Pharmacia AB
Uppsala, Sweden
For Pharmacia Inc. Ophthalmics
Monrovia, CA 91017-7136
Revised: July 1991
Healon is covered by
U.S. patent 4,141,973, 1979

HEALON GV™ ℞
(sodium hyaluronate)

Product Information

Description: Healon GV is a sterile, nonpyrogenic, transparent viscoelastic preparation of a highly purified, noninflammatory, high molecular weight (average = 5 million daltons) fraction of sodium hyaluronate. Healon GV contains 14 mg/ml of sodium hyaluronate 7000, dissolved in a physiological sodium chloride-phosphate buffer (pH 7.0–7.5). This polymer consists of repeating disaccharide units of N-acetylglucosamine and sodium glucuronate linked by glycosidic bonds.

Sodium hyaluronate is a physiological substance that is widely distributed in the extracellular matrix of connective tissues in both animals and man. For example, it is present in the vitreous and aqueous humor of the eye, the synovial fluid, the skin and the umbilical cord. Sodium hyaluronate derived from various human or animal tissues do not differ chemically.

Indications: Healon GV is indicated for use in anterior segment ophthalmic surgical procedures.

Healon GV creates and maintains a deep anterior chamber, to facilitate manipulation inside the eye with reduced trauma to the corneal endothelium and other ocular tissues. Healon GV also can be used to efficiently maneuver, separate and control ocular tissues.

Contraindications: There are no known contraindications to the use of Healon GV when used as recommended.

Precautions: Precautions normally considered during ophthalmic surgical procedure should be taken.

Postoperative intraocular pressure may be increased if Healon GV is left in the eye. Due to the greater viscosity of Healon GV, this increase in postoperative IOP may be higher than that caused by leaving the same amount of other sodium hyaluronate viscoelastic products, with lower zero shear viscosity, in the anterior chamber. Since rises in postoperative intraocular pressure, including cases of significant elevation and subsequent complications, have been reported, the following precautions are strongly recommended.

—Special care should be taken to ensure as complete removal as possible by continuing to irrigate/aspirate after you see displacement of the initial bolus of viscoelastic from the eye; continued irrigation/aspiration should facilitate removal of viscoelastic which may remain in the anterior segment.

—Pre-existing glaucoma, other causes of compromised outflow, higher preoperative intraocular pressure and complications in surgical procedures also may lead to increased intraocular pressure; consequently, extra care should be taken in patients with these conditions.

—Carefully monitor intraocular pressure, particularly during the early postoperative period.

—Treat with appropriate intraocular pressure lowering therapy, if required.

Healon GV is a highly purified fraction extracted from avian tissues which may contain minute amounts of protein. The potential risks associated with the injection of biological material should be considered.

Express a small amount of Healon GV from the syringe prior to use and carefully examine it during use to avoid injecting minute rubber particles which may be released when the syringe diaphragm is punctured.

Sodium hyaluronate solution may appear cloudy or form precipitates when it is injected. Based on *in vitro* laboratory studies, this phenomenon may be related to interactions with concomitantly used ophthalmic medications or detergents which remain in reused cannulas. Avoid reuse of cannulas.

Adverse Events: Increased intraocular pressure has been reported after use of Healon GV:

—Increased intraocular pressure is likely to occur if Healon GV is not removed as completely as possible. Clinical judgment concerning the use of this product should be considered in cases where thorough removal may not be possible. The Precautions noted above should be taken to manage any increased postoperative intraocular pressure and to reduce the likelihood of occurence of related postoperative complications such as optic neuropathy, pupillary atonia and dilation, and iris atrophy.

Rarely, postoperative, inflammatory reactions (iritis, hypopyon, endophthalmitis) following the use of sodium hyaluronate, as well as incidents of corneal edema and corneal decompensation, have been reported. Their relationship to sodium hyaluronate has not been established.

How Supplied: Healon GV is a sterile, nonpyrogenic viscoelastic preparation supplied in disposable 0.85 ml and 0.55 ml glass syringes.

Each ml of Healon GV contains:

14mg	sodium hyaluronate 7000
8.5mg	sodium chloride
0.28mg	disodium hydrogen phosphate dihydrate
0.04mg	sodium dihydrogen phosphate monohydrate
q.s.	water for injection USP

Healon GV syringes are terminally sterilized and aseptically packaged. A sterile single-use, 27 gauge cannula is included with each syringe.

Preparation and Storage

Refrigerated Healon GV should be held at room temperature for approximately 30 minutes before use. Protect from freezing and exposure to light.

For intraocular use.

Store between 2–8°C.

References:

1. Balazs, E.A.: Ultrapure hyaluronic acid and the use thereof. U.S. patent 4,141,973 (1979).
2. Fry L.L. & Yee R.W. (1993): Healon GV in extracapsular cataract extraction with intraocular lens implantation. Cataract Refract. Surg, 19:409–412.
3. Gaskel A. & Haining W. (1991): A double blind randomized multicentre clinical trial of "Healon GV," compared with "Healon" in ECCE with IOL implantation. Eur J. Implant Ref. Surg. 3:241.

Caution: Federal (US) law restricts this device to sale by or on the order of a physician.

Manufactured By:
Pharmacia AB
Sweden
Manufactured For:
Pharmacia Inc. Ophthalmics
Monrovia, CA 91017-7136
U.S. patent 4,141,973, 1979.
 February 1994.

HEALON YELLOW™ ℞
(sodium hyaluronate)

Information listed for Healon® also applies to Healon Yellow with the following exceptions.
Description: Healon Yellow Sodium hyaluronate is a sterile, nonpyrogenic, yellow viscoelastic preparation of a highly purified, noninflammatory, high molecular weight fraction of sodium hyaluronate and fluorescein sodium.
Healon Yellow contains 10 mg/ml of sodium hyaluronate and 0.005 mg/ml of fluorescein sodium, dissolved in physiological sodium chloride-phosphate buffer (pH 7.0–7.5). This high molecular weight polymer is made up of repeating disaccharide units of N-acetylglucosamine and sodium glucuronate linked by β1–3 and β1–4 glycosidic bonds.
It is yellow and transparent.
The fluorescein sodium in Healon Yellow facilitates the visualization of the product during the surgical procedure.
How Supplied: Healon Yellow is a sterile, nonpyrogenic viscoelastic preparation supplied in disposable glass syringes, delivering either 0.55 ml or 0.85 ml sodium hyaluronate (10 mg/ml) and fluorescein sodium (0.005 mg/ml) dissolved in physiological sodium chloride-phosphate buffer (pH 7.0–7.5). Each ml of Healon Yellow contains 10 mg of sodium hyaluronate, 0.005 mg of fluorescein sodium, 8.5 mg sodium chloride, 0.28 mg of disodium hydrogen phosphate dihydrate, 0.04 mg of sodium dihydrogen phosphate hydrate and q.s. water for injection USP.
A sterile single-use 27G cannula is enclosed in each box.

Pharmavite Corporation
15451 SAN FERNANDO MISSION BLVD.
MISSION HILLS, CA 91346-9606

NATURE MADE® OXY-VISION™ OTC
[*ăk 'sə-vizh 'ən*]
High Potency Zinc with Antioxidants
Multivitamin/Multimineral Formula

Description: Oxy-Vision™ is manufactured to contain no artificial colors, no artificial flavors, no preservatives, no chemical solvents, no yeast and no sodium. Tablets are clear coated for ease of swallowing.
Each Oxy-Vision tablet provides:
[See table above.]
Each Oxy-Vision tablet meets or exceeds USP (United States Pharmacopeia) standards for purity, potency, and release (disintegration and dissolution).
Inactive Ingredients: (in descending order of predominance) Dibasic Calcium Phosphate, Cellulose, Gelatin, Corn Starch, Crospovidone, Glucose, Magnesium Stearate, Hydroxypropyl Methylcellulose, Acetylated Monoglycerides, Ethylcellulose, Polyethylene Glycol, Carnauba Wax.
Benefit: Oxy-Vision is a specialized formula developed to supplement the diet of those persons who may have or be at an increased risk for nutritional deficiencies due to diet, age, and/or medications. Antioxidant vitamins and minerals (Beta Carotene, Vitamin C, Vitamin E, Selenium) may help protect cells against the damaging effects of free radicals. Free radicals are highly reactive oxygen molecules created by environmental factors such as ultraviolet light, pollution, X-rays and alcohol, as well as by normal body processes.

NATURE MADE® OXY-VISION™

Vitamin/Mineral	Source	Amount	Adult US RDA*
Zinc	Zinc Oxide	40 mg	267%
Vitamin C	Ascorbic Acid	120 mg	200%
Vitamin E	d,l-Alpha Tocopheryl Acetate	60 I.U.	200%
Vitamin A	Beta-Carotene	5,000 I.U.	100%
Copper	Cupric Oxide	2 mg	100%
Selenium	Sodium Selenate	50 mcg	**
Folic Acid		200 mcg	50%
Vitamin D		100 I.U.	25%

* Percentage of the U.S. Recommended Daily Allowance for adults.
** No U.S. RDA established.

Suggested Use: One tablet, one or two times daily, or as directed by physician.
How Supplied: Clear coated oval tablet in bottles of 60.
Store at room temperature.
Shelf life: 24 months
Shown in Product Identification Guide, page 105

Roche Laboratories
A Member of the Roche Group

Hoffmann-La Roche Inc.
340 KINGSLAND STREET
NUTLEY, NEW JERSEY 07110-1199

GANTRISIN® ℞
[*gan 'trĭ-sin*]
brand of
sulfisoxazole diolamine
OPHTHALMIC SOLUTION

The following text is complete prescribing information based on official labeling in effect June 1994.
Description: Gantrisin (sulfisoxazole diolamine) Ophthalmic Solution is an antibacterial sulfonamide preparation specifically intended for topical ophthalmic use. The solution is a sterile, isotonic preparation containing 4% (40 mg/mL) sulfisoxazole in the form of the diolamine salt, and phenylmercuric nitrate 1:100,000 as a preservative. The solution has a physiologic pH, and does not cause significant stinging or burning on application.
Chemically, sulfisoxazole diolamine is N^1-(3,4-dimethyl-5-isoxazolyl) sulfanilamide compound with 2,2′-iminodiethanol (1:1). It is a white to off-white, odorless, crystalline powder that is freely soluble in water and soluble in alcohol. Sulfisoxazole diolamine has a molecular weight of 372.44.
Clinical Pharmacology: Sulfonamides do not appear to be appreciably absorbed from mucous membranes.
Microbiology: Sulfonamides exert a bacteriostatic effect against a wide range of gram-positive and gram-negative microorganisms. Sulfonamides inhibit bacterial synthesis of dihydrofolic acid by competing with *para*-aminobenzoic acid (PABA). Resistant strains are capable of utilizing folic acid precursors or preformed folic acid. Currently, the increasing frequency of resistant organisms is a limitation of the usefulness of antibacterial agents, including the sulfonamides.
Indications: For the treatment of conjunctivitis, corneal ulcers and other superficial ocular infections due to susceptible microorganisms, and as an adjunct in systemic sulfonamide therapy of trachoma.
Contraindications: Hypersensitivity to sulfonamides or to other ingredients in the formulation. Infants less than 2 months of age. Pregnancy at term and during the nursing period because sulfonamides pass the placenta and are excreted in the milk and may cause kernicterus.
Precautions: ***General:*** Nonsusceptible organisms, including fungi, may proliferate with the use of this preparation. Sulfonamides are inactivated by the *para*-aminobenzoic acid present in purulent exudates. Should undesirable reactions occur, discontinue Gantrisin immediately.
Information for Patients: Patients using Gantrisin Ophthalmic Solution should be instructed not to touch the dropper tip to any surface, since contamination of the solution may result.
Drug Interactions: Gantrisin Ophthalmic Solution is incompatible with preparations containing silver. *In vitro* antagonism with sulfisoxazole diolamine and gentamicin sulfate (Garamycin) has been reported.
Carcinogenesis, Mutagenesis, Impairment of Fertility: *Carcinogenesis:* Carcinogenic studies have not been performed with ophthalmic preparations of sulfisoxazole. Sulfisoxazole was not carcinogenic in either sex when administered by gavage for 103 weeks at dosages up to 2000 mg/kg/day in mice or 400 mg/kg/day in rats.
Mutagenesis: Bacterial mutagenic studies have not been performed with sulfisoxazole. However, Gantrisin was not observed to be mutagenic in *E. coli* Sd-4-73 when tested in the absence of a metabolic activating system.
Impairment of Fertility: Fertility studies have not been performed with ophthalmic preparations of sulfisoxazole. No effects on mating behavior, conception rate or fertility index (percent pregnant) were observed in a reproduction study in rats given oral dosages of 800 mg/kg/day sulfisoxazole.
Pregnancy: Teratogenic Effects: Pregnancy Category C. Teratogenic studies of ophthalmic preparations of sulfisoxazole have not been performed in laboratory animals. Sulfisoxazole was not teratogenic in either rats or rabbits at oral dosages of 800 mg/kg/day. However, in another teratogenicity study, cleft palates developed in both rats and mice after oral administration of 1000 mg/kg/day sulfisoxazole;

Continued on next page

Roche—Cont.

skeletal defects were also observed in rats. This dose is 9 to 18 times the usual adult dosage for oral Gantrisin.

There are no adequate and well-controlled studies of Gantrisin in pregnant women. Gantrisin Ophthalmic Solution should be used during pregnancy only if the potential benefit justifies the potential risk to the fetus.

Nursing Mothers: See CONTRAINDICATIONS section.

Pediatric Use: Gantrisin Ophthalmic Solution is not recommended for use in infants younger than 2 months of age.

Adverse Reactions: Topical application of the sulfonamides may produce sensitization and preclude later systemic use of these drugs. In addition, patients who have been sensitized by systemic sulfonamide administration may exhibit hypersensitivity reactions following topical application of the drugs.

Ophthalmic: Ocular irritation, chemosis, itching.

Included in the listing that follows are adverse reactions that have not been reported with this dosage form but have been reported for the systemically absorbed sulfonamides.

Hematologic: Agranulocytosis, aplastic anemia, thrombocytopenia, leukopenia, hemolytic anemia, purpura, hypoprothrombinemia and methemoglobinemia.

Allergic Reactions: Erythema multiforme (Stevens-Johnson syndrome), generalized skin eruptions, epidermal necrolysis, urticaria, serum sickness, pruritus, exfoliative dermatitis, anaphylactoid reactions, periorbital edema, conjunctival and scleral injection, photosensitization, arthralgia and allergic myocarditis.

Gastrointestinal Reactions: Nausea, emesis, abdominal pain, hepatitis, hepatocellular necrosis, diarrhea, anorexia, pancreatitis and stomatitis.

C.N.S. Reactions: Headache, peripheral neuritis, mental depression, convulsions, ataxia, hallucinations, tinnitus, vertigo and insomnia.

Miscellaneous Reactions: Drug fever, chills, and toxic nephrosis with oliguria and anuria. Periarteritis nodosa and L.E. phenomenon have occurred.

Endocrine: The sulfonamides bear certain chemical similarities to some goitrogens, diuretics (acetazolamide and the thiazides) and oral hypoglycemic agents. Goiter production, diuresis and hypoglycemia have occurred rarely in patients receiving sulfonamides. Cross sensitivity may exist with these agents.

Dosage and Administration: *Solution:* Instill 2 or 3 drops in the eye 3 or more times daily. Care should be taken not to touch dropper tip to any surface, since contamination of the solution may result.

How Supplied: *Gantrisin Ophthalmic Solution,* containing 4% (40 mg/mL) sulfisoxazole in the form of the diolamine salt–½ oz bottles with dropper (NDC 0004-1702-39).

Solution is stable at room temperature and does not require refrigeration.

Revised: May 1993

Shown in Product Identification Guide, page 106

Refer to contents page
for information on
Instruments and Equipment.

Ross Products Division
Abbott Laboratories
COLUMBUS, OHIO 43215-1724

CLEAR EYES® OTC
[klēr īz]

Lubricating Eye Redness Reliever Drops

Description: Clear Eyes is a sterile, isotonic buffered solution containing the active ingredients naphazoline hydrochloride (0.012%) and glycerin (0.2%). It also contains boric acid, purified water and sodium borate. Edetate disodium and benzalkonium chloride are added as preservatives. Clear Eyes is a lubricating, decongestant ophthalmic solution specially designed for temporary relief of redness and drying due to minor eye irritation caused by dust, smoke, smog, sun glare, wearing contact lenses, allergies or swimming. Clear Eyes contains laboratory-tested and scientifically blended ingredients, including an effective vasoconstrictor which narrows swollen blood vessels and rapidly whitens reddened eyes in a formulation which also contains a lubricant and produces a refreshing, soothing effect. Clear Eyes is a sterile, isotonic solution compatible with the natural fluids of the eye.

Indications: For the temporary relief of redness due to minor eye irritation AND for protection against further irritation or dryness of the eye.

Warnings: To avoid contamination, do not touch tip of container to any surface. Replace cap after using. If you experience eye pain, changes in vision, continued redness or irritation of the eye, or if the condition worsens or persists for more than 72 hours, discontinue use and consult a doctor. If you have glaucoma, do not use this product except under the advice and supervision of a doctor. Overuse of this product may produce increased redness of the eye. If solution changes color or becomes cloudy, do not use. Keep this and all drugs out of the reach of children.

Dosage and Administration: Instill 1 or 2 drops in the affected eye(s) up to four times daily.

How Supplied: In 0.5-fl-oz (15 mL) and 1.0-fl-oz (30 mL) plastic dropper bottles.
(FAN 2393)

CLEAR EYES® ACR OTC
[klēr īz]

Astringent/Lubricating Eye Redness Reliever Drops

Description: Clear Eyes ACR is a sterile, isotonic buffered solution containing the active ingredients naphazoline hydrochloride (0.012%), zinc sulfate (0.25%) and glycerin (0.2%). It also contains boric acid, purified water, sodium chloride and sodium citrate. Edetate disodium and benzalkonium chloride are added as preservatives. Clear Eyes ACR is a triple-action formula that: (1) has an extra ingredient to clear away mucus buildup and relieve itching associated with allergies and colds, (2) immediately removes redness and (3) moisturizes irritated eyes. Clear Eyes ACR contains laboratory-tested and scientifically blended ingredients, including an effective vasoconstrictor which narrows swollen blood vessels and rapidly whitens reddened eyes in a formulation which also contains a lubricant and produces a refreshing, soothing effect. Clear Eyes ACR also contains an ocular astringent (zinc sulfate) that precipitates the sticky mucus buildup on the eye often associated with hay fever, allergies and colds, and this helps clear the mucus from the outer surface of the eye. Clear Eyes ACR is a sterile, isotonic solution compatible with the natural fluids of the eye.

Indications: For the temporary relief of redness due to minor eye irritation AND for protection against further irritation or dryness of the eye.

Warnings: To avoid contamination, do not touch tip of container to any surface. Replace cap after using. If you experience eye pain, changes in vision, continued redness or irritation of the eye, or if the condition worsens or persists for more than 72 hours, discontinue use and consult a doctor. If you have glaucoma, do not use this product except under the advice and supervision of a doctor. Overuse of this product may produce increased redness of the eye. If solution changes color or becomes cloudy, do not use. Keep this and all drugs out of the reach of children.

Dosage and Administration: Instill 1 or 2 drops in the affected eye(s) up to four times daily.

How Supplied: In 0.5-fl-oz (15 mL) and 1.0-fl-oz (30 mL) plastic dropper bottles.
(FAN 2393)

MURINE® OTC
[mur'ēn]

Lubricating Eye Drops

Description: Murine eye lubricant is a sterile buffered solution containing the active ingredients 0.5% polyvinyl alcohol and 0.6% povidone. Also contains benzalkonium chloride, dextrose, disodium edetate, potassium chloride, purified water, sodium bicarbonate, sodium chloride, sodium citrate and sodium phosphate (mono- and dibasic). Murine is a sterile, hypotonic solution formulated to more closely match the natural fluid of the eye for gentle, soothing relief from minor eye irritation while moisturizing and relieving dryness. Use as desired to temporarily relieve minor eye irritation, dryness and burning.

Indications: For the temporary relief or prevention of further discomfort due to minor eye irritations and symptoms related to dry eyes.

Warnings: To avoid contamination, do not touch tip of container to any surface. Replace cap after using. If you experience eye pain, changes in vision, continued redness or irritation of the eye, or if the condition worsens or persists for more than 72 hours, discontinue use and consult a doctor. If solution changes color or becomes cloudy, do not use. Keep this and all drugs out of the reach of children.

Dosage and Administration: Instill 1 or 2 drops in the affected eye(s) as needed.

How Supplied: In 0.5-fl-oz (15 mL) and 1.0-fl-oz (30 mL) plastic dropper bottles.
(FAN 2393)

MURINE® PLUS OTC
[mur'ēn]

Lubricating Redness Reliever Eye Drops

Description: Murine Plus is a sterile, nonstaining buffered solution containing the active ingredients 0.5% polyvinyl alcohol, 0.6% povidone and 0.05% tetrahydrozoline hydrochloride. Also contains benzalkonium chloride, dextrose, disodium edetate, potassium chloride, purified water, sodium bicarbonate, sodium chloride, sodium citrate and sodium phosphate (mono- and dibasic). Murine Plus is a sterile, hypotonic, ophthalmic solution formulated to more closely match the natural fluid of the eye. It contains demulcents for gentle, soothing relief from minor eye irritation as well as the sympathomimetic agent, tetrahydrozoline hydrochloride, which produces local vasoconstriction in the eye. Thus, the drug effectively narrows swollen blood vessels locally and provides symptomatic relief of edema and hyperemia of conjunctival tissues due to eye allergies, minor local irritations and conjunctivitis. Use up to four times daily, to remove redness due to minor eye irritation. The effect of Murine Plus is prompt (apparent within minutes) and sustained.

Indications: For the temporary relief or prevention of further discomfort due to minor eye irritations and symptoms related to dry eyes PLUS removal of redness.

Warnings: To avoid contamination, do not touch tip of container to any surface. Replace cap after using. If you experience eye pain, changes in vision, continued redness or irritation of the eye, or if the condition worsens or persists for more than 72 hours, discontinue use and consult a doctor. If you have glaucoma, do not use this product except under the advice and supervision of a doctor. Overuse of this product may produce increased redness of the eye. If solution changes color or becomes cloudy, do not use. Keep this and all drugs out of the reach of children.

Dosage and Administration: Instill 1 or 2 drops in the affected eye(s) **up to four times daily.**

How Supplied: In 0.5-fl-oz (15 mL) and 1.0-fl-oz (30 mL) plastic dropper bottles.
(FAN 2393)

Storz Ophthalmics

3365 TREE COURT INDUSTRIAL BLVD.
ST. LOUIS, MO 63122-6694

Products manufactured by:

Lederle Laboratories
A Division of American Cyanamid Co.
One Cyanamid Plaza
Wayne, NJ 07470

Lederle Parenterals, Inc.
Carolina, Puerto Rico 00987

LEDERMARK® Product Identification Code
Many Lederle tablets and capsules bear an identification code. A current listing appears in the Product Information Section of the 1995 PDR for Prescription Drugs.

ACHROMYCIN® ℞

[ak 'ro-mi "sin]
tetracycline hydrochloride
Ophthalmic Ointment, USP,
1% Sterile

Description: ACHROMYCIN Ophthalmic Ointment, USP, Sterile contains 10 mg of tetracycline hydrochloride per gram with Light Mineral Oil, White Petrolatum and Anhydrous Lanolin as inactive ingredients.

Chemically, ACHROMYCIN is: [4S-(4α, 4aα,5aα,6β,12aα)]-4-(dimethylamino)-1, 4, 4a, 5,5a,6,11,12a-octahydro-3, 6, 10, 12, 12a-pentahydroxy-6-methyl-1, 11-dioxo-2-naphthacenecarboxamide monohydrochloride.

Indications: For the treatment of superficial ocular infections susceptible to ACHROMYCIN.

For prophylaxis of ophthalmia neonatorum due to *Neisseria gonorrhoeae* or *Chlamydia trachomatis.* The Centers for Disease Control (USPHS) and the Committee on Drugs, the Committee on Fetus and Newborn, and the Committee on Infectious Diseases of the American Academy of Pediatrics recommend 1 percent silver nitrate solution in single-dose ampoules or single-use tubes of an ophthalmic ointment containing 0.5 percent erythromycin or 1 percent tetracycline as "effective and acceptable regimens for prophylaxis of gonococcal ophthalmia neonatorum."[1] (For infants born to mothers with clinically apparent gonorrhea, intravenous or intramuscular injections of aqueous crystalline penicillin G should be given: a single dose of 50,000 units for term infants or 20,000 units for infants of low birth weight. Topical prophylaxis alone is inadequate for these infants.[1])

The following organisms have demonstrated susceptibility to ACHROMYCIN:

- *Staphylococcus aureus*
- Streptococci including *Streptococcus pneumoniae*
- *Escherichia coli*
- *Neisseria* species
- *Chlamydia trachomatis*

When treating trachoma a concomitant oral tetracycline is helpful.

Other organisms, not known to cause superficial eye infections, but with demonstrated susceptibility to ACHROMYCIN, have been omitted from the above list.

ACHROMYCIN does not provide adequate coverage against:

- *Haemophilus influenzae*
- *Klebsiella/Enterobacter* species
- *Pseudomonas aeruginosa*
- *Serratia marcescens*

Contraindications: This product is contraindicated in persons who have shown hypersensitivity to any of the tetracyclines.

Precautions: The use of antibiotics occasionally may result in overgrowth of nonsusceptible organisms. Constant observation of the patient is essential. If new infections appear during therapy, appropriate measures should be taken.

Adverse Reactions: Dermatitis and allied symptomatology have been reported.

If adverse reaction or idiosyncrasy occurs, discontinue medication and institute appropriate therapy.

Dosage and Administration: Apply directly to the affected area every 2 hours or more often, as the severity of the infection and the degree of response indicate. Severe or stubborn ocular infections may require treatment for many days, and may also require oral therapy. Mild infections may respond within 48 hours.

How Supplied: ACHROMYCIN *tetracycline HCl* Ophthalmic Ointment, USP, 1%:
NDC 0005-3501-51—⅛ oz. tube.

Store at Controlled Room Temperature 15°–30°C (59°–86°F).

Reference: 1. American Academy of Pediatrics. Prophylaxis and treatment of neonatal gonococcal infections. *Pediatrics.* 1980; 65:1047.

LEDERLE LABORATORIES DIVISION
American Cyanamid Company
Pearl River, NY 10965 Rev. 8/86
12157

ACHROMYCIN® ℞

[ak 'ro-mi "sin]
tetracycline hydrochloride
Ophthalmic Suspension, USP,
1% Sterile

Description: ACHROMYCIN Ophthalmic Suspension, USP, Sterile contains 10 mg of tetracycline hydrochloride per mL with Plastibase 50W and Light Mineral Oil as inactive ingredients.

Chemically, ACHROMYCIN is: [4S-(4α,4aα, 5aα,6β,12aα)]-4-(dimethylamino)-1, 4, 4a, 5, 5a, 6, 11, 12a-octahydro-3, 6, 10, 12, 12a-pentahydroxy-6-methyl-1, 11-dioxo-2-naphthacenecarboxamide monohydrochloride.

Indications: For the treatment of superficial ocular infections susceptible to ACHROMYCIN.

For prophylaxis of ophthalmia neonatorum due to *Neisseria gonorrhoeae* or *Chlamydia trachomatis.* The Centers for Disease Control (USPHS) and the Committee on Drugs, the Committee on Fetus and Newborn, and the Committee on Infectious Diseases of the American Academy of Pediatrics recommend 1 percent silver nitrate solution in single-dose ampoules or single-use tubes of an ophthalmic ointment containing 0.5 percent erythromycin or 1 percent tetracycline as "effective and acceptable regimens for prophylaxis of gonococcal ophthalmia neonatorum."[1] (For infants born to mothers with clinically apparent gonorrhea, intravenous or intramuscular injections of aqueous crystalline penicillin G should be given: a single dose of 50,000 units for term infants or 20,000 units for infants of low birth weight. Topical prophylaxis alone is inadequate for these infants.[1])

The following organisms have demonstrated susceptibility to ACHROMYCIN:

- *Staphylococcus aureus*
- Streptococci including *Streptococcus pneumoniae*
- *Escherichia coli*
- *Neisseria* species
- *Chlamydia trachomatis*

When treating trachoma, a concomitant oral tetracycline is helpful.

Other organisms, not known to cause superficial eye infections, but with demonstrated susceptibility to ACHROMYCIN, have been omitted from the above list.

ACHROMYCIN does not provide adequate coverage against:

- *Haemophilus influenzae*
- *Klebsiella/Enterobacter* species
- *Pseudomonas aeruginosa*
- *Serratia marcescens*

Contraindications: This product is contraindicated in persons who have shown hypersensitivity to any of the tetracyclines.

Precautions: The use of antibiotics occasionally may result in overgrowth of nonsusceptible organisms. Constant observation of the patient is essential. If new infections appear during therapy, appropriate measures should be taken.

Adverse Reactions: Dermatitis and allied symptomatology have been reported.

If adverse reaction or idiosyncrasy occurs, discontinue medication and institute appropriate therapy.

Dosage and Administration: For most susceptible bacterial infections shake well, then gently squeeze the plastic dropper bottle to instill 2 drops in the affected eye, or if necessary, in both eyes, 2 or 4 times daily, or more frequently, depending upon the severity of the infection. Very severe infections may require days of treatment, whereas other cases may be cured by instillation with much less frequency for 48 hours.

In acute and chronic trachoma, instill 2 drops in each eye 2 to 4 times daily. This treatment should be continued for 1 to 2 months, except that certain individual or complicated cases may require a longer duration. A concomitant oral tetracycline is helpful.

For unit dose administration and convenience, the DISPENSER may be used. Immediately prior to use, simultaneously roll, invert and squeeze DISPENSER between thumb and fingers. Repeat several times to mix contents well. Use aseptic technique to cut the tip of the DISPENSER, thereby maintaining sterility. Discard first two drops before instilling drops

Continued on next page

Information on Storz products listed on these pages is the full Prescribing Information from product literature or package inserts effective in June 1994. Information concerning all Storz products may be obtained from the Professional Services Department, Lederle Laboratories, Pearl River, New York 10965

Storz Ophthalmics, Inc.—Cont.

in eye(s). Instill two drops in eye(s), then discard DISPENSER.

How Supplied: ACHROMYCIN *tetracycline hydrochloride* Ophthalmic Suspension, USP, 1% Sterile is supplied as follows:

NDC 0005-3505-18—4 mL plastic dropper type bottle

Store at Controlled Room Temperature 15°–30°C (59°–86° F).

Reference: 1. American Academy of Pediatrics. Prophylaxis and treatment of neonatal gonococcal infections. *Pediatrics.* 1980; 65:1047.

LEDERLE LABORATORIES DIVISION
American Cyanamid Company
Pearl River, NY 10965 Rev. 1/90
25727

Shown in Product Identification Guide, page 106

AUREOMYCIN® ℞
chlortetracycline HCl
Ophthalmic Ointment 1.0%
Sterile

Description: AUREOMYCIN Ointment (Ophthalmic) (sterile) contains 10 mg of Chlortetracycline HCl per gram in an anhydrous lanolin-petrolatum base.

Indications: For the treatment of superficial ocular infections susceptible to AUREOMYCIN.

The following organisms have demonstrated susceptibility to AUREOMYCIN:

Staphylococcus aureus,
Streptococcus pyogenes,
N. gonorrhoeae,
D. pneumoniae,
H. influenzae,
H. ducreyi,
Klebsiella pneumoniae,
Past. tularensis,
Past. pestis,
E. coli,
B. anthracis,
Lymphogranuloma venereum.

In the treatment of trachoma (in conjunction with oral therapy).

Contraindications: This product is contraindicated in persons who have shown hypersensitivity to any of the tetracyclines.

Precautions: The use of antibiotics occasionally may result in overgrowth of nonsusceptible organisms. Constant observation of the patient is essential. If new infections appear during therapy, appropriate measures should be taken.

Adverse Reactions: Dermatitis and allied symptomatology have been reported.

If adverse reaction or idiosyncrasy occurs, discontinue medication and institute appropriate therapy.

Dosage and Administration: Apply to the infected eye every 2 hours or oftener as the condition and response indicate. Severe or stubborn infections may require treatment for many days or oral administration in addition to local treatment. Mild infections may respond in as little as 48 hours.

How Supplied:
NDC 0005-3511-51—1/8 oz tubes

LEDERLE LABORATORIES DIVISION
American Cyanamid Company
Pearl River, NY 10965

Rev. 11/81
03680

DIAMOX® ℞
[di 'ah-moks]
Acetazolamide Tablets USP and
DIAMOX Sterile Acetazolamide Sodium USP Intravenous

Description: DIAMOX, an inhibitor of the enzyme carbonic anhydrase, is a white to faintly yellowish white crystalline, odorless powder, weakly acidic, very slightly soluble in water and slightly soluble in alcohol. The chemical name for DIAMOX is *N*-(5-Sulfamoyl-1,3,4-thiadiazol-2yl)-acetamide. Its chemical formula is $C_4H_6N_4O_3S_2$. Its molecular weight is 222.24.

DIAMOX is available as oral tablets containing 125 mg and 250 mg of acetazolamide, respectively, and the following inactive ingredients: Corn Starch, Dibasic Calcium Phosphate, Magnesium Stearate, Povidone, and Sodium Starch Glycolate.

DIAMOX is also available for intravenous use, and is supplied as a sterile powder requiring reconstitution. Each vial contains an amount of acetazolamide sodium equivalent to 500 mg of acetazolamide. The bulk solution is adjusted to pH 9.2 using sodium hydroxide and, if necessary, hydrochloric acid prior to lyophilization.

Clinical Pharmacology: DIAMOX is a potent carbonic anhydrase inhibitor, effective in the control of fluid secretion (eg, some types of glaucoma), in the treatment of certain convulsive disorders (eg, epilepsy), and in the promotion of diuresis in instances of abnormal fluid retention (eg, cardiac edema).

DIAMOX is not a mercurial diuretic. Rather, it is a nonbacteriostatic sulfonamide possessing a chemical structure and pharmacological activity distinctly different from the bacteriostatic sulfonamides.

DIAMOX is an enzyme inhibitor that acts specifically on carbonic anhydrase, the enzyme that catalyzes the reversible reaction involving the hydration of carbon dioxide and the dehydration of carbonic acid. In the eye, this inhibitory action of acetazolamide decreases the secretion of aqueous humor and results in a drop in intraocular pressure, a reaction considered desirable in cases of glaucoma and even in certain nonglaucomatous conditions. Evidence seems to indicate that DIAMOX has utility as an adjuvant in the treatment of certain dysfunctions of the central nervous system (eg, epilepsy). Inhibition of carbonic anhydrase in this area appears to retard abnormal, paroxysmal, excessive discharge from central nervous system neurons. The diuretic effect of DIAMOX is due to its action in the kidney on the reversible reaction involving hydration of carbon dioxide and dehydration of carbonic acid. The result is renal loss of HCO_3 ion, which carries out sodium, water, and potassium. Alkalinization of the urine and promotion of diuresis are thus effected. Alteration in ammonia metabolism occurs due to increased reabsorption of ammonia by the renal tubules as a result of urinary alkalinization.

Placebo-controlled clinical trials have shown that prophylactic administration of DIAMOX at a dose of 250 mg every 8 to 12 hours (or a 500 mg controlled-release capsule once daily) before and during rapid ascent to altitude results in fewer and/or less severe symptoms (such as headache, nausea, shortness of breath, dizziness, drowsiness, and fatigue) of acute mountain sickness (AMS). Pulmonary function (eg, minute ventilation, expired vital capacity, and peak flow) is greater in the DIAMOX treated group, both in subjects with AMS and asymptomatic subjects. The DIAMOX treated climbers also had less difficulty in sleeping.

Indications and Usage: For adjunctive treatment of: edema due to congestive heart failure; drug-induced edema; centrencephalic epilepsies (petit mal, unlocalized seizures); chronic simple (open-angle) glaucoma, secondary glaucoma, and preoperatively in acute angle-closure glaucoma where delay of surgery is desired in order to lower intraocular pressure. DIAMOX is also indicated for the prevention or amelioration of symptoms associated with acute mountain sickness in climbers attempting rapid ascent and in those who are very susceptible to acute mountain sickness despite gradual ascent.

Contraindications: DIAMOX *acetazolamide* therapy is contraindicated in situations in which sodium and/or potassium blood serum levels are depressed, in cases of marked kidney and liver disease or dysfunction, in suprarenal gland failure, and in hyperchloremic acidosis. It is contraindicated in patients with cirrhosis because of the risk of development of hepatic encephalopathy.

Long-term administration of DIAMOX is contraindicated in patients with chronic noncongestive angle-closure glaucoma since it may permit organic closure of the angle to occur while the worsening glaucoma is masked by lowered intraocular pressure.

Warnings: Fatalities have occurred, although rarely, due to severe reactions to sulfonamides including Stevens-Johnson syndrome, toxic epidermal necrolysis, fulminant hepatic necrosis, agranulocytosis, aplastic anemia, and other blood dyscrasias. Sensitizations may recur when a sulfonamide is readministered irrespective of the route of administration. If signs of hypersensitivity or other serious reactions occur, discontinue use of this drug.

Caution is advised for patients receiving concomitant high-dose aspirin and DIAMOX, as anorexia, tachypnea, lethargy, coma and death have been reported.

Precautions: General: Increasing the dose does not increase the diuresis and may increase the incidence of drowsiness and/or paresthesia. Increasing the dose often results in a decrease in diuresis. Under certain circumstances, however, very large doses have been given in conjunction with other diuretics in order to secure diuresis in complete refractory failure.

Information for Patients: Adverse reactions common to all sulfonamide derivatives may occur: anaphylaxis, fever, rash (including erythema multiforme, Stevens-Johnson syndrome, toxic epidermal necrolysis), crystalluria, renal calculus, bone marrow depression, thrombocytopenic purpura, hemolytic anemia, leukopenia, pancytopenia, and agranulocytosis. Precaution is advised for early detection of such reactions, and the drug should be discontinued and appropriate therapy instituted.

In patients with pulmonary obstruction or emphysema where alveolar ventilation may be impaired, DIAMOX, which may precipitate or aggravate acidosis, should be used with caution.

Gradual ascent is desirable to try to avoid acute mountain sickness. If rapid ascent is undertaken and DIAMOX *acetazolamide* is used, it should be noted that such use does not obviate the need for prompt descent if severe forms of high altitude sickness occur, ie, high altitude pulmonary edema (HAPE) or high altitude cerebral edema.

Caution is advised for patients receiving concomitant high-dose aspirin and DIAMOX, as anorexia, tachypnea, lethargy, coma and death have been reported (see **Warnings**).

Laboratory Tests: To monitor for hematologic reactions common to all sulfonamides, it is recommended that a baseline CBC and platelet count be obtained on patients prior to initiating DIAMOX therapy and at regular intervals during therapy. If significant changes occur, early discontinuance and institution of appropriate therapy are important. Periodic monitoring of serum electrolytes is recommended.

Carcinogenesis, Mutagenesis, Impairment of Fertility: Long-term studies in animals to evaluate the carcinogenic potential of DIAMOX have not been conducted. In a bacterial mutagenicity assay, DIAMOX was not mutagenic when evaluated with and without metabolic activation.

The drug had no effect on fertility when administered in the diet to male and female rats at a daily intake of up to four times the recommended human dose of 1000 mg in a 50 kg individual.

Pregnancy: Pregnancy Category C: Acetazolamide, administered orally or parenterally, has been shown to be teratogenic (defects of the limbs) in mice, rats, hamsters, and rabbits. There are no adequate and well-controlled studies in pregnant women. Acetazolamide should be used in pregnancy only if the potential benefit justifies the potential risk to the fetus.

Nursing Mothers: Because of the potential for serious adverse reaction in nursing infants from DIAMOX, a decision should be made whether to discontinue nursing or to discontinue the drug, taking into account the importance of the drug to the mother.

Pediatric Use: The safety and effectiveness of DIAMOX *acetazolamide* in children have not been established.

Adverse Reactions: Adverse reactions, occurring most often early in therapy, include paresthesias, particularly a "tingling" feeling in the extremities, hearing dysfunction or tinnitus, loss of appetite, taste alteration and gastrointestinal disturbances such as nausea, vomiting and diarrhea; polyuria, and occasional instances of drowsiness and confusion. Metabolic acidosis and electrolyte imbalance may occur.

Transient myopia has been reported. This condition invariably subsides upon diminution or discontinuance of the medication.

Other occasional adverse reactions include urticaria, melena, hematuria, glycosuria, hepatic insufficiency, flaccid paralysis, photosensitivity and convulsions. Also see **Precautions, Information for Patients,** for possible reactions common to sulfonamide derivatives. Fatalities have occurred although rarely, due to severe reactions to sulfonamides including Stevens-Johnson syndrome, toxic epidermal necrolysis, fulminant hepatic necrosis, agranulocytosis, aplastic anemia and other blood dyscrasias (see **Warnings**).

Overdosage: No data are available regarding DIAMOX overdosage in humans as no cases of acute poisoning with this drug have been reported. Animal data suggest that DIAMOX is remarkably nontoxic. No specific antidote is known. Treatment should be symptomatic and supportive.

Electrolyte imbalance, development of an acidotic state, and central nervous effects might be expected to occur. Serum electrolyte levels (particularly potassium) and blood pH levels should be monitored.

Supportive measures are required to restore electrolyte and pH balance. The acidotic state can usually be corrected by the administration of bicarbonate.

Despite its high intraerythrocytic distribution and plasma protein binding properties, DIAMOX may be dialyzable. This may be particularly important in the management of DIAMOX overdosage when complicated by the presence of renal failure.

Dosage and Administration: *Preparation and Storage of Parenteral Solution:* Each 500 mg vial containing DIAMOX parenteral should be reconstituted with at least 5 mL of Sterile Water for Injection prior to use. Reconstituted solutions retain their physical and chemical properties for 3 days under refrigeration at 2° to 8°C (36° to 46°F), or 12 hours at room temperature 15° to 30°C (59° to 86°F). CONTAINS NO PRESERVATIVE. The direct intravenous route of administration is preferred. Intramuscular administration is not recommended.

Glaucoma: DIAMOX *acetazolamide* should be used as an adjunct to the usual therapy. The dosage employed in the treatment of *chronic simple (open-angle) glaucoma* ranges from 250 mg to 1 g of DIAMOX per 24 hours, usually in divided doses for amounts over 250 mg. It has usually been found that a dosage in excess of 1 g per 24 hours does not produce an increased effect. In all cases, the dosage should be adjusted with careful individual attention both to symptomatology and ocular tension. Continuous supervision by a physician is advisable.

In treatment of secondary glaucoma and in the preoperative treatment of some cases of *acute congestive (closed-angle) glaucoma,* the preferred dosage is 250 mg every 4 hours, although some cases have responded to 250 mg twice daily on short term therapy. In some acute cases, it may be more satisfactory to administer an initial dose of 500 mg followed by 125 or 250 mg every 4 hours depending on the individual case. Intravenous therapy may be used for rapid relief of ocular tension in acute cases. A complementary effect has been noted when DIAMOX has been used in conjunction with miotics or mydriatics as the case demanded.

Epilepsy: It is not clearly known whether the beneficial effects observed in epilepsy are due to direct inhibition of carbonic anhydrase in the central nervous system or whether they are due to the slight degree of acidosis produced by the divided dosage. The best results to date have been seen in petit mal in children. Good results, however, have been seen in patients, both children and adult, in other types of seizures such as grand mal, mixed seizure patterns, myoclonic jerk patterns, etc. The suggested total daily dose is 8 to 30 mg per kg in divided doses. Although some patients respond to a low dose, the optimum range appears to be from 375 to 1000 mg daily. However, some investigators feel that daily doses in excess of 1 g do not produce any better results than a 1 g dose. When DIAMOX is given in combination with other anticonvulsants, it is suggested that the starting dose should be 250 mg once daily in addition to the existing medications. This can be increased to levels as indicated above.

The change from other medications to DIAMOX should be gradual and in accordance with usual practice in epilepsy therapy.

Congestive Heart Failure: For diuresis in congestive heart failure, the starting dose is usually 250 to 375 mg once daily in the morning (5 mg/kg). If, after an initial response, the patient fails to continue to lose edema fluid, do not increase the dose but allow for kidney recovery by skipping medication for a day. DIAMOX *acetazolamide* yields best diuretic results when given on alternate days, or for 2 days alternating with a day of rest.

Failures in therapy may be due to overdosage or too frequent dosage. The use of DIAMOX does not eliminate the need for other therapy such as digitalis, bed rest, and salt restriction.

Drug-Induced Edema: Recommended dosage is 250 to 375 mg of DIAMOX once a day for 1 or 2 days, alternating with a day of rest.

Acute Mountain Sickness: Dosage is 500 mg to 1000 mg daily, in divided doses using tablets or sustained-release capsules as appropriate. In circumstances of rapid ascent, such as in rescue or military operations, the higher dose level of 1000 mg is recommended. It is preferable to initiate dosing 24 to 48 hours before ascent and to continue for 48 hours while at high altitude, or longer as necessary to control symptoms.

Note: The dosage recommendations for glaucoma and epilepsy differ considerably from those for congestive heart failure, since the first two conditions are not dependent upon carbonic anhydrase inhibition in the kidney which requires intermittent dosage if it is to recover from the inhibitory effect of the therapeutic agent.

Parenteral drug products should be inspected visually for particulate matter and discoloration prior to administration, whenever solution and container permit.

How Supplied: *DIAMOX acetazolamide Tablets:* 125 mg–Round, flat-faced, beveled, white tablets engraved with DIAMOX and 125 on one side and scored in half on the other side. Engraved with LL on the right of the score and D1 on the left, are supplied as follows:

NDC 57706-754-23—Bottle of 100

250 mg—Round, convex, white tablets engraved with DIAMOX and 250 on one side and scored in quarters on the other side. Engraved with LL in the upper right quadrant and D2 in the lower left quadrant, are supplied as follows:

NDC 57706-755-23—Bottle of 100
NDC 57706-755-34—Bottle of 1000
NDC 57706-755-60—Unit Dose 10 × 10s

Store at Controlled Room Temperature 15°–30°C (59°–86°F).

Manufactured for
STORZ OPHTHALMICS
St. Louis, MO 63122
by
LEDERLE LABORATORIES DIVISION
American Cyanamid Company
Pearl River, NY 10965

DIAMOX Sterile acetazolamide sodium, Intravenous: Sterile intravenous (lyophilized) powder.

NDC 57706-762-96–500 mg vial

Store at Controlled Room Temperature 15°–30°C (59°–86° F).

Manufactured for
STORZ OPHTHALMICS
St. Louis, MO 63122
by
LEDERLE PARENTERALS, INC.
Carolina, Puerto Rico 00987 Rev. 11/93
31916-93

Shown in Product Identification Guide, page 106

DIAMOX® Acetazolamide SEQUELS® Sustained-Release Capsules ℞

Description: DIAMOX is an inhibitor of the enzyme carbonic anhydrase.

DIAMOX is a white to faintly yellowish white crystalline, odorless powder, weakly acidic, very slightly soluble in water and slightly soluble in alcohol. The chemical name for DIAMOX is *N*-(5-Sulfamoyl-1,3,4-thiadiazol-2-yl)-acetamide.

DIAMOX SEQUELS are sustained-release capsules, for oral administration, each containing 500 mg of acetazolamide and the following inactive ingredients: Benzoin, Ethylcellulose, Ethyl Vanillin, FD&C Blue No. 1, FD&C Yellow No. 6, Gelatin, Glycerin, Magnesium Stearate, Methylparaben, Mineral Oil, Mono- and Diglycerides, Propylene Glycol, Propylpara-

Continued on next page

Information on Storz products listed on these pages is the full Prescribing Information from product literature or package inserts effective in June 1994. Information concerning all Storz products may be obtained from the Professional Services Department, Lederle Laboratories, Pearl River, New York 10965

Storz Ophthalmics, Inc.—Cont.

ben, Silicon Dioxide, Sucrose, Talc, Terpene Resin, Vanillin, and White Wax.

Clinical Pharmacology: DIAMOX is a potent carbonic anhydrase inhibitor, effective in the control of fluid secretion (eg, some types of glaucoma), in the treatment of certain convulsive disorders (eg, epilepsy), and in the promotion of diuresis in instances of abnormal fluid retention (eg, cardiac edema).

DIAMOX is not a mercurial diuretic. Rather it is a nonbacteriostatic sulfonamide possessing a chemical structure and pharmacological activity distinctly different from the bacteriostatic sulfonamides.

DIAMOX is an enzyme inhibitor that acts specifically on carbonic anhydrase, the enzyme that catalyzes the reversible reaction involving the hydration of carbon dioxide and the dehydration of carbonic acid. In the eye, this inhibitory action of acetazolamide decreases the secretion of aqueous humor and results in a drop in intraocular pressure, a reaction considered desirable in cases of glaucoma and even in certain nonglaucomatous conditions. Evidence seems to indicate that DIAMOX has utility as an adjuvant in the treatment of certain dysfunctions of the central nervous system (eg, epilepsy). Inhibition of carbonic anhydrase in this area appears to retard abnormal, paroxysmal, excessive discharge from central nervous system neurons. The diuretic effect of DIAMOX is due to its action in the kidney on the reversible reaction involving hydration of carbon dioxide and dehydration of carbonic acid. The result is renal loss of HCO_3 ion, which carries out sodium, water, and potassium. Alkalinization of the urine and promotion of diuresis are thus effected. Alteration in ammonia metabolism occurs due to increased reabsorption of ammonia by the renal tubules as a result of urinary alkalinization.

DIAMOX SEQUELS sustained-release capsules provide prolonged action to inhibit aqueous humor secretion for 18 to 24 hours after each dose, whereas tablets act for only 8 to 12 hours. The prolonged continuous effect of SEQUELS permits a reduction in dosage frequency.

Plasma concentrations of acetazolamide peak between 3 to 6 hours after administration of DIAMOX SEQUELS, compared to 1 to 4 hours with tablets.

Placebo-controlled clinical trials have shown that prophylactic administration of DIAMOX at a dose of 250 mg every 8 to 12 hours (or a 500 mg controlled-release capsule once daily) before and during rapid ascent to altitude results in fewer and/or less severe symptoms (such as headache, nausea, shortness of breath, dizziness, drowsiness, and fatigue) of acute mountain sickness (AMS). Pulmonary function (eg, minute ventilation, expired vital capacity, and peak flow) is greater in the DIAMOX treated group, both in subjects with AMS and asymptomatic subjects. The DIAMOX treated climbers also had less difficulty in sleeping.

Indications and Usage: For adjunctive treatment of: chronic simple (open-angle) glaucoma, secondary glaucoma, and preoperatively in acute angle-closure glaucoma where delay of surgery is desired in order to lower intraocular pressure. DIAMOX is also indicated for the prevention or amelioration of symptoms associated with acute mountain sickness in climbers attempting rapid ascent and in those who are very susceptible to acute mountain sickness despite gradual ascent.

Contraindications: Acetazolamide therapy is contraindicated in situations in which sodium and/or potassium blood serum levels are depressed, in cases of marked kidney and liver disease or dysfunction, in suprarenal gland failure, and in hyperchloremic acidosis. It is contraindicated in patients with cirrhosis because of the risk of development of hepatic encephalopathy.

Long-term administration of DIAMOX *acetazolamide* is contraindicated in patients with chronic noncongestive angle-closure glaucoma since it may permit organic closure of the angle to occur while the worsening glaucoma is masked by lowered intraocular pressure.

Warnings: Fatalities have occurred, although rarely, due to severe reactions to sulfonamides including Stevens-Johnson syndrome, toxic epidermal necrolysis, fulminant hepatic necrosis, agranulocytosis, aplastic anemia, and other blood dyscrasias. Sensitizations may recur when a sulfonamide is readministered irrespective of the route of administration. If signs of hypersensitivity or other serious reactions occur, discontinue use of this drug.

Caution is advised for patients receiving concomitant high-dose aspirin and DIAMOX, as anorexia, tachypnea, lethargy, coma, and death have been reported.

Precautions: General: Increasing the dose does not increase the diuresis and may increase the incidence of drowsiness and/or paresthesia. Increasing the dose often results in a decrease in diuresis. Under certain circumstances, however, very large doses have been given in conjunction with other diuretics in order to secure diuresis in complete refractory failure.

Information for Patients: Adverse reactions common to all sulfonamide derivatives may occur: anaphylaxis, fever, rash (including erythema multiforme, Stevens-Johnson syndrome, toxic epidermal necrolysis), crystalluria, renal calculus, bone marrow depression, thrombocytopenic purpura, hemolytic anemia, leukopenia, pancytopenia, and agranulocytosis. Precaution is advised for early detection of such reactions, and the drug should be discontinued and appropriate therapy instituted.

In patients with pulmonary obstruction or emphysema, where alveolar ventilation may be impaired, DIAMOX *acetazolamide,* which may aggravate acidosis, should be used with caution.

Gradual ascent is desirable to try to avoid acute mountain sickness. If rapid ascent is undertaken and DIAMOX is used, it should be noted that such use does not obviate the need for prompt descent if severe forms of high altitude sickness occur, ie, high altitude pulmonary edema (HAPE) or high altitude cerebral edema.

Caution is advised for patients receiving concomitant high-dose aspirin and DIAMOX, as anorexia, tachypnea, lethargy, coma, and death have been reported (see **Warnings**).

Laboratory Tests: To monitor for hematologic reactions common to all sulfonamides, it is recommended that a baseline CBC and platelet count be obtained on patients prior to initiating DIAMOX therapy and at regular intervals during therapy. If significant changes occur, early discontinuance and institution of appropriate therapy are important. Periodic monitoring of serum electrolytes is recommended.

Carcinogenesis, Mutagenesis, Impairment of Fertility: Long-term studies in animals to evaluate the carcinogenic potential of DIAMOX have not been conducted. In a bacterial mutagenicity assay, DIAMOX was not mutagenic when evaluated with and without metabolic activation. The drug had no effect on fertility when administered in the diet to male and female rats at a daily intake of up to four times the maximum recommended human dose of 1000 mg in a 50 kg individual.

Pregnancy Category C. Acetazolamide, administered orally or parenterally, has been shown to be teratogenic (defects of the limbs) in mice, rats, hamsters, and rabbits. There are no adequate and well-controlled studies in pregnant women. Acetazolamide should be used in pregnancy only if the potential benefit justifies the potential risk to the fetus.

Nursing Mothers: Because of the potential for serious adverse reactions in nursing infants from DIAMOX, a decision should be made whether to discontinue nursing or to discontinue the drug, taking into account the importance of the drug to the mother.

Pediatric Use: The safety and effectiveness of DIAMOX in children have not been established.

Adverse Reactions: Adverse reactions, occurring most often early in therapy, include paresthesias, particularly a "tingling" feeling in the extremities, hearing dysfunction or tinnitus, loss of appetite, taste alteration and gastrointestinal disturbances such as nausea, vomiting, and diarrhea; polyuria, and occasional instances of drowsiness and confusion. Metabolic acidosis and electrolyte imbalance may occur.

Transient myopia has been reported. This condition invariably subsides upon diminution or discontinuance of the medication.

Other occasional adverse reactions include urticaria, melena, hematuria, glycosuria, hepatic insufficiency, flaccid paralysis, photosensitivity, and convulsions. Also see **Precautions: Information for Patients** for possible reactions common to sulfonamide derivatives. Fatalities have occurred although rarely, due to severe reactions to sulfonamides including Stevens-Johnson syndrome, toxic epidermal necrolysis, fulminant hepatic necrosis, agranulocytosis, aplastic anemia, and other blood dyscrasias (see **Warnings**).

Overdosage: No data are available regarding DIAMOX *acetazolamide* overdosage in humans as no cases of acute poisoning with this drug have been reported. Animal data suggest that DIAMOX is remarkably nontoxic. No specific antidote is known. Treatment should be symptomatic and supportive.

Electrolyte imbalance, development of an acidotic state, and central nervous effects might be expected to occur. Serum electrolyte levels (particularly potassium) and blood pH levels should be monitored.

Supportive measures are required to restore electrolyte and pH balance. The acidotic state can usually be corrected by the administration of bicarbonate.

Despite its high intraerythrocytic distribution and plasma protein binding properties, DIAMOX may be dialyzable. This may be particularly important in the management of DIAMOX overdosage when complicated by the presence of renal failure.

Dosage and Administration: Glaucoma: The recommended dosage is one capsule (500 mg) two times a day. Usually one capsule is administered in the morning and one capsule in the evening. It may be necessary to adjust the dose, but it has usually been found that dosage in excess of two capsules (1 g) does not produce an increased effect. The dosage should be adjusted with careful individual attention both to symptomatology and intraocular tension. In all cases, continuous supervision by a physician is advisable.

In those unusual instances where adequate control is not obtained by the twice-a-day administration of DIAMOX *acetazolamide* SEQUELS sustained-release capsules, the desired control may be established by means of DIAMOX (tablets or parenteral). Use tablets or parenteral in accordance with the more frequent dosage schedules recommended for these dosage forms, such as 250 mg every 4 hours, or an initial dose of 500 mg followed by 250 mg or 125 mg every 4 hours, depending on the case in question.

Acute Mountain Sickness: Dosage is 500 mg to 1000 mg daily, in divided doses using tablets or sustained-release capsules as appropriate. In circumstances of rapid ascent, such as in rescue or military operations, the higher dose level of 1000 mg is recommended. It is preferable to initiate dosing 24 to 48 hours before ascent and to continue for 48 hours while at high altitude, or longer, as necessary to control symptoms.

How Supplied:
DIAMOX SEQUELS, 500 mg orange capsules printed with DIAMOX over D3, are supplied as follows:

NDC 57706-753-23—Bottle of 100

Store at Controlled Room Temperature 15°–30°C (59°–86°F).

WARNING: Manufactured with trichloroethane, a substance that harms public health and environment by destroying ozone in the upper atmosphere.

Manufactured for
STORZ OPHTHALMICS
St. Louis, MO 63122
by
LEDERLE LABORATORIES DIVISION
American Cyanamid Company
Pearl River, NY 10965 Rev. 3/94
40713-94

Shown in Product Identification Guide, page 106

NEPTAZANE® ℞

[*nĕp-ta 'zāne*]
Methazolamide Tablets, USP

Description: NEPTAZANE, a sulfonamide derivative, is a white crystalline powder, weakly acidic, slightly soluble in water, alcohol and acetone. The chemical name for methazolamide is: *N*-[5-(aminosulfonyl)-3-methyl-1,3,4-thiadiazol-2 (3*H*)-ylidene]-acetamide.

NEPTAZANE is available for oral administration as 25 mg and 50 mg tablets containing the following inactive ingredients: Acacia, Alginic Acid, Corn Starch, Dibasic Calcium Phosphate, Gelatin, and Magnesium Stearate.

Clinical Pharmacology: NEPTAZANE is a potent inhibitor of carbonic anhydrase.

NEPTAZANE is well absorbed from the gastrointestinal tract. Peak plasma concentrations are observed 1 to 2 hours after dosing. In a multiple-dose, pharmacokinetic study, administration of NEPTAZANE 25 mg bid, 50 mg bid, and 100 mg bid demonstrated a linear relationship between plasma methazolamide levels and NEPTAZANE dose. Peak plasma concentrations (C_{max}) for the 25 mg, 50 mg, and 100 mg bid regimens were 2.5 mcg/mL, 5.1 mcg/mL, and 10.7 mcg/mL, respectively. The areas under the plasma concentration-time curves (AUC) were 1130 mcg.min/mL, 2571 mcg.min/mL, and 5418 mcg.min/mL for the 25 mg, 50 mg, and 100 mg dosage regimens, respectively.

NEPTAZANE is distributed throughout the body including the plasma, cerebrospinal fluid, aqueous humor of the eye, red blood cells, bile and extracellular fluid. The mean apparent volume of distribution (V_{area}/F) ranges from 17 L to 23 L. Approximately 55% is bound to plasma proteins. The steady-state NEPTAZANE red blood cell: plasma ratio varies with dose and was found to be 27:1, 16:1, and 10:1 following the administration of NEPTAZANE 25 mg bid, 50 mg bid, and 100 mg bid, respectively.

The mean steady-state plasma elimination half-life for NEPTAZANE is approximately 14 hours. At steady state approximately 25% of the dose is recovered unchanged in the urine over the dosing interval. Renal clearance accounts for 20% to 25% of the total clearance of drug. After repeated bid-tid dosing, NEPTAZANE accumulates to steady-state concentrations in 7 days.

Methazolamide's inhibitory action on carbonic anhydrase decreases the secretion of aqueous humor and results in a decrease in intraocular pressure. The onset of the decrease in intraocular pressure generally occurs within 2 to 4 hours, has a peak effect in 6 to 8 hours, and a total duration of 10 to 18 hours.

NEPTAZANE *methazolamide* is a sulfonamide derivative; however, it does not have any clinically significant antimicrobial properties. Although NEPTAZANE achieves a high concentration in the cerebrospinal fluid, it is not considered an effective anticonvulsant.

NEPTAZANE has a weak and transient diuretic effect; therefore use results in an increase in urinary volume, with excretion of sodium, potassium, and chloride. The drug should not be used as a diuretic. Inhibition of renal bicarbonate reabsorption produces an alkaline urine. Plasma bicarbonate decreases, and a relative, transient metabolic acidosis may occur due to a disequilibrium in carbon dioxide transport in the red cell. Urinary citrate excretion is decreased by approximately 40% after doses of 100 mg every 8 hours. Uric acid output has been shown to decrease 36% in the first 24 hour period.

Indications and Usage: NEPTAZANE is indicated in the treatment of ocular conditions where lowering intraocular pressure is likely to be of therapeutic benefit, such as chronic open-angle glaucoma, secondary glaucoma, and preoperatively in acute angle-closure glaucoma where lowering the intraocular pressure is desired before surgery.

Contraindications: NEPTAZANE therapy is contraindicated in situations in which sodium and/or potassium serum levels are depressed, in cases of marked kidney or liver disease or dysfunction, in adrenal gland failure, and in hyperchloremic acidosis. In patients with cirrhosis, use may precipitate the development of hepatic encephalopathy.

Long-term administration of NEPTAZANE is contraindicated in patients with angle-closure glaucoma, since organic closure of the angle may occur in spite of lowered intraocular pressure.

Warnings: Fatalities have occurred, although rarely, due to severe reactions to sulfonamides including Stevens-Johnson syndrome, toxic epidermal necrolysis, fulminant hepatic necrosis, agranulocytosis, aplastic anemia, and other blood dyscrasias. Hypersensitivity reactions may recur when a sulfonamide is readministered, irrespective of the route of administration.

If hypersensitivity or other serious reactions occur, the use of this drug should be discontinued.

Caution is advised for patients receiving high-dose aspirin and NEPTAZANE concomitantly, as anorexia, tachypnea, lethargy, coma, and death have been reported with concomitant use of high-dose aspirin and carbonic anhydrase inhibitors.

Precautions

General: Potassium excretion is increased initially upon administration of NEPTAZANE *methazolamide* and in patients with cirrhosis or hepatic insufficiency could precipitate a hepatic coma.

In patients with pulmonary obstruction or emphysema, where alveolar ventilation may be impaired, NEPTAZANE should be used with caution because it may precipitate or aggravate acidosis.

Information for Patients: Adverse reactions common to all sulfonamide derivatives may occur: anaphylaxis, fever, rash (including erythema multiforme, Stevens-Johnson syndrome, toxic epidermal necrolysis), crystalluria, renal calculus, bone marrow depression, thrombocytopenic purpura, hemolytic anemia, leukopenia, pancytopenia, and agranulocytosis. Precaution is advised for early detection of such reactions, and the drug should be discontinued and appropriate therapy instituted.

Caution is advised for patients receiving high-dose aspirin and NEPTAZANE concomitantly.

Laboratory Tests: To monitor for hematologic reactions common to all sulfonamides, it is recommended that a baseline CBC and platelet count be obtained on patients prior to initiating NEPTAZANE therapy and at regular intervals during therapy. If significant changes occur, early discontinuance and institution of appropriate therapy are important. Periodic monitoring of serum electrolytes is also recommended.

Drug Interactions: NEPTAZANE should be used with caution in patients on steroid therapy because of the potential for developing hypokalemia.

Caution is advised for patients receiving high-dose aspirin and NEPTAZANE concomitantly, as anorexia, tachypnea, lethargy, coma, and death have been reported with concomitant use of high-dose aspirin and carbonic anhydrase inhibitors (see **WARNINGS**).

Carcinogenesis, Mutagenesis, Impairment of Fertility: Long-term studies in animals to evaluate the carcinogenic potential of NEPTAZANE and its effect on fertility have not been conducted. NEPTAZANE was not mutagenic in the Ames bacterial test.

Pregnancy: *Teratogenic effects.* Pregnancy Category C. NEPTAZANE has been shown to be teratogenic (skeletal anomalies) in rats when given in doses approximately 40 times the human dose. There are no adequate and well-controlled studies in pregnant women. NEPTAZANE should be used during pregnancy only if the potential benefit justifies the potential risk to the fetus.

Nursing Mothers: It is not known whether this drug is excreted in human milk. Because many drugs are excreted in human milk and because of the potential for serious adverse reactions in nursing infants from NEPTAZANE *methazolamide*, a decision should be made whether to discontinue nursing or to discontinue the drug, taking into account the importance of the drug to the mother.

Pediatric Use: The safety and effectiveness of NEPTAZANE in children have not been established.

Adverse Reactions: Adverse reactions, occurring most often early in therapy, include paresthesias, particularly a "tingling" feeling in the extremities; hearing dysfunction or tinnitus; fatigue; malaise; loss of appetite; taste alteration; gastrointestinal disturbances such as nausea, vomiting, and diarrhea; polyuria; and occasional instances of drowsiness and confusion.

Metabolic acidosis and electrolyte imbalance may occur.

Transient myopia has been reported. This condition invariably subsides upon diminution or discontinuance of the medication.

Other occasional adverse reactions include urticaria, melena, hematuria, glycosuria, hepatic insufficiency, flaccid paralysis, photosensitivity, convulsions, and rarely, crystalluria and renal calculi. Also see **PRECAUTIONS, Information for Patients** for possible reactions common to sulfonamide derivatives. Fatalities have occurred, although rarely, due to

Continued on next page

Information on Storz products listed on these pages is the full Prescribing Information from product literature or package inserts effective in June 1994. Information concerning all Storz products may be obtained from the Professional Services Department, Lederle Laboratories, Pearl River, New York 10965

Storz Ophthalmics, Inc.—Cont.

severe reactions to sulfonamides including Stevens-Johnson syndrome, toxic epidermal necrolysis, fulminant hepatic necrosis, agranulocytosis, aplastic anemia, and other blood dyscrasias (see **WARNINGS**).

Overdosage: No data are available regarding NEPTAZANE overdosage in humans as no cases of acute poisoning with this drug have been reported. Animal data suggest that even a high dose of NEPTAZANE is nontoxic. No specific antidote is known. Treatment should be symptomatic and supportive.

Electrolyte imbalance, development of an acidotic state, and central nervous system effects might be expected to occur. Serum electrolyte levels (particularly potassium) and blood pH levels should be monitored.

Supportive measures may be required to restore electrolyte and pH balance.

Dosage and Administration: The effective therapeutic dose administered varies from 50 mg to 100 mg two to three times daily. The drug may be used concomitantly with miotic and osmotic agents.

How Supplied: NEPTAZANE methazolamide Tablets, USP, 25 mg, are square white tablets with engraved N2 on one side and embossed large N on the other side, supplied as follows:

NDC 57706-756-23—Bottle of 100

NEPTAZANE methazolamide Tablets, USP, 50 mg, are round white scored tablets engraved with LL on one side and N above and 1 below the score on the other side, supplied as follows:

NDC 57706-757-23—Bottle of 100

NEPTAZANE is not available for parenteral use.

Store at Controlled Room Temperature 15° to 30°C (59° to 86°F).

National Stock Number:

NSN 6505-00-065-4205—Bottle of 100

Marketed by
STORZ OPHTHALMICS
St. Louis, MO 63122

40648-94
Rev. 2/94

Shown in Product Identification Guide, page 106

OCUCOAT™

2% Hydroxypropylmethylcellulose

Description: OCUCOAT is a sterile, isotonic, nonpyrogenic viscoelastic solution of highly purified, noninflammatory, 2% hydroxypropylmethylcellulose with a high molecular weight greater than 80,000 daltons. OCUCOAT is supplied in 1 mL syringes. Each mL provides 20 mg/mL of hydroxypropylmethylcellulose dissolved in a physiological balanced salt solution containing 0.49% sodium chloride, 0.075% potassium chloride, 0.048% calcium chloride, 0.03% magnesium chloride, 0.39% sodium acetate, 0.17% sodium citrate and water for injection. The osmolarity of OCUCOAT is 285±32 mOsM, the viscosity is 4000±1500 cst, and the pH is 7.2±0.4.

Characteristics: OCUCOAT is an ophthalmic surgical aid for use in anterior segment surgery.

OCUCOAT:

1. Is a space occupying, tissue protective substance
2. Exhibits excellent flow properties
3. Is completely transparent
4. Is nonantigenic
5. Is easily removed from the anterior chamber
6. Contains no proteins which may cause inflammation or foreign body reactions
7. Requires no refrigeration or restrictive storage conditions
8. Does not interfere with normal wound healing process
9. Clears the trabecular meshwork in 24 hours (98% clearance rate)

Indications: OCUCOAT is indicated for use as an ophthalmic surgical aid in anterior segment surgical procedures, including cataract extraction and intraocular lens implantation. OCUCOAT maintains a deep chamber during anterior segment surgery and thereby allows for more efficient manipulation with less trauma to the corneal endothelium and other ocular tissues. The viscoelasticity of OCUCOAT helps the vitreous face to be pushed back, thus preventing formation of a postoperative flat chamber.

Contraindications: At present, there are no known contraindications to the use of OCUCOAT when used as recommended.

Precautions: Precautions are limited to those normally associated with the ophthalmic surgical procedure being performed.

There may be transient increased intraocular pressure following surgery because of pre-existing glaucoma or due to the surgery itself. For these reasons, the following precautions should be considered:

- OCUCOAT should be removed from the anterior chamber at the end of surgery.
- If the postoperative intraocular pressure increases above expected values, appropriate therapy should be administered.

Adverse Reactions: Clinical testing of OCUCOAT showed it to be extremely well tolerated after injection into the human eye.

A transient rise in intraocular pressure postoperatively has been reported in some cases. Rarely, postoperative inflammatory reactions (iritis, hypopyon), as well as incidents of corneal edema and corneal decompensation, have been reported with viscoelastic agents. Their relationship to OCUCOAT has not been established.

Clinical Applications: In anterior segment surgery, OCUCOAT should be carefully introduced into the anterior chamber using a 20 gauge or smaller cannula. OCUCOAT may be injected into the chamber prior to or following delivery of the crystalline lens. Injection of OCUCOAT prior to lens delivery will provide additional protection to the corneal endothelium and other ocular tissues. Injection of the material at this point is significant in that a coating of OCUCOAT may protect the corneal endothelium from possible damage arising from surgical instrumentation during the cataract extraction surgery.

OCUCOAT *2% hydroxypropylmethylcellulose* may also be used to coat an intraocular lens as well as tips of surgical instruments prior to implantation surgery. Additional OCUCOAT may be injected during anterior segment surgery to fully maintain the chamber, or to replace fluid lost during the surgical procedure. OCUCOAT should be removed from the anterior chamber at the end of surgery. Rather than aspirate OCUCOAT from the eye with the OCUCOAT syringe, it is recommended that OCUCOAT be aspirated using an automated I/A device, or irrigated using an irrigation syringe or a BSS squeeze bottle.

How Supplied: OCUCOAT is a sterile, nonpyrogenic, viscoelastic preparation supplied in a 1 mL single use glass syringe with a Luer tip and a Luer lock cannula. OCUCOAT syringes are aseptically packaged and terminally sterilized. The sterility expiration date is on the outer package.

Store at room temperature; avoid excessive heat (60°C). Protect from light. For intraocular use.

Warning: Manufactured with CFC-12, a substance which harms public health and environment by destroying ozone in the upper atmosphere.

Directions for Use—Syringe Assembly:

Use sterile opening technique.

Open pouch and drop sterile contents onto sterile field.

Assembly:

Insert glass carpule into plastic holder and push carpule until spike penetrates rubber tip.

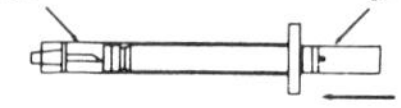

Screw plunger rod clockwise into rubber stopper.

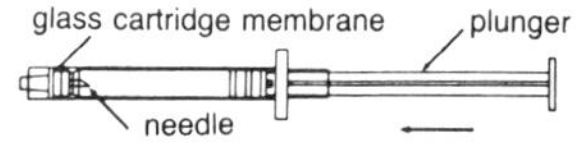

Connect Luer lock cannula to syringe tip, twist firmly in place, and check for proper function. Allow air bubbles, if any, to rise to the surface, and push plunger rod slightly to release any air bubbles from syringe tip and cannula.

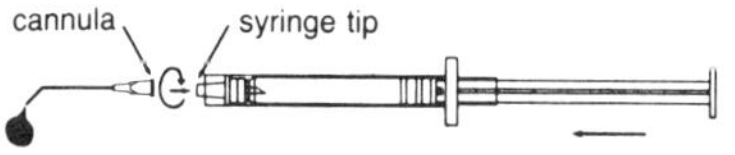

* NOTE: It is recommended that the cannula hub be partially or totally filled with BSS prior to attaching to the syringe. This will further reduce the introduction of air bubbles into the anterior chamber.

Caution: Federal (USA) law restricts this device to sale by or on the order of a physician. For intraocular use only. Discard unused contents of OCUCOAT *2% hydroxypropylmethylcellulose* syringe after each use. Do not resterilize.

References:

1. Fechner PU, Fechner MU. Methylcellulose and lens implantation. *Br J Ophthalmol.* 1983;67.
2. Aron-Rosa D, et al. Methylcellulose instead of Healon® in extracapsular surgery with intraocular lens implantation. *Ophthalmology.* 1983;90:10.
3. Smith SG, et al. Safety and efficacy of 2% methylcellulose in cat and monkey cataract-implant surgery. *Am Intraocular Implant Soc J.* 1984:10.
4. Liesegang TJ, et al. The use of hydroxypropyl methylcellulose in extracapsular cataract extraction with intraocular lens implantation. *Am J Ophthalmol.* 1986:102.

Manufactured for:
STORZ OPHTHALMICS
21 Park Place Blvd. N.
Clearwater, FL 34619-3917

14361G
4/93

Shown in Product Identification Guide, page 106

OCUCOAT™ and OCUCOAT™ PF OTC

Lubricating Eye Drops

Description: Multidose: Dextran 70 (0.1%), hydroxypropyl methylcellulose 2910 (0.8%), monobasic sodium phosphate, dibasic sodium phosphate, potassium chloride, sodium chlo-

ride, dextrose and purified water. Preserved with benzalkonium chloride (0.01%). May also contain hydrochloric acid and/or sodium hydroxide to adjust the pH.
Unit Dose: Dextran 70 (0.1%), hydroxypropyl methylcellulose 2910 (0.8%), monobasic sodium phosphate, dibasic sodium phosphate, potassium chloride, sodium chloride, dextrose and purified water. May also contain hydrochloric acid and/or sodium hydroxide to adjust the pH.
Indications: For use as a lubricant to prevent further irritation or to relieve dryness of the eye.
Directions: Multidose: Carefully tilt container over the open eye. Without touching the eye or eyelid, squeeze one or two drops into the affected eye(s) as needed or as directed by a doctor.
Unit Dose: Detach a single-dose container from the strip. Be sure each container is intact before using it. Do not use if container is not intact.
To open, gently twist off the tip.
With thumb and finger on either side of the bubble, carefully tilt the container over the open eye. Without touching the tip to the eye or eyelid, squeeze one or two drops into the affected eye(s) as needed or as directed by a doctor.
Do not reuse. Once opened, discard.
Warnings: Keep this and all drugs out of the reach of children. In case of accidental ingestion, seek professional assistance or contact a Poison Control Center immediately.
If you experience eye pain, changes in vision, continued redness or irritation of the eye, or if the condition worsens or persists for more than 72 hours, discontinue use and consult a doctor.
If solution changes color or becomes cloudy, do not use.
To avoid contamination, do not touch tip of container to any surface.
For multidose units, replace cap immediately after using.
For unit dose units, discard after single use.
How Supplied:
OCUCOAT:
NDC 0005-0769-09—15 mL bottle
OCUCOAT PF:
NDC 0005-0768-65—28 single-dose containers
FOR OPHTHALMIC USE ONLY.
STORE AT ROOM TEMPERATURE.
Marketed by
STORZ OPHTHALMICS
St. Louis, MO 63122
Distributed by
LEDERLE LABORATORIES DIVISION
American Cyanamid Company
Pearl River, NY 10965

Shown in Product Identification Guide, page 106

OCUVITE®

Vitamin and Mineral Supplement

Description: Each tablet contains:

For Adults—Percentage of US Recommended Daily Allowance (US RDA)

Zinc (as Zinc Oxide)	40 mg (elemental)	267%
Copper (as Cupric Oxide)	2 mg (elemental)	100%
Vitamin C	60 mg	100%
Vitamin E	30 IU	100%
Vitamin A (as Beta Carotene)	5000 IU	100%
Selenium	40 mcg* (elemental)	

*No US RDA established.

Inactive Ingredients: Crospovidone, FD&C Yellow No. 6, hydroxypropyl methylcellulose, lactose, magnesium stearate, microcrystalline cellulose, modified food starch, povidone, silica gel, and titanium dioxide.
Indications: OCUVITE is specifically formulated to supplement the diets of people who may have or be at risk of deficiencies of the vitamins and minerals found in the OCUVITE formulation.
Recommended Intake: Adults: One tablet, one or two times daily or as directed by their doctor.
How Supplied: Two-tone peach, eye shaped, film coated tablet engraved LL on one side, 04 on the other side.
NDC 0005-4550-19—Bottle of 60
NDC 0005-4550-24—Bottle of 120
Store at Room Temperature.
Distributed by
LEDERLE LABORATORIES DIVISION
American Cyanamid Company
Pearl River, NY 10965
Marketed by
STORZ OPHTHALMICS
St. Louis, MO 63122

32398–93

Shown in Product Identification Guide, page 106

R̄EV-EYES® ℞

[reev-eyes]
dapiprazole hydrochloride
Ophthalmic Eyedrops, 0.5%—Sterile

Description: For ophthalmic use only.
R̄EV-EYES is an alpha-adrenergic blocking agent.
Dapiprazole hydrochloride is 5,6,7,8-tetrahydro-3-[2-(4-*o*-tolyl-1-piperazinyl) ethyl]-*s*-triazolo[4,3-a]pyridine hydrochloride.
Dapiprazole hydrochloride has the empirical formula $C_{19}H_{27}N_5$ HCl and a molecular weight of 361.93.
Dapiprazole hydrochloride is a sterile, white, lyophilized powder soluble in water.
R̄EV-EYES Eyedrops is a clear, colorless, slightly viscous solution for topical application. Each mL (when reconstituted as directed) contains 5 mg of dapiprazole hydrochloride as the active ingredient.
The reconstituted solution has a pH of approximately 6.6 and an osmolarity of approximately 415 mOsm.
The inactive ingredients include: mannitol (2%), sodium chloride, hydroxypropyl methylcellulose (0.4%), edetate sodium (0.01%), sodium phosphate dibasic, sodium phosphate monobasic, water for injection, and benzalkonium chloride (0.01%) as a preservative.
R̄EV-EYES Eyedrops, 0.5% is supplied in a kit consisting of one vial of dapiprazole hydrochloride (25 mg), one vial of diluent (5 mL) and one dropper for dispensing.
Clinical Pharmacology: Dapiprazole acts through blocking the alpha-adrenergic receptors in smooth muscle. Dapiprazole produces miosis through an effect on the dilator muscle of the iris.
Dapiprazole does not have any significant activity on ciliary muscle contraction and, therefore, does not induce a significant change in the anterior chamber depth or the thickness of the lens.
Dapiprazole has demonstrated safe and rapid reversal of mydriasis produced by phenylephrine and to a lesser degree tropicamide. In patients with decreased accommodative amplitude due to treatment with tropicamide, dapiprazole partially restores the accommodative amplitude. This activity is not only due to its miotic effect but also to a direct effect on accommodation.
Eye color affects the rate of pupillary constriction. In individuals with brown irides, the rate of pupillary constriction may be slightly slower than in individuals with blue or green irides. Eye color does not appear to affect the final pupil size.
Dapiprazole does not significantly alter intraocular pressure in normotensive or in eyes with elevated intraocular pressure.
Indications and Usage: Dapiprazole is indicated in the treatment of iatrogenically induced mydriasis produced by adrenergic (phenylephrine) or parasympatholytic (tropicamide) agents. Dapiprazole is not indicated for the reduction of intraocular pressure or in the treatment of open angle glaucoma.
Contraindications: Miotics are contraindicated where constriction is undesirable, such as acute iritis, and in those subjects showing hypersensitivity to any component of this preparation.
Warning: For Topical Ophthalmic Use Only. NOT FOR INJECTION. Do not touch the dropper up to lids or any surface, as this may contaminate the solution. Dapiprazole should not be used in the same patient more frequently than once a week.
Precautions:
Information to Patients: Miosis may cause difficulty in dark adaptation and may reduce the field of vision. Patients should exercise caution when involved in night driving or other activities in poor illumination.
Carcinogenesis, Mutagenesis, Impairment of Fertility: Dapiprazole has been shown to significantly increase the incidence of liver tumors in rats after continuous dietary administration for 104 weeks. This effect was found only in male rats treated with the highest dose administered in the study, ie, 300 mg/kg/day (80,000 times the human dose) and was not observed in male and female rats at doses of 30 and 100 mg/kg/day and female rats at doses of 300 mg/kg/day.
Negative results have been reported on the mutagenicity and impairment of fertility studies with dapiprazole.
Pregnancy: *Pregnancy Category B:* Reproduction studies have been performed in rats and rabbits at doses up to 128,000 (rat) and 27,000 (rabbit) times the human ophthalmic dose and revealed no evidence of impaired fertility or harm to the fetus due to dapiprazole. There are, however, no adequate and well-controlled studies in pregnant women. Because animal reproduction studies are not always predictive of human response, this drug should be used during pregnancy only if clearly needed.
Nursing Mothers: It is not known whether this drug is excreted in human milk. Because many drugs are excreted in human milk, caution should be exercised when dapiprazole is administered to a nursing woman.
Pediatric Use: Safety and effectiveness in children have not been established.
Adverse Reactions: In controlled studies the most frequent reaction to dapiprazole was conjunctival injection lasting 20 minutes in over 80% of patients. Burning on instillation of dapiprazole was reported in approximately half of all patients. Reactions occurring in 10% to 40% of patients included ptosis, lid erythema, lid edema, chemosis, itching, punctate keratitis, corneal edema, brow ache, photophobia and headaches. Other reactions reported less frequently included dryness of eyes, tearing, and blurring of vision.
Dosage and Administration: Two drops followed 5 minutes later by an additional 2

Continued on next page

Information on Storz products listed on these pages is the full Prescribing Information from product literature or package inserts effective in June 1994. Information concerning all Storz products may be obtained from the Professional Services Department, Lederle Laboratories, Pearl River, New York 10965

Storz Ophthalmics, Inc.—Cont.

drops applied topically to the conjunctiva of each eye should be administered after the ophthalmic examination to reverse the diagnostic mydriasis. Dapiprazole should not be used in the same patient more frequently than once per week.

Directions for Preparing Eyedrops:

1. Use aseptic technique.
2. Tear off aluminum seals, remove and discard rubber plugs from both drug and diluent vials.
3. Pour diluent into drug vial.
4. Remove dropper assembly from its sterile wrapping and attach to the drug vial.
5. Shake container for several minutes to ensure mixing.

How Supplied: RĒV-EYES *dapiprazole hydrochloride* Eyedrops, 0.5%
NDC 57706-761-62
Each package contains RĒV-EYES (25 mg), diluent (5 mL) and dropper for dispensing.

Storage and Stability of Eyedrops: Once the eyedrops have been reconstituted they may be stored at room temperature 15°–30°C (59°–86°F) for 21 days. Discard any solution that is not clear and colorless.
Patented U.S. Patent No. 4,252,721
Caution: Federal (USA) law prohibits dispensing without prescription.

Manufactured by
ABBOTT LABORATORIES
North Chicago, IL 60064
For
ANGELINI PHARMACEUTICALS INC.
River Edge, NJ 07661
Marketed by
STORZ OPHTHALMICS
Storz Division
American Cyanamid Company
Pearl River, NY 10965

Rev. 5/92
01-2508-R1
20438-92

Information on Storz products listed on these pages is the full Prescribing Information from product literature or package inserts effective in June 1994. Information concerning all Storz products may be obtained from the Professional Services Department, Lederle Laboratories, Pearl River, New York 10965.

Vision Pharmaceuticals, Inc.
1022 N. MAIN STREET
MITCHELL, SD 57301

VIVA-DROPS® — OTC
Lubricant Eye Drops

Description: VIVA-DROPS® is a preservative-free, non-oily, sterile ophthalmic lubricant for relief from irritation due to dryness of the eye or discomfort caused by exposure to wind, sun or dry air. The patented formulation of VIVA-DROPS® includes antioxidants that protect the active ingredient from autoxidation.

Contains: Active: polysorbate 80.
Inactives: purified water, sodium chloride, citric acid, edetate disodium, with retinyl palmitate, mannitol, sodium citrate, and pyruvate as antioxidants.

FDA APPROVED USES

Indications: FOR USE AS A LUBRICANT TO PREVENT FURTHER IRRITATION OR TO RELIEVE DRYNESS OF THE EYE.

Warnings: If you experience eye pain, changes in vision, continued redness or irritation of the eye, or if the condition persists for more than 72 hours, discontinue use and consult a doctor. If solution changes color or becomes cloudy, do not use. Keep this and all drugs out of the reach of children.

Directions: Instill 1 or 2 drops in the affected eye(s) as needed.

How Supplied: In 10mL (NDC 54891-001-02) and 15mL (NDC 54891-001-01) bottles.
Store at room temperature.
U.S. Patent No. 5,032,392

Walker Pharmacal Company
4200 LACLEDE AVENUE
ST. LOUIS, MO 63108

SUCCUS CINERARIA MARITIMA — ℞
[*suk 'us si-ne 'ra "ria mar "i-te 'ma*]
(Senecio Cineraria Compound Solution)
SCM—WALKER™
Sterile—Ophthalmic

Description: Succus Cineraria Maritima is an aqueous and glycerin solution of the total extractives of the fresh Senecio Cineraria USPH 8th (Senecio Compositae) with extract of Hamamelis V. (Witch Hazel) and boric acid USP. The Alkaloids included in the total extract include Senecine and Senecionine. Total nonvolatiles are approximately 20%. The pH is adjusted to 4.1 pH; osmotic pressure is 5.5 osmols.

Actions and Uses: Succus Cineraria Maritima applied locally to the eyes acts as a safe lymphagogue, increasing circulation in the intraocular tissues, also stimulating collateral circulation and normal metabolism, functions so necessary from the standpoint of the physiology of the eye. Clinical observation indicates the definite value of local applications of Succus Cineraria Maritima in checking, or even aborting existing opacities. The benefits attained are obviously more satisfactory when treatment is instituted in the early stage of cataract. In cases of well advanced opacity, and where pathological changes caused by the deterioration of the metabolic functions have occurred, as is characteristic in senility, less favorable results can be expected.
The use of Succus Cineraria Maritima, however, is justified in certain cases well past the incipient stage, particularly when an operation is not contemplated or is contraindicated. It gives comfort to the patient to know that something potentially beneficial is being done. Clinical studies of advanced stages of cataract treated with Succus Cineraria Maritima indicated that in 22.5% of these cases beneficial results were obtained. In many of the cases which did not show improvement the process of the opacity was retarded or checked. In certain cases Succus Cineraria Maritima only gives temporary relief or serves to postpone the surgical removal.

Indications: Succus Cineraria Maritima is indicated in the treatment of various cases of optic opacity caused by cataract.

Contraindications: A history of a previous hypersensitivity reaction to any of the Senecio Alkaloids or to Hamamelis V. is a contraindication.

Warning: The possibility of sensitivity reactions should be considered in patients with a history of allergy. If excessive irritation occurs it may be advisable to dilute the dosage, or discontinue treatment. (pH of 4.1 may cause minor irritation.) For topical ophthalmic use only. If excessive irritation should develop, patient should consult the prescribing physician.

Caution: Federal Law prohibits dispensing without prescription.

Caution: Not intended for use in glaucoma.

Dosage and Administration: Succus Cineraria Maritima should be instilled in the affected eye, two drops morning and evening, or as directed by physician. Do not touch dropper tip to any surface, since this may contaminate the solution.

Supplied: In sterile ¼ oz. dropper vial (7cc).
NDC 619-4021-38.

Wyeth-Ayerst Laboratories
Division of American Home Products Corporation
P.O. BOX 8299
PHILADELPHIA, PA 19101

As a result of a merger of Wyeth Laboratories and Ayerst Laboratories, all prescription products of both companies and all nonprescription products formerly of Wyeth are products of Wyeth-Ayerst Laboratories. All nonprescription products formerly of Ayerst Laboratories are products of Whitehall Laboratories.

COLLYRIUM for FRESH EYES — OTC
[*ko-lir 'e-um*]
EYE WASH
A neutral borate solution

Description: Soothing Collyrium Eye Wash for Fresh Eyes is specially formulated to soothe, refresh, and cleanse irritated eyes.
Collyrium Eye Wash is a neutral borate solution that contains boric acid, sodium borate, benzalkonium chloride as a preservative, and water.

Indications: Patients are advised of the following. Use Collyrium Eye Wash to cleanse the eye, loosen foreign material, air pollutants or chlorinated water.

Recommended Uses:
Home—For emergency flushing of foreign bodies or whenever a soothing eye rinse is necessary.
Hospitals, dispensaries and clinics—For emergency flushing of chemicals or foreign bodies from the eye.

Directions: Patients are advised of the following. Remove the eyecup from blister. Puncture bottle by twisting threaded eyecup down onto bottle; then remove it from the bottle. Rinse eyecup with clean water immediately before and after each use. Avoid contamination of rim and interior surfaces of eyecup. Fill eyecup one-half full with Collyrium Eye Wash. Apply cup tightly to the affected eye to prevent escape of the liquid and tilt head backward. Open eyelid wide and rotate eyeball to thoroughly wash eye. Rinse cup with clean water after use and recap by twisting threaded eyecup on the bottle for storage.

Warnings: Patients are advised of the following. Do not use if solution changes color or becomes cloudy, or with a wetting solution for contact lenses or other eye care products containing polyvinyl alcohol.
This product contains benzalkonium chloride as a preservative. Do not use this product if you are sensitive to benzalkonium chloride.
To avoid contamination do not touch tip of container to any surface. Replace cap after using. If you experience eye pain, changes in vision, continued redness, irritation of the eye, or if the condition worsens or persists, consult a doctor. Obtain immediate medical treatment for all open wounds in or near the eyes.

The Collyrium for Fresh Eyes bottle is sealed for your protection. Prior to first use, remove cap and squeeze bottle. If bottle leaks, do not use.
Keep this and all medication out of the reach of children.
Keep bottle tightly closed at Room Temperature, Approx. 77° F (25° C).
How Supplied: Bottles of 4 FL. OZ. (118 mL) with eyecup.

Shown in Product Identification Guide, page 106

COLLYRIUM FRESH™ OTC
[*ko-lir 'e-um*]
Sterile Eye Drops
Lubricant • Redness Reliever

Description: Collyrium Fresh is a specially formulated sterile eye drop which can be used up to 4 times daily, to relieve redness and discomfort due to minor eye irritations caused by dust, smoke, smog, swimming, or sun glare.
The active ingredients are tetrahydrozoline HCl (0.05%) and glycerin (1.0%). Other ingredients include benzalkonium chloride (0.01%) and edetate disodium (0.1%) as preservatives, boric acid, hydrochloric acid and sodium borate.
Indications: Patients are advised of the following. For the temporary relief of redness due to minor eye irritations or discomfort due to burning or exposure to wind or sun.
Directions: Patients are advised of the following. Tilt head back and squeeze 1 to 2 drops into each eye up to 4 times daily, or as directed by a physician.
Warnings: Patients are advised of the following. Do not use if solution changes color or becomes cloudy. Remove contact lenses before using. If you have glaucoma, do not use this product except under the advice and supervision of a physician. Overuse of this product may produce increased redness of the eye. To avoid contamination, do not touch tip of container to any surface. Replace cap after using. If you experience eye pain, changes in vision, continued redness or irritation of the eye, or if the condition worsens or persists for more than 72 hours, discontinue use and consult a physician.
Keep this and all medication out of the reach of children. The product's carton should be retained for complete product information.
Keep bottle tightly closed at Room Temperature, Approx. 77° F (25° C).
How Supplied: Bottles of 0.5 FL. OZ. (15 mL) with built-in eye dropper.

Shown in Product Identification Guide, page 106

FLUOR-I-STRIP® ℞
[*floo-or 'a "strip*]
(Fluorescein Sodium Ophthalmic Strips)

Composition (per strip):

Fluorescein Sodium 9 mg	diagnostic dye
Chlorobutanol (chloral derivative) 0.5%	preservative
Polysorbate 80	surface active agent
Potassium Chloride	
Boric Acid	buffering agents
Sodium Carbonate	

Description: FLUOR-I-STRIP is a specially prepared sterile ophthalmic strip for diagnostic use.
Indications: For staining the anterior segment of the eye when:

a) delineating a corneal injury, herpetic lesion or foreign body,
b) determining the site of an intraocular injury,
c) fitting contact lenses,
d) making the fluorescein test to ascertain postoperative closure of the sclerocorneal (also referred to as corneoscleral) wound in delayed anterior chamber reformation,
e) making the lacrimal drainage test.

Directions for Use: To open envelope, grasp pull-tabs firmly and separate slowly. Separate the two strips by tearing off white tab end. Moisten end of strip with a drop of sterile water. Place moistened strip at the fornix in the lower cul-de-sac close to the punctum. For best results, patient should close lid tightly over strip until desired amount of staining is obtained. Another method is to retract upper lid and touch tip of strip to the bulbar conjunctiva on the temporal side until an adequate amount of stain is available for a clearly defined end point reading.
Warning: Never use fluorescein while the patient is wearing *soft contact lenses* because the lenses may become stained. Whenever fluorescein is used, flush the eyes with sterile, normal saline solution, and wait at least one hour before replacing the lenses.
Storage: Store at room temperature (approximately 25°C).
How Supplied: Boxes of 300 strips in individual envelopes (NDC 0046-1028-83).

Shown in Product Identification Guide, page 106

FLUOR-I-STRIP® -A.T. ℞
[*floo-or 'a "strip*]
(Fluorescein Sodium Ophthalmic Strips)
For Applanation Tonometry

Composition (Per Strip):

Fluorescein Sodium 1 mg	diagnostic dye
Chlorobutanol (chloral derivative) 0.5%	preservative
Polysorbate 80	surface active agent
Boric Acid	
Potassium Chloride	buffering agents
Sodium Carbonate	

Description: FLUOR-I-STRIP-A.T. consists of sterile ophthalmic strips, specially prepared for diagnostic use in applanation tonometry.
Indications: For staining the anterior segment of the eye when:

a) delineating a corneal injury, herpetic lesion or foreign body,
b) determining the site of an intraocular injury,
c) fitting contact lenses,
d) making the fluorescein test to ascertain postoperative closure of the sclerocorneal (also referred to as corneoscleral) wound in delayed anterior chamber reformation,
e) making the lacrimal drainage test.

Directions for Use: To open envelope, grasp pull-tabs firmly and separate slowly. Separate the two strips by tearing off white tab end. Anesthetize the eyes. Retract upper lid and touch tip of strip to the bulbar conjunctiva on the temporal side until an adequate amount of stain is available for a clearly defined end-point reading.
Warning: Never use fluorescein while the patient is wearing *soft contact lenses* because the lenses may become stained. Whenever fluorescein is used, flush the eyes with sterile, normal saline solution, and wait at least one hour before replacing the lenses.
Storage: Store at room temperature (approximately 25°C).
How Supplied: Boxes of 300 strips, 2 in each envelope (NDC 0046-1048-83).

Shown in Product Identification Guide, page 106

OPHTHALGAN® ℞
[*of"thal 'găn*]
(glycerin ophthalmic solution)*
STERILE

Caution: Federal law prohibits dispensing without prescription.
Description: Glycerin is 1,2,3-propanetriol:

$$CH_2OH—CHOH—CH_2OH$$

It is a clear, colorless, viscous liquid.
OPHTHALGAN is a sterile glycerin ophthalmic solution.

---

*OPHTHALGAN contains not more than 1.0% water. Chlorobutanol (chloral derivative) 0.55% is incorporated as preservative. The pH of this solution may differ from that specified in the U.S.P.

Clinical Pharmacology: OPHTHALGAN (glycerin ophthalmic solution) is used only for topical application to the cornea. By virtue of its osmotic action, it promptly reduces edema and causes clearing of corneal haze. The action of OPHTHALGAN is transient, and it is, therefore, used primarily for diagnostic purposes.
Indications and Usage: OPHTHALGAN is indicated to clear an edematous cornea in order to facilitate ophthalmoscopic and gonioscopic examination especially in acute glaucoma, bullous keratitis, Fuchs's endothelial dystrophy, and so forth. In gonioscopy of an edematous cornea, additional OPHTHALGAN may be used as the lubricant. A local anesthetic should be instilled shortly before use of OPHTHALGAN.
Contraindications: Hypersensitivity to the active or inactive ingredients.
Precautions: Because OPHTHALGAN (glycerin ophthalmic solution) is an irritant and may cause pain, a local anesthetic should be instilled shortly before its use.
Carcinogenesis, Mutagenesis, Impairment of Fertility: No long-term studies in animals or humans have been conducted.
Pregnancy Category C: Animal reproduction studies have not been conducted with OPHTHALGAN. It is also not known whether OPHTHALGAN can cause fetal harm when administered to a pregnant woman or can affect reproduction capacity. OPHTHALGAN should be given to a pregnant woman only if clearly needed.
Nursing Mothers: It is not known whether this drug is excreted in human milk. Because many drugs are excreted in human milk, caution should be exercised when OPHTHALGAN is administered to a nursing woman.
Pediatric Use: Safety and effectiveness in children have not been established.
Adverse Reactions: Some pain and/or irritation may occur upon instillation.
Dosage and Administration: One or two drops prior to examination. In gonioscopy of an edematous cornea, additional OPHTHALGAN (glycerin ophthalmic solution) may be used as the lubricant.
DISCARD THIS PRODUCT SIX MONTHS AFTER DROPPER IS FIRST PLACED IN THE DRUG SOLUTION.
How Supplied: OPHTHALGAN is available in dropper-screw cap bottles of 7.5 mL (NDC 0046-1013-07).
Store at room temperature (approximately 25°C).
Note: Keep bottle tightly closed.

Shown in Product Identification Guide, page 106

Continued on next page

Wyeth-Ayerst—Cont.

PHOSPHOLINE IODIDE® ℞

[fos"fo'lĭn i"o-dīd]

(echothiophate iodide for ophthalmic solution)

Caution: Federal law prohibits dispensing without prescription.

Description: Chemical name: (2-mercaptoethyl) trimethylammonium iodide O,O-diethyl phosphorothioate.

PHOSPHOLINE IODIDE occurs as a white, crystalline, water-soluble, hygroscopic solid having a slight mercaptan-like odor. When freeze-dried in the presence of potassium acetate, the mixture appears as a white amorphous deposit on the walls of the bottle.

Each package contains materials for dispensing 5 mL of eyedrops: (1) bottle containing sterile PHOSPHOLINE IODIDE in one of four potencies [1.5 mg (0.03%), 3 mg (0.06%), 6.25 mg (0.125%), or 12.5 mg (0.25%)] as indicated on the label, with 40 mg potassium acetate in each case. Sodium hydroxide or acetic acid may have been incorporated to adjust pH during manufacturing; (2) a 5 mL bottle of sterile diluent containing chlorobutanol (chloral derivative), 0.55%; mannitol, 1.2%; boric acid, 0.06%; and exsiccated sodium phosphate, 0.026%; (3) sterilized dropper.

Clinical Pharmacology: PHOSPHOLINE IODIDE is a long-acting cholinesterase inhibitor for topical use which enhances the effect of endogenously liberated acetylcholine in iris, ciliary muscle, and other parasympathetically innervated structures of the eye. It thereby causes miosis, increase in facility of outflow of aqueous humor, fall in intraocular pressure, and potentiation of accommodation.

PHOSPHOLINE IODIDE (echothiophate iodide) will depress both plasma and erythrocyte cholinesterase levels in most patients after a few weeks of eyedrop therapy.

Indications and Usage: GLAUCOMA—Chronic open-angle glaucoma. Subacute or chronic angle-closure glaucoma after iridectomy or where surgery is refused or contraindicated. Certain non-uveitic secondary types of glaucoma, especially glaucoma following cataract surgery.

ACCOMMODATIVE ESOTROPIA—Concomitant esotropias with a significant accommodative component.

Contraindications:

1. Active uveal inflammation.
2. Most cases of angle-closure glaucoma, due to the possibility of increasing angle block.
3. Hypersensitivity to the active or inactive ingredients.

Warnings:

1. Succinylcholine should be administered only with great caution, if at all, prior to or during general anesthesia to patients receiving anticholinesterase medication because of possible respiratory or cardiovascular collapse.
2. Caution should be observed in treating glaucoma with PHOSPHOLINE IODIDE (echothiophate iodide) in patients who are at the same time undergoing treatment with systemic anticholinesterase medications for myasthenia gravis, because of possible adverse additive effects.

(See "Precautions—Drug Interactions" for further information.)

Precautions:

General

1. Gonioscopy is recommended prior to initiation of therapy. Routine examination to detect lens opacity should accompany clinical use of PHOSPHOLINE IODIDE.
2. Where there is a quiescent uveitis or a history of this condition, anticholinesterase therapy should be avoided or used cautiously because of the intense and persistent miosis and ciliary muscle contraction that may occur.
3. While systemic effects are infrequent, proper use of the drug requires digital compression of the nasolacrimal ducts for a minute or two following instillation to minimize drainage into the nasal chamber with its extensive absorption area. To prevent possible skin absorption, hands should be washed following instillation.
4. Temporary discontinuance of medication is necessary if cardiac irregularities occur.
5. Anticholinesterase drugs should be used with extreme caution, if at all, in patients with marked vagotonia, bronchial asthma, spastic gastrointestinal disturbances, peptic ulcer, pronounced bradycardia and hypotension, recent myocardial infarction, epilepsy, parkinsonism, and other disorders that may respond adversely to vagotonic effects.
6. Anticholinesterase drugs should be employed prior to ophthalmic surgery only as a considered risk because of the possible occurrence of hyphema.
7. PHOSPHOLINE IODIDE (echothiophate iodide) should be used with great caution, if at all, where there is a prior history of retinal detachment.
8. Temporary discontinuance of medication is necessary if salivation, urinary incontinence, diarrhea, profuse sweating, muscle weakness, or respiratory difficulties occur.
9. Patients receiving PHOSPHOLINE IODIDE who are exposed to carbamate- or organophosphate-type insecticides and pesticides (professional gardeners, farmers, workers in plants manufacturing or formulating such products, etc.) should be warned of the additive systemic effects possible from absorption of the pesticide through the respiratory tract or skin. During periods of exposure to such pesticides, the wearing of respiratory masks, and frequent washing and clothing changes may be advisable.

Drug Interactions: PHOSPHOLINE IODIDE potentiates other cholinesterase inhibitors such as succinylcholine or organophosphate and carbamate insecticides. Patients undergoing systemic anticholinesterase treatment should be warned of the possible additive effects of PHOSPHOLINE IODIDE.

Carcinogenesis, Mutagenesis, Impairment of Fertility: No data is available regarding carcinogenesis, mutagenesis, and impairment of fertility.

Pregnancy:

Teratogenic Effects—Pregnancy Category C: Animal reproduction studies have not been conducted with PHOSPHOLINE IODIDE. It is also not known whether PHOSPHOLINE IODIDE can cause fetal harm when administered to a pregnant woman or can affect reproduction capacity. PHOSPHOLINE IODIDE (echothiophate iodide) should be given to a pregnant woman only if clearly needed.

Nursing Mothers:

Because of the potential for serious adverse reactions in nursing infants from PHOSPHOLINE IODIDE, a decision should be made whether to discontinue nursing or to discontinue the drug, taking into account the importance of the drug to the mother.

Adverse Reactions:

1. Although the relationship, if any, of retinal detachment to the administration of PHOSPHOLINE IODIDE has not been established, retinal detachment has been reported in a few cases during the use of PHOSPHOLINE IODIDE in adult patients without a previous history of this disorder.
2. Stinging, burning, lacrimation, lid muscle twitching, conjunctival and ciliary redness, browache, induced myopia with visual blurring may occur.
3. Activation of latent iritis or uveitis may occur.
4. Iris cysts may form, and if treatment is continued, may enlarge and obscure vision. This occurrence is more frequent in children. The cysts usually shrink upon discontinuance of the medication, reduction in strength of the drops or frequency of instillation. Rarely, they may rupture or break free into the aqueous. Regular examinations are advisable when the drug is being prescribed for the treatment of accommodative esotropia.
5. Prolonged use may cause conjunctival thickening, obstruction of nasolacrimal canals.
6. Lens opacities occurring in patients under treatment for glaucoma with PHOSPHOLINE IODIDE have been reported and similar changes have been produced experimentally in normal monkeys. Routine examinations should accompany clinical use of the drug.
7. Paradoxical increase in intraocular pressure may follow anticholinesterase instillation. This may be alleviated by prescribing a sympathomimetic mydriatic such as phenylephrine.
8. Cardiac irregularities.

Dosage and Administration:

Directions for Preparing Eyedrops

1. Use aseptic technique.
2. Tear off aluminum seals, and remove and discard rubber plugs from both drug and diluent containers.
3. Pour diluent into drug container.
4. Remove dropper assembly from its sterile wrapping. Holding dropper assembly by the screw cap and, WITHOUT COMPRESSING RUBBER BULB, insert into drug container and screw down tightly.
5. Shake for several seconds to ensure mixing.
6. Do not cover nor obliterate instructions to patient regarding storage of eyedrops.

GLAUCOMA

Selection of Therapy—The *medication prescribed* should be that which will control the intraocular pressure around-the-clock with the least risk of side effects or adverse reactions. "Tonometric glaucoma" (ocular hypertension without other evidence of the disease) is frequently not treated with any medication, and PHOSPHOLINE IODIDE (echothiophate iodide) is certainly not recommended for this condition. In early chronic simple glaucoma with field loss or disc changes, pilocarpine is generally used for initial therapy and can be recommended so long as control is thereby maintained over the 24 hours of the day.

When this is not the case, PHOSPHOLINE IODIDE 0.03% may be effective and probably has no greater potential for side effects. If this dosage is inadequate, epinephrine and a carbonic anhydrase inhibitor may be added to the regimen. When still more effective medication is required, the higher strengths of PHOSPHOLINE IODIDE may be prescribed with the recognition that the control of the intraocular pressure should have priority regardless of potential side effects. In secondary glaucoma following cataract surgery, the higher strengths of the drug are frequently needed and are ordinarily very well tolerated.

The *dosage regimen* prescribed should call for the lowest concentration that will control the intraocular pressure around-the-clock. Where tonometry around-the-clock is not feasible, it is suggested that appointments for tension-taking be made at different times of the day so that inadequate control may be more readily detected. Two doses a day are preferred to one in order to maintain as smooth a diurnal tension curve as possible, although a single dose per day or every other day has been used with satisfactory results. Because of the long duration of action of the drug, it is never necessary or desirable to exceed a schedule of twice a day. The daily dose or one of the two daily doses should always be instilled just before retiring to avoid inconvenience due to the miosis.

Early Chronic Simple Glaucoma—PHOSPHOLINE IODIDE (echothiophate iodide) 0.03% instilled twice a day, just before retiring and in the morning, may be prescribed advantageously for cases of early chronic simple glaucoma that are not controlled around-the-clock with other less potent agents. Because of prolonged action, control during the night and early morning hours may then sometimes be obtained. A change in therapy is indicated if, at any time, the tension fails to remain at an acceptable level on this regimen.

Advanced Chronic Simple Glaucoma and *Glaucoma Secondary to Cataract Surgery*—These cases may respond satisfactorily to PHOSPHOLINE IODIDE 0.03% twice a day as above. When the patient is being transferred to PHOSPHOLINE IODIDE (echothiophate iodide) because of unsatisfactory control with pilocarpine, carbachol, epinephrine, etc., one of the higher strengths, 0.06%, 0.125%, or 0.25% will usually be needed. In this case, a brief trial with the 0.03% eyedrops will be advantageous in that the higher strengths will then be more easily tolerated.

Concomitant Therapy—PHOSPHOLINE IODIDE may be used concomitantly with epinephrine, a carbonic anhydrase inhibitor, or both.

Technique—Good technique in the administration of PHOSPHOLINE IODIDE requires that finger pressure at the inner canthus should be exerted for a minute or two following instillation of the eyedrops, to minimize drainage into the nose and throat. Excess solution around the eye should be removed with tissue and any medication on the hands should be rinsed off.

ACCOMMODATIVE ESOTROPIA (PEDIATRIC USE)

In Diagnosis—One drop of 0.125% may be instilled once a day in both eyes on retiring, for a period of two or three weeks. If the esotropia is accommodative, a favorable response will usually be noted which may begin within a few hours.

In Treatment—PHOSPHOLINE IODIDE (echothiophate iodide) is prescribed at the lowest concentration and frequency which gives satisfactory results. After the initial period of treatment for diagnostic purposes, the schedule may be reduced to 0.125% every other day or 0.06% every day. These dosages can often be gradually lowered as treatment progresses. The 0.03% strength has proven to be effective in some cases. The maximum usually recommended dosage is 0.125% once a day, although more intensive therapy has been used for short periods.

Technique—(See "Dosage and Administration—Glaucoma.")

Duration of Treatment—In diagnosis, only a short period is required and little time will be lost in instituting other procedures if the esotropia proves to be unresponsive. In therapy, there is no definite limit so long as the drug is well tolerated. However, if the eyedrops, with or without eyeglasses, are gradually withdrawn after about a year or two and deviation recurs, surgery should be considered. As with other miotics, tolerance may occasionally develop after prolonged use. In such cases, a rest period will restore the original activity of the drug.

How Supplied: Each package contains sterile PHOSPHOLINE IODIDE (echothiophate iodide), sterile diluent, and dropper for dispensing 5 mL eyedrops of the strength indicated on the label. Four potencies are available:

NDC 0046-1062-05..............1.5 mg package for 0.03%
White amorphous deposit on bottle walls. Aluminum crimp seal is blue.

NDC 0046-1064-05.....3 mg package for 0.06%
White amorphous deposit on bottle walls. Aluminum crimp seal is red.

NDC 0046-1065-05 ....6.25 mg package for 0.125%
White amorphous deposit on bottle walls. Aluminum crimp seal is green.

NDC 0046-1066-05 ....12.5 mg package for 0.25%
White amorphous deposit on bottle walls. Aluminum crimp seal is yellow.

Handling and Storage:

Store at or below room temperature (approximately 25°C).

After reconstitution, keep eyedrops in refrigerator to obtain maximum useful life of 6 months. Room temperature is acceptable if drops will be used within a month.

Shown in Product Identification Guide, page 106

Ocumed, Inc.
119 HARRISON AVENUE
ROSELAND, NJ 07068

(UNIT DOSE) PRODUCTS

OCU-TEARS PF™
in Ophtha-Dose™ unit dispenser Preservative Free, (Polyvinyl Alcohol ocular lubricant), Sterile Ophthalmic Solution.
How Supplied: 60 Ophtha-Dose™ Single Use Container NDC #51944-4485-01
120 Ophtha-Dose™ Single Use Container NDC #51944-4485-02

(MULTI-DOSE) PRODUCTS

EYE-ZINE
(tetrahydrozoline hydrochloride 0.05%)
Sterile eye drops
How Supplied: In 0.5 fl. oz. plastic dropper bottle.

IRI-SOL
(irrigating eye wash)
Sterile isotonic buffered solution
How Supplied: In 0.5 fl. oz., 1 fl. oz. and 4 fl. oz. plastic dispenser bottle.

OCU-CAINE ℞
(proparacaine hydrochloride 0.5%)
Sterile Ophthalmic Solution
How Supplied: In 2 ml and 15 ml plastic dropper bottle.

OCU-CARPINE ℞
(pilocarpine hydrochloride)
(0.5%, 1%, 2%, 3%, 4%. 5% and 6%)
Sterile Ophthalmic Solution
How Supplied: 15 ml Plastic Dropper Bottles.

OCU-LUBE
(white petrolatum base ocular lubricant)
Sterile ophthalmic Ointment
How Supplied: In 3.5 g tube with ophthalmic tip.

OCU-MYCIN ℞
(gentamicin sulfate—equiv. 3.0 mg)
Sterile Ophthalmic Ointment
How Supplied: In 3.5 g tubes with ophthalmic tip.

OCU-MYCIN ℞
(gentamicin sulfate—equiv. 3.0 mg)
Sterile Ophthalmic Solution
How Supplied: In 5 ml and 15 ml plastic dropper bottle.

OCU-PENTOLATE ℞
(cyclopentolate hydrochloride 1%)
Sterile Ophthalmic Solution
How Supplied: In 2 ml, 5 ml and 15 ml plastic dropper bottle.

OCU-PHRIN
(phenylephrine hydrochloride 0.12%)
Sterile Eye Drops
How Supplied: In 0.5 fl. oz. plastic dropper bottle.

OCU-PHRIN ℞
(phenylephrine hydrochloride 2.5% and 10%)
Sterile Ophthalmic Solution
How Supplied: In 5 ml and 15 ml plastic dropper bottle.

OCU-TEARS
(polyvinyl alcohol ocular lubricant)
Sterile Ophthalmic Solution
How Supplied: In 0.5 fl. oz. plastic dropper bottle.

OCU-TROL ℞
(polymyxin B sulfate 10,000 u/g)
(neomycin sulfate—equiv. 3.5 mg/g)
(dexamethasone 0.1%)
Sterile Ophthalmic Ointment
How Supplied: In 3.5 g tube with ophthalmic tip.

OCU-TROL ℞
(polymyxin B sulfate 10,000 u/g)
(neomycin sulfate—equiv. 3.5 mg/g)
dexamethesone 0.1%)
Sterile Ophthalmic Suspension
How Supplied: In 5 ml plastic dropper bottle.

OCU-TROPIC ℞
(tropicamide 0.5% and 1.0%)
Sterile Ophthalmic Solution
How Supplied: In 15 ml plastic dropper bottle.

OCU-TROPINE ℞
(atropine sulfate 1%)
Sterile Ophthalmic Ointment
How Supplied: In 3.5 g tubes with ophthalmic tip.

OCU-TROPINE ℞
(atropine sulfate 1%)
Sterile Ophthalmic Solution
How Supplied: In 15 ml plastic dropper bottle.

OCU-SPOR-B ℞
(polymyxin B sulfate—10,000 u/cc)
(neomycin sulfate—equiv. 3.5 mg/g)
(zinc bacitracin 400 u/g)
Sterile Ophthalmic Ointment
How Supplied: In 3.5 g tubes with ophthalmic tip.

OCU-SPOR-G ℞
(polymyxin B sulfate—10,000 u/cc)
(neomycin sulfate—equiv. 1.75 mg/cc)
(gramicidin 0.025%)
Sterile Ophthalmic Solution
How Supplied: In 10 cc plastic dropper bottle.

MEDICAL ECONOMICS

SECTION 9

LENSES AND LENS CARE PRODUCT INFORMATION

Included in this section is manufacturers' information on a variety of contact and intraocular lenses, as well as leading lens care products. The listings are organized in three parts:

Part 1 - Contact Lenses (Hard and Soft)

Vistakon
Johnson & Johnson Vision Products, Inc.
4500 SALISBURY ROAD
JACKSONVILLE, FL 32216

ACUVUE®
(etafilcon A)
Soft Hydrophilic Contact Lens

Description: The **ACUVUE**® (etafilcon A) Contact Lens, clear and with visibility tint, is a soft hydrophilic lens which is available as a spherical lens. The lens is intended to be used within the Vistakon system for planned lens replacement. This sytem allows flexiblity to prescribe the lens replacement and wearing schedule that best meets the needs of the patient. The lens may be prescribed for either Disposable Wear or Frequent Replacement Wear.

The **ACUVUE** (etafilcon A) Contact Lens, clear and with visibility tint, has the following properties and parameters:

- **Lens Material:** 58% water and 42% etafilcon A polymer (2-hydroxyethyl methacrylate and methacrylic acid crosslinked with 1, 1, 1 -trimethylol propane trimethacrylate and ethylene glycol dimethacrylate).

- **Lens Properties:**

• wet refractive index	1.40 ± .01
• visible light transmittance	
—visibility tinted	85% minimum
—clear	95% minimum

	VALUE	METHOD
• oxygen permeability (Dk)	$28.0 \pm 2.0 \times 10^{-11}$ (cm^2/sec) (ml O_2/ml × mm Hg) at 35°C	• Fatt method (boundary corrected, non-edge corrected)
	$21.4 \pm 1.5 \times 10^{-11}$ (cm^2/sec) (ml O_2/ml × mm Hg) at 35°C	• Fatt method (boundary corrected, edge corrected)

The ACUVUE (etafilcon A) Contact Lens with visibility tint is tinted blue using Reactive Blue Dye #4 to make the lens more visible for handling.

- **Available Lens Parameters:**

Parameters	Minus Lens	Plus Lens
• power range (increments)	−0.50 D to −6.00 D (in 0.25 D increments) −6.50 D to −9.00 D (in 0.50 D increments)	+0.50 D to +6.00 D (in 0.25 D increments)
• base curves	8.4mm 8.8mm 9.3mm	9.1mm
• diameter	14.0mm 14.0mm 14.4mm	14.4mm
• center thickness range (varies with power)	.07mm to .11mm	.12mm to .23mm

[See table above.]

Actions: In its hydrated state, the ACUVUE (etafilcon A) Contact Lens, when placed on the cornea, acts as a refracting medium to focus light rays on the retina.

- **How Supplied:**

Each sterile lens is supplied in a foil-sealed plastic package containing buffered saline solution. The plastic package is marked with the lens power, manufacturing expiration date, base curve/diameter series identification and manufacturing lot number.

Indications: The **ACUVUE** (etafilcon A) Contact Lens is indicated for the correction of visual acuity in not-aphakic persons with non-diseased eyes who are myopic or hyperopic and may have 1.00 diopter or less of astigmatism that does not interfere with visual acuity.

The lens may be prescribed for either daily wear or for extended wear from 1 to 7 days between removals for cleaning and disinfection or disposal, as recommended by the eye care practitioner (See LENS REPLACEMENT section for an additional description of these wear schedules). The lens ranges in power from −0.50 to −9.00 and +0.50 to +6.00 diopters.

Contraindications: The **ACUVUE** (etafilcon A) Contact Lens is contraindicated by the presence of any of the following conditions:

1. Acute and subacute inflammation of the anterior segment of the eye.
2. Any eye disease which affects the cornea or conjunctiva.
3. Insufficiency of lacrimal secretion (dry eye).
4. Corneal hypoesthesia (reduced corneal sensitivity).
5. Any systemic disease or allergy which may affect the eye or be exaggerated by wearing contact lenses.
6. Ocular irritation due to allergic reactions which may be caused by or exaggerated by the wearing of contact lenses and/or the use of contact lens solutions that may contain chemicals or preservatives such as thimerosal or other mercury compounds to which some people may be allergic.
7. Any medication that contraindicates contact lens wear.

Warnings: Problems with contact lenses or lens care products could result in serious injury to the eye. Patients should be cautioned that proper use and care of contact lenses and lens care products, including lens cases, are essential for the safe use of these products.

Eye problems, including corneal ulcers, can develop rapidly and lead to loss of vision. The results of a study[1] indicate the following:

- The overall annual incidence of ulcerative keratitis in daily wear contact lens users is estimated to be about 4.1 per 10,000 persons and about 20.9 per 10,000 persons in extended wear contact lens users.
- The risk of ulcerative keratitis is 4 to 5 times greater for extended wear contact lens users than for daily wear users. When daily wear users who wear their lenses overnight and extended wear users who wear their lenses on a daily basis are excluded from the comparison, the risk among extended wear users is 10 to 15 times greater than among daily wear users.
- The risk among extended wear lens users increases with the number of consecutive days that lenses are worn between removals, beginning with the first overnight use.
- The overall risk of ulcerative keratitis may be reduced by carefully following directions for emergency lens care, including cleaning of the lens case (for Disposable Wear) and for routine lens care, including cleaning of the lens case (for Scheduled Replacement Wear).
- The risk of ulcerative keratitis among contact lens users who smoke is estimated to be 3 to 8 times greater than among nonsmokers.

If patients experience eye discomfort, excessive tearing, vision changes, redness of the eye or other problems, they should be instructed to immediately remove their lenses and promptly contact their eye care practitioner. It is recommended that contact lens wearers see their eye care practitioners routinely as directed.

[1] New England Journal of Medicine, September 21, 1989.

Precautions: These precautions should be carefully observed when prescribing contact lenses.

- The lens must move sufficiently on the eye to help assure proper fit.
- Before leaving the eye care practitioner's office, the patient should demonstrate the ability to properly insert and remove the lens.
- The patient should be instructed against the use of tweezers or other tools to remove the lens from the lens container to avoid damaging the lens.

Continued on next page

Vistakon—Cont.

- The patient should be instructed to promptly remove the lens in the event that dust, a foreign body or other contaminant gets between the lens and the eye to avoid any serious injury.
- The patient should be instructed to replace any lens which becomes dehydrated or damaged.
- The patient should be informed that eye irritation may result if cosmetics, lotions, soaps, creams and deodorants come in contact with the lens or the lens is contaminated through some other means.
- The patient should be instructed to avoid using aerosol products such as hair spray while wearing lenses. If sprays are used, eyes should be kept closed until the spray has settled.
- The patient who is prescribed **ACUVUE** (etafilcon A) Contact Lenses on a Daily Wear schedule should be cautioned to remove the lenses before sleeping.
- Not every patient is able to wear a lens on an extended wear basis, even if he or she is able to wear the same lens on a daily wear basis.
- Periodic eye examinations are extremely important, especially for a patient on an extended wear schedule.
- The patient should be instructed to remove the lenses before getting into a hot tub, going swimming or in the presence of noxious or irritating vapors. The patient who swims frequently may be placed on Frequent Replacement Wear.
- The patient should be instructed to inform his or her employer that contact lenses are worn, as some jobs may require the use of eye protection equipment or that contact lenses not be worn.
- The patient should be instructed to inform his or her physician that contact lenses are worn and to consult his or her eye care practitioner before using any medication in the eye.
- Certain medications such as antihistamines, decongestants, diuretics, muscle relaxants, transquilizers, and those for motion sickness may cause dryness of the eye, increased lens awareness or blurred vision. Should such conditions exist proper remedial measures should be prescribed. Depending on the severity, this could include the use of lubricating drops that are indicated for use with soft contact lenses or the temporary discontinuance of contact lens wear while such medication is being used.
- Oral contraceptive users could develop visual changes or changes in lens tolerance when using contact lenses. Patients should be cautioned accordingly.
- Regular fluorescein should not be used while the lenses are on the patient's eyes. When fluorescein is used, the patient's eyes should be flushed with a sterile normal saline solution following such use.

Adverse Reactions: The following problems may occur when wearing contact lenses:

- The eye may burn, sting or itch.
- There may be less comfort than when the lens was first placed on the eye.
- There may be a feeling of something in the eye (foreign body, scratched area).
- There may be the potential for some temporary impairment due to peripheral infiltrates, peripheral corneal ulcers, and corneal erosion. There may be the potential for other physiological observations such as local or generalized edema, corneal neovascularization, corneal staining, injection, tarsal abnormalities, iritis and conjunctivitis, some of which are clinically acceptable in low amounts.
- There may also be excessive watering, unusual eye secretions, or redness of the eye.
- Poor visual acuity, blurred vision, rainbows or halos around objects, photophobia, or dry eyes may also occur if the lenses are worn continuously for too long a time.
- The patient should be instructed to conduct a simple 3-part self examination at least once a day. They should ask themselves:
  - How do the lenses feel on my eyes?
  - How do my eyes look?
  - Do I continue to see well?

If the patient reports any problems, he or she should be instructed to IMMEDIATELY REMOVE THE LENS.

If the discomfort or problem stops, the patient should then look closely at the lens.

If the lens is in any way damaged, the patient SHOULD NOT put the lens back on the eye. The patient should discard the lens and insert a new fresh lens on the eye.

If the patient is on a frequent replacement schedule and the lens has dirt, an eyelash, or foreign body on it, or the problem stops and the lens appears undamaged, he or she should be instructed to thoroughly clean, rinse and disinfect the lens; then reinsert it.

Fitting: Conventional methods of fitting soft contact lenses to the **ACUVUE** (etafilcon A) Contact Lens. For a detailed description of the fitting technique, refer to the **ACUVUE** Lens Fitting and Patient Management Guide for the Professional, copies of which are available from:

Vistakon
P.O. Box 10157
Jacksonville, Florida 32247-0157

CAUTION: FEDERAL LAW PROHIBITS DISPENSING WITHOUT A PRESCRIPTION FROM AN EYE CARE PRACTITIONER.

Lens Replacement: The **ACUVUE** (etafilcon A) Contact Lens may be prescribed for either Disposable Wear or Frequent Replacement Wear within the Vistakon system for planned lens replacement.

- **Disposable Wear**—This includes only single-use wear of the product. The lens is not recommended for routine cleaning and disinfection (see wear schedule below).
- **Frequent Replacement Wear**—This includes reuse of the product and planned replacement wear. The lens is to be cleaned, rinsed and disinfected each time it is removed from the patient's eye and discarded after the wearing period prescribed by the eye care practitioner. It is recommended that lenses be replaced at least every 2 weeks (see wear schedule below).

Wear Schedule: DAILY WEAR (periods less than 24 hours while awake)—The maximum suggested wearing time each day for the **ACUVUE** (etafilcon A) Contact Lens when worn on a daily wear basis should be determined by the eye care practitioner based upon the patient's physiological eye condition, because individual response to contact lenses vary.

EXTENDED WEAR (periods greater than 24 hours, including while asleep)—The **ACUVUE** (etafilcon A) Contact Lens for extended wear is recommended for 1 to 7 days/6 nights of continuous wear. Once the lens is removed, it is recommended that the patient's eye should have a rest period of overnight or longer.

It is recommended that the new contact lens wearer first be evaluated on a daily wear schedule. If, in the opinion of the eye care practitioner, the patient is determined to be an acceptable extended wear candidate, the eye care practitioner is encouraged to determine a wearing schedule based upon the response of the patient.

LENS CARE DIRECTIONS (FOR FREQUENT REPLACEMENT WEAR AND ON AN EMERGENCY BASIS FOR DISPOSABLE WEAR)

For Frequent Replacement Wear, lenses must be cleaned, rinsed and disinfected according to the labeling instructions specified with the solutions recommended by the eye care practitioner. The chemical method of disinfection, including hydrogen peroxide, is recommended. The heat method of disinfection is generally not advised. For Disposable Wear the lenses should only be cleaned and disinfected on an emergency basis when replacement lenses are not available.

The eye care practitioner should review the following instructions with the patients:

- Always wash and rinse hands before handling lenses.
- Only use fresh sterile cleaning, disinfecting and rinsing solutions which are indicated for use with soft contact lenses according to the labeling instructions provided.
- Never use conventional hard contact lens solutions unless also indicated for use with soft contact lenses.
- Do not use saliva, tap water, homemade saline solution, or anything other than the recommended solutions to wet lenses.
- To help avoid serious eye injury from contamination, always empty and rinse the lens case with fresh sterile rinsing solution and allow to air dry.
- If a lens lubricant is required, use one that is recommended for use with soft (hydrophilic) contact lenses according to the directions on the product labeling.
- If the lens is off the eye and exposed to air from 30 minutes to 1 hour or more, its surface will become dry and gradually become non-wetting. If this should occur, discard the lens and use a new one.

FOR ADDITIONAL INFORMATION

For additional information concerning the **ACUVUE** (etafilcon A) Contact Lens, call us toll free at 1-800-843-2020.

A-02-94-09 March, 1994

SUREVUE®
(etafilcon A)
Soft Hydrophilic Contact Lens

Description: The **SUREVUE®** (etafilcon A) Soft Hydrophilic Contact Lens, clear and with visibility tint, is a soft hydrophilic contact lens which is available as a spherical lens. The lens is intended to be used as a Daily Wear lens for frequent replacement.

The **SUREVUE** (etafilcon A) Contact Lens, clear and with visibility tint, has the following properties and parameters:

- **Lens Material:** 58% water and 42% etafilcon A polymer (2-hydroxyethyl methacrylate and methacrylic acid crosslinked with 1, 1, 1 -trimethylol propane trimethacrylate and ethylene glycol dimethacrylate).

[See table on next page.]

Actions: In its hydrated state, the SUREVUE (etafilcon A) Contact Lens, when placed on the cornea, acts as a refracting medium to focus light rays on the retina.

- **How Supplied:**

Each sterile lens is supplied in a foil-sealed plastic package containing buffered saline solution. The plastic package is marked with the lens power, manufacturing expiration date, base curve, diameter and manufacturing lot number.

Indications:

DAILY WEAR

The **SUREVUE** (etafilcon A) Contact Lens is indicated for Daily Wear (less than 1 day while awake) for the correction of visual acuity in non-aphakic persons with nondiseased eyes who are myopic and may have 1.00 diopter or less of astigmatism that does not interfere with visual acuity. The **SUREVUE** Contact Lens is indicated for scheduled replacement as recommended by the eye care practitioner. The lens ranges in power from −0.50 to −9.00 and +0.50 to +6.00 diopters.

Contraindications: The **SUREVUE** (etafilcon A) Contact Lens is contraindicated by the presence of any of the following conditions:

1. Acute and subacute inflammation of the anterior segment of the eye.
2. Any eye disease which affects the cornea or conjunctiva.
3. Insufficiency of lacrimal secretion (dry eye).
4. Corneal hypoesthesia (reduced corneal sensitivity).
5. Any systemic disease or allergy which may affect the eye or be exaggerated by wearing contact lenses.
6. Ocular irritation due to allergic reactions which may be caused by or exaggerated by the wearing of contact lenses and/or the use of contact lens solutions that may contain chemicals or preservatives such as thimerosal or other mercury compounds to which some people may be allergic.
7. Any medication that contraindicates contact lens wear.

Warnings: Problems with contact lenses or lens care products could result in serious injury to the eye. Patients should be cautioned that proper use and care of contact lenses and lens care products, including lens cases, are essential for the safe use of these products.

Eye problems, including corneal ulcers, can develop rapidly and lead to loss of vision. The results of a study[1] indicate the following:

- The overall annual incidence of ulcerative keratitis in daily wear contact lens users is estimated to be about 4.1 per 10,000 persons and about 20.9 per 10,000 persons in extended wear contact lens users.
- The risk of ulcerative keratitis is 4 to 5 times greater for extended wear contact lens users than for daily wear users. When daily wear users who wear their lenses overnight and extended wear users who wear their lenses on a daily basis are excluded from the comparison, the risk among extended wear users is 9 to 15 times greater than among daily wear users.
- When daily wear users wear their lenses overnight (outside the approved indication), the risk of ulcerative keratitis is nine times greater than among those who do not wear them overnight.
- The overall risk of ulcerative keratitis may be reduced by carefully following directions for lens care, including cleaning of the lens case.
- The risk of ulcerative keratitis among contact lens users who smoke is estimated to be 3 to 8 times greater than among nonsmokers.

If patients experience eye discomfort, excessive tearing, vision changes, redness of the eye or other problems, they should be instructed to immediately remove their lenses and promptly contact their eye care practitioner. It is recommended that contact lens wearers see their eye care practitioners routinely as directed.

[1] New England Journal of Medicine, September 21, 1989.

Precautions: These precautions should be carefully observed when prescribing contact lenses.

- The lens must move sufficiently on the eye to help assure proper fit.
- Before leaving the eye care practitioner's office, the patient should demonstrate the ability to properly insert and remove the lenses.
- The patient should be instructed against the use of tweezers or other tools to remove the lens from the lens container to avoid damaging the lens.

- **Lens Properties:**

• wet refractive index	1.40 ± .01	
• visible light transmittance		
—visibility tinted	85% minimum	
—clear	95% minimum	

	VALUE	METHOD
• oxygen permeability (Dk)	• $28.0 \pm 2.0 \times 10^{-11}$ (cm^2/sec) (ml O_2/ml × mm Hg) at 35°C	• Fatt method (boundary corrected, non-edge corrected)
	• $21.4 \pm 1.5 \times 10^{-11}$ (cm^2/sec) (ml O_2/ml × mm Hg) at 35°C	• Fatt method (boundary corrected edge corrected)

The SUREVUE (etafilcon A) Contact Lens with visibility tint is tinted blue using Reactive Blue Dye #4 to make the lens more visible for handling.

- **Available Lens Parameters:**

Parameters	Minus Lens	Plus Lens
• power range (increments)	−0.50D to −6.00D (in 0.25D increments) −6.50D to −9.00D (in 0.50D increments)	+0.50D to +6.00D (in 0.25D increments)
• base curve	8.8mm, 8.4mm	9.1mm
• diameter	14.0mm, 14.0mm	14.4mm
• center thickness range (varies with power)	.10mm to .16mm	16mm to 24mm

- The patient should be instructed to promptly remove the lens in the event that dust, a foreign body or other contaminant gets between the lens and the eye to avoid any serious injury.
- The patient should be instructed to replace any lens which becomes dehydrated or damaged.
- The patient should be informed that eye irritation may result if cosmetics, lotions, soaps, creams and deodorants come in contact with the lens or the lens is contaminated through some other means.
- The patient should be instructed to avoid using aerosol products such as hair spray while wearing lenses. If sprays are used, eyes should be kept closed until the spray has settled.
- The patient who is prescribed **SUREVUE** (etafilcon A) Contact Lenses should be cautioned to remove the lenses before sleeping.
- Periodic eye examinations are extremely important.
- The patient should be instructed to remove the lenses before getting into a hot tub, going swimming or in the presence of noxious or irritating vapors. The patient who swims frequently may be placed on Frequent Replacement Wear.
- The patient should be instructed to inform his or her employer that contact lenses are worn, as some jobs may require the use of eye protection equipment or that contact lenses not be worn.
- The patient should be instructed to inform his or her physician that contact lenses are worn and to consult his or her eye care practitioner before using any medication in the eye.
- Certain medications such as antihistamines, decongestants, diuretics, muscle relaxants, tranquilizers, and those for motion sickness may cause dryness of the eye, increased lens awareness or blurred vision. Should such conditions exist proper remedial measures should be prescribed. Depending on the severity, this could include the use of lubricating drops that are indicated for use with soft contact lenses or the temporary discontinuance of contact lens wear while such medication is being used.
- Oral contraceptive users could develop visual changes or changes in lens tolerance when using contact lenses. Patients should be cautioned accordingly.
- Regular fluorescein should not be used while the lenses are on the patient's eyes. When fluorescein is used, the patient's eyes should be flushed with a sterile normal saline solution following such use.

Adverse Reactions: The following problems may occur when wearing contact lenses:

- The eye may burn, sting or itch.
- There may be less comfort than when the lens was first placed on the eye.
- There may also be excessive watering, unusual eye secretions, or redness of the eye.
- Poor visual acuity, blurred vision, rainbows or halos around objects, photophobia, or dry eyes may also occur if the lenses are worn continuously for too long a time.

The patient should be instructed to conduct a simple 3-part self examination at least once a day. They should ask themselves:

—How do the lenses feel on my eyes?
—How do my eyes look?
—Do I continue to see well?

If the patient reports any problems, he or she should be instructed to IMMEDIATELY REMOVE THE LENS.

If the discomfort or problem stops, the patient should then look closely at the lens.

If the lens is in any way damaged, the patient SHOULD NOT put the lens back on the eye. The patient should discard the lens and insert a new fresh lens on the eye.

If the lens has dirt, an eyelash, or foreign body on it, or the problem stops and the lens appears undamaged, he or she should be instructed to thoroughly clean, rinse and disinfect the lens; then reinsert it.

If the problem continues, the patient SHOULD NOT put the lens back on the eye but IMMEDIATELY CONSULT HIS OR HER EYE CARE PRACTITIONER.

The patient should be advised that when any of the above symptoms occur, a serious condition such as infection, corneal ulcer, neovascularization, or iritis may be present. He or she should be instructed to seek immediate professional identification of the problem and prompt treatment to avoid serious eye damage.

Fitting: Conventional methods of fitting soft contact lenses apply to the **SUREVUE** (etafilcon A) Contact Lens. For a detailed description of the fitting technique, refer to the **SUREVUE** Fitting and Patient Management Guide for the

Continued on next page

Vistakon—Cont.

Professional, copies of which are available from:

VISTAKON
Johnson & Johnson Vision Products, Inc.
P.O. Box 10157
Jacksonville, Florida 32247-0157

CAUTION: FEDERAL LAW PROHIBITS DISPENSING WITHOUT A PRESCRIPTION FROM AN EYE CARE PRACTITIONER.

Lens Replacement: The **SUREVUE** (etafilcon A) Contact Lens is to be prescribed within the Vistakon system for planned lens replacement. The lens is to be cleaned and disinfected each time it is removed from the patient's eye, and discarded after the wearing period prescribed by the eye care practitioner. It is recommended that lenses be replaced at least every two weeks (see wear schedule below).

Wear Schedule: DAILY WEAR (periods less than 1 day while awake)—The maximum suggested wearing time each day for the **SUREVUE** (etafilcon A) Contact Lens worn on a daily wear basis should be determined by the eye care practitioner based upon the patient's physiological eye condition, because individual response to contact lenses vary.

Lens Care Directions: Lenses must be both cleaned and disinfected according to the labeling instructions specified with the solutions recommended by the eye care practitioner. The chemical method of disinfection is recommended. The heat method of disinfection is generally not advised.

The eye care practitioner should review the following instructions with the patients:

- Always wash and rinse hands before handling lenses.
- Only use fresh sterile lens care solutions which are indicated for use with soft contact lenses according to the labeling instructions provided.
- Never use conventional hard contact lens solutions unless also indicated for use with soft contact lenses.
- Do not use saliva, tap water, homemade saline solution, or anything other than the recommended solutions to wet lenses.
- To help avoid serious eye injury from contamination, always empty and rinse the lens case with fresh sterile rinsing solution and allow to air dry.
- If a lens lubricant is required, use one that is recommended for use with soft (hydrophilic) contact lenses according to the directions on the product labeling.
- If the lens is off the eye and exposed to air from 30 minutes to 1 hour or more, its surface will become dry and gradually become non-wetting. If this should occur, discard the lens and use a new one.

For Additional Information: For additional information concerning the **SUREVUE** (etafilcon A) Contact Lens, call us toll free at 1-800-843-2020.

Printed in U.S.A. December, 1993
SV 12-93-01

Part 2 - Intraocular Lenses

Alcon Surgical

6201 SOUTH FREEWAY
FT. WORTH, TX 76134

Address Inquiries to:
Marketing Department (817) 293-0450
1-800-TO-ALCON
(1-800-862-5266)

IOLAB Corporation

a Johnson & Johnson Company
500 IOLAB DRIVE
CLAREMONT, CA 91711

Address inquiries to:
Marketing Services (800) 423-1871
CA only (800) 352-1891

IOLAB, a Johnson & Johnson company, manufactures a complete line of ophthalmic products including Intraocular Lenses, Microsurgical Equipment, Viscoelastics and Pharmaceuticals.

IOLAB intraocular lens products include the new SLIMFIT™ Small Incision Lenses and EZVUE™ Violet Haptic Lenses. IOLAB also distributes AMVISC® and AMVISC® Plus Sodium Hyaluronate.

IOLAB provides the widest selection of Pre-Market Approved lenses available for the posterior and anterior chamber. IOLs are available in many styles including one-piece designs and special high and low diopter powers. All models are available with class I UV filtration. Many models are available with or without positioning holes as well as a variety of optic sizes. These range from 5.5 mm & 5.0 mm round, 5 × 6 mm to 7mm round.

For current information on intraocular lenses or any other product please contact your IOLAB Sales Representative or IOLAB directly.

AMVISC® PLUS ℞
(sodium hyaluronate)

Description: AMVISC® PLUS is a sterile nonpyrogenic solution of sodium hyaluronate. AMVISC® PLUS contains 16 mg/mL of sodium hyaluronate adjusted to yield approximately 55,000 centistokes dissolved in physiological saline and exhibits an osmolality of approximately 340 milliosmoles.

Characteristics: Sodium hyaluronate is a high molecular weight polysaccharide composed of sodium glucuronate and N-acetylglucosamine. Sodium hyaluronate is ubiquitously distributed throughout the tissues of the body and is present in high concentrations in such tissues as vitreous humor, synovial fluid, umbilical cord and the dermis of rooster combs. Sodium hyaluronate functions as a tissue lubricant (1,2) and it is thought to play an important role in modulating the interactions between adjacent tissues. It can also act as a viscoelastic support maintaining a separation between tissues. Sodium hyaluronates prepared from different tissues may have different molecular weights but are thought to have the same chemical structure. The sodium hyaluronate in AMVISC® PLUS is prepared from the dermis of rooster combs (3). It has a molecular weight greater than 1,000,000, is reported to be nonantigenic (4,5), does not cause foreign body reactions, is nonpyrogenic and is well tolerated in human eyes (6). AMVISC® PLUS does not interfere with normal wound healing processes.

Indications: AMVISC® PLUS is indicated for use as a surgical aid in ophthalmic anterior (7) and posterior (6) segment procedures including • glaucoma filtering surgery • surgical procedures to reattach the retina • implantation of an intraocular lens (IOL) • extraction of a cataract • corneal transplantation surgery. Due to its lubricating and viscoelastic properties, transparency and ability to protect corneal endothelial cells (8), AMVISC® PLUS helps maintain anterior chamber depth and visibility, minimizes interaction between tissues, and acts as a tamponade and vitreous substitute during retina reattachment surgery. AMVISC® PLUS also preserves tissue integrity and good visibility when used to fill the anterior and posterior segments of the eye following open sky procedures.

Contraindications: At the present time there are no contraindications to the use of AMVISC® PLUS when used as recommended as an intraocular implant.

Applications:

1. Cataract surgery and IOL implantation—The required amount of AMVISC® PLUS is slowly infused through a needle or cannula into the anterior chamber. The protective effect of AMVISC® PLUS as an aid is optimized when the injection is performed prior to cataract extraction and insertion of the IOL and is effective for both intra- and extracapsular cataract procedures. AMVISC® PLUS may be applied to the IOL prior to insertion. Additional AMVISC® PLUS can be injected as required to facilitate surgical procedures (SEE PRECAUTIONS).
2. Corneal transplant surgery—The corneal button is removed and the anterior chamber filled with AMVISC® PLUS until it is level with the surface of the cornea. The donor graft is then placed on top of the AMVISC® PLUS and sutured into place. Additional AMVISC® PLUS can be used as required to aid in surgical procedures (SEE PRECAUTIONS).
3. Glaucoma filtration surgery—AMVISC® PLUS is injected through a corneal paracentesis to restore and maintain anterior chamber volume during the performance of the trabeculectomy. Additional AMVISC® PLUS can be used as required to aid in the surgical procedures (SEE PRECAUTIONS).
4. Intraocular injection in conjunction with scleral buckling procedures for retina reattachment—After release of subretinal fluid and development of buckling by tying the mattress sutures, air is injected into the vitreous cavity and then exchanged with AMVISC® PLUS injected through a needle (22 to 30 gauge) passed via the pars plana epithelium. The volume of AMVISC® PLUS injected (2–4 mL) will vary with the volume of the subretinal fluid released and the space occupied by the buckle.

Precautions: Those precautions normally considered during anterior segment and retina reattachment procedures are recommended.

There may be increased intraocular pressure following surgery (9) caused by preexisting glaucoma or by the surgery itself. For these reasons the following precautions should be considered.

- An excess quantity of AMVISC® PLUS should not be used. • AMVISC® PLUS should be removed from the anterior chamber at the end of surgery. • If the postoperative intraocular pressure increases above expected values, correcting therapy should be administered. • AMVISC® PLUS is prepared from a biological source and the physician should be aware of the possible effects of using any biological materials. • Reuse of cannula should be avoided. Even after cleaning and rinsing, resterilized cannula could release particulate matter as AMVISC® PLUS is injected. It is recommended that disposable cannula be used when administering AMVISC® PLUS. • There have been isolated reports of diffuse particulates or haziness appearing after injection of AMVISC® PLUS into the eye. While such reports are infrequent and seldom associated with any effects on ocular tissues, the physician should be aware of this occurrence. If observed, the particulate matter should be removed by irrigation and/or aspiration.

Adverse Reactions: Sodium hyaluronate is a natural component of the tissues of the body and is extremely well tolerated in human eyes. Transient postoperative inflammatory reactions were reported in clinical trials (6) and oral and topical steroid preparations were administered. AMVISC® PLUS is tested in animals to determine that each batch is essentially noninflammatory. Since sodium hyaluronate molecules are noninflammatory, any phlogistic response is considered to be caused by the surgical procedures. The best index of the degree of phlogistic response is the postoperative clarity of the vitreous cavity. As outlined above a transient postoperative increase in intraocular pressure has been observed following the use of sodium hyaluronate in anterior segment surgery. On rare occasions postoperative reactions including inflammation, corneal edema and corneal decompensation have been reported. The relationship to the use of AMVISC® PLUS has not been established.

How Supplied: AMVISC® PLUS is a sterile viscoelastic preparation supplied in a disposable glass syringe delivering either 0.5 mL or 0.8 mL of sodium hyaluronate dissolved in physiological saline. Each mL of AMVISC® PLUS contains 16 mg of sodium hyaluronate adjusted to yield approximately 55,000 centistokes, 9 mg of Sodium Chloride and q.s. Sterile Water for Injection USP. AMVISC® PLUS exhibits an osmolality of approximately 340 milliosmoles. Sodium hydroxide and/or hydrochloric acid are added to adjust pH (if necessary). AMVISC® PLUS syringes are terminally sterilized and aseptically packaged. Contents of unopened and undamaged pouches are sterile. Refrigerated AMVISC® PLUS should be allowed to reach room temperature (approximately 20 to 45 minutes, depending on volume) prior to use.

For Intraocular Use: Store at 2–8°C. Protect from freezing.

Caution: Federal law restricts this device to sale by or on the order of a physician.

References:

1. Swann DA, Radin El, Nazimiec, Weisser PA, Curran N, Lewinneck G. Role of hyaluronic acid in joint lubrication. Ann Rheum Dis 1974; 33:318.
2. Radin EL, Paul IL, Swann DA, Schottstaedt ES. Lubrication of synovial membrane. Ann Rheum Dis 1971; 30:322.
3. Swann DA, Studies of Hyaluronic Acid. I. The preparation and properties of rooster comb hyaluronic acid. Biochim Biophys Acta 1968; 156:17.
4. Richter W. Non-immunogenicity of purified hyaluronic acid preparations tested by passive cutaneous anaphylaxis. Int Arch Allergy 1974; 47:211.
5. Richter, W, Ryde EM, Zetterstrom EO. Non-immunogenicity of a purified sodium hyaluronate preparation in man. Int Arch Appl Immunol 1979; 59:45.
6. Pruett RC, Schepens CL, Swann DA, Hyaluronic acid vitreous substitute. A six-year clinical evaluation. Arch Ophthalmol 1979; 97:2325.
7. Pape LG, Balazs EA. The use of sodium hyaluronate (Healon®) in human anterior segment surgery. Ophthalmol 1980; 87:699.
8. Miller D, Stegmann R. Use of Na-hyaluronate in anterior segment eye surgery. Am Intra-Ocular Implant Soc J 1980; 6:13.
9. Miller D, Stegmann R. The use of Healon® in intraocular lens implantation. Int Ophthalmol Clinics 1982; 22:177.

Size	Reorder #
0.5 mL	60051
0.8 mL	60081

Distributed by:
IOLAB CORPORATION
a Johnson & Johnson company
500 Iolab Drive
Claremont, CA 91711
Toll-free: 800/423-1871 • In CA: 800/352-1891
Revised June 1991

For more information regarding AMVISC Plus or AMVISC viscoelastics contact: IOLAB, 500 IOLAB Drive, Claremont, California 91711. Toll free: 800-423-1871 ext. 1225. • In California: 800-352-1891 ext. 1225.

AMVISC® ℞

Information listed for AMVISC Plus also applies to AMVISC with the following exceptions.

- AMVISC contains 12 mg/mL sodium hyaluronate adjusted to yield approximately 40,000cs dissolved in physiological saline.
- AMVISC is a sterile viscoelastic preparation supplied in a disposable glass syringe delivering either 0.50mL or 0.80mL sodium hyaluronate dissolved in physiological saline. Each mL of AMVISC contains 12mg sodium hyaluronate adjusted to yield approximately 40,000cs, 9.0mg of sodium chloride and sterile water for injection. U.S.P.q.s.

For more information regarding AMVISC Plus or AMVISC viscoelastics contact: IOLAB, 500 IOLAB Drive, Claremont, California 91711. Toll free: 800-423-1871 ext. 1225. • In California: 800-352-1891 ext. 1225.

Part 3 - Lens Care Products

Allergan, Inc.

Optical Division
2525 DUPONT DRIVE
P.O. BOX 19534
IRVINE, CA 92713-9534

ALLERGAN® HYDROCARE® CLEANING AND DISINFECTING SOLUTION

For use with clear and tinted SOFT (hydrophilic) contact lenses in a chemical (not heat) lens care system.

Description: (Ingredients): ALLERGAN® HYDROCARE® Cleaning and Disinfecting Solution is a sterile, isotonic, buffered solution that contains sodium bicarbonate; sodium phosphate, dibasic, anhydrous; sodium phosphate, monobasic; propylene glycol; polysorbate 80; special soluble polyhema; and hydrochloric acid with tris (2-hydroxyethyl) tallow ammonium chloride (0.013%); thimerosal (0.002%); and bis (2-hydroxyethyl) tallow ammonium chloride as preservatives.

Actions: ALLERGAN® HYDROCARE® Cleaning and Disinfecting Solution loosens and removes accumulations of film, deposits and debris from your lenses and destroys harmful microorganisms on the surface of your lenses.

Indications (Uses): Use ALLERGAN® HYDROCARE® Cleaning and Disinfecting Solution to clean, disinfect and store your soft (hydrophilic) contact lenses.

Contraindications (Reasons Not to Use): If you are allergic to any ingredient in ALLERGAN® HYDROCARE® Cleaning and Disinfecting Solution, do not use.

Warnings: PROBLEMS WITH CONTACT LENSES AND LENS CARE PRODUCTS COULD RESULT IN SERIOUS INJURY TO THE EYE. It is essential that you follow your eye care practitioner's directions and all labeling instructions for proper use and care of your lenses and lens care products, including the lens case. **EYE PROBLEMS, INCLUDING CORNEAL ULCERS, CAN DEVELOP RAPIDLY AND LEAD TO LOSS OF VISION.**

Daily wear lenses are not indicated for overnight wear and should not be worn while sleeping. Clinical studies have shown the risk of serious adverse reactions is increased when these lenses are worn overnight.

Extended wear lenses should be regularly removed for cleaning and disinfection or for disposal and replacement on the schedule prescribed by your eye care practitioner. Clinical studies have shown that there is an increased incidence of serious adverse reactions in extended wear contact lens users as compared to daily wear contact lens users. Studies have also shown that the risk of serious adverse reactions increases the longer extended wear lenses are worn before removal for cleaning and disinfection or for disposal and replacement.

Studies have also shown that smokers had a higher incidence of adverse reactions.

If you experience eye discomfort, excessive tearing, vision changes, or redness of the eye, immediately remove your lenses and promptly contact your eye care practitioner.

It is recommended that contact lens wearers see their eye care practitioner twice each year or if directed, more frequently.

This product contains thimerosal (0.002%) as a preservative. Do not use this product if you are sensitive to thimerosal or any other ingredient containing mercury.

To avoid contamination, do not touch tip of container to any surface. Replace cap after using.

Precautions:

- Do not put this product in the eye. **The red tip is to remind you not to put this product in your eye.**
- Never reuse this solution.
- Keep out of the reach of children.
- Always wash, rinse and dry hands before handling lenses.
- After reapplying your lenses, always empty your lens storage case, rinse with sterile rinsing solution and allow to air dry.
- After using **ALLERGAN® ENZYMATIC** Contact Lens Cleaner for soft (hydrophilic) lenses each week to remove accumulated protein deposits, thoroughly rinse your lenses with **LENS PLUS®** Sterile Saline Solution, **ALLERGAN® HYDROCARE®** Preserved Saline Solution, or other appropriate saline solution before disinfecting.

Continued on next page

Allergan Optical—Cont.

- Do not let **ALLERGAN® HYDROCARE®** Cleaning and Disinfecting Solution dry on the lenses.
- Store at room temperature.
- Use before the expiration date marked on the bottle and carton.

Note: This product is not recommended for use with crofilcon A (CSI® and AZTECH™)* lenses.

Adverse Reactions and What to Do:
The following may occur:

- Eyes stinging, burning, or itching (irritation)
- Excessive watering (tearing) of the eyes
- Unusual eye secretions
- Redness of the eyes
- Reduced sharpness of vision (visual acuity)
- Blurred vision
- Sensitivity to light (photophobia)
- Dry eyes

If you notice any of the above, immediately remove and examine your lenses. If a lens appears to be damaged, do not reapply; consult your eye care practitioner. If the symptom stops and the lenses appear to be undamaged, thoroughly clean, rinse and disinfect the lenses and reapply them. If the symptom continues, immediately remove your lenses and consult your eye care practitioner.

If any of the above symptoms occur, a serious condition such as infection, corneal ulcer, neovascularization, or iritis may be present. Immediately remove your lenses and seek immediate professional identification of the problem and begin treatment, if necessary, to avoid serious eye damage. For more information, see your **Instructions for Wearers** booklet for your specific contact lens type.

Directions For Use:

- Clean, rinse and disinfect your lenses each time you remove them.
- Always wash, rinse and dry your hands before handling lenses.
- Always remove and clean the same lens first to avoid any mix-ups.

Prepare The Storage Case For Lens Disinfection:

- Fill each chamber of your lens storage case with **ALLERGAN® HYDROCARE®** Cleaning and Disinfecting Solution.

Clean and Rinse Your Lenses:

- After you remove one lens, place it in the palm of your hand. Place 3 drops of **LENS PLUS®** Daily Cleaner or **ALLERGAN® HYDROCARE®** Cleaning and Disinfecting Solution on each lens surface and rub for 20 seconds in the palm with your forefinger or between your thumb and forefinger. Then rinse the lens with **LENS PLUS®** Sterile Saline Solution. Place the lens in the appropriate chamber of your lens storage case. Repeat the cleaning and rinsing procedure with your other lens and place it in the proper chamber.

Disinfect and Store Your Lenses:

- Allow your lenses to soak a minimum of 4 hours in the cleaning and disinfecting solution for proper disinfection.
- Your lenses should always be stored in **ALLERGAN® HYDROCARE®** Cleaning and Disinfecting Solution when you are not wearing them.

  If you do not intend to wear your lenses immediately following disinfection, you may store them in the unopened storage case until ready to wear later in the day.

  If the lenses have been stored in the unopend case for more than 24 hours, disinfect before wearing. Put fresh solution inside the lens storage case, completely covering the lenses, before disinfecting.

  If lenses will be stored for longer periods of time, disinfect once a week and before wearing.

Rinse and Wear:

- Since **ALLERGAN® HYDROCARE®** Cleaning and Disinfecting Solution is not intended for use directly in the eye, lenses should be rinsed thoroughly with **LENS PLUS®** Sterile Saline Solution, **ALLERGAN® HYDROCARE®** Preserved Saline Solution or other appropriate saline solution before wearing.

  To prevent contamination and to help avoid serious eye injury, always empty and rinse lens case with sterile rinsing solution and allow to air dry.

How Supplied:
ALLERGAN® HYDROCARE® Cleaning and Disinfecting Solution is supplied in sterile 4 fl oz, 8 fl oz and 12 fl oz plastic bottles. The bottles and cartons are marked with lot number and expiration date.

Lenses: ALLERGAN® HYDROCARE® Cleaning and Disinfecting Solution is for use with clear and tinted soft (hydrophilic) contact lenses.

* Trademarks of Pilkington/Barnes-Hind.

ALLERGAN® HYDROCARE® PRESERVED SALINE SOLUTION

For rinsing in conjunction with chemical disinfection and for rinsing, heat disinfection and storage of soft (hydrophilic) contact lenses. Regular use in your heat disinfection unit prevents calcium deposits from forming on soft contact lenses.

Description: ALLERGAN® HYDROCARE® Preserved Saline Solution is a sterile, buffered, isotonic solution containing sodium chloride, sodium hexametaphosphate, boric acid and sodium borate with edetate disodium (0.01%) and thimerosal (0.001%) as preservatives and sodium hydroxide to adjust the pH.

Actions: Rinsing lenses with ALLERGAN® HYDROCARE® Preserved Saline Solution after cleaning will remove loosened debris and traces of daily cleaning products. Disinfection of lenses is accomplished by immersing your lenses in ALLERGAN® HYDROCARE® Preserved Saline Solution in an appropriate carrying case and heating them in your heat disinfection (heating) unit.

When used with your heat disinfection unit, the special sequestering agent in ALLERGAN® HYDROCARE® Preserved Saline Solution prevents inorganic deposits such as calcium and rust from attaching to your soft contact lenses.

Indications (Uses): ALLERGAN® HYDROCARE® Preserved Saline Solution is for use with soft (hydrophilic) contact lenses. It can be used for rinsing, heat disinfection, and storage. It may also serve as a rinsing solution in conjunction with chemical disinfection.

Regular use in your heat disinfection unit prevents calcium deposits from forming on soft contact lenses.

Contraindications (Reasons Not to Use):
If you are allergic to mercury, which is in thimerosal, or to any other ingredient in ALLERGAN® HYDROCARE® Preserved Saline Solution, do not use this product.

Warnings: PROBLEMS WITH CONTACT LENSES AND LENS CARE PRODUCTS COULD RESULT IN SERIOUS INJURY TO THE EYE. It is essential that you follow your eye care practitioner's directions and all labeling instructions for proper use of your lenses and lens care products, including the lens case. **EYE PROBLEMS, INCLUDING CORNEAL ULCERS, CAN DEVELOP RAPIDLY AND LEAD TO LOSS OF VISION.**

Daily wear lenses are not indicated for overnight wear and should not be worn while sleeping. Clinical studies have shown the risk of serious adverse reactions is increased when these lenses are worn overnight.

Extended wear lenses should be regularly removed for cleaning and disinfection or for disposal and replacement on the schedule prescribed by your eye care practitioner. Clinical studies have shown that there is an increased incidence of serious adverse reactions in extended wear contact lens users as compared to daily wear contact lens users. Studies have also shown that the risk of serious adverse reactions increases the longer extended wear lenses are worn before removal for cleaning and disinfection or for disposal and replacement.

Studies have also shown that smokers had a higher incidence of adverse reactions.

If you experience eye discomfort, excessive tearing, vision changes or redness of the eye, immediately remove your lenses and promptly contact your eye care practitioner.

It is recommended that contact lens wearers see their eye care practitioner twice each year or if directed, more frequently.

To avoid contamination, do not touch tip of container to any surface. Replace cap after using.

Precautions:

- Always wash, rinse and dry your hands thoroughly before handling your lenses.
- Fresh ALLERGAN® HYDROCARE® Preserved Saline Solution should be used daily. **Never reuse the solution.**
- To prevent buildup of calcium deposits which can damage lenses, this solution should be used daily. Do not wait until buildup occurs, since removal of established calcium deposits may reveal that permanent damage to your lenses has already occurred.
- After reapplying your lenses, always empty your lens storage case, rinse with sterile rinsing solution, and allow to air dry.
- Store at room temperature.
- Use before the expiration date marked on bottle and carton.

Adverse Reactions and What to Do:
The following may occur:

- Eyes stinging, burning, or itching (irritation)
- Excessive watering (tearing) of the eye
- Unusual eye secretions
- Redness of the eyes
- Reduced sharpness of vision (visual acuity)
- Blurred vision
- Sensitivity to light (photophobia)
- Dry eyes

If you notice any of the above, immediately remove and examine your lenses. If a lens appears to be damaged, do not reapply; consult your eye care practitioner. If the symptom stops and the lenses appear to be undamaged, thoroughly clean, rinse and disinfect the lenses and reapply them. If the symptom continues, immediately remove your lenses and consult your eye care practitioner.

If any of the above symptoms occur, a serious condition such as infection, corneal ulcer, neovascularization, or iritis may be present. Seek immediate professional identification of the problem and begin treatment, if necessary, to avoid serious eye damage. For more information, see your **Instructions for Wearers** booklet for your specific contact lens type.

Directions For Use:

- Always wash, rinse and dry your hands before you handle your lenses.
- Clean, rinse, and disinfect your lenses each time you remove them.
- Clean and rinse one lens first (always the same lens first to avoid mix-ups) and put that lens into the correct chamber (section) of the lens storage case. Then repeat the procedure for the second lens.
- After you clean your lens, rinse it thoroughly with ALLERGAN® HYDROCARE® Preserved Saline Solution by holding the lens between the forefinger

and thumb of one hand and directing a steady stream onto the lens or placing the lens in the palm of one hand and directing a steady stream of ALLERGAN® HYDROCARE® Preserved Saline Solution onto the lens.

Chemical Disinfection (Not Heat)

- Disinfect and store your lenses as directed by your eye care practitioner.
- Before reapplying your lenses, rinse the lenses thoroughly with ALLERGAN® HYDROCARE® Preserved Saline Solution.
- After you remove your lenses from the lens case, empty and rinse your lens storage case with sterile rinsing solution and allow it to air dry. When you next use the case, refill it with fresh disinfecting solution.

Heat (Thermal) Disinfection

- Prepare the empty lens storage case. Wet the chambers of the case with ALLERGAN® HYDROCARE® Preserved Saline Solution.
- Place each lens in its correct chamber of the storage case.
- Fill the chamber using enough ALLERGAN® HYDROCARE® Preserved Saline Solution to completely cover the lens.
- Tightly close the top on the chamber.
- Repeat the above procedure for the second lens.
- Put the lens storage case into the disinfection unit and follow the directions for operating your unit.

Emergency (Alternate) Method for Heat (Thermal) Disinfection

If your heat disinfection unit is not available, place the tightly closed lens storage case which contains the lenses into a pan of already boiling water. Leave the closed lens case in the pan of boiling water for at least 10 minutes. (Above an altitude of 7,000 feet, boil for at least 15 minutes.) Be careful not to allow the water to boil away. Remove the pan from the heat and allow it to cool for 30 minutes to complete the disinfection of the lenses.

NOTE: USE OF THE HEAT DISINFECTION UNIT SHOULD BE RESUMED AS SOON AS POSSIBLE.

- Leave the lenses in the unopened storage case until ready to put on your eyes. Before reapplying the lenses, rinsing is not necessary unless your eye care practitioner recommends rinsing.
- To prevent contamination and to help avoid serious eye injury, always empty and rinse lens case with sterile rinsing solution and allow to air dry.

  Clean soft contact lenses weekly with ALLERGAN® ENZYMATIC Contact Lens Cleaner to remove tear protein deposits which can damage your lenses, impair your vision and reduce comfort.

How Supplied:
ALLERGAN® HYDROCARE® Preserved Saline Solution is supplied in 8 fl oz and 12 fl oz plastic bottles. Bottles and cartons are marked with lot number and expiration date.

Lenses: ALLERGAN® HYDROCARE® Preserved Saline Solution is for use with soft (hydrophilic) contact lenses.

U.S. Patent No. 4,395,346

A product of Allergan Research.

ALLERGAN® ENZYMATIC

Contact Lens Cleaner

For weekly use with soft (hydrophilic) contact lenses.

Description: ALLERGAN® ENZYMATIC Contact Lens Cleaner is a round tablet containing the enzyme papain, sodium chloride, sodium carbonate, sodium borate, and edetate disodium.

Action: ALLERGAN® ENZYMATIC Contact Lens Cleaner removes protein deposits from the surface of daily wear and extended wear soft (hydrophilic) contact lenses. It safely and effectively removes protein and reduces its buildup on your lenses when used as directed.

Indications: Use **ALLERGAN® ENZYMATIC** Contact Lens Cleaner prepared with sterile saline solution once a week to reduce protein buildup for clear vision and comfortable lens wear.

Contraindications: Do not use this product if you are allergic to any of its ingredients. If you are allergic to any ingredient in one sterile saline solution, use another appropriate sterile saline solution for soft contact lenses to prepare the enzymatic cleaning solution.

Warnings: This product contains the enzyme papain. Do not use this product if you are allergic to papain.

LENSES MUST BE RINSED AND DISINFECTED FOLLOWING EACH ENZYMATIC CLEANING CYCLE. FAILURE TO DISINFECT MAY CAUSE IRRITATION AND DISCOMFORT. DO NOT INSTILL THE ENZYMATIC CLEANING SOLUTION DIRECTLY INTO THE EYE.

NEVER USE DISTILLED WATER TO DISSOLVE THE TABLETS. DISTILLED WATER IS NOT STERILE. USE OF A NON-STERILE PRODUCT IN THE PREPARATION OF SOFT CONTACT LENS SOLUTIONS MAY LEAD TO MICROBIAL CONTAMINATION OF LENSES WHICH CAN CAUSE SERIOUS EYE INFECTIONS.

PROBLEMS WITH CONTACT LENSES AND LENS CARE PRODUCTS COULD RESULT IN SERIOUS INJURY TO THE EYE. It is essential that you follow your eye care practitioner's directions and all labeling instructions for proper use of your lenses and lens care products, including the lens case. **EYE PROBLEMS, INCLUDING CORNEAL ULCERS, CAN DEVELOP RAPIDLY AND LEAD TO LOSS OF VISION.** Daily wear lenses are not indicated for overnight wear and should not be worn while sleeping. Clinical studies have shown the risk of serious adverse reactions is increased when these lenses are worn overnight.

Extended wear lenses should be regularly removed for cleaning and disinfection or for disposal and replacement on the schedule prescribed by your eye care practitioner. Clinical studies have shown that there is an increased incidence of serious adverse reactions in extended wear contact lens users as compared to daily wear contact lens users. Studies have also shown that the risk of serious adverse reactions increases the longer extended wear lenses are worn before removal for cleaning and disinfection or for disposal and replacement.

Studies have also shown that smokers had a higher incidence of adverse reactions. If you experience eye discomfort, excessive tearing, vision changes or redness of the eye, immediately remove your lenses and promptly contact your eye care practitioner.

It is recommended that contact lens wearers see their eye care practitioner twice each year or if directed, more frequently.

Precautions:

- Do not soak low water content (less than 55%) contact lenses longer than 12 hours. If you are unsure of the type of lens you wear, consult your eye care practitioner.
- Do not soak high water content (55% or more) contact lenses longer than 2 hours, otherwise ocular irritation may result. Should ocular irritation occur, immediately remove your contact lenses, clean and disinfect the lenses again and reapply. If irritation continues, remove your lenses and consult your eye care practitioner.
- KEEP OUT OF THE REACH OF CHILDREN.
- Do not take tablets internally.
- Do not use brown or otherwise discolored tablets.
- Avoid excessive heat.
- Always wash, rinse and dry hands before handling lenses.
- Lenses should **never** be placed on the eye directly from the enzymatic cleaning solution.
- **Use only sterile saline solution and the special vials provided to prepare the enzymatic cleaning solution. Do not use anything else to dissolve the tablets or any other containers.**
- Use only freshly prepared enzymatic cleaning solution and discard immediately after use.
- Use before expiration date on foil wrapper and unit carton.

Adverse Reactions and What to Do:
The following may occur:

- Eyes stinging, burning or itching (irritation)
- Excessive watering (tearing) of the eyes
- Unusual eye secretions
- Redness of the eyes
- Reduced sharpness of vision (visual acuity)
- Blurred vision
- Sensitivity to light (photophobia)
- Dry eyes

If you notice any of the above, a serious condition such as infection, corneal ulcer, neovascularization or iritis may be present. IMMEDIATELY remove and examine your lenses. If your lenses appear to be damaged, do not reapply; consult your eye care practitioner. If the symptom stops and the lenses appear to be undamaged, thoroughly clean, rinse and disinfect the lenses and reapply them. If the symptom continues, immediately remove the lenses and consult your eye care practitioner for identification of the problem and, if necessary, obtain treatment to avoid serious eye damage.

Directions: Your lenses must be cleaned using the special vials included in the cleaning kit. If you are using a refill package, transfer the vials from the previous kit. Do not use any other containers.

Clean your lenses with **ALLERGAN® ENZYMATIC** Contact Lens Cleaner once a week, or more often if needed, as follows.

USE ONLY STERILE SALINE SOLUTION TO DISSOLVE THE TABLETS.

1. Vigorously rinse each vial with sterile saline solution. Then examine for cleanliness. Next, fill with sterile saline solution up to the fill line indicated on the vial. Drop one tablet into each vial. The tablet will effervesce (fizz) and quickly dissolve. Always use fresh solution for each enzymatic cleaning cycle.
2. Remove one lens at a time and clean with daily cleaner or sterile saline solution in the manner recommended by your eye care practitioner. Then rinse each lens thoroughly with sterile saline solution.
3. Place each lens in the appropriate vial (R for right. L for left lens).
4. Place the caps on the vials and shake to ensure thorough mixing.

   Low Water Content (less than 55%) Contact Lenses

   Soak lenses a minimum of 2 hours. Do not soak lenses in the enzymatic cleaning solution for more than 12 hours. (See Precautions)

   High Water Content (55% or more) Contact Lenses

   Soak lenses for 15 minutes to a maximum of 2 hours. (See Precautions)

   The enzymatic cleaning solution is not intended for the storage of lenses.
5. After the required soaking interval, remove the lenses from the enzymatic cleaning solution. **Rinse the lenses thoroughly with sterile saline solution and rub gently with your fingertips to remove debris and traces**

Continued on next page

Allergan Optical—Cont.

of the enzymatic cleaning solution. Disinfect lenses as directed by your eye care practitioner.
6. Pour out the remaining solution, rinse the vials thoroughly with sterile saline solution and allow to air dry. **Do not use soap or detergent.**

Note: The enzymatic cleaning solution has a characteristic odor. This odor is normal. More than one enzymatic cleaning cycle may be required to adequately clean your lenses. Lenses must be disinfected in the usual way prior to reapplication.

How Supplied: In kits of 12 and 48 tablets including vials. (Promotional packages of tablets may not contain vials.) Also in refill packages of 24 and 36 tablets.
Avoid excessive heat.

Lenses: **ALLERGAN® ENZYMATIC** Contact Lens Cleaner is for use with soft (hydrophilic) contact lenses.
U.S. Patent 3,910,296

CLEAN-N-SOAK®
Hard Contact Lens Cleaning and Soaking Solution

Description: **CLEAN-N-SOAK®** Hard Contact Lens Cleaning and Soaking Solution removes dirt and residue and provides an antiseptic soaking and conditioning solution for hard contact lenses.

Contains: Cleaning agent, phenylmercuric nitrate (0.004%) in a sterile, buffered solution.

Directions: Wash and rinse hands thoroughly before handling lenses. Fill storage case with enough solution to completely cover lenses. Soak lenses at least four hours. Rinse lenses with running tap water and wet with **LIQUIFILM®** Wetting Solution.
Solution should be changed daily.
Use **LC-65®** Daily Contact Lens Cleaner as a super cleaner for stubborn deposits.

Warnings: To avoid contamination, do not touch tip of container to any surface. Replace cap after using. Not for use with soft (hydrophilic) contact lenses. Do not put this product in the eye. The red tip is to remind you not to put this product in your eye.

How Supplied: 4 fl oz bottle.

COMPLETE® OTC
All-In-One Solution

COMPLETE® All-In-One Solution is a cleaning, disinfecting, rinsing, and storing solution formulated specifically for use with any soft (hydrophilic) contact lenses. It is designed to work effectively in as little as 4 hours.

Description (Ingredients): COMPLETE® All-In-One Solution is a sterile, isotonic, buffered solution containing purified water, sodium chloride, TrisChem™ (polyhexamethylene biguanide), tromethamine, Tyloxapol and edetate disodium. COMPLETE® All-In-One Solution contains no chlorhexidine or thimerosal.

Actions:
- COMPLETE® All-In-One Solution cleans, loosens and removes accumulations of film, deposits, and debris from soft (hydrophilic) contact lenses.
- COMPLETE® All-In-One Solution destroys and prevents the growth of harmful microorganisms on the surface of the lenses.
- COMPLETE® All-In-One Solution can be effectively used as both a rinsing and storing solution for any soft (hydrophilic) contact lenses.

Indications:
- Use COMPLETE® All-In-One Solution to clean, disinfect, rinse and store your soft (hydrophilic) contact lenses.
- Use COMPLETE® All-In-One Solution to destroy and prevent the growth of harmful microorganisms that may cause infections.
- Use COMPLETE® All-In-One Solution every day for daily wear lenses and weekly for extended wear lenses.

Contraindications: DO NOT USE if you are allergic to any ingredient in this product.

Warnings: PROBLEMS WITH CONTACT LENSES AND LENS CARE PRODUCTS COULD RESULT IN SERIOUS INJURY TO THE EYE. It is essential that you follow your eye care practitioner's directions and all labeling instructions for proper use and care of your lenses and lens care products, including the lens case. EYE PROBLEMS, INCLUDING CORNEAL ULCERS, CAN DEVELOP RAPIDLY AND LEAD TO LOSS OF VISION.
Daily wear lenses are not indicated for overnight wear and should not be worn while sleeping. Clinical studies have shown that the risk of serious adverse reactions is increased when these lenses are worn overnight.
Extended wear lenses should be regularly removed for cleaning and disinfection or for disposal and replacement on the schedule prescribed by your eye care practitioner.
Clinical studies have shown that there is an increased incidence of serious adverse reactions in extended wear contact lens users as compared to daily wear contact lens users. Studies have also shown that the risk of serious adverse reactions increases the longer extended wear lenses are worn before removal for cleaning and disinfection or for disposal and replacement.
Studies have also shown that smokers had a higher incidence of adverse reactions.
It is recommended that contact lens wearers see their eye care practitioner twice each year or if directed, more frequently.
To avoid contamination do not touch the tip of the COMPLETE® All-In-One Solution bottle to any surface. Replace cap after using.

Precautions:
- Always wash, rinse and dry your hands before handling lenses.
- Always clean and disinfect your lenses each time they are removed.
- Never reuse solution.
- Keep the bottle tightly closed when not in use.
- After reapplying your lenses, empty the lens case, rinse with COMPLETE® All-In-One Solution and allow to air dry.
- Store at room temperature.
- Use before the expiration date marked on the bottle and carton.
- Never use COMPLETE® All-In-One Solution with a heat disinfection unit.
- Keep out of reach of children.

Adverse Reactions and What to Do:
The following may occur:
- Eyes stinging, burning, or itching
- Excessive watering (tearing) of the eyes
- Unusual eye secretions
- Redness of the eyes
- Reduced sharpness of vision (visual acuity)
- Blurred vision
- Sensitivity to light (photophobia)
- Dry eyes

If you notice any of the above, IMMEDIATELY remove and examine your lenses.
If a lens appears to be damaged, do not reapply; consult your eye care practitioner. If the problem stops and the lenses appear to be undamaged, follow the "Directions for Use" below, before reapplying the lens.
If the problem continues, IMMEDIATELY remove your lenses, discontinue use of all lens care products that contact the eye, and consult your eye care practitioner.
If any of the above occur, a serious condition such as an infection, corneal ulcer, neovascularization, or iritis may be present. Seek immediate professional identification of the problem and obtain treatment if necessary, to avoid serious eye damage.

Directions: Please read carefully and follow these instructions.

Clean and Rinse:
- Apply three drops of COMPLETE® All-In-One Solution to each lens surface in the palm of your hand and rub each side of the lens gently with a finger of your other hand for at least 10 seconds. No separate daily cleaner is necessary.
- Rinse both lens surfaces with a sufficient amount of COMPLETE® All-In-One Solution to remove all debris.

Disinfect and Store:
- Place cleaned lenses in the lens case, fill with fresh COMPLETE® All-In-One Solution and secure the cap on the lens case.
- Soak the lenses for a minimum of four hours.
- After disinfecting, your lenses are ready to wear. If any debris remains on the lenses, rinse again with sufficient amounts of COMPLETE® All-In-One Solution.
- You may store your lenses in the unopened case until ready to wear, up to a maximum of 7 days. If your lenses are stored for longer than 7 days they must be cleaned and disinfected again with fresh solution prior to wear.

How Supplied: COMPLETE® All-In-One Solution is supplied in 2 fl. oz., 4 fl. oz. and 12 fl. oz. plastic bottles.

Lenses: COMPLETE® All-In-One Solution is for use with any soft (hydrophilic) contact lenses including daily wear disposables.

LC–65®
Daily Contact Lens Cleaner
For use with gas permeable*, hard and soft (hydrophilic) contact lenses.

Description: **LC-65®** Daily Contact Lens Cleaner is a sterile, surface active, buffered solution containing cocoamphocarboxyglycinate (and) sodium lauryl sulfate (and) hexylene glycol, sodium chloride, sodium phosphate and edetate disodium.

Actions: **LC-65®** Daily Contact Lens Cleaner is formulated for gentle but efficient cleaning of gas permeable, hard and soft (hydrophilic) contact lenses. It safely removes undesirable film and deposits within seconds. Use of **LC-65®** Daily Contact Lens Cleaner leaves lenses optically clear, more wettable and more comfortable.

Indications (Uses): Use **LC-65®** Daily Contact Lens Cleaner every time you remove your lenses to clean your gas permeable*, hard and soft (hydrophilic) contact lenses before rinsing and disinfection.

Contraindications (Reasons Not to Use): If you are allergic to any ingredient in **LC-65®** Daily Contact Lens Cleaner, do not use this product.
LC-65® Daily Contact Lens Cleaner is useful for lens wearers with a history of sensitivity to mercury (thimerosal) or other preservatives present in other daily cleaners.

Warnings: **PROBLEMS WITH CONTACT LENSES AND LENS CARE PRODUCTS COULD RESULT IN SERIOUS INJURY TO THE EYE.** It is essential that you follow your eye care practitioner's directions and all labeling instructions for proper use of your lenses and lens care products, including the lens case. **EYE PROBLEMS, INCLUDING CORNEAL ULCERS, CAN DEVELOP RAPIDLY AND LEAD TO LOSS OF VISION.** Daily wear lenses are not indicated for overnight wear and should not be worn while sleeping. Clinical studies have shown the risk of serious adverse reactions is increased when these lenses are worn overnight.

Extended wear lenses should be regularly removed for cleaning and disinfection or for disposal and replacement on the schedule prescribed by your eye care practitioner. Clinical studies have shown that there is an increased incidence of serious adverse reactions in extended wear contact lens users as compared to daily wear contact lens users. Studies have also shown that the risk of serious adverse reactions increases the longer extended wear lenses are worn before removal for cleaning and disinfection or for disposal and replacement.

Studies have also shown that smokers had a higher incidence of adverse reactions.

If you experience eye discomfort, excessive tearing, vision changes, or redness of the eye, immediately remove your lenses and promptly contact your eye care practitioner.

It is recommended that contact lens wearers see their eye care practitioner twice each year or if directed, more frequently.

To avoid contamination, do not touch tip of container to any surface. Replace cap after using.

Precautions:

- Do not put this product in the eye. The red tip is to remind you not to put this product in your eye.
- Always wash, rinse and dry your hands thoroughly before handling your lenses.
- Do not allow **LC-65**® Daily Contact Lens Cleaner to dry on your lenses.
- Keep out of the reach of children.
- Store at room temperature.
- Use before the expiration date stamped on the bottle.
- Never wet contact lenses with saliva or place lenses in your mouth.
- Soft (hydrophilic) contact lenses should never be rinsed with water.

Adverse Reactions and What to Do: The following may occur:

- Eyes stinging, burning, or itching (irritation)
- Excessive watering (tearing) of the eye
- Unusual eye secretions
- Redness of the eyes
- Reduced sharpness of vision (visual acuity)
- Blurred vision
- Sensitivity to light (photophobia)
- Dry eyes

If you notice any of the above symptoms, immediately remove and examine your lenses. If a lens appears to be damaged, do not reapply; consult your eye care practitioner. If the symptom stops and the lenses appear to be undamaged, thoroughly clean, rinse and disinfect the lenses and reapply them. If the symptom continues, immediately remove your lenses and consult your eye care practitioner.

If any of the above symptoms occur, a serious condition such as infection, corneal ulcer, neovascularization, or iritis may be present. Immediately remove your lenses and seek immediate professional identification of the problem and, if necessary, obtain treatment to avoid serious eye damage. For more information, see your **Instructions for Wearers** booklet for your specific contact lenses.

Directions For Use:

- Clean, rinse and disinfect your lenses each time you remove them.
- Always wash, rinse and dry your hands thoroughly before handling contact lenses.
- Always remove and clean the same lens first to avoid mix-ups.

Gas Permeable* And Hard Contact Lenses

Prepare The Storage Case For Lens Disinfection:

- Fill each chamber of your lens storage case with **WET-N SOAK PLUS**® Wetting and Soaking Solution or other appropriate soaking solution.

Clean and Rinse Your Lenses:

- After you remove one lens, place it in the palm of your hand. Place three drops of **LC-65**® Daily Contact Lens Cleaner on each lens surface and rub for 20 seconds in the palm with your forefinger or between your thumb and forefinger. Rinse hard and gas permeable lenses with **WET-N-SOAK PLUS**® Wetting and Soaking Solution or other appropriate rinsing solution. Place the lens in the appropriate chamber of your lens case. Repeat the cleaning and rinsing procedure with your other lens and place it in the proper chamber.

Disinfect And Store Your Lenses:

- Be sure the lenses are completely covered with soaking solution before firmly tightening the caps. Disinfect and store your lenses as recommended by your eye care practitioner.

Clean gas permeable lenses** weekly with **PROFREE/GP**® Weekly Enzymatic Cleaner to reduce the buildup of tear-protein deposits which can impair vision and reduce comfort.

Soft (Hydrophilic) Contact Lenses

Prepare The Storage Case For Lens Disinfection:

- For HEAT DISINFECTION, fill each chamber of your lens storage case with fresh **LENS PLUS**® Sterile Saline Solution or other appropriate saline solution. FOR CHEMICAL DISINFECTION, fill lens case with **ALLERGAN**® **HYDROCARE**® Cleaning and Disinfecting Solution or other appropriate disinfecting solution.

Clean and Rinse Your Lenses:

- After you remove one lens, place it in the palm of your hand. Place 3 drops of **LC-65**® Daily Contact Lens Cleaner on each lens surface and rub for 20 seconds in the palm with your forefinger or between your thumb and forefinger. Rinse thoroughly with **LENS PLUS**® Sterile Saline Solution, other appropriate saline solution, or your disinfecting solution. Place the lens in the appropriate chamber of your lens storage case. Repeat the cleaning and rinsing procedure with your other lens and place it in the proper chamber.

Disinfect And Store Your Lenses:

- Be sure the lenses are completely covered with solution before firmly tightening the caps. Disinfect and store lenses as directed by your eye care practitioner.
- After lens application, always empty and rinse lens case with sterile rinsing solution and allow to air dry, to prevent contamination and to help avoid serious eye injury.

Clean soft (hydrophilic) lenses weekly with **ALLERGAN**® **ENZYMATIC** Contact Lens Cleaner to reduce the buildup of tear-protein deposits which can damage your lenses, impair vision and reduce comfort.

How Supplied: **LC-65**® Daily Contact Lens Cleaner is supplied in ½ fl oz (15 mL) and 2 fl oz (60 mL) plastic bottles. The bottles and cartons are marked with lot number and expiration date.

Lenses: **LC-65**® Daily Contact Lens Cleaner is for use with gas permeable*, hard and soft (hydrophilic) contact lenses.

*The following gas permeable lenses are recommended for use with **LC-65**® Daily Contact Lens Cleaner: FluoroPerm® and silicone acrylate lenses, such as Boston®, Paraperm® and Polycon®.

**See product labeling for list of lenses.

FluoroPerm, Boston, Paraperm and Polycon are registered trademarks of other companies.

LENS PLUS®
DAILY CLEANER

For use with SOFT (hydrophilic) contact lenses.

Preservative Free.

Description: **LENS PLUS**® Daily Cleaner is a sterile, surface-active buffered solution containing cocoamphocarboxyglycinate (and) sodium lauryl sulfate (and) hexylene glycol, sodium chloride and sodium phosphate.

Actions: **LENS PLUS**® Daily Cleaner is specially formulated for gentle but efficient cleaning of SOFT (hydrophilic) contact lenses. It safely removes the day's accumulation of undesirable film and deposits within seconds. Daily use of **LENS PLUS**® Daily Cleaner leaves lenses optically clear, more wettable and more comfortable.

Indications (Uses): Use **LENS PLUS**® Daily Cleaner every day to clean your SOFT (hydrophilic) contact lenses, before rinsing and disinfection.

LENS PLUS® Daily Cleaner is useful for lens wearers with a history of sensitivity to mercury (thimerosal) or other preservatives present in other daily cleaners.

Contraindications (Reasons Not To Use): If you are allergic to any ingredient in **LENS PLUS**® Daily Cleaner, do not use this product.

Warnings: **PROBLEMS WITH CONTACT LENSES AND LENS CARE PRODUCTS COULD RESULT IN SERIOUS INJURY TO THE EYE.** It is essential that you follow your eye care practitioner's directions and all labeling instructions for proper use of your lenses and lens care products, including the lens case. **EYE PROBLEMS, INCLUDING CORNEAL ULCERS, CAN DEVELOP RAPIDLY AND LEAD TO LOSS OF VISION.**

Daily wear lenses are not indicated for overnight wear and should not be worn while sleeping. Clinical studies have shown the risk of serious adverse reactions is increased when these lenses are worn overnight.

Extended wear lenses should be regularly removed for cleaning and disinfection or for disposal and replacement on the schedule prescribed by your eye care practitioner. Clinical studies have shown that there is an increased incidence of serious adverse reactions in extended wear contact lens users as compared to daily wear contact lens users. Studies have also shown that the risk of serious adverse reactions increases the longer extended wear lenses are worn before removal for cleaning and disinfection or for disposal and replacement.

Studies have also shown that smokers had a higher incidence of adverse reactions.

If you experience eye discomfort, excessive tearing, vision changes, or redness of the eye, immediately remove your lenses and promptly contact your eye care practitioner.

It is recommended that contact lens wearers see their eye care practitioner twice each year or if directed, more frequently.

To avoid contamination, do not touch tip of container to any surface. Replace cap after using.

Precautions:

- Do not put this product in the eye. The red tip is to remind you not to put this product in your eye.
- Always wash, rinse and dry hands before handling lenses.
- Do not allow **LENS PLUS**® Daily Cleaner to dry on your lenses.
- Keep out of the reach of children.
- Store at room temperature.
- Use before the expiration date stamped on the bottle.
- Never wet contact lenses with saliva or place lenses in your mouth.
- SOFT (hydrophilic) contact lenses should never be rinsed with water.

Adverse Reactions And What To Do: The following may occur:

- Eyes stinging, burning, or itching (irritation)
- Excessive watering (tearing) of the eye
- Unusual eye secretions
- Redness of the eyes

Continued on next page

Allergan Optical—Cont.

- Reduced sharpness of vision (visual acuity)
- Blurred vision
- Sensitivity to light (photophobia)
- Dry eyes

If you notice any of the above, immediately remove and examine your lenses. If a lens appears to be damaged, do not reapply; consult your eye care practitioner. If the symptom stops and the lenses appear to be undamaged, thoroughly clean, rinse and disinfect the lenses and reapply them. If the symptom continues, immediately remove your lenses and consult your eye care practitioner.

If any of the above symptoms occur, a serious condition such as infection, corneal ulcer, neovascularization, or iritis may be present. Immediately remove your lenses and seek immediate professional identification of the problem and, if necessary, obtain treatment to avoid serious eye damage. For more information, see your Instructions for Wearers booklet for your specific contact lenses.

Directions For Use:

- Clean, rinse and disinfect your lenses each time you remove them.
- Always wash, rinse and dry hands before handling contact lenses.
- Always remove and clean the same lens first to avoid any mix-ups.

Prepare The Storage Case For Lens Disinfection:

- For HEAT DISINFECTION, fill each chamber of your lens storage case with fresh **LENS PLUS®** Sterile Saline Solution or other appropriate saline solution. For CHEMICAL DISINFECTION, fill lens case with your disinfecting solution.

Clean And Rinse Your Lenses:

- After you remove one lens, place it in the palm of your hand. Place 3 drops of **LENS PLUS®** Daily Cleaner on each lens surface and rub for 20 seconds in the palm with your forefinger or between your thumb and forefinger. Rinse thoroughly with **LENS PLUS®** Sterile Saline Solution, other appropriate saline solution or your disinfecting solution. Place the lens in the appropriate chamber of your lens storage case. Repeat the cleaning and rinsing procedure with your other lens and place it in the proper chamber.

Disinfect And Store Your Lenses:

- Be sure the lenses are completely covered with solution before firmly tightening the caps. Disinfect and store lenses as directed by your eye care practitioner.
- To prevent contamination and to help avoid serious eye injury, always empty and rinse lens case with sterile rinsing solution and allow to air dry.

Clean SOFT (hydrophilic) lenses weekly with **ALLERGAN® ENZYMATIC** Contact Lens Cleaner to reduce the buildup of tear-protein deposits which can damage your lenses, impair vision and reduce comfort. For hydrogen peroxide disinfection systems, use **ULTRAZYME®** Enzymatic Cleaner.

How Supplied: **LENS PLUS®** Daily Cleaner is supplied in ½ fl oz (15 mL) and 1 fl oz (30 mL) plastic bottles. The bottles and cartons are marked with lot number and expiration date.

Lenses: **LENS PLUS®** Daily Cleaner is for use with SOFT (hydrophilic) contact lenses.

LENS PLUS® Rewetting Drops

Preservative free

For use with soft (hydrophilic) contact lenses while the lenses are on the eyes.

Description: **LENS PLUS®** Rewetting Drops is a sterile, preservative-free, buffered, isotonic, aqueous solution containing sodium chloride and boric acid. **LENS PLUS®** Rewetting Drops contains no thimerosal, other mercury-containing ingredients, chlorhexidine or other preservatives.

Actions: **LENS PLUS®** Rewetting Drops rehydrates and rewets soft (hydrophilic) contact lenses and helps to remove particulate material that may cause irritation and/or discomfort.

Indications (Uses): Use **LENS PLUS®** Rewetting Drops while wearing your lenses to moisten and rehydrate them. Also, use **LENS PLUS®** Drops to relieve minor irritation, discomfort and/or blurring which may occur while wearing your lenses.

Contraindications (Reasons Not To Use): Do not use this product if you are allergic to any ingredient.

Warnings: Use only if tab and single-use container are intact.

To avoid contamination, do not touch tip of container to any surface. **Discard container after each use. Do not touch tip of container directly to the eye.**

PROBLEMS WITH CONTACT LENSES AND LENS CARE PRODUCTS COULD RESULT IN SERIOUS INJURY TO THE EYE. It is essential that you follow your eye care practitioner's directions and all labeling instructions for proper use of your lenses and lens care products, including the lens case. **EYE PROBLEMS, INCLUDING CORNEAL ULCERS, CAN DEVELOP RAPIDLY AND LEAD TO LOSS OF VISION.**

Daily wear lenses are not indicated for overnight wear and should not be worn while sleeping. Clinical studies have shown the risk of serious adverse reactions is increased when these lenses are worn overnight.

Extended wear lenses should be regularly removed for cleaning and disinfection or for disposal and replacement on the schedule prescribed by your eye care practitioner. Clinical studies have shown that there is an increased incidence of serious adverse reactions in extended wear contact lens users as compared to daily wear contact lens users. Studies have also shown that the risk of serious adverse reactions increases the longer extended wear lenses are worn before removal for cleaning and disinfection or for disposal and replacement.

Studies have also shown that smokers had a higher incidence of adverse reactions.

If you experience eye discomfort, excessive tearing, vision changes, or redness of the eye, immediately remove your lenses and promptly contact your eye care practitioner.

It is recommended that contact lens wearers see their eye care practitioner twice each year or, if directed, more frequently.

Precautions: Use immediately after opening. Do not store opened container. Store solution at room temperature. Use before the expiration date marked on the container tab and carton.

Adverse Reactions And What To Do:

The following may occur:

- Eyes stinging, burning or itching (irritation)
- Excessive watering (tearing) of the eye
- Unusual eye secretions
- Redness of the eyes
- Reduced sharpness of vision (visual acuity)
- Blurred vision
- Sensitivity to light (photophobia)
- Dry eyes

If you notice any of the above, immediately remove and examine your lenses. If a lens appears to be damaged, do not reapply; consult your eye care practitioner. If the symptom stops and the lenses appear to be undamaged, thoroughly clean, rinse, and disinfect the lenses and reapply them. If the symptom continues after replacing your lens, immediately remove the lens and consult your eye care practitioner.

If any of the above symptoms occur, a serious condition such as infection, corneal ulcer, neovascularization or iritis may be present. Immediately remove your lenses and seek immediate professional identification of the problem and, if necessary, obtain treatment to avoid serious eye damage. For more information, see your **Instructions for Wearers** booklet for your specific contact lenses.

Directions: To use **LENS PLUS®** Rewetting Drops while you wear your lenses, twist the tab off of the convenient single-use container.

To rewet and rehydrate your lenses and to relieve minor irritation, discomfort and/or blurring, apply one or two drops to each eye on each lens. **Discard container after each use.**

Additional units of **LENS PLUS®** Rewetting Drops can be used as needed throughout the day.

How Supplied: **LENS PLUS®** Rewetting Drops is supplied in sterile 0.01 fl oz (0.35 mL) disposable single-use plastic containers that are packaged in cartons of 30 units each.

The containers and cartons are marked with lot number and expiration date.

Lenses: **LENS PLUS®** Rewetting Drops is for use with soft (hydrophilic) contact lenses.

LENS PLUS®

Sterile Saline Solution

PRESERVATIVE-FREE: Gentle Buffered Formula

SOFT (hydrophilic) Contact Lenses:

FOR: Rinsing, heat disinfection, storage after heat disinfection or rinsing in conjunction with chemical disinfection.

- Dissolving enzyme tablets

RIGID GAS PERMEABLE* CONTACT LENSES:

FOR: Rinsing after daily cleaning.

- Dissolving enzyme tablets

Description: **LENS PLUS®** Sterile Saline Solution is a sterile, preservative-free, buffered, isotonic solution containing sodium chloride, boric acid and nitrogen,** as an aerosol propellant in an aerosol container.

Indications (Uses):

SOFT (hydrophilic) Contact Lenses:

- For rinsing, heat disinfection and storage after heat disinfection.
- For rinsing in conjunction with chemical disinfection.
- For dissolving enzyme tablets.

Rigid Gas Permeable* Contact Lenses:

- For rinsing after daily cleaning.
- For dissolving enzyme tablets.

LENS PLUS® Saline is useful for patients with a history of sensitivity to mercury (thimerosal) or other substances present in preserved saline solutions.

Contraindications (Reasons Not to Use): Do not use this product if you are allergic to any ingredient.

Warnings: **CONTENTS UNDER PRESSURE. DO NOT APPLY DIRECTLY TO EYE AS INJURY MAY RESULT.**

PROBLEMS WITH CONTACT LENSES AND LENS CARE PRODUCTS COULD RESULT IN SERIOUS INJURY TO THE EYE. It is essential that you follow your eye care practitioner's directions and all labeling instructions for proper use of your lenses and lens care products, including the lens case. **EYE PROBLEMS, INCLUDING CORNEAL ULCERS, CAN DEVELOP RAPIDLY AND LEAD TO LOSS OF VISION.**

Daily wear lenses are not indicated for overnight wear and should not be worn while sleeping. Studies have shown the risk of serious adverse reactions is increased when these lenses are worn overnight.

Extended wear lenses should be regularly removed for cleaning and disinfection or for disposal and replacement on the schedule prescribed by your eye care practitioner. Studies have shown that there is an increased incidence of serious adverse reactions in extended wear contact lens users as compared to daily wear contact lens users. Studies have also shown that the risk of serious adverse reactions increases the longer extended wear lenses are worn before removal for cleaning and disinfection or for disposal and replacement.

Studies have also shown that smokers had a higher incidence of adverse reactions.

If you experience eye discomfort, excessive tearing, vision changes, or redness of the eye, immediately remove your lenses and promptly contact your eye care practitioner.

It is recommended that contact lens wearers see their eye care practitioner twice each year or if directed, more frequently.

To avoid contamination, do not touch tip of container to any surface or transfer the solution to any other storage bottle prior to use. Replace cap after using.

Precautions:

- Always wash, rinse and dry hands before handling lenses.
- Fresh **LENS PLUS®** Saline should be used daily. **Never reuse the solution.**
- DO NOT USE SOLUTION THAT HAS NOT BEEN HEAT DISINFECTED FOR STORAGE OF LENSES.
- Keep out of the reach of children.
- Do not puncture or incinerate. Do not store at temperatures above 120°F.
- **LENS PLUS®** Saline should be used before the expiration date stamped on the container.
- After reapplying your lenses, always empty your lens case, rinse with sterile rinsing solution, and allow to air dry.

Adverse Reactions and What to Do: The following may occur:

- Eyes stinging, burning, or itching (irritation)
- Excessive watering (tearing) of the eye
- Unusual eye secretions
- Redness of the eye
- Reduced sharpness of vision (visual acuity)
- Blurred vision
- Sensitivity to light (photophobia)
- Dry eyes

If you notice any of the above, immediately remove and examine your lenses. If a lens appears to be damaged, do not reapply; consult your eye care practitioner. If the symptom stops and the lenses appear to be undamaged, thoroughly clean, rinse and disinfect the lenses and reapply them. If the symptom continues, immediately remove your lenses and consult your eye care practitioner.

If any of the above symptoms occur, a serious condition such as infection, corneal ulcer, neovascularization, or iritis may be present. Immediately remove your lenses and seek immediate professional identification of the problem and begin treatment, if necessary, to avoid serious eye damage. For more information, see your **Instructions for Wearers** booklet for your specific contact lenses.

Directions:

SOFT (HYDROPHILIC) CONTACT LENSES:

Heat (Thermal) Disinfection

- Always wash, rinse and dry hands before handling lenses.
- Clean, rinse, and disinfect your lenses each time you remove them.
- Use can with nozzle directed at dot on rim. DO NOT TILT CAN BEYOND HORIZONTAL.
- To dispense solution, aim nozzle and press. Before each use, always expel a short stream of **LENS PLUS®** Saline from tube to clear nozzle.
- Prepare the empty lens case. Wet the chambers of the case with **LENS PLUS®** saline.
- Clean and rinse one lens first (always the same lens first to avoid mix-ups).
- After you clean your lens, rinse it thoroughly with **LENS PLUS®** saline by holding the lens between the forefinger and thumb of one hand, and directing a steady stream onto the lens or placing the lens in the palm of one hand, and directing a steady stream of **LENS PLUS®** saline onto the lens.
- Put that lens into the correct chamber (section) of the lens case.
- Fill the chamber using enough **LENS PLUS®** saline to completely cover the lens.
- Tightly close the top on the chamber.
- Repeat the above procedure for the second lens.
- Put the lens case into the disinfection unit and follow the directions for operating your heat disinfection unit.

Emergency (Alternate) Method for Heat (Thermal) Disinfection

If your heat disinfection unit is not available, place the tightly closed lens case which contains the lenses into a pan of already boiling water. Leave the closed lens case in the pan of boiling water for at least 10 minutes. (Above an altitude of 7,000 feet, boil for at least 15 minutes.) Be careful not to allow the water to boil away. Remove the pan from the heat and allow it to cool for 30 minutes to complete the disinfection of the lenses.

NOTE: USE OF THE HEAT DISINFECTION UNIT SHOULD BE RESUMED AS SOON AS POSSIBLE.

- Leave the lenses in the unopened lens case until ready to wear. Before lens reapplication rinsing is not necessary unless your eye care practitioner recommends rinsing.

Chemical Disinfection (not heat)

- Always wash, rinse and dry hands before handling lenses.
- Disinfect and store lenses as directed by your eye care practitioner.
- Before reapplying lenses that are chemically disinfected, expel a short stream of **LENS PLUS®** Saline from the tube to clear nozzle, then rinse the lenses thoroughly with **LENS PLUS®** Saline.

RIGID GAS PERMEABLE* CONTACT LENSES:

- After cleaning with an appropriate daily cleaner, rinse lenses with **LENS PLUS®** Saline.
- Disinfect the lenses as recommended by your eye care practitioner.

LENS PLUS® Sterile Saline Solution can be used to dissolve **ALLERGAN® ENZYMATIC** Contact Lens Cleaner for soft (hydrophilic) contact lenses and **PROFREE/GP®** Enzymatic Cleaner for rigid gas permeable*** lenses or other enzymatic cleaning tablets designed to be dissolved in saline.

To prevent contamination and to help avoid serious eye injury, always empty and rinse lens case with sterile rinsing solution and allow to air dry.

How Supplied: LENS PLUS® Sterile Saline Solution is supplied in sterile 3 fl oz, 8 fl oz, 12 fl oz and 15 fl oz aerosol containers. The containers are marked with lot number and expiration date.

Lenses: LENS PLUS® Sterile Saline Solution is recommended for use with soft (hydrophilic) and rigid gas permeable* contact lenses.

*Fluorosilicone acrylate, silicone acrylate and polyperfluoroether.

**Nonflammable.

***See product packaging for list of lenses.

LIDS & LASHES™
HYGIENIC CLEANSING PADS

Gently And Effectively Removes Oily Debris Or Buildup As Well As Eye Makeup From Eyelids And Eyelashes

LIDS & LASHES™ premoistened ready-to-use cleansing pads:

- Unique formula combines three ingredients to safely and effectively remove oily debris or buildup around the eyelids and eyelashes.
- Can be used daily to gently and effectively remove eye makeup, especially in conjunction with contact lens wear.
- Simple to use — eliminates the mess and waste of other products.

LIDS & LASHES™ Pads have been scientifically formulated for cleansing the delicate area around the eyes. They are hypoallergenic, pH-balanced, and non-irritating. And because they are oil-free, alcohol-free and fragrance-free they're an excellent choice for sensitive eyes.

LIDS & LASHES™ premoistened ready-to-use pads are safe and recommended for contact lens wearers.

Directions For Use: For external use only. Do not use directly in the eye. Before following these steps, thoroughly wash and rinse your hands.

Cleansing: Remove one ready-to-use pad from the LIDS & LASHES™ container. Using a well-lit mirror, expose the edge of the lower eyelid and rub it several times with the LIDS & LASHES™ Pad. Avoid rubbing the surface of the eye. Repeat the process on the edge of the upper eyelid. Close the eye and rub the LIDS & LASHES™ Pad thoroughly over the eyelid and eyelashes. Discard the used pad. Open the cleansed eye and repeat the process on the other eye with a clean LIDS & LASHES™ Pad.

Rinse: Thoroughly rinse both lids with clean, warm water and pat dry.

For those with especially heavy buildup of oil and debris: Prepare the eyelid by applying a warm compress (washcloth soaked in warm water) to the closed eyes for several minutes before cleansing.

NOTE: Do not add liquid of any kind to the container or pads. Store away from heat.

How Supplied: LIDS & LASHES™ Pads are supplied in jars containing 70 pads. The jars and cartons are marked with lot number and expiration date.

Contains: Cocoamphodiacetate (and) sodium trideceth sulfate (and) hexylene glycol; PPG-10 methyl glucose ether; PEG-20 methyl glucose sesquisterate; boric acid; quaternium-15; purified water USP.

LIQUIFILM® Wetting Solution
for comfortable hard contact lens wear

LIQUIFILM® Wetting Solution wets and lubricates hard contact lenses with a clear antiseptic film to increase wearing time and comfort.

Contains: Polyvinyl alcohol with hydroxypropyl methylcellulose, edetate disodium, sodium chloride, potassium chloride and benzalkonium chloride (0.004%).

Directions: Wash hands well. Apply to both surfaces of the lens. Rub gently between thumb and forefinger. Rinse with water. Apply another drop to inner surface and apply lens.

Warnings: To avoid contamination, do not touch tip of container to any surface. Replace cap after using. Keep out of the reach of children.

Note: Not for use with soft (hydrophilic) contact lenses.

How Supplied: 2 fl oz plastic bottles.

Continued on next page

Allergan Optical—Cont.

OxyCup®
Lens Case
for use in the
Oxysept®
DISINFECTION SYSTEM
for use with daily wear
and extended wear
soft (hydrophilic)
contact lenses

OXYCUP® Lens Case for use in the **OXYSEPT®** DISINFECTION SYSTEM

Directions: Always wash and rinse your hands before handling contact lenses. Use **OXYSEPT® 1** Disinfecting Solution to disinfect lenses. Always use **OXYSEPT® 2** Rinse and Neutralizer to neutralize lenses after disinfection. Use only the **OXYCUP®** Lens Case for proper disinfection, neutralization, and storage of your lenses. The **OXYCUP®** Lens Case should NOT be overfilled or cap overtightened.

SEE PACKAGE INSERT ACCOMPANYING THE **OXYSEPT®** DISINFECTION SYSTEM PRODUCTS FOR IMPORTANT SAFETY INFORMATION.

Note: Use **ULTRAZYME®** Enzymatic Cleaner weekly to remove protein and reduce its buildup on your soft (hydrophilic) contact lenses.

OXYSEPT® 2
Neutralizing Tablets
For use in the OXYSEPT® DISINFECTION SYSTEM—A disinfecting, neutralizing and storage system for daily wear and extended wear soft (hydrophilic) contact lenses* in a chemical (not heat) lens care system.

The OXYSEPT® DISINFECTION SYSTEM consists of:

- **OXYSEPT® 1 Disinfecting Solution,** a sterile 3% hydrogen peroxide solution for lens disinfection.
- **OXYSEPT® 2 Neutralizing Tablets,** a neutralizer in a tablet form designed specifically for use with **OXYSEPT® 1** Disinfecting Solution.
- **OXYTAB® Cup,** a specially designed lens case that ***must be used with this lens care system.***

Description (Ingredients):

- **OXYSEPT® 1 Disinfecting Solution** is a sterile solution that contains microfiltered hydrogen peroxide 3% (stabilized with sodium stannate and sodium nitrate, and buffered with phosphates) and purified water.
- **OXYSEPT® 2 Neutralizing Tablets** are smooth, round, off-white to bluish-gray, slightly mottled tablets that contain catalase, with buffering and tableting agents.
- **OXYTAB® Cup** is a specially designed lens case that must be used with this system. It consists of a single flared cup and a lens holder attached to the cap.

Actions:

- **OXYSEPT® 1 Disinfecting Solution** destroys and prevents the growth of harmful microorganisms on the surface of the lenses in a minimum of 10 minutes.
- **OXYSEPT® 2 Neutralizing Tablets** are used to neutralize the **OXYSEPT® 1** Disinfecting Solution, in a minimum of 10 minutes, after disinfection.
- **OXYTAB® Cup** is a specially designed case that ***must be used*** with the **OXYSEPT®** DISINFECTION SYSTEM for proper disinfection, neutralization and storage of soft (hydrophilic) contact lenses.

Indications (Uses):
Use the **OXYSEPT® DISINFECTION SYSTEM** to disinfect, neutralize and store soft (hydrophilic) contact lenses.

- Use **OXYSEPT® 1 Disinfecting Solution** to destroy and prevent the growth of harmful microorganisms which may cause infections.
- Use **OXYSEPT® 2 Neutralizing Tablets** to neutralize the **OXYSEPT® 1** Disinfecting Solution after disinfection.
- Use the **OXYTAB® Cup** to hold the lenses during disinfection, neutralization and storage.

Contraindications (Reasons Not To Use):
If you are allergic to any ingredient in the **OXYSEPT®** DISINFECTION SYSTEM, do not use this system.

Warnings:

- **KEEP OXYSEPT® 1 Disinfecting Solution (HYDROGEN PEROXIDE) OUT OF THE EYES.** The red tip is to remind you not to put this product in your eye. If **OXYSEPT® 1** Disinfecting Solution accidentally comes in contact with the eyes, it may cause burning, stinging or redness. Immediately remove the lenses and flush your eyes with water. If burning or irritation continues, seek professional assistance. **ALWAYS NEUTRALIZE LENSES WITH OXYSEPT® 2 Neutralizing Tablets BEFORE APPLYING LENSES TO YOUR EYES.**
- To avoid lens case cracking from excessive pressure, use only the **OXYTAB®** Cup. The **OXYTAB®** Cup is specially designed for use with **OXYSEPT® 2** Neutralizing Tablets to allow venting of pressure during neutralization. Other lens cases may not have this venting feature.
- Do not use **OXYSEPT® 2** Neutralizing Tablets that do not bubble (effervesce) when added to **OXYSEPT® 1** Disinfecting Solution. Bubbling indicates that the solution is being neutralized. If the tablet does not bubble, refer to the "Directions For Use" for what to do.
- Keep **OXYSEPT® 1** Disinfecting Solution out of the reach of children. If accidentally swallowed, an upset stomach and vomiting may result. Seek immediate professional medical assistance or contact a poison control center.

PROBLEMS WITH CONTACT LENSES AND LENS CARE PRODUCTS COULD RESULT IN SERIOUS INJURY TO THE EYE. It is essential that you follow your eye care practitioner's directions and all labeling instructions for proper use of your lenses and lens care products, including the lens case. **EYE PROBLEMS, INCLUDING CORNEAL ULCERS, CAN DEVELOP RAPIDLY AND LEAD TO LOSS OF VISION.**

Daily wear lenses are not indicated for overnight wear and should not be worn while sleeping. Clinical studies have shown the risk of serious adverse reactions is increased when these lenses are worn overnight.

Extended wear lenses should be regularly removed for cleaning and disinfection or for disposal and replacement on the schedule prescribed by your eye care practitioner. Clinical studies have shown that there is an increased incidence of serious adverse reactions in extended wear contact lens users as compared to daily wear contact lens users. Studies have also shown that the risk of serious adverse reactions increases the longer extended wear lenses are worn before removal for cleaning and disinfection or for disposal and replacement.

Studies have also shown that smokers had a higher incidence of adverse reactions.

If you experience eye discomfort, excessive tearing, vision changes, or redness of the eye, immediately remove your lenses and promptly contact your eye care practitioner.

It is recommended that contact lens wearers see their eye care practitioner twice each year or if directed, more frequently.

To avoid contamination, do not touch the **OXYSEPT® 2** Neutralizing Tablets. Do not touch the tip of the **OXYSEPT® 1** Disinfecting Solution bottle to any surface. Replace the **OXYSEPT® 1** Disinfecting Solution cap after using.

Precautions:

- Always wash, rinse and dry hands before handling lenses.
- Always clean, disinfect, and neutralize your lenses each time they are removed.
- Use only **OXYSEPT® 1** Disinfecting Solution for disinfection and **OXYSEPT® 2** Neutralizing Tablets for neutralization.
- Use only the **OXYTAB®** Cup with this system.
- Fill the **OXYTAB®** Cup exactly to the fill line. Do not overfill. Tighten the cap firmly.
- Use only **OXYSEPT®** DISINFECTION SYSTEM components; do not substitute.
- Never reuse solutions.
- Do not use tablets that appear to be broken or chipped.
- Do not take tablets internally.
- After adding the **OXYSEPT® 2** Neutralizing Tablet, do not allow lenses to soak in the solution for longer than 24 hours without disinfecting and neutralizing again before wearing.
- After reapplying your lenses, always empty the **OXYTAB®** Cup, rinse with sterile rinsing solution, and allow to air dry.
- Store solution and tablets at room temperature.
- Use before the expiration date marked on the bottle, foil pouch, blister card and cartons.
- Never use **OXYSEPT® 1** Disinfecting Solution or **OXYSEPT® 2** Neutralizing Tablets in a heat disinfection unit as these products are not designed for use with heat disinfection.

Adverse Reactions And What To Do:
The following may occur:

- Eyes stinging, burning, or itching (irritation)
- Excessive watering (tearing) of the eyes
- Unusual eye secretions
- Redness of the eyes
- Reduced sharpness of vision (visual acuity)
- Blurred vision
- Sensitivity to light (photophobia)
- Dry eyes

If you notice any of the above, IMMEDIATELY remove and examine your lenses. If a lens appears to be damaged, do not reapply; consult your eye care practitioner. If the symptom stops and the lenses appear to be undamaged, follow the complete "Directions For Use," below, before reapplying them. If the symptom continues, IMMEDIATELY remove the lenses, discontinue use of all lens care products that contact the eye, and consult your eye care practitioner.

If any of the above symptoms occur, a serious condition such as infection, corneal ulcer, neovascularization, or iritis may be present. Seek immediate professional identification of the problem, and obtain treatment, if necessary, to avoid serious eye damage. For more information, see your *Instructions for Wearers* booklet for your specific contact lens type.

Directions For Use:
Follow the instructions below each time you remove your contact lenses. Always wash, rinse and dry hands before handling contact lenses. Always remove the same lens first to avoid mix-ups.

1. **PREPARE THE OXYTAB® Cup FOR LENS DISINFECTION**
   Remove the cap of the **OXYTAB®** Cup. Fill the **OXYTAB®** Cup exactly to the fill line with **OXYSEPT® 1** Disinfecting Solution. Do not overfill.
2. **RINSE, CLEAN AND RINSE YOUR LENSES**
   Remove and handle one lens at a time. Rinse with an appropriate sterile saline solution, such as **LENS PLUS®** Sterile Saline Solution, then gently rub with an appropri-

ate daily cleaner, such as **LENS PLUS®** Daily Cleaner. Rinse **thoroughly** with more sterile saline solution. Place the lens in the appropriate basket of the lens holder attached to the cap and close the basket lid. Repeat with the remaining lens.

3. **DISINFECT YOUR LENSES**
Place the lens holder into the **OXYTAB®** Cup filled with **OXYSEPT® 1** Disinfecting Solution. Tighten the cap (do not overtighten). Allow the lenses to soak for a minimum of 10 minutes to overnight.

4. **NEUTRALIZE YOUR LENSES**
After soaking the lenses in **OXYSEPT® 1** Disinfecting Solution, open the **OXYTAB®** Cup and place the lens holder aside without allowing the lens basket to come in contact with any surface. DO NOT DISCARD the **OXYSEPT® 1** Disinfecting Solution remaining in the case.

- Bend the blister card containing the tablets along the perforations and remove one section.
- Hold the section over the **OXYTAB®** Cup, with the tablet side facing up.
- Grasp the foil backing underneath, at the corner where it is not sealed to the plastic.
- Then, carefully peel back the foil to allow the tablet to fall directly into the cup.
- To avoid contamination, DO NOT TOUCH THE TABLET. If you touch the tablet or the tablet misses the cup, discard the tablet and dispense a new tablet into the cup.
- Replace the lens holder in the cup, tighten the cap (do not overtighten) and allow the lenses to soak for a minimum of 10 minutes to overnight. Some foaming will occur. This means that the neutralizing tablet is working and is normal. In order to keep the foaming to a minimum, do not agitate or transport lens case during the first 10 minutes of neutralization.
- Keep lens case in upright position.

If the tablet does not vigorously bubble (effervesce) in the OXYSEPT® 1 Disinfecting Solution, or, if you are not sure whether you have neutralized your lenses, discard the solution and repeat steps 3 and 4.

5. **RINSE AND WEAR**
When you are ready to wear your lenses, remove one lens at a time. Rinse briefly (2 to 3 seconds) with an appropriate sterile saline solution, such as **LENS PLUS®** Sterile Saline Solution, then apply lenses.

- To prevent contamination and to help avoid serious eye injury, always empty and rinse lens case with sterile rinsing solution and allow to air dry.

6. **STORE YOUR LENSES**
Keep the **OXYTAB®** Cup closed until you are ready to wear your lenses. If you do not intend to wear your lenses immediately following disinfection and neutralization, you may store them in the *unopened* **OXYTAB®** Cup until ready to wear later in the day. However, lenses should not remain in the solution for longer than 24 hours.
If the lenses have been stored in the unopened **OXYTAB®** Cup for more than 24 hours, disinfect and neutralize again before wearing (repeat steps 3 and 4). If the lenses are left in the **OXYTAB®** Cup for longer periods of time, disinfect and neutralize once a week and again before wearing.

Note: Use an enzymatic cleaner such as **ULTRAZYME®** Enzymatic Cleaner, weekly to reduce the buildup of protein on your soft contact lenses. For further information, see the **ULTRAZYME®** package insert, or ask your eye care practitioner.

How Supplied: OXYSEPT® 1 Disinfecting Solution is supplied in sterile 8 and 12 fl oz plastic bottles.
OXYSEPT® 2 Neutralizing Tablets are supplied in cartons of 12 and 36 tablets.
OXYTAB® Cup is available in the 12-tablet size of **OXYSEPT® 2** Neutralizing Tablets.
The bottles, foil pouches, blister cards and cartons are marked with lot number and expiration date.
Store **OXYSEPT® 1** Disinfecting Solution and **OXYSEPT® 2** Neutralizing Tablets at room temperature.

Lenses: The **OXYSEPT®** DISINFECTION SYSTEM is for use with daily wear and extended wear soft (hydrophilic) contact lenses.
***NOTE:** This product is not recommended for use with ILLUSIONS® (tefilcon) lenses. Use of this product may cause lens damage.
ILLUSIONS is a registered trademark of CIBA Vision Corporation.

OXYSEPT® 1 — OTC
Disinfecting Solution

For use in the **OXYSEPT®** DISINFECTION SYSTEM, a disinfecting, neutralizing and storage system for daily wear and extended wear soft (hydrophilic) contact lenses* in a chemical (not heat) lens care system.
The **OXYSEPT® DISINFECTION SYSTEM** consists of:

- **OXYSEPT® 1 Disinfecting Solution** for lens disinfection and a choice of either:
- **OXYSEPT® 2 Rinse and Neutralizer** for neutralization and rinsing and the **OXYCUP® Lens Case.**

OR

- **OXYSEPT® 2 Neutralizing Tablets**—a neutralizer in a tablet form designed specifically for use with **OXYSEPT® 1** Disinfecting Solution and the **OXYTAB® Cup,** a specially designed lens case that must be used when using the **OXYSEPT® 2 Neutralizing Tablets** to neutralize **OXYSEPT® 1 Disinfecting Solution.**

Description (Ingredients):

- **OXYSEPT® 1** Disinfecting Solution is a sterile solution that contains microfiltered hydrogen peroxide 3% (stabilized with sodium stannate, sodium nitrate, and buffered with phosphates) and purified water.

Actions:

- **OXYSEPT® 1** Disinfecting Solution destroys and prevents the growth of harmful microorganisms on the surface of the lenses in a minimum of 10 minutes.

Indications (Uses):

- Use **OXYSEPT® 1** Disinfecting Solution to destroy and prevent the growth of harmful microorganisms which may cause infections.

Contraindications (Reasons not to use): If you are allergic to any ingredient in **OXYSEPT® 1** Disinfecting Solution, do not use this product.

Warnings:

- **KEEP OXYSEPT® 1 Disinfecting Solution (HYDROGEN PEROXIDE) OUT OF THE EYES.** The red tip is to remind you not to put this product in your eye. If **OXYSEPT® 1** Disinfecting Solution accidentally comes in contact with eyes, it may cause burning, stinging or redness. Immediately remove the lenses and flush your eyes with water. If burning or irritation continues, seek professional assistance.
  ALWAYS NEUTRALIZE LENSES WITH OXYSEPT® 2 Rinse and Neutralizer or OXYSEPT® 2 Neutralizing Tablets BEFORE APPLYING LENSES TO YOUR EYES.
- **KEEP OUT OF THE REACH OF CHILDREN. If OXYSEPT® 1 Disinfecting Solution is accidentally swallowed, an upset stomach and vomiting may result. Seek immediate professional medical assistance or contact a poison control center.**
  PROBLEMS WITH CONTACT LENSES AND LENS CARE PRODUCTS COULD RESULT IN SERIOUS INJURY TO THE EYE. It is essential that you follow your eye care practitioner's directions and all labeling instructions for proper use and care of your lenses and lens care products, including the lens case. **EYE PROBLEMS, INCLUDING CORNEAL ULCERS, CAN DEVELOP RAPIDLY AND LEAD TO LOSS OF VISION.**
  Daily wear lenses are not indicated for overnight wear and should not be worn while sleeping. Clinical studies have shown the risk of serious adverse reactions is increased when these lenses are worn overnight.
  Extended wear lenses should be regularly removed for cleaning and disinfection or for disposal and replacement on the schedule prescribed by your eye care practitioner. Clinical studies have shown that there is an increased incidence of serious adverse reactions in extended wear contact lens users as compared to daily wear contact lens users. Studies have also shown that the risk of serious adverse reactions increases the longer extended wear lenses are worn before removal for cleaning and disinfection or for disposal and replacement.
  Studies have also shown that smokers had a higher incidence of adverse reactions.

If you experience eye discomfort, excessive tearing, vision changes, or redness of the eye, immediately remove your lenses and promptly contact your eye care practitioner.
It is recommended that contact lens wearers see their eye care practitioner twice each year or, if directed, more frequently.

- To avoid contamination, do not touch tip of container to any surface. Replace cap after using.

Precautions:

- Always wash, rinse and dry hands before handling contact lenses.
- Always clean, disinfect and neutralize your lenses each time they are removed.
- Fill the **OXYCUP®** Lens Case or **OXYTAB®** Cup exactly to the fill line. Do not overfill or overtighten the cap.
- Use only **OXYSEPT®** DISINFECTION SYSTEM components; do not substitute.
- Never reuse solution.
- After reapplying your lenses, always empty the **OXYCUP®** Lens Case or **OXYTAB®** Cup, rinse with sterile rinsing solution, and allow to air dry.
- Store solution at room temperature.
- Use before the expiration date marked on the bottle and carton.
- Never use **OXYSEPT® 1** Disinfecting Solution in a heat disinfection unit, as this product is not designed for use with heat disinfection.

Adverse Reactions and What To Do: The following may occur:

- Eyes stinging, burning, or itching (irritation)
- Excessive watering (tearing) of the eyes
- Unusual eye secretions
- Redness of the eyes
- Reduced sharpness of vision (visual acuity)
- Blurred vision
- Sensitivity to light (photophobia)
- Dry eyes

If you notice any of the above, **IMMEDIATELY** remove and examine your lenses. If a lens appears to be damaged, do not reapply; consult your eye care practitioner. If the symptom stops and the lenses appear to be undamaged, follow the complete **Directions for Use,** below, before reapplying them. If the symptom continues, **IMMEDIATELY** remove the lenses, discontinue use of all lens care products that contact the eye, and consult your eye care practitioner.
If any of the above symptoms occur, a serious condition such as infection, corneal ulcer, neovascularization, or iritis may be present. Seek

Continued on next page

Allergan Optical—Cont.

immediate professional identification of the problem, and obtain treatment, if necessary, to avoid serious eye damage. For more information, see your **Instructions for Wearers Booklet** for your specific contact lens type.

Directions For Use: Follow the instructions below each time you remove your lenses. Always wash, rinse and dry hands before handling contact lenses. Always remove the same lens first to avoid mix-ups.

1. **Prepare Your Lens Case for Lens Disinfection**
   If you will be using the **OXYSEPT® 2 Rinse and Neutralizer** to neutralize your lenses **after disinfection**, prepare your **OXYCUP® Lens Case** for lens disinfection.
   If you will be neutralizing your lenses with **OXYSEPT® 2 Neutralizing Tablets**, prepare your **OXYTAB® Cup** for lens disinfection.
   Fill the lens case cup exactly to the fill line with **OXYSEPT® 1 Disinfecting Solution.** Do not overfill.
2. **Rinse, Clean, and Rinse Your Lenses**
   Remove and handle one lens at a time. Rinse with a sterile solution such as **LENS PLUS®** Sterile Saline Solution, then gently rub with **LENS PLUS®** Daily Cleaner or other recommended daily cleaner. Rinse thoroughly with more saline solution. Place the lens in the appropriate basket and close the basket lid. Repeat with the remaining lens.
3. **Disinfect Your Lenses**
   Place the lens holder into the lens case filled with **OXYSEPT® 1 Disinfecting Solution** and tighten the cap. **Do not overtighten.** Allow the lenses to soak for a **minimum of 10 minutes** to overnight.
4. **Neutralize Your Lenses**
   After soaking the lenses in **OXYSEPT® 1** Disinfecting Solution, hold the lens case over the sink, unscrew and remove the cap.
   ALWAYS USE OXYSEPT® 2 Rinse and Neutralizer OR OXYSEPT® 2 Neutralizing Tablets FOR A MINIMUM OF 10 MINUTES TO OVERNIGHT TO NEUTRALIZE LENSES AFTER DISINFECTION.
   Follow the Directions For Use contained in the package insert of **either OXYSEPT® 2** Rinse and Neutralizer or **OXYSEPT® 2** Neutralizing Tablets to neutralize your lenses.
5. **Store Your Lenses**
   Keep the lens case closed until you are ready to wear your lenses. If you do not intend to wear your lenses immediately following disinfection and neutralization, you may store them in the **unopened** lens case until ready to wear later in the day.
   See the **Directions For Use** in the package insert of **either OXYSEPT® 2** Rinse and Neutralizer or **OXYSEPT® 2** Neutralizing Tablets for additional storage directions.
   If lenses have been stored in the unopened lens case for more than the recommended time, disinfect and neutralize again before wearing. If lenses are left in the lens case for longer periods of time, disinfect and neutralize once a week and before wearing.
6. **Rinse and Wear**
   When you are ready to wear your lenses, remove one lens at a time. Rinse briefly (2 to 3 seconds) with **LENS PLUS®** Sterile Saline Solution, or other sterile saline solution, then apply lenses.
   To prevent contamination and to help avoid serious eye injury, always empty and rinse lens case with sterile rinsing solution and allow to air dry.

Note: Use an enzymatic cleaner, such as **ULTRAZYME®** Enzymatic Cleaner, weekly to reduce the buildup of protein on your soft contact lenses. For further information, see the **ULTRAZYME®** package insert or ask your eye care practitioner.

How Supplied:
OXYSEPT® 1 Disinfecting Solution is supplied in sterile 8 fl oz and 12 fl oz plastic bottles. The bottles and cartons are marked with lot number and expiration date. Store **OXYSEPT® 1** Disinfecting Solution at room temperature.

Lenses:
OXYSEPT® 1 Disinfecting Solution and the **OXYSEPT®** DISINFECTION SYSTEM are for use with daily wear and extended wear soft (hydrophilic) contact lenses.

***NOTE:** This product is not recommended for use with ILLUSIONS® (tefilcon) lenses. Use of this product may cause lens damage.

ILLUSIONS is a registered trademark of CIBA Vision Corporation.

OXYSEPT® DISINFECTION SYSTEM

A sterile, preservative-free disinfecting and storage system for daily wear and extended wear soft (hydrophilic) contact lenses* in a chemical (not heat) lens care system.

The OXYSEPT® DISINFECTION SYSTEM consists of:

- **OXYSEPT® 1** Disinfecting Solution for lens disinfection
- **OXYSEPT® 2** Rinse and Neutralizer for neutralization and rinsing
- **OXYCUP®** Lens Case, a specially designed lens case to hold your lenses during disinfection, neutralization and storage.

Weekly use of **ULTRAZYME®** Enzymatic Cleaner for soft (hydrophilic) lenses will reduce the buildup of protein deposits on your lenses for clear, comfortable soft contact lens wear.

Description (Ingredients):

- **OXYSEPT® 1 Disinfecting Solution** is a preservative-free, sterile solution that contains microfiltered hydrogen peroxide 3% (stabilized with sodium stannate, sodium nitrate, and buffered with phosphates) and purified water.
- **OXYSEPT® 2 Rinse and Neutralizer** is a preservative-free, sterile, isotonic, buffered product that contains catalase (catalytic neutralizing agent), edetate disodium, purified water, sodium chloride, and mono- and dibasic sodium phosphates.
  The catalytic neutralizing agent may have a white particulate appearance.
- **OXYCUP® Lens Case** is a specially designed case for use with this system. It consists of a single cup and a lens holder attached to the cap.

Actions:

- **OXYSEPT® 1 Disinfecting Solution** destroys and prevents the growth of harmful microorganisms on the surface of the lenses in a minimum of 10 minutes.
- **OXYSEPT® 2 Rinse and Neutralizer** is used to neutralize any remaining hydrogen peroxide on the lenses in a minimum of 10 minutes, and to rinse lenses before neutralization.
- **OXYCUP® Lens Case** is a specially designed case that must be used with the **OXYSEPT®** DISINFECTION SYSTEM for proper disinfection, neutralization and storage.

Indications (Uses):
Use the **OXYSEPT® DISINFECTION SYSTEM** to disinfect, neutralize and store soft contact lenses.

- Use **OXYSEPT® 1 Disinfecting Solution** to destroy and prevent the growth of harmful microorganisms which may cause infections.
- Use **OXYSEPT® 2 Rinse and Neutralizer** to neutralize any remaining **OXYSEPT® 1** Disinfecting Solution (hydrogen peroxide) on the lenses and to rinse lenses before neutralization. Neutralization converts the hydrogen peroxide into water and oxygen, eliminating potential irritation.
- Use the **OXYCUP® Lens Case** to hold the lenses during disinfection, neutralization and storage.

Contraindications (Reasons Not To Use):
If you are allergic to any ingredient in the **OXYSEPT®** DISINFECTION SYSTEM, do not use this system.

Warnings:

- **KEEP OXYSEPT® 1 Disinfecting Solution (HYDROGEN PEROXIDE) OUT OF THE EYES.** If **OXYSEPT® 1** Disinfecting Solution accidentally comes in contact with the eyes, it may cause burning, stinging or redness. Immediately remove the lenses and flush your eyes with water. If burning or irritation continues, seek professional assistance. **ALWAYS NEUTRALIZE LENSES WITH OXYSEPT® 2 Rinse and Neutralizer BEFORE APPLYING LENSES TO YOUR EYES.**
- Keep out of the reach of children. If **OXYSEPT® 1** Disinfecting Solution is accidentally swallowed, an upset stomach and vomiting may result. Seek immediate professional medical assistance or contact a poison control center.

PROBLEMS WITH CONTACT LENSES AND LENS CARE PRODUCTS COULD RESULT IN SERIOUS INJURY TO THE EYE. It is essential that you follow your eye care practitioner's directions and all labeling instructions for proper use of your lenses and lens care products, including the lens case. **EYE PROBLEMS, INCLUDING CORNEAL ULCERS, CAN DEVELOP RAPIDLY AND LEAD TO LOSS OF VISION.**

Daily wear lenses are not indicated for overnight wear and should not be worn while sleeping. Clinical studies have shown the risk of serious adverse reactions is increased when these lenses are worn overnight.

Extended wear lenses should be regularly removed for cleaning and disinfection or for disposal and replacement on the schedule prescribed by your eye care practitioner. Clinical studies have shown that there is an increased incidence of serious adverse reactions in extended wear contact lens users as compared to daily wear contact lens users. Studies have also shown that the risk of serious adverse reactions increases the longer extended wear lenses are worn before removal for cleaning and disinfection or for disposal and replacement.

Studies have also shown that smokers had a higher incidence of adverse reactions.

If you experience eye discomfort, excessive tearing, vision changes, or redness of the eye, immediately remove your lenses and promptly contact your eye care practitioner.

It is recommended that contact lens wearers see their eye care practitioner twice each year or if directed, more frequently.

- To avoid contamination, do not touch tips of containers to any surface. Replace cap of **OXYSEPT® 1** Disinfecting Solution after using.
- **Discard the OXYSEPT® 2 Rinse and Neutralizer single-use container IMMEDIATELY after use. DO NOT SAVE UNUSED CONTENTS.**

Precautions:

- Always wash, rinse and dry your hands before handling lenses.
- Always clean, disinfect and neutralize your lenses each time they are removed.
- Use only **OXYSEPT® 1** Disinfecting Solution for disinfection and **OXYSEPT® 2** Rinse and Neutralizer for neutralization.
- Fill the **OXYCUP®** Lens Case exactly to the fill line. Do not overfill the cup or overtighten the cap.
- Use only **OXYSEPT®** DISINFECTION SYSTEM components; do not substitute.
- Never reuse solutions.

- Do not allow lenses to soak in **OXYSEPT® 2** Rinse and Neutralizer for longer than 12 hours without disinfecting and neutralizing again before wearing.
- After reapplying your lenses, always empty the **OXYCUP®** Lens Case, rinse with sterile rinsing solution and allow to air dry.
- Store solutions at room temperature.
- Use before the expiration dates marked on the bottles and cartons.
- Never use **OXYSEPT® 1** Disinfecting Solution or **OXYSEPT® 2** Rinse and Neutralizer in a heat disinfection unit as these products are not designed for use with heat disinfection.

Adverse Reactions and What To Do:
The following may occur:

- Eyes stinging, burning, or itching (irritation)
- Excessive watering (tearing) of the eyes
- Unusual eye secretions
- Redness of the eyes
- Reduced sharpness of vision (visual acuity)
- Blurred vision
- Sensitivity to light (photphobia)
- Dry eyes

If you notice any of the above, **IMMEDIATELY** remove and examine your lenses. If a lens appears to be damaged, do not reapply; consult your eye care practitioner. If the symptom stops and the lenses appear to be undamaged, follow the complete Directions For Use, below, before reapplying them. If the problem continues, **IMMEDIATELY** remove the lenses, discontinue use of all lens care products that contact the eye, and consult your eye care practitioner.

If any of the above symptoms occur, a serious condition such as infection, corneal ulcer, neovascularization, or iritis may be present. Seek immediate professional identification of the problem, and obtain treatment, if necessary, to avoid serious eye damage. For more information. see your **Instructions for Wearers Booklet** for your specific contact lens type.

Directions For Use:
Follow the instructions below each time you remove your lenses. Always wash, rinse and dry your hands before handling contact lenses. Always remove the same lens first to avoid mix-ups.

1. **Prepare The OXYCUP® Lens Case for Lens Disinfection**
   Remove the cap of the **OXYCUP®** Lens Case. Fill the **OXYCUP®** Lens Case cup **exactly to the fill line with OXYSEPT® 1 Disinfecting Solution.** Do not overfill.
2. **Rinse, Clean, And Rinse Your Lenses**
   Remove and handle one lens at a time. Rinse with **LENS PLUS® Sterile Saline Solution, then gently rub with LENS PLUS®** Daily Cleaner or other recommended daily cleaner. Rinse thoroughly with more saline solution. Place the lens in the appropriate basket and close the basket lid. Repeat with the remaining lens.
3. **Disinfect Your Lenses**
   Place the lens holder into the **OXYCUP®** Lens Case filled with **OXYSEPT® 1 Disinfecting Solution.** Tighten the cap (do not overtighten). Allow the lenses to soak for a minimum of 10 minutes to overnight.
4. **Rinse and Neutralize Your Lenses**
   After soaking the lenses in **OXYSEPT® 1** Disinfecting Solution, hold the **OXYCUP®** Lens Case over the sink, unscrew and remove the cap. Discard the **OXYSEPT® 1** Disinfecting Solution from the **OXYCUP®** Lens Case and fill to the line with **OXYSEPT® 2 Rinse and Neutralizer.** Do not overfill. Do not remove the lenses from the lens holder. Hold the cap and shake the lens holder downward to remove the excess **OXYSEPT® 1** Disinfecting Solution. Rinse the lens holder containing the lenses for 2 to 3 seconds with **OXYSEPT® 2 Rinse and Neutralizer.** Place the lens holder containing the lenses in the **OXYCUP®** Lens Case, replace the cap **but do not overtighten,** then shake gently for a few seconds. (Note: Bubbling is a signal that the remaining **OXYSEPT® 1** Disinfecting Solution is being neutralized.) Allow lenses to soak in **OXYSEPT® 2 Rinse and Neutralizer for a minimum of 10 minutes to a maximum of 12 hours (overnight).** Note: If ever you are not sure whether you have neutralized your lenses, rinse and neutralize again with **Oxysept® 2** Rinse and Neutralizer.
5. **Store Your Lenses**
   Keep the OXYCUP® Lens Case closed until you are ready to wear your lenses. If you do not intend to wear your lenses immediately following disinfection and neutralization, you may store them in the **unopened OXYCUP®** Lens Case until ready to wear later in the day. **However, lenses should not remain in OXYSEPT® 2 Rinse and Neutralizer longer than 12 hours.**
   If the lenses have been stored in the unopened **OXYCUP®** Lens Case for more than 12 hours, disinfect and neutralize again before wearing. If lenses are left in the **OXYCUP®** Lens Case for longer periods of time, disinfect once a week and before wearing.
6. **Rinse and Wear**
   When you are ready to wear your lenses remove one lens at a time. Rinse briefly (2 to 3 seconds) with **LENS PLUS®** Sterile Saline Solution, or sterile saline solution, then apply lenses.
   To prevent contamination and to help avoid serious eye injury, always empty and rinse lens case with sterile rinsing solution and allow to air dry.

Note: Use **ULTRAZYME®** Enzymatic Cleaner weekly to reduce the buildup of protein on your soft contact lenses. For further information, see the **ULTRAZYME®** Enzymatic Cleaner package insert or ask your eye care practitioner.

How Supplied: OXYSEPT® 1 Disinfecting Solution is supplied in sterile 8 and 12 fl oz plastic bottles.

OXYSEPT® 2 Rinse and Neutralizer is supplied in sterile ½ fl oz single-use containers, packaged in cartons of 15 and 25.

The bottles and cartons are marked with lot number and expiration date. Store **OXYSEPT® 1** Disinfecting Solution and **OXYSEPT® 2** Rinse and Neutralizer at room temperature.

OXYCUP® Lens Case for use with the **OXYSEPT®** DISINFECTION SYSTEM is available separately.

Lenses: The **OXYSEPT®** DISINFECTION SYSTEM is for use with daily wear and extended wear soft (hydrophilic) contact lenses.

*NOTE: This product is not recommended for use with ILLUSIONS® (tefilcon) lenses. Use of this product may cause lens damage. ILLUSIONS is a registered trademark of CIBA Vision Corporation.

ProFree/GP®
Weekly Enzymatic Cleaner
For use with rigid gas permeable contact lenses.*

Description: PROFREE/GP® Weekly Enzymatic Cleaner is a round tablet containing the enzyme papain, sodium chloride, sodium carbonate, sodium borate, and edetate disodium.

Action: PROFREE/GP® Weekly Enzymatic Cleaner removes protein deposits from the surface of rigid gas permeable contact lenses.* It safely and effectively removes protein and reduces its buildup on your lenses when used as directed.

Indications: Use **PROFREE/GP®** Weekly Enzymatic Cleaner once a week for as little as 2 hours to reduce protein buildup for clear vision and comfortable lens wear.

Contraindications: Do not use **PROFREE/GP®** Weekly Enzymatic Cleaner if you are allergic to any of the ingredients in the tablet. If you are allergic to any ingredient in one sterile saline solution, use another sterile saline solution as recommended by your eye care practitioner to prepare the enzymatic cleaning solution.

Warnings: This product contains the enzyme papain. Do not use this product if you are allergic to papain.

Lenses must be rinsed and disinfected following each enzymatic cleaning cycle. DO NOT INSTILL THE ENZYMATIC CLEANING SOLUTION DIRECTLY INTO THE EYE.

NEVER USE DISTILLED WATER TO DISSOLVE THE TABLETS. DISTILLED WATER IS NOT STERILE. USE OF A NON-STERILE PRODUCT IN THE PREPARATION OF CONTACT LENS SOLUTIONS MAY LEAD TO MICROBIAL CONTAMINATION OF LENSES WHICH CAN CAUSE SERIOUS EYE INFECTIONS.

PROBLEMS WITH CONTACT LENSES AND LENS CARE PRODUCTS COULD RESULT IN SERIOUS INJURY TO THE EYE. It is essential that you follow your eye care practitioner's directions and all labeling instructions for proper use of your lenses and lens care products. **EYE PROBLEMS, INCLUDING CORNEAL ULCERS, CAN DEVELOP RAPIDLY AND LEAD TO LOSS OF VISION; THEREFORE, IF YOU EXPERIENCE EYE DISCOMFORT, EXCESSIVE TEARING, VISION CHANGES, OR REDNESS OF THE EYE, IMMEDIATELY REMOVE YOUR LENSES AND PROMPTLY CONTACT YOUR EYE CARE PRACTITIONER.**

All contact lens wearers must see their eye care practitioner as directed. If your lenses are for extended wear, your eye care practitioner may prescribe more frequent visits.

Precautions:

- KEEP OUT OF THE REACH OF CHILDREN.
- Do not take tablets internally.
- Do not use brown or otherwise discolored tablets.
- Avoid excessive heat.
- Always wash, rinse and dry hands before handling lenses.
- **Lenses must be disinfected following each enzymatic cleaning cycle. The enzymatic cleaning cycle is NOT a substitute for disinfection of your lenses.** After enzymatic cleaning, lenses must be gently rubbed, then rinsed with an appropriate solution and disinfected in the usual way prior to reapplication.
- Do not soak lenses longer than 12 hours.
- Lenses should **never** be placed on the eye directly from the enzymatic cleaning solution.
- Use only the special vials provided to prepare enzymatic cleaning solution. Do not use any other container.
- Use only freshly prepared enzymatic cleaning solution and discard immediately after use.
- Use before expiration date on foil wrapper and unit carton.

Adverse Reactions and What to Do: The following may occur:

- Eyes stinging, burning, or itching (irritation)
- Excessive watering (tearing) of the eyes
- Unusual eye secretions
- Redness of the eyes
- Reduced sharpness of vision (visual acuity)
- Blurred vision
- Sensitivity to light (photophobia)
- Dry eyes

Continued on next page

Allergan Optical—Cont.

If you notice any of the above, a serious condition such as infection, corneal ulcer, neovascularization or iritis may be present. Immediately remove and examine your lenses. If a lens appears to be damaged, do not reapply; consult your eye care practitioner. If the symptom stops and the lenses appear to be undamaged, thoroughly clean, rinse and disinfect the lenses and reapply them. If the symptom continues, immediately remove the lenses and consult your eye care practitioner for identification of the problem and, if necessary, obtain treatment to avoid serious eye damage.

Directions: Your lenses must be enzymatically cleaned using the special vials included in the cleaning kit. If you are using a refill package, transfer the vials from the previous kit you received to the receptacle in this package. Do not use any other containers.

Clean your lenses with **PROFREE/GP®** Weekly Enzymatic Cleaner once a week, or more often if needed, as follows:

1. Rinse vials thoroughly with sterile saline solution. Then examine for cleanliness. Next, fill with sterile saline solution up to the fill line indicated on the vial. **Use only sterile saline solution to dissolve the tablets.** Drop one tablet into each vial. The tablet will effervesce (fizz) and quickly dissolve. Always prepare fresh solution for each enzymatic cleaning cycle.
2. After removing the lenses from your eyes, clean each lens with **RESOLVE/GP®** Daily Cleaner, **LC-65®** Daily Contact Lens Cleaner or other appropriate cleaner.** Rinse each lens thoroughly with **WET-N-SOAK PLUS®** Wetting and Soaking Solution or other appropriate rinsing solution** as directed by your eye care practitioner.
3. Place each lens in the appropriate vial.
4. Place the caps on the vials and shake to ensure thorough mixing. Soak lenses a minimum of 2 hours. **The enzymatic cleaning solution is not intended for the storage of lenses.** Do not soak lenses in the enzymatic cleaning solution for more than twelve (12) hours.
5. After soaking your lenses, remove them from the vials. Thoroughly clean each lens and rinse as directed in Step 2. Then disinfect your lenses as directed by your eye care practitioner.
6. Pour out the remaining solution, rinse the vials thoroughly with sterile saline solution and allow to air dry. **Do not use soap or detergent.**

Note: The enzymatic cleaning solution has a characteristic odor. This odor is normal. In the case of unusually heavy protein deposits, more than one complete enzymatic cleaning cycle may be required to adequately clean your lenses. Lenses must be disinfected in the usual way prior to reapplication.

How Supplied: In cartons of 16 and 24 tablets including vials.

Avoid excessive heat.

Lenses: PROFREE/GP® Weekly Enzymatic Cleaner is for use with rigid gas permeable contact lenses.*

*The following rigid gas permeable lenses are recommended for use with **PROFREE/GP®** Weekly Enzymatic Cleaner: FluoroPerm® and silicone acrylate lenses (including Boston®, Paraperm®, Polycon®, Ocusil® and Optacryl). Consult your eye care practitioner to identify the type of lens you wear.

FluoroPerm, Boston, Paraperm, and Polycon are registered trademarks of other companies.

**See individual product packaging for list of lenses.

U.S. Patent 3,910,296.

RESOLVE/GP®
Daily Cleaner
For use with rigid gas permeable* and hard contact lenses.
PRESERVATIVE FREE**

Description: RESOLVE/GP® Daily Cleaner is a sterile, buffered solution with a combination of cocoamphocarboxyglycinate, sodium lauryl sulfate, hexylene glycol, alkyl ether sulfate and fatty acid amide surfactant cleaning agents.

Actions: RESOLVE/GP® Daily Cleaner effectively cleans by removing lipids, mucus and other undesirable film and surface deposits from rigid gas permeable and hard contact lenses. The combination of surfactant cleaning agents also provides antimicrobial activity to eliminate the need to add potentially sensitizing preservatives.

Indications (Uses): Use **RESOLVE/GP®** Daily Cleaner to clean your rigid gas permeable* and hard contact lenses before rinsing and disinfection.

Contraindications (Reasons Not To Use): Do not use this product if you are allergic to any ingredient.

Warnings: PROBLEMS WITH CONTACT LENSES AND LENS CARE PRODUCTS COULD RESULT IN SERIOUS INJURY TO THE EYE. It is essential that you follow your eye care practitioner's directions and all labeling instructions for proper use of your lenses and lens care products. **EYE PROBLEMS, INCLUDING CORNEAL ULCERS, CAN DEVELOP RAPIDLY AND LEAD TO LOSS OF VISION; THEREFORE, IF YOU EXPERIENCE EYE DISCOMFORT, EXCESSIVE TEARING, VISION CHANGES, OR REDNESS OF THE EYE, IMMEDIATELY REMOVE YOUR LENSES AND PROMPTLY CONTACT YOUR EYE CARE PRACTITIONER.**

All contact lens wearers must see their eye care practitioner as directed. If your lenses are for extended wear, your eye care practitioner may prescribe more frequent visits.

To avoid contamination, do not touch tip of container to any surface. Replace cap after using.

Precautions:

- DO NOT PUT THIS PRODUCT IN THE EYE. The red tip is to remind you not to put this product in your eye.
- NOT FOR USE WITH SOFT (hydrophilic) CONTACT LENSES.
- Always wash, rinse and dry hands before handling lenses.
- Keep out of the reach of children.
- Store at room temperature.
- Use before the expiration date stamped on the bottle.
- Never wet contact lenses with saliva or place lenses in your mouth.

Adverse Reactions And What To Do:

The following may occur:

- Eyes stinging, burning, or itching (irritation)
- Excessive watering (tearing) of the eye
- Unusual eye secretions
- Redness of the eyes
- Reduced sharpness of vision (visual acuity)
- Blurred vision
- Sensitivity to light (photophobia)
- Dry eyes

If you notice any of the above, IMMEDIATELY remove and examine your lenses. If a lens appears to be damaged, do not reapply; consult your eye care practitioner. If the symptom stops and your lenses appear to be undamaged, thoroughly clean, rinse and disinfect the lenses; then reapply. If the symptom continues, IMMEDIATELY remove your lenses, discontinue use of all lens care products that contact the eye, and consult your eye care practitioner.

If any of the above symptoms occur, a serious condition such as infection, corneal ulcer, neovascularization, or iritis may be present. Immediately remove your lenses and seek immediate professional identification of the problem. Obtain treatment, if necessary, to avoid serious eye damage. For more information, see your Instructions for Wearers booklet for your specific contact lens type.

Directions For Use:

- Clean, rinse and disinfect your lenses each time you remove them.
- Always wash, rinse and dry hands before handling contact lenses.
- Always remove and clean the same lens first to avoid any mix-ups.

Prepare The Storage Case For Lens Disinfection:

- Fill each chamber of your lens storage case with **WET-N-SOAK PLUS®** Wetting and Soaking Solution or other appropriate soaking solution.

Clean And Rinse Your Lenses:

- After you remove one lens, place it in the palm of your hand. Place 3 drops of **RESOLVE/GP®** Daily Cleaner on each lens surface and rub for 20 seconds in the palm with your forefinger or between your thumb and forefinger. Rinse thoroughly with an appropriate rinsing solution as recommended by your eye care practitioner. Place the lens in the appropriate chamber of your lens case. Repeat the cleaning and rinsing procedure with your other lens and place it in the proper chamber.

Disinfect And Store Your Lenses:

- Be sure the lenses are completely covered with soaking solution before tightening the caps. Disinfect and store your lenses as recommended by your eye care practitioner.

Clean silicone acrylate and FluoroPerm® rigid gas permeable contact lenses weekly with **PROFREE/GP®** Weekly Enzymatic Cleaner to reduce the buildup of tear-protein deposits which can impair vision and reduce comfort.

How Supplied: RESOLVE/GP® Daily Cleaner is supplied in sterile 1 fl oz (30 mL) plastic bottles. The bottles and cartons are marked with lot number and expiration date.

Lenses: RESOLVE/GP® Daily Cleaner is for use with rigid gas permeable* and hard contact lenses.

* The following rigid gas permeable lenses are recommended for use with **RESOLVE/GP®** Daily Cleaner: silicone acrylate, including Boston®, Paraperm®, Polycon®, Ocusil®, and Optacryl; fluorosilicone acrylate, including FluoroPerm® and Equalens®. Consult your eye care practitioner to identify the type of lenses you wear.

** The combination of surfactant cleaning agents provides antimicrobial activity which eliminates the need to add potentially sensitizing preservatives.

Boston, Paraperm, Polycon, FluoroPerm and Equalens are registered trademarks of other companies.

Style Keeper®
Contact Lens Carrying Case

Directions For Use:

- Always wash and rinse hands thoroughly before handling lenses.
- Rinse the lens case with tap water before each use and allow to air dry. Do not use soaps or detergents.
- Always follow the lens care procedures recommended by your eye care practitioner. For complete information on the use of a particular lens solution, consult the package insert accompanying the product, or ask your eye care practitioner.

- Use fresh solutions daily.
- For easy identification, both the left cap and outer base of left lens well are marked with a raised "L".

Warning: If you experience any unexplained eye discomfort, watering, vision change, or redness of the eye, immediately remove your lenses and consult your eye care practitioner to identify the cause.

FOR HEAT DISINFECTION OF SOFT (HYDROPHILIC) LENSES: Use LENS PLUS® Daily Cleaner and LENS PLUS® Sterile Saline Solution.

FOR CHEMICAL DISINFECTION OF SOFT (HYDROPHILIC) LENSES: Use ALLERGAN® HYDROCARE® Cleaning and Disinfecting Solution.

FOR HARD AND RIGID GAS PERMEABLE LENSES: Use EASYCLEAN/GP® Daily Cleaner and WET-N-SOAK PLUS® Wetting and Soaking Solution.

CAUTION: Never heat lenses in **ALLERGAN® HYDROCARE®** Cleaning and Disinfecting Solution. Do not use hard contact lens solutions with soft (hydrophilic) lenses. Do not use hydrogen peroxide disinfecting solutions with the **STYLE KEEPER®** Lens Case.

TOTAL®

The All-In-One Hard Contact Lens Solution

TOTAL® Solution is an all-purpose solution to wet, cushion, clean and soak hard contact lenses.

Contains: Polyvinyl alcohol, edetate disodium and benzalkonium chloride in a sterile, buffered, isotonic solution.

Directions: Wash hands thoroughly.

To clean and wet lenses before wearing, cover lens surface with a few drops of **TOTAL®** Solution. Rub gently, then rinse with an appropriate rinsing solution as recommended by your eye care practitioner. Place a drop of **TOTAL®** Solution on inner lens surface and apply lens.

To store lenses, fill storage case with enough **TOTAL®** Solution to completely cover lenses. Soak overnight.

Keep case tightly closed while storing lenses. Change solution every day.

Warnings: To avoid contamination, do not touch dropper tip to any surface. Replace cap after using. Not for use with soft contact lenses.

For those stubborn, hard-to-remove deposits, use **LC-65® Daily Contact Lens Cleaner,** the super-cleaner.

How Supplied: 2 fl oz, 4 fl oz

ULTRACARE® SYSTEM

A disinfecting, neutralizing and storage system for daily and extended wear soft (hydrophilic) contact lenses* in a chemical (not heat) lens care system. Included in the **ULTRACARE® System is ULTRACARE® Disinfecting Solution/Neutralizer.**

ULTRACARE® Disinfecting Solution/Neutralizer consists of:

- **ULTRACARE®** Disinfecting Solution — a sterile 3% hydrogen peroxide solution for lens disinfection.
- **ULTRACARE®** Neutralizing Tablets — a delayed-release neutralizing tablet that is added at the beginning of the disinfection cycle. This tablet allows disinfection to occur before neutralizing the solution all in one easy step.
- **ALLERGAN®** Cup — a specially designed lens cup that **must be used with this system.** (Not included in the 12 fl. oz/36 tablet size)

Description (Ingredients):

- **ULTRACARE®** Disinfecting Solution is a sterile solution that contains micro-filtered hydrogen peroxide 3% (stabilized with sodium stannate and sodium nitrate, and buffered with phosphates) and purified water.
- **ULTRACARE®** Neutralizing Tablets are smooth, round, off-white to bluish-gray, slightly mottled tablets that contain catalase and hydroxypropyl methylcellulose, with buffering and tableting agents.
- **ALLERGAN®** Cup is a specially designed lens cup that **must be used with this system** It consists of a single flared cup and a lens holder attached to the cap. The left lens basket and the gasket inside the top of the cap are blue. This will distinguish this cup from other lens cases.

Actions:

- **ULTRACARE®** Disinfecting Solution destroys and prevents the growth of harmful microorganisms on the surface of the lenses.
- **ULTRACARE®** Neutralizing Tablets, in a delayed-release manner, neutralize the **ULTRACARE®** Disinfecting Solution after disinfection occurs.
- **ALLERGAN®** Cup is a specially designed cup that must be used with this system for proper disinfection, neutralization and storage.

Indications (Uses):

Use **ULTRACARE®** Disinfecting Solution/Neutralizer to disinfect, neutralize and store your soft (hydrophilic) contact lenses.

- Use **ULTRACARE®** Disinfecting Solution to destroy and prevent the growth of harmful microorganisms that may cause infections.
- Use **ULTRACARE®** Neutralizing Tablets to neutralize the **ULTRACARE®** Disinfecting Solution. **ULTRACARE®** Neutralizing Tablets are added at the beginning of the disinfection cycle so that disinfection and neutralization occur without any additional steps.
- Use the **ALLERGAN®** Cup to hold the lenses during disinfection, neutralization and storage.

Contraindications (Reasons Not to Use): If you are allergic to any ingredient in **ULTRACARE®** Disinfecting Solution/Neutralizer, do not use this system.

Warnings:

- KEEP **ULTRACARE®** Disinfecting Solution (HYDROGEN PEROXIDE) OUT OF THE EYES. The red tip is to remind you not to put this product in your eyes. ALWAYS USE AN **ULTRACARE®** Neutralizing Tablet WITH **ULTRACARE®** Disinfecting Solution TO NEUTRALIZE YOUR LENSES BEFORE APPLYING THEM TO YOUR EYES. If **ULTRACARE®** Disinfecting Solution accidentally comes in contact with the eyes, it may cause burning, stinging or redness. Immediately flush your eyes with water and remove the lenses. If burning or irritation continues, seek professional assistance.
- Do not crush the **ULTRACARE®** Neutralizing Tablet. If a crack occurs in the coating, the tablet may begin to neutralize the **ULTRACARE®** Disinfecting Solution before adequate disinfection occurs.
- The **ALLERGAN®** Cup is specially designed with a shortened lens holder to allow room for the **ULTRACARE®** Neutralizing Tablet at the bottom of the cup. The left lens basket and the inner cap gasket of the **ALLERGAN®** Cup are blue for identification of the correct cup. Use only this cup as other lens cases may not allow enough room for the tablet. Replace your **ALLERGAN®** Cup every 6 months or more frequently as recommended by your eye care practitioner.
- Keep **ULTRACARE®** Disinfecting Solution out of the reach of children. If accidentally swallowed, an upset stomach and vomiting may result. Seek immediate professional medical assistance or contact a poison control center.

PROBLEMS WITH CONTACT LENSES AND LENS CARE PRODUCTS COULD RESULT IN SERIOUS INJURY TO THE EYE. It is essential that you follow your eye care practitioner's directions and all labeling instructions for proper use and care of your lenses and lens care products, including the lens case.

EYE PROBLEMS, INCLUDING CORNEAL ULCERS, CAN DEVELOP RAPIDLY AND LEAD TO LOSS OF VISION.

Daily wear lenses are not indicated for overnight wear and should not be worn while sleeping. Clinical studies have shown that the risk of serious adverse reactions is increased when these lenses are worn overnight.

Extended wear lenses should be regularly removed for cleaning and disinfection or for disposal and replacement on the schedule prescribed by your eye care practitioner. Clinical studies have shown that there is an increased incidence of serious adverse reactions in extended wear contact lens users as compared to daily wear contact lens users. Studies have also shown that the risk of serious adverse reactions increases the longer extended wear lenses are worn before removal for cleaning and disinfection or for disposal and replacement.

Studies have also shown that smokers had a higher incidence of adverse reactions.

It is recommended that contact lens wearers see their eye care practitioner twice each year, or if directed, more frequently.

To avoid contamination, do not touch the tip of the **ULTRACARE®** Disinfecting Solution to any surface. Replace cap after using.

Precautions:

- Always wash, rinse and dry hands before handling lenses.
- Always clean, disinfect and neutralize your lenses each time they are removed.
- If any tablet appears discolored, brownish in color, or the blister card appears damaged in any way, **DO NOT USE** any tablet from that card. Use a tablet from another card to neutralize the peroxide.
- Use only **ULTRACARE®** Disinfecting Solution/Neutralizer components; do not substitute.
- Never reuse solutions.
- Do not use tablets that appear to be broken or chipped.
- Do not take tablets internally.
- After reapplying your lenses, always empty the **ALLERGAN®** Cup, rinse with sterile rinsing solution, such as LENS PLUS® Sterile Saline Solution, and allow to air dry.
- Store solutions and tablets at room temperature.
- Use before the expiration date marked on the bottle, foil pouch, blister card and cartons.
- Never use **ULTRACARE®** Disinfecting Solution or **ULTRACARE®** Neutralizing Tablets in a heat disinfection unit as these products are not designed for use with heat disinfection.

Adverse Reactions And What To Do:

The following may occur:

- Eyes stinging, burning, or itching (irritation)
- Excessive watering (tearing) of the eyes
- Unusual eye secretions
- Redness of the eyes
- Reduced sharpness of vision (visual acuity)
- Blurred vision
- Sensitivity to light
- Dry eyes

If you notice any of the above, IMMEDIATELY remove and examine your lenses. If a lens appears to be damaged, do not reapply; consult your eye care practitioner. If the symptom stops and the lenses appear to be undamaged,

Continued on next page

Allergan Optical—Cont.

follow the complete "Directions for Use", below, before reapplying them. If the symptom continues, IMMEDIATELY remove your lenses, discontinue use of all lens care products that contact the eye, and consult your eye care practitioner.

If any of the above symptoms occur, a serious condition such as infection, corneal ulcer, neovascularization, or iritis may be present. Seek immediate professional identification of the problem, and obtain treatment, if necessary, to avoid serious eye damage.

Directions for Use:

Follow the instructions below each time you remove your contact lenses. Always wash, rinse and dry hands before handling contact lenses. Always remove the same lens first to avoid mix-ups.

1. Clean and Rinse Your Lenses
   Remove and handle one lens at a time. Gently rub each lens with an appropriate daily cleaner, such as LENS PLUS® Daily Cleaner. Rinse thoroughly with sterile saline solution, such as LENS PLUS® Sterile Saline Solution. Place the lens in the appropriate basket of the lens holder attached to the cap and close the basket lid. For easy identification, the left lens basket is blue.
2. Disinfect and Neutralize Your Lenses
   Fill the **ALLERGAN®** Cup to the fill line with **ULTRACARE®** Disinfecting Solution. With dry hands, remove one **ULTRACARE®** Neutralizing Tablet from the blister card, drop it into the solution and **immediately** place the lens holder containing the lenses into the **ALLERGAN®** Cup. Tighten the cap.

Gently turn the **ALLERGAN®** Cup upside down, then right side up 3 consecutive times to wet the upper surfaces of the cup and the inside of the cap. Make sure that the tablet is in the solution. You will see a few bubbles or some light bubbling. If the tablet immediately begins to bubble **vigorously,** causing foam to form on the solution surface, the tablet is neutralizing the solution too quickly for disinfection to take place. Discard the solution and tablet, fill the cup with fresh solution, add another tablet and immediately tighten the cap. Allow the lenses to soak for a minimum of 2 hours to overnight.

The delayed-release **ULTRACARE®** Neutralizing Tablet will allow disinfection to occur before it neutralizes the solution. During the neutralization process, the tablet will begin to bubble vigorously and will completely dissolve.

3. Wear
   After soaking, apply the lenses directly to your eyes. If desired, rinse your lenses with sterile saline solution, such as **LENS PLUS®** Sterile Saline Solution, before lens application. Do not use **ULTRACARE®** Disinfecting Solution (hydrogen peroxide) to rinse your lenses before wearing.

If you do not intend to wear your lenses immediately after disinfection, you may store them in the **unopened ALLERGAN®** Cup for up to 7 days. If stored for longer than 7 days, disinfect and neutralize before applying the lenses to your eye.

To prevent contamination and to help avoid serious eye injury, always empty and rinse cup with sterile rinsing solution and allow to air dry. Once a week, **while you are wearing your lenses,** fill the **ALLERGAN®** Cup with fresh **ULTRACARE®** Disinfecting Solution. Tighten the cap. Turn the cup upside down to allow the solution to cover the inside of the cap and the top part of the cup. Leave the cup in this position until you are ready to remove your lenses from your eyes and disinfect.

Note: Once a week, simply add an **ULTRAZYME®** Enzymatic Cleaner tablet to the **ULTRACARE®** Disinfecting Solution at the same time that you add the **ULTRACARE®** Neutralizing Tablet. You will simultaneously reduce the buildup of protein on your soft (hydrophilic) contact lenses as you disinfect and neutralize them. For more information, see the **ULTRAZYME®** Enzymatic Cleaner package insert, or ask your eye care practitioner.

How Supplied: **ULTRACARE®** Disinfecting Solution/Neutralizer is supplied in a travel size package containing a 4 fl oz bottle of **ULTRACARE®** Disinfecting Solution, 12 **ULTRACARE®** Neutralizing Tablets, and an **ALLERGAN®** Cup.

ULTRACARE® Disinfecting Solution/Neutralizer is also supplied in a package containing a 12 fl oz bottle of **ULTRACARE®** Disinfecting Solution and 36 **ULTRACARE®** Neutralizing Tablets.

The bottle, foil pouches, blister cards and carton are marked with lot number and expiration date. Store **ULTRACARE®** Disinfecting Solution and **ULTRACARE®** Neutralizing Tablets at room temperature.

Lenses: **ULTRACARE®** Disinfecting Solution/Neutralizer is for use with soft (hydrophilic) contact lenses.

***NOTE:** This product is not recommended for use with ILLUSIONS® (tefilcon) lenses. Use of this product may cause lens damage.

ILLUSIONS is a registered trademark of CIBA Vision Corporation.

ULTRAZYME® Enzymatic Cleaner
for use with soft (hydrophilic) contact lenses in combination with OXYSEPT® 1 Disinfecting Solution and other* (see instructions at the end of this insert) 3% hydrogen peroxide disinfecting solutions.

Description (Ingredients): **ULTRAZYME®** Enzymatic Cleaner is an effervescent, smooth, oval, white tablet that contains the enzyme subtilisin A, with effervescing, buffering, and tableting agents.

Actions: **ULTRAZYME®** Enzymatic Cleaner, dissolved in **OXYSEPT® 1** Disinfecting Solution or other* 3% hydrogen peroxide disinfecting solutions, simultaneously removes protein deposits while lenses are being disinfected. When used as directed, one **ULTRAZYME®** Enzymatic Cleaner tablet safely and effectively removes protein and reduces its buildup on your lenses while enhancing the disinfection capability of your hydrogen peroxide disinfecting solution.

Indications (Uses): **ULTRAZYME®** Enzymatic Cleaner is indicated for use in a recommended 3% hydrogen peroxide disinfecting solution such as **OXYSEPT® 1** Disinfecting Solution, to remove protein and reduce its buildup on soft (hydrophilic) contact lenses.

Contraindications (Reasons Not To Use): Do not use **ULTRAZYME®** Enzymatic Cleaner tablets if you are allergic to the enzyme subtilisin A.

Warnings:

- After the enzymatic/disinfection and neutralization cycles, **lenses must be gently rubbed and rinsed with an appropriate rinsing solution before applying to your eyes.**
- **KEEP THE ENZYMATIC/DISINFECTING SOLUTION OUT OF YOUR EYES.** If the solution accidentally comes in contact with eyes, it may cause burning, stinging or redness. Immediately remove your lenses and flush your eyes with water. If burning or irritation continues, seek professional assistance.
- **ALL ENZYMATIC/DISINFECTION, NEUTRALIZATION AND RINSING CYCLES MUST BE COMPLETED BEFORE REAPPLYING YOUR LENSES.**

PROBLEMS WITH CONTACT LENSES AND LENS CARE PRODUCTS COULD RESULT IN SERIOUS INJURY TO THE EYE. It is essential that you follow your eye care practitioner's directions and all labeling instructions for proper use of your lenses and lens care products, including the lens case. **EYE PROBLEMS, INCLUDING CORNEAL ULCERS, CAN DEVELOP RAPIDLY AND LEAD TO LOSS OF VISION.**

Daily wear lenses are not indicated for overnight wear and should not be worn while sleeping. Clinical studies have shown the risk of serious adverse reactions is increased when these lenses are worn overnight.

Extended wear lenses should be regularly removed for cleaning and disinfection or for disposal and replacement on the schedule prescribed by your eye care practitioner. Clinical studies have shown that there is an increased incidence of serious adverse reactions in extended wear contact lens users as compared to daily wear contact lens users. Studies have also shown that the risk of serious adverse reactions increases the longer extended wear lenses are worn before removal for cleaning and disinfection or for disposal and replacement.

Studies have also shown that smokers had a higher incidence of adverse reactions.

If you experience eye discomfort, excessive tearing, vision changes, or redness of the eye, immediately remove your lenses and promptly contact your eye care practitioner.

It is recommended that contact lens wearers see their eye care practitioner twice each year or if directed, more frequently.

Precautions:

- KEEP OUT OF THE REACH OF CHILDREN.
- Always wash, rinse and dry hands before handling lenses.
- Use the lens case recommended for your disinfection system.
- Never interchange or reuse solutions.
- Do not use tablets that are soft and sticky or irregular in appearance.
- Do not take tablets internally.
- The weekly enzymatic/disinfection cycle is not a substitute for cleaning and disinfecting.
- After reapplying your lenses, always empty the lens case, rinse with sterile saline solution, and allow to air dry.
- Use before the expiration date on the foil, blister package and carton.
- Never use **ULTRAZYME®** Enzymatic Cleaner in a heat disinfection unit as this product is not designed for use with heat disinfection.
- Store at room temperature, 15°–30°C (59°–86°F), in a dry place.

Adverse Reactions And What To Do:

The following may occur:

- Eyes stinging, burning, or itching (irritation)
- Excessive watering (tearing) of the eyes
- Unusual eye secretions
- Redness of the eyes
- Reduced sharpness of vision (visual acuity)
- Blurred vision
- Sensitivity to light (photophobia)
- Dry eyes

If you notice any of the above, IMMEDIATELY remove and examine your lenses. If a lens appears to be damaged, do not reapply; consult your eye care practitioner. If the symptom stops and your lenses appear to be undamaged, thoroughly clean, rinse, and disinfect the lenses; then reapply. If the symptom continues, IMMEDIATELY remove your lenses, discontinue use of all lens care products that contact the eye, and consult your eye care practitioner.

If any of the above symptoms occur, a serious condition such as infection, corneal ulcer, neovascularization or iritis may be present. Immediately remove your lenses and seek immediate professional identification of the problem, and obtain treatment, if necessary, to avoid serious eye damage. For more information, see your **Instructions for Wearers** Booklet for your specific contact lens type.

Directions For Use With The OXYSEPT® DISINFECTION SYSTEM: Use **ULTRAZYME®** Enzymatic Cleaner once a week or more often as recommended by your eye care practitioner.

Always wash, rinse and dry hands before handling contact lenses. Always remove the same lens first to avoid mix-ups.

Follow the instructions below each time you use the **ULTRAZYME®** Enzymatic Cleaner tablet with the **OXYSEPT®** DISINFECTION SYSTEM.

- If your disinfection system consists of **OXYSEPT® 1 Disinfecting Solution** and **OXYSEPT® 2 Rinse and Neutralizer,** use only the **OXYCUP® Lens Case** for weekly enzymatic cleaning/disinfection and neutralization. Do not substitute any other lens case.
- If your disinfection system consists of **OXYSEPT® 1 Disinfecting Solution** and **OXYSEPT® 2 Neutralizing Tablets,** use only the **OXYTAB® Cup** for weekly enzymatic cleaning/disinfection and neutralization. Do not substitute any other lens case.

1. **PREPARE THE LENS CASE (OXYCUP® or OXYTAB® Cup) FOR WEEKLY ENZYMATIC CLEANING/DISINFECTION.**
Fill the cup of the lens case exactly to the fill line with **OXYSEPT® 1 Disinfecting Solution.** Do not overfill. Next, place one (1) **ULTRAZYME®** Enzymatic Cleaner tablet in the cup. The tablet will fizz and quickly dissolve.
2. **CLEAN AND RINSE YOUR LENSES.**
Remove one lens at a time and clean with **LENS PLUS®** Daily Cleaner or other recommended daily cleaner. Rinse thoroughly with a sterile saline solution such as **LENS PLUS®** Sterile Saline Solution. Place the lenses in the proper lens baskets of the lens holder and close the basket lids.
3. **ENZYMATICALLY CLEAN AND DISINFECT YOUR LENSES.**
Place the lens holder in the lens case (**OXYCUP®** or **OXYTAB®** Cup) and tighten the cap (do not overtighten). Allow the lenses to soak for **at least 15 minutes to a maximum of overnight.** Increasing the soak time up to a maximum of overnight will allow for increased protein removal. Consult your eye care practitioner to determine the best soak time for you, as individuals vary in the amount of protein they deposit.

FOLLOW THE NEUTRALIZATION STEPS FOR EITHER **OXYSEPT® 2** Rinse and Neutralizer or **OXYSEPT® 2** Neutralizing Tablets.

DIRECTIONS FOR NEUTRALIZING WITH **OXYSEPT® 2** Rinse and Neutralizer:

4. **RINSE AND NEUTRALIZE YOUR LENSES.**
After the required soaking time, open the **OXYCUP®** over a sink. DISCARD the enzymatic/disinfecting solution from the cup and fill exactly to the line with **OXYSEPT® 2** Rinse and Neutralizer. Do not overfill. Do not remove the lenses from the lens holder. Hold the cap and shake the baskets downward to remove the excess enzymatic/disinfecting solution. Then rinse the lens baskets containing the lenses for 2 to 3 seconds with the remaining **OXYSEPT® 2** Rinse and Neutralizer.
Replace the lens holder containing the lenses in the **OXYCUP®**, tighten the cap (do not overtighten) and shake gently for a few seconds. (Note: Bubbling is a signal that the remaining **OXYSEPT® 1** Disinfecting Solution is being neutralized.) Allow the lenses to soak in **OXYSEPT® 2** Rinse and Neutralizer for a minimum of 10 minutes to a maximum of 12 hours.
NOTE: If ever you are not sure whether you have neutralized your lenses, rinse and neutralize again with **OXYSEPT® 2** Rinse and Neutralizer.

OR

DIRECTIONS FOR NEUTRALIZING WITH **OXYSEPT® 2** Neutralizing Tablets:

4. **NEUTRALIZE YOUR LENSES.** After the required soaking time, open the **OXYTAB®** Cup and place the lens holder aside without allowing the baskets to come in contact with any surface. DO NOT DISCARD the **OXYSEPT® 1** Disinfecting Solution remaining in the case.
Detach one section of the blister card containing the **OXYSEPT® 2** Neutralizing Tablets. Hold the section over the **OXYTAB®** Cup with the tablet side facing up. Grasp and peel back the foil to allow the tablet to fall directly into the cup. To avoid contamination, DO NOT TOUCH THE TABLET. If you touch the tablet or the tablet misses the cup, discard that tablet and dispense a new tablet into the cup.
Replace the lens holder in the cup, tighten the cap (do not overtighten) and soak for a minimum of 10 minutes to overnight.
5. **RUB, RINSE AND WEAR.**
When you are ready to wear your lenses, remove one lens at a time and gently rub and rinse thoroughly with **LENS PLUS®** Sterile Saline Solution, or other appropriate sterile rinsing solution; then apply lenses.
To prevent contamination and to help avoid serious eye injury, always empty and rinse lens case with sterile rinsing solution and allow to air dry.

***DIRECTIONS FOR OTHER 3% HYDROGEN PEROXIDE SYSTEMS:**
(AOSept®, Lensept®, MiraSept™, CONSEPT™, Quik-Sept™ and PureSept™)

Follow the directions for your particular disinfection system. Use the lens case designed for use with your 3% hydrogen peroxide disinfecting solution.

- Place one (1) **ULTRAZYME®** Enzymatic Cleaner tablet in your 3% hydrogen peroxide disinfecting solution.
- Allow lenses to soak as usual in your disinfecting solution. However, if your disinfecting solution calls for a disinfection soak time less than 15 minutes, **increase the soak time to a minimum of 15 minutes when using ULTRAZYME® Enzymatic Cleaner.** Increasing the soak time up to a maximum of overnight will allow for increased protein removal. Consult your eye care practitioner to determine the best soak time for you, as individuals vary in the amount of protein they deposit.
NOTE: FAILURE TO FOLLOW THE INSTRUCTIONS SPECIFIED FOR YOUR HYDROGEN PEROXIDE DISINFECTING SOLUTION MAY RESULT IN SERIOUS EYE INFECTION. THE MINIMUM SOAK TIME WITH ULTRAZYME ENZYMATIC CLEANER SHOULD NEVER BE LESS THAN THE MINIMUM RECOMMENDED DISINFECTION SOAK TIME FOR YOUR HYDROGEN PEROXIDE DISINFECTING SOLUTION.
- After your lenses have been enzymatically cleaned/disinfected and neutralized (following the directions for your particular disinfection system), they **must be gently rubbed and rinsed** with **LENS PLUS®** Sterile Saline Solution or other appropriate sterile rinsing solution before wearing.

How Supplied: ULTRAZYME® Enzymatic Cleaner is supplied in packages of 5, 10, 15 and 20 tablets. The foil packages and cartons are marked with lot number and expiration date.

Lenses: ULTRAZYME® Enzymatic Cleaner is for use with soft (hydrophilic) contact lenses. U.S. Patent 3,910,296, 4,585,488 and Re. 32,672.

AOSept, Lensept, MiraSept, CONSEPT, Quik-Sept and PureSept are trademarks of other companies.

WET–N–SOAK PLUS®

Wetting and Soaking Solution
For use with gas permeable contact lenses* and hard contact lenses

Description: WET-N-SOAK PLUS® Wetting and Soaking Solution is a sterile, buffered isotonic solution that contains polyvinyl alcohol, edetate disodium and benzalkonium chloride (0.003%) as the preservative.

Actions: WET-N-SOAK PLUS® disinfects your lenses by destroying harmful microorganisms on the surface of the lens. Use **WET-N-SOAK PLUS®** to store your lenses after disinfection. **WET-N-SOAK PLUS®** also wets and provides cushioning of the lens when placed on the eye.

Indications (Uses): WET-N-SOAK PLUS® is indicated for chemical disinfection and storage of gas permeable lenses* and hard contact lenses. Use **WET-N-SOAK PLUS®** to wet and cushion your lenses before applying them to your eyes.

Contraindications (Reasons Not to Use): Do not use if you are allergic to any ingredient in this product.

Warnings: PROBLEMS WITH CONTACT LENSES AND LENS CARE PRODUCTS COULD RESULT IN SERIOUS INJURY TO THE EYE. It is essential that you follow your eye care practitioner's directions and all labeling instructions for proper use of your lenses and lens care products. **EYE PROBLEMS, INCLUDING CORNEAL ULCERS, CAN DEVELOP RAPIDLY AND LEAD TO LOSS OF VISION; THEREFORE, IF YOU EXPERIENCE EYE DISCOMFORT, EXCESSIVE TEARING, VISION CHANGES, OR REDNESS OF THE EYE, IMMEDIATELY REMOVE YOUR LENSES AND PROMPTLY CONTACT YOUR EYE CARE PRACTITIONER.**

All contact lens wearers must see their eye care practitioner as directed. If your lenses are for extended wear, your eye care practitioner may prescribe more frequent visits.

To avoid contamination, do not touch tip of container to any surface. Replace cap after using.

Precautions:

- Always wash, rinse and dry hands before handling contact lenses.
- Always use fresh solution daily.
- Not for use with soft (hydrophilic) contact lenses.
- Keep out of the reach of children.
- Store solution at room temperature.
- Use before the expiration date marked on the bottle and carton.

Adverse Reactions and What to Do: The following may occur:

- Eyes stinging, burning, or itching (irritation)
- Excessive watering (tearing) of the eye
- Unusual eye secretions
- Redness of the eye
- Reduced sharpness of vision (visual acuity)
- Blurred vision
- Sensitivity to light (photophobia)
- Dry eyes

If you notice any of the above, IMMEDIATELY remove and examine your lenses. If a lens appears to be damaged, do not reapply; consult your eye care practitioner. If the symptom stops and the lenses appear to be undamaged, thoroughly clean, rinse and disinfect the lenses and reapply them. If the symptom continues, IMMEDIATELY remove your lenses and consult your eye care practitioner.

If any of the above symptoms occur, a serious condition such as infection, corneal ulcer, neo-

Continued on next page

Allergan Optical—Cont.

vascularization or iritis may be present. Immediately remove your lenses and seek immediate practitioner identification of the problem and obtain treatment, if necessary, to avoid serious eye damage. For more information, see your Instructions for Wearers booklet for your specific contact lenses.

Directions:

- Clean, rinse and disinfect your lenses each time you remove them.
- Always wash, rinse and dry hands before handling contact lenses.
- Always remove the same lens first to avoid any mix-ups.

Prepare The Storage Case For Lens Disinfection:

- Fill each chamber of your lens storage case with **WET-N-SOAK PLUS®** Wetting and Soaking Solution.

Clean And Rinse Your Lenses:

- Remove one lens and clean it with an appropriate daily cleaner as directed by your eye care practitioner. Rinse thoroughly with an appropriate rinsing solution. Place the lens in the appropriate chamber of your lens storage case. Be sure the lens is completely covered with **WET-N-SOAK PLUS®** before firmly tightening the cap. Repeat the entire procedure with your other lens.

Disinfect And Store Your Lenses:
Allow lenses to soak overnight or for a minimum of 4 hours in **WET-N-SOAK PLUS®**.

Apply Your Lenses

- After soaking, lenses may be removed from the case and placed directly on the eyes. For cushioning, place one drop of **WET-N-SOAK PLUS®** on the inner surface of each lens before applying.
  Note: Use **PROFREE/GP®** Weekly Enzymatic Cleaner once a week to remove protein and reduce its buildup on your silicone acrylate or FluoroPerm® rigid gas permeable lenses. For further information, see the **PROFREE/GP®** package insert accompanying the product or ask your eye care practitioner.

If you do not intend to wear your lenses immediately following disinfection you may store them in the unopened lens case.
If the lenses have been stored in the unopened lens case for more than 1 week, put fresh solution in the lens case and disinfect before wearing. If left in the lens case for longer periods of time, disinfect once a week and before wearing.
After reapplying lenses, empty the lens case, rinse with fresh rinsing solution, and allow to air dry.

How Supplied: **WET-N-SOAK PLUS®** Wetting and Soaking Solution is supplied in sterile 4 fl oz and 6 fl oz plastic bottles. The bottles and cartons are marked with lot number and expiration date.

Lenses: **WET-N-SOAK PLUS®** is for use with gas permeable contact lenses* and hard contact lenses.

*The following gas permeable lenses are recommended for use with **WET-N-SOAK PLUS®**: silicone acrylate lenses (including Boston®, Paraperm®, Polycon®, Ocusil® and Optacryl) and fluorosilicone acrylate lenses. Consult your eye care practitioner to identify the lens you wear.

Boston, FluoroPerm, Paraperm and Polycon are registered trademarks of other companies.

WET–N–SOAK®
Rewetting Drops

For use with rigid gas permeable* contact lenses.

Description: **WET-N-SOAK®** Rewetting Drops is a sterile, isotonic, borate buffered solution containing hydroxyethyl cellulose and WSCP (poly[oxyethylene(dimethyliminio) ethylene (dimethyliminio)ethylene dichloride]) 0.0060% as the preservative.

Actions: **WET-N-SOAK®** Rewetting Drops lubricate and rewet your lenses while you are wearing them.

Indications: Use **WET-N-SOAK®** Rewetting Drops to lubricate and rewet your rigid gas permeable* contact lenses.

Contraindications: Do not use this product if you are allergic to any of its ingredients.

Warnings:
PROBLEMS WITH CONTACT LENSES AND LENS CARE PRODUCTS COULD RESULT IN SERIOUS INJURY TO THE EYE. It is essential that you follow your eye care practitioner's directions and all labeling instructions for proper use and care of your lenses and lens care products, including the lens case. **EYE PROBLEMS, INCLUDING CORNEAL ULCERS, CAN DEVELOP RAPIDLY AND LEAD TO LOSS OF VISION; THEREFORE, IF YOU EXPERIENCE EYE DISCOMFORT, EXCESSIVE TEARING, VISION CHANGES, OR REDNESS OF THE EYE, IMMEDIATELY REMOVE YOUR LENSES AND PROMPTLY CONTACT YOUR EYE CARE PRACTITIONER.**
It is recommended that contact lens wearers see their eye care practitioner twice each year or, if directed, more frequently.
To avoid contamination, do not touch tip of container to any surface. Replace cap and keep tightly closed when not in use.

Precautions:

- Always wash, rinse and dry hands before handling lenses.
- Store solution at room temperature.
- Use before the expiration date marked on the bottle and carton.
- Keep out of the reach of children.
- Not for use with soft (hydrophilic) contact lenses.

ADVERSE REACTIONS AND WHAT TO DO
The following may occur:

- Eyes stinging, burning, or itching (irritation)
- Excessive watering (tearing) of the eyes
- Unusual eye secretions
- Redness of the eyes
- Reduced sharpness of vision (visual acuity)
- Blurred vision
- Sensitivity to light (photophobia)
- Dry eyes

If you notice any of the above, immediately remove and examine your lenses. If a lens appears to be damaged, do not reapply, consult your eye care practitioner. If the symptom stops and the lenses appear to be undamaged, thoroughly clean, rinse and disinfect the lenses and reapply them. If the symptom continues, immediately remove your lenses and consult your eye care practitioner.
If any of the above symptoms occur, a serious condition such as infection, corneal ulcer, neovascularization or iritis may be present. Immediately remove your lenses and seek immediate practitioner identification of the problem and obtain treatment, if necessary, to avoid serious eye damage.

Directions:

1. With the lenses on the eye, apply 1 to 2 drops to each eye as needed, or as directed by your eye care practitioner.
2. Blink several times.

To avoid contamination, be careful not to touch the dropper tip to your eye or eyelid.

How Supplied: **WET-N-SOAK®** Rewetting Drops is supplied in sterile ½ fl oz plastic bottles. The bottles and cartons are marked with the lot number and expiration date.

***Lenses:** Use **WET-N-SOAK®** Rewetting Drops with the following rigid gas permeable lenses:
silicone acrylate (such as Boston®, Paraperm® and Polycon®), and fluorosilicone acrylate (such as FluoroPerm®).

Boston, Paraperm, Polycon and FluoroPerm are registered trademarks of other companies.

SECTION 10

INSTRUMENTATION AND EQUIPMENT PRODUCT INFORMATION

Participating companies have supplied product information by category and/or specific model or brand. For more information, contact the manufacturer at the address or telephone number shown.

Alcon Surgical

6201 SOUTH FREEWAY
FT. WORTH, TX 76134

Address Inquiries to:
Marketing Department (817) 293-0450
1-800-TO-ALCON
(1-800-862-5266)

BSS® AND BSS PLUS® IRRIGATION ADMINISTRATION SET

This is a sterile inside and out administration set for recommended use in ophthalmic surgical irrigation with BSS® and BSS PLUS® Sterile Irrigating Solutions. It may also be used in a variety of other surgical procedures where administration set tubing interfaces with a sterile field.

In addition to its sterility, the BSS® and BSS PLUS® Irrigation Solution Administration Set is 96″ in length and contains a terminal male luer connector and guard which adapts to most operative uses. Other features include a vented spike, drip chamber with 5 micron filter, and in-line ball check control. The set is packaged in a tyvek chevron pouch for optimum security and delivery onto the sterile field. Each box contains fifty product pouches.

Endo Optiks, Inc.

39 SYCAMORE AVE.
LITTLE SILVER, NJ 07739

MicroProbe™

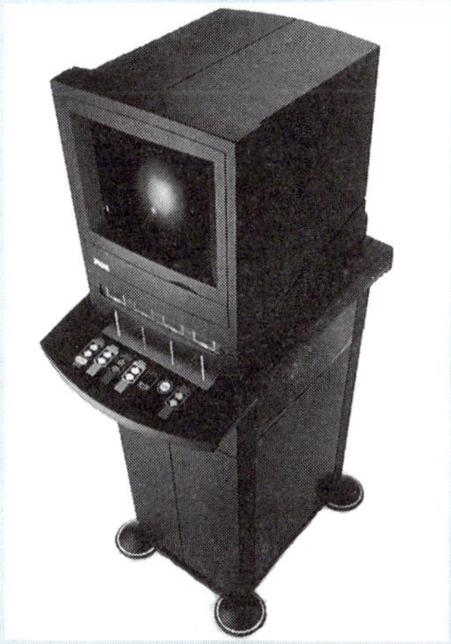

The MicroProbe™ Integrated Laser Endoscope System is a unique breakthrough technology engineered to overcome many of the limitations imposed by current surgical technologies. The MicroProbe™ combines a brilliant light source, solid state laser delivery, and video imaging capability in one 20 gauge probe. With a 70° field of vision in the standard probe and a 110° field of vision in the wide field probe, the MicroProbe™ can view all the structures of the eye that are now inaccessible to conventional technology producing a video image not available with current probes or viewing devices. The MicroProbe™ can be used for treatment of glaucoma or management of Vitreo Retinal disorders. For more information or to arrange for a surgical evaluation contact Endo Optiks®, Inc. directly at 800-756-3636.

Interzeag Inc.

100 OTIS STREET
NORTHBORO, MA 01532

HEIDELBERG RETINA TOMOGRAPH

Computerized imaging system performs confocal laser scanning to capture 32 two-dimensional images of the optic nerve head or macular region in less than two seconds, then converts results into a topographic map. Contour line can be drawn around area of investigation, which will then provide various stereometric results and calculations. Data can be stored for a change analysis follow-up over time. System's accuracy is less than 30 microns.

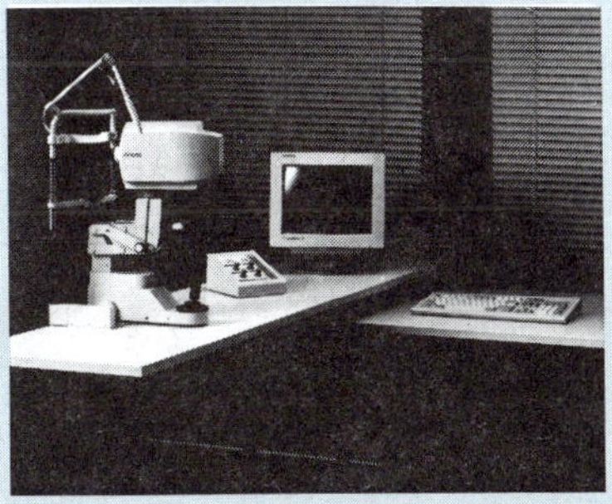

For more information contact Intezeag Inc. 1-800-627-6286

IFA EYE CARE SOFTWARE

[ē′-fa″]

ifa Software is designed to address the clinical aspects of practice management and to automate the patient record. It is new to the US, but has been in use in Europe for over 7 years managing over 15 million patients. Data input devices range from a standard keyboard to serial interfaces with instruments (LM, AR, PH, NCT, Perimeters). Images from bio-indirect, fundus cameras, video slit-lamps and B-Scans can be stored in the patient's file and recalled for review or comparison to "real time" images or transmitted to colleagues via modem. Findings, diagnoses, procedures and medications and other critical data can be entered by a single-touch pre-programmed digitizer or digitized voice input delivering the information to the patient's file. The software is preloaded with all appropriate CPT codes, ICD9's, findings, diagnoses, procedures and medications files. It has the ability to interface with many existing billing packages.

OCTOPUS 1-2-3 Direct Projection Perimeter

Direct projection perimeter analyzes central 30 degree with full library of screening and thresholding programs performed in multiple stages with statistical analysis standard. Compact, uses automatic left/right eye determination, joystick patient alignment, and direct pupil image analysis for continuous fixation monitoring. Connects to personal computer for data handling and storage with PeriData software.

M2X Macular Program offers high resolution threshold testing of the central 5° and 10° fields. CT Custom Test Program allows the user to create or emulate any visual field program. Very user and patient friendly and does not require darkened room for testing.

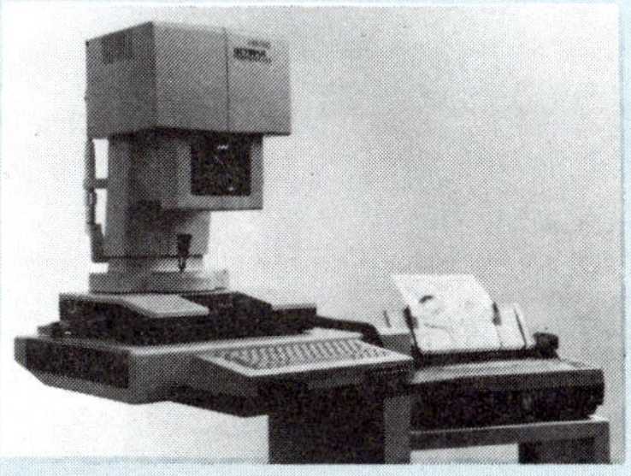

For more information contact Interzeag Inc. at 800-627-6286.

Continued on next page

Interzeag—Cont.

OCTOPUS

The OCTOPUS PERIMETER 101

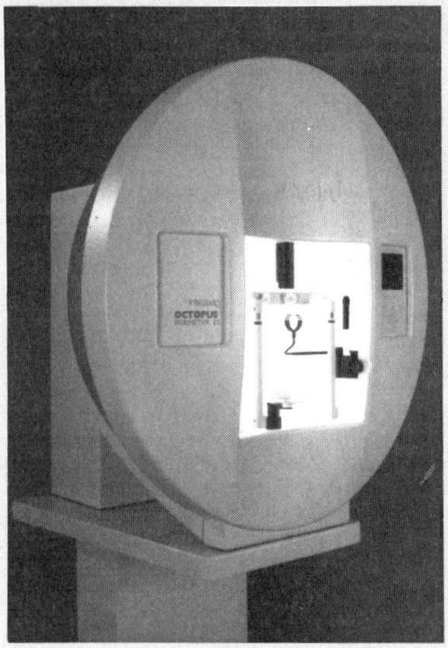

The Octopus Perimeter 101 is a modular full bowl system operating through a personal computer with full color Windows software using Goldmann size I-V stimulus. The design of the Octopus 101 focuses on ergonomic flexibility for both the patient and the operator. Continuous 100% eye fixation check, remote patient realignment, automatic left/right eye registration, silent projection with acoustic patient alert and auto pupil alignment for simple patient set up. The Octopus 101 offers a complete library of diagnostic programs including full field tests, Glaucoma, Macula, Neurological, Diabetes, Low Vision Central Field, Low Vision Peripheral Field, Thresholding, Screening, Custom Test capabilities and Program Tool. Multi-stage examination programs with on-line Defect Level Indicator allow user to finish exams in as little as 3 minutes for screening or 6 minutes for thresholding. Choice of printouts for easy field interpretation. PeriData Software performs statistical analysis and accepts data from all Octopus and Humphrey perimeters. Provides global and point to point statistical trend analysis of up to 25 examinations with a 3D color screen display.
Contact Interzeag Inc. 800-627-6286

PERIDATA STATISTICAL ANALYSIS SOFTWARE

This statistical analysis software package for use with the OCTOPUS and Humphrey visual field information on a personal computer provides single field analysis, right/left eye comparisons, regression analysis, hemifield and topographic analysis and long-term fluctuation analysis. System can provide for a direct comparison between the standard indices of OCTOPUS and Humphrey fields.
For more information contact Interzeag Inc. 1-800-627-6286.

IOLAB Corporation

Site Microsurgical Systems
135 GIBRALTAR ROAD
HORSHAM, PA 19044

SITE TXR® SYSTEM

The SITE TXR® Microsurgical System is a totally modular, precision instrument intended for surgical use in the human eye for both anterior and posterior segment surgery. The SITE TXR System is available in two different pump versions; Peristaltic or Diaphragm. Each TXR System console accepts up to four different modules. Each system may be tailored to meet the specific needs of a particular hospital or surgeon, and easily upgrades to keep pace with changing needs. The SITE TXR 2200 (Diaphragm) system or 2300 (Peristaltic) system includes both I/A and cutting (Vitrectomy) modules. Other available modules include the Linear/Pulse Phaco Module, Fiberoptic and Bipolar Modules. The Phaco Module features an exceptionally straight tip excursion path minimizing turbulence while virtually eliminating bubble formation. The autoclavable air cooled piezoelectric handpiece is quiet, lightweight and designed to sit well in the surgeons hand. The module features precise sensitive linear control of Phaco power as well as pulse mode automatic load compensation and selftuning. Both TXR systems feature easy to setup disposables as well as a variety of fluid-dynamic controls that will meet the needs of novice through expert surgeons.
Contact your local IOLAB/SITE representative or SITE Microsurgical directly for price information at 1-800-445-SITE.

Marco Ophthalmic, Inc.

11825 CENTRAL PARKWAY
P.O. BOX 16938
JACKSONVILLE, FL 32245-6938

TOLL FREE NUMBER:
U.S. (800) 874-5274
(904) 642-9330
Telex: 756172

CHAIRS AND STANDS

Marco's complete line of chairs and stands offers a wide range of combinations to choose from. Each chair shares the same proven hydraulic elevation system and is built identical, to the same quality specifications. The Marco Tilt Chair is a classic, all-steel design that adjusts from fully upright to nearly prone without changing patient position. Its unusually wide range of height makes it well suited to examining both children and adults. Elevation adjustments include both hand and foot controls with a convenient auto-return feature which automatically lowers the chair. The electronically adjustable, reclining Encore Automatic Chair also features auto-return, as well as a refined control system for easy positioning at any point between upright and horizontal. The Marco Standard Encore Chair is an ideal unit for those who do not require the electronic-reclining feature of the Automatic model, but prefer a basic, simple chair with manual recline. The Marco Deluxe Stand features convenient counterbalanced, locking instrument arms and groups all controls and three rechargeable instrument wells within fingertip reach. A non-console model is available for installations where rechargeable instrument wells are not needed.

KERATOMETERS

The availability of two models provides you with the choice between the standard external reading model, or our internal reading unit. Both models utilize our unique split mire target system, millimeter and diopeter measurement scales, an internal fixation light for aphakic patients and a comfortable rubber eye cup for the practitioner. Brass and stainless steel construction insures long term durability.

LENSMETERS

Marco's line of lensmeters provides you with a choice of standard, digital projection, or completely automated. The standard models 101 and 201 offer such features as full 90-degree inclination to facilitate measurement of contact lenses, a standard prism compensator, and an American cross-line target. The 201 includes all of the same features as the 101, but is an internal reading lensmeter. The LM-770 digital projection lensmeter features black-screen technology which provides the most crisp, clear imaging from any angle and under any lighting conditions. Instant digital readout displays the actual prescription with a built-in printer ready for hard copies. The new LM-820A Automatic Lensmeter provides instantaneous measurements at the touch of a button. Simple for even an untrained operator to master, the LM-820A utilizes a dot matrix target which helps the operator better understand accurate lens centering. Each measurement can be stored or instantly printed out. Progressive lenses are also easily read by using the strain gauge feature which indicates proper additive lens alignment or the new progressive "chanel" display which shows the path of the progressive lens. Prism values are also easily measured at the touch of a button.

MARCO RADIUSGAUGES

The selection of Marco Radiusgauges include Standard monocular and binocular units, as well as digital models. All Marco Radiusgauges perform two critical functions in measuring contact lenses. In addition to the standard measurement of contact lens curvature, lens thickness can also be easily measured. A large external dial gauge is standard with 100X magnification, coarse and fine focusing knobs, and a built-in transformer enhance the quality of Marco Radiusgauges.

MARCO SURGISCOPE III OPERATION MICROSCOPE

The new Marco Surgiscope III operation microscope combines a simple, compact design with uncompromising optical quality necessary for in-offical microsurgical techniques. The unit offers the practitioner a built-in three-step magnification drum, motorized fine focusing, dual coaxial illumination, and a variety of optional accessories which includes video and 35mm photographic kits. Mounting options include wall, table, unit, and floor stand.

SLIT LAMPS

MARCO Slit Lamps have earned a well-deserved reputation for having the best quality in the industry. To assure consistent, uniform quality, every component is manufactured in-house by Marco. Each Slit Lamp model is conveniently controlled by a single-handed joystick for easy elevation and focusing. These competitively priced models are available in a variety to suit every need, including extreme high power, parallel optics and photo documentation.

Compact and economical, the Marco G-II offers you a choice of standard parallel or optional converging optics. The model G-IV is similar to the G-II but offers a wider range of magnification powers. The model II-B Slit Lamp is ideal for general examinations and contact lens work and represents extremely high value. The light source tilting feature of the models V and V-G make them popular among many practitioners, with the V offering converging optics and the V-G featuring parallel optics and photo capability.

MARCO CHART PROJECTORS

Marco chart projectors offers the practitioner a choice of manual halogen, or automatic, remote operation. The CP-600 Automatic Chart Projector is a programmable unit with a wireless remote control that makes refracting easy and efficient. The CP-600's full complement of 26 charts can be conveniently programmed or selected by random access with the hand held remote control. Vertical, horizontal, and single letter presentation can be quickly accomplished as well as the capability of Red/green masking on appropriate charts. Four separate 20/20 lines are also standard. The manually operated Standard Chart Projector accomodates a wide variety of slides and offers a variable-focus objective barrel for accurate testing at any distance from ten to twenty feet. A flow-through "chimney" is used to dissipate heat with a built-in thermistor to also help reduce electrical surges to the bulb. The new Everlight halogen chart projector incorporates many of the same features as the manual unit, but utilizes a halogen illumination for longer bulb life.

TRIAL SETS AND FRAMES

Marco's trial frame and lens sets are equally constructed to withstand even the heaviest daily use for years. The full diameter trial lens set offers an even distribution of bi-convex and bi-concave lenses from the lowest to the highest powers. Metal rims are engraved with power designations on both sides of the handles, which are satin-finished for an easier, more sure grip. Also with a maximum selection of powers, the Custom Deluxe Lens Set meets the needs of practitioners who prefer corrected-curve Lenses. These Lenses are available in a deluxe or limited lens selection with color-coded handles for easy recognition. Popular among doctors who perform out-of-office refraction is the Perimeter Lens set, which contains a more modest, specialized range of Lenses. The MTL Trial Frame can be used with all trial sets, offering fingertip control of a full range of adjustments. Its lightweight aluminum construction means greater comfort for the patient as well.

Marco Technologies

11825 CENTRAL PARKWAY
P.O. BOX 16938
JACKSONVILLE, FL 32245-6938

TOLL FREE NUMBER:
U.S. (800) 874-5274
(904) 642-9330
Telex: 756172

MARCO AUTOMATIC REFRACTORS

Highly sophisticated, state of the art technology is what separates the Marco line of autorefractors from all the rest. Sold and serviced exclusively in the United States by Marco Technologies, the line begins with the rapid fire objective measurements of the AR-800. For the practitioner who just wants quick, accurate objective measurements and a machine that requires very little operator training, the AR-800 is by far the best objective automatic refractor. Next, comes the ARK-900 combination auto-refractor/keratometer. In one instrument, the ARK-900 combines the speed and accuracy of automated refraction with the split second measurement of the eye's central curvature in both millimeters and diopters. Finally comes the AR-820. The same quick objective measurements are combined with subjective capability. Near vision testing is also possible with the AR-820. An extremely high-resolution television monitor is standard on all units with an automatic fogging system to eliminate patient accomodation.

MARCO COS-1000

The new Compact Optical System 1000 from Marco Technologies creates a true 20-foot exam lane in fewer than 30 square feet. The COS 1000 incorporates the TRS electronic refraction system and any Marco Automatic Refractor for a complete electronic refraction "Lane". Two COS-1000 units can fit into a single-lane space, doubling the exam capabilities.

MARCO LASERON YAG LASER

The full featured Yag Laser from Marco is designed specifically for doctors to use in their own offices. The Marco Laseron is built into the head of a Marco II-L slit lamp and is controlled from a console attached to the slit lamp power table. Compact but powerful and flexible, the Laseron features dual "He Ne" aiming beams and can be used in either a single pulse or a burst mode. The laser output is continuously variable up to 10 millijoules and is digitally displayed on the face of the instrument as well as on the console. Special safety features include a Q-switch verification system; a fail-safe shutter, and tamper-proof system interlocks.

MARCO TRS–1200 TOTAL REFRACTION SYSTEM

The TRS-1200 is an electronically operated refractor independently controlled by a comfortably positioned keyboard panel. Fingertip lens selections are simple and fast and can be performed in a sitting or standing position. Although the TRS-1200 can be used as an individual refractor, the full benefits are realized when the system is completely interfaced with a Marco automatic refractor and CP-600 automatic chart projector. An automatic refractor measurement is transferred to the TRS-1200 which is automatically loaded into the refractor and simultaneously signals the CP-600 automated chart projector to display the appropriate viewing chart. Refining the refractive results then becomes a relaxed process by using the TRS-1200 instrument control panel. The user can also "pre-program" the system to automatically follow a certain sequence of lens and chart selections or perform random selections.

MS–30 AUTOMATIC PERIMETER

The new Marco MS-30 Automated Perimeter provides the operator with a lightweight, compact field machine that offers single-stimulus perimetry as well as a new multistimulus testing program. With a very simple setup procedure, the MS-30 quickly allows the operator to administer any selected screening or full threshold test. The MS-30 is powered by its own built-in computer. When enhancements become available, the computer can easily be upgraded right in the office.

Topcon America Corporation

65 W. CENTURY ROAD
PARAMUS, NEW JERSEY
07652

Address inquiries to:
MEDICAL INSTRUMENT DIVISION
(201) 261-9450
(800) 223-1130

AUTO REFRACTOMETERS

The model RM-A2000 provides automatic objective results while the model RM-A2300G extends versatility by combining objective and subjective modes with glare testing ability. Our new KR-3000 combines both refraction measurements and keratometer readings in one instrument. Also, our new PR-2000 provides strabismus detection for infants from a 1 meter working distance.

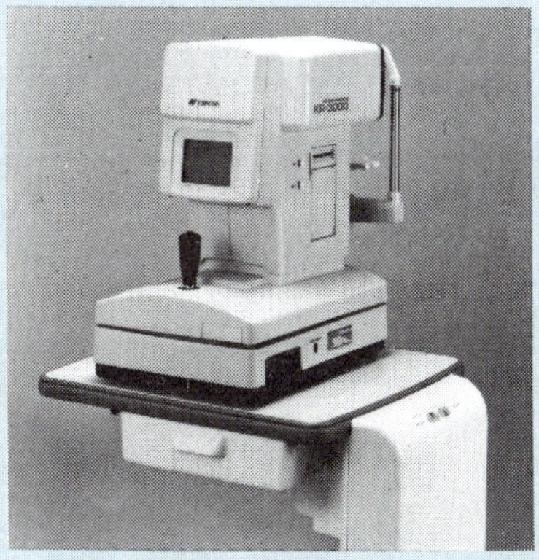

Continued on next page

Topcon—Cont.

BINOCULAR INDIRECTS AND ASPHERICAL LENSES

The model ID-5 is a compact lightweight instrument with halogen illumination. In addition, the model ID-10 provides small pupil capability and built-in filters and apertures. A wide range of accessories are available, including TOPCON aspherical lenses with their unique hard lens coating which eliminates surface reflections and produces accurate retinal images. Three powers are available: 14D, 20D and 30D, each with its own hard shell case.

CHAIRS AND STANDS

Topcon now offers four ophthalmic chairs designed with patient comfort and operator convenience in mind. Manual chairs include the 1800M, 2000M and the OC-20T. The 2000A automatic chair features streamlined design with automated convenience. Manual and automatic chairs are available in a choice of colors and styles which are sure to coordinate with any office setting.
Topcon's stands include the IS-80 and IS-1000. Complete catalogs may be ordered for color and style choices.

CHART PROJECTORS

Select either our model CP-5D with its traditional styling and variable focus lens, or our extremely fast automatic models ACP-7S and ACP-7R. Each has a wireless remote control for quick access to 30 built-in slides. The model ACP-7R also provides one-touch random access chart selection and programming capabilities as well as single letter isolation.

COMPUTERIZED TONOMETER

The model CT-20 is a contemporary styled non contact tonometer featuring a built-in TV monitor for alignment ease, reduced air pressure for increased patient comfort, an automatic measuring mode which minimizes measurement time, a built-in printer and automatic shut off.

COMPUTERIZED VISION TESTER

The model CV-2000 is a sealed instrument with all controls located on the instruments' remote controller. Spherical power range from −19.00 diopters to +16.75 diopters; cylindrical range from 0.00 to 8.00 diopters; electrical rotary prism is incorporated for binocular test. Can be connected to the TOPCON Auto Refractometer to accept the refraction measurements and set lenses accordingly.

DIGITAL IMAGING EQUIPMENT

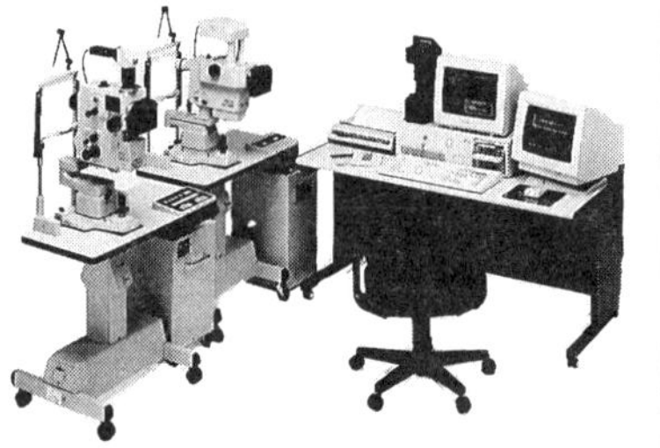

The IMAGEnet Digital Imaging System captures and digitizes retinal images through a video camera adapted to your fundus camera. Complete software programs are available for ICG and fluorescein angiography, optic disc analysis and endothelial cell counting. Connects to fundus camera, slit lamp and can analyze images from slides. Measurement functions, enhancement functions, magnification ability, and other image processing techniques are included. Systems for both 512 or 1024 resolution imaging.

LENSMETERS

Four models are available to choose from. The selections range from the economical and traditional monocular styled instruments with either corona dot or cross line targets, to the semi-automatic digital model LM-P6 with an optional printer and our most advanced fully automatic computerized lensmeter model CL-2000.

OPERATION MICROSCOPES

Three models, the OMS-60, OMS-75, and OMS-600 are designed to fulfill all your surgical needs. Ideal for the clinic, examining and emergency rooms and the outpatient surgical suite or hospital. All models feature fine optical quality, variable magnification, halogen illumination and a complete range of accessories.

RETINAL CAMERAS

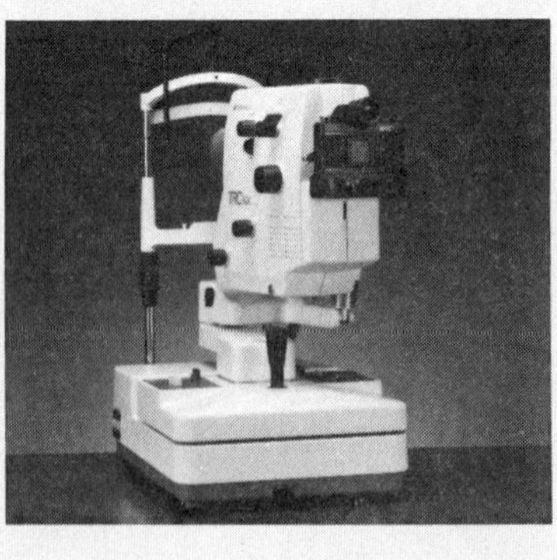

As the world's leading manufacturer of retinal cameras, TOPCON offers the widest selection of cameras currently available. If you only require color documentation, you may choose either a conventional mydratic model-TRC-50XF or a 20° & 45° field non-mydriatic model TRC-NW5. A more advanced system designed for both color documentation and fluorescein angiography is available in the form of our model TRC-50X. In addition, our model TRC-SS2 retinal camera makes it possible to obtain simultaneous stereo photographs on a single 35mm exposure.

SLIT LAMPS

TOPCON offers five models from which to choose, each designed to fulfill specific requirements. Whether you require the economy and simplicity of our dispensing type instrument, superior diagnostic capabilities of our more advanced models or the versatility found in the extensive selection of accessories in our photographic model, there is a TOPCON slit lamp suitable for your needs.

TRIAL LENS SET & FRAME

Available in a full diamter version or with a special corrective curve additive design which compensates for thickness and air spacing between lenses. Choose from our deluxe model with plus and minus cylinders or our deluxe model with one set of cylinders. If you require a smaller selection of lenses, we offer a limited version.

VISION TESTERS

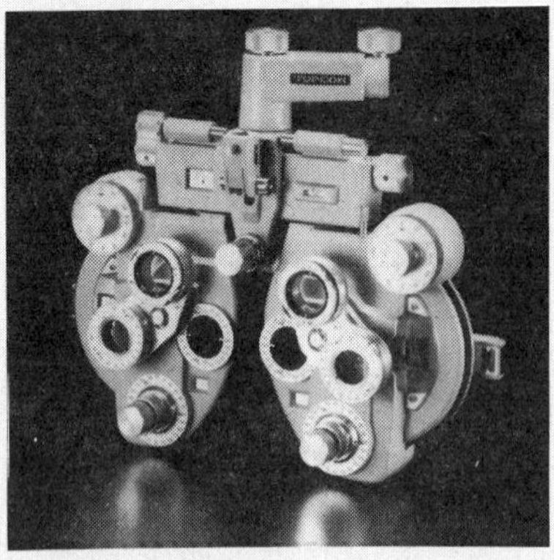

Our VT-10 vision tester combines precision and convenience in a design that guarantees accuracy in refraction measurements. This instrument is available in either plus or minus cylinder formats and light grey or black enameled finishes.

NOTES

NOTES